Molecular Cytogenetics: Methods and Protocols

Molecular Cytogenetics: Methods and Protocols

Edited by Camila Blair

hayle
medical

New York

Hayle Medical,
750 Third Avenue, 9th Floor,
New York, NY 10017, USA

Visit us on the World Wide Web at:
www.haylemedical.com

ISBN: 978-1-63241-799-2

Cataloging-in-Publication Data

Molecular cytogenetics : methods and protocols / edited by Camila Blair.
p. cm.
Includes bibliographical references and index.
ISBN 978-1-63241-799-2
1. Cytogenetics. 2. Molecular genetics. 3. Human cytogenetics. 4. Medical genetics. I. Blair, Camila.
RB155 .M65 2019
616.042--dc23

Table of Contents

Preface

The purpose of the book is to provide a glimpse into the dynamics and to present opinions and studies of some of the scientists engaged in the development of new ideas in the field from very different standpoints. This book will prove useful to students and researchers owing to its high content quality.

The branch of genetics, which studies how chromosomes relate to cell behavior and their behavior during mitosis and meiosis, is known as cytogenetics. Molecular cytogenetics is a field involving the combination of cytogenetics and molecular biology. It uses several reagents and focuses on identifying and distinguishing normal and cancer-causing cells. It acts as a vital tool for the treatment of malignancies like brain tumors and hematological malignancies. It includes techniques and methods, like fluorescence in situ hybridization (FISH) and comparative genomic hybridization (CGH). This book is compiled in such a manner, that it will provide in-depth knowledge about the theory and practice of molecular cytogenetics. From theories to research to practical applications, case studies related to all contemporary topics of relevance to this field have been included in it. This book aims to equip students and experts with the advanced topics and upcoming concepts in this area.

At the end, I would like to appreciate all the efforts made by the authors in completing their chapters professionally. I express my deepest gratitude to all of them for contributing to this book by sharing their valuable works. A special thanks to my family and friends for their constant support in this journey.

Editor

3C and 3C-based techniques: the powerful tools for spatial genome organization deciphering

Jinlei Han[1], Zhiliang Zhang[1] and Kai Wang[1,2]* (iD)

Abstract

It is well known that the chromosomes are organized in the nucleus and this spatial arrangement of genome play a crucial role in gene regulation and genome stability. Different techniques have been developed and applied to uncover the intrinsic mechanism of genome architecture, especially the chromosome conformation capture (3C) and 3C-derived methods. 3C and 3C-derived techniques provide us approaches to perform high-throughput chromatin architecture assays at the genome scale. However, the advantage and disadvantage of current methodologies of C-technologies have not been discussed extensively. In this review, we described and compared the methodologies of C-technologies used in genome organization studies with an emphasis on Hi-C method. We also discussed the crucial challenges facing current genome architecture studies based on 3C and 3C-derived technologies and the direction of future technologies to address currently outstanding questions in the field. These latest news contribute to our current understanding of genome structure, and provide a comprehensive reference for researchers to choose the appropriate method in future application. We consider that these constantly improving technologies will offer a finer and more accurate contact profiles of entire genome and ultimately reveal specific molecular machines govern its shape and function.

Keywords: Chromosome conformation capture (3C), Topologically associating domains (TADs), Hi-C, C-technologies, Chromosome territory

Background

During the higher eukaryotic cell cycle, the spatial volumes of each chromosome are not random but are organized into specific patterns, in which individual chromosomes occupy defined, mutually exclusive regions of the nuclear volume that represent a structural unit referred to as a chromosome territory (CT) [1–4]. With extensive effort, the spatial organizations of individual chromosomes and the entire genome, with resolutions down to 1kbp, have been described [5–12]. It has now been widely accepted that genome architecture is a crucial aspect of gene regulation and genome stability [1, 5, 13–20] because the highly ordered chromatin arrangement facilitates communication between genes and their regulatory elements [21–26].

Early studies of genomic conformation were largely based on cytological techniques, such as fluorescence in situ hybridization (FISH), which allows direct evaluation of the proximity between genetic loci using probes. Observations of genome architecture by FISH have revealed the existence of CTs [27–29], looping out from CTs [30–32], and the tendency for clustering of active chromatin domains [33, 34]. While this method has been a widely used tool to study topography of chromosomes or DNA fragments of interest in individual cells, and allow us to determine how the chromosomes are organized by directly viewing their position with microscopy [35, 36]. However, technical limitations such as low throughput, low resolution and probe sequence specificity make it unsuitable for elaborate genome-wide studies of chromosomal topology [37–39]. Recently, chromosome conformation capture (3C) and 3C-based techniques using high-throughput sequencing data have emerged as powerful tools to reconstruct the spatial topology at regional, whole chromosome and genome levels [40–45]. These techniques have become the most effective

* Correspondence: kwang5@126.com
[1]Key Laboratory of Genetics, Breeding and Multiple Utilization of Corps, Ministry of Education, Fujian Provincial Key Laboratory of Haixia Applied Plant Systems Biology, Center for Genomics and Biotechnology, Fujian Agriculture and Forestry University, Fuzhou, Fujian, China
[2]National Engineering Research Center of Sugarcane, Fujian Agriculture and Forestry University, Fuzhou, China

way to elucidate the functional impact and the potential mechanisms establishing and maintaining spatial genome organization. In this review, we describe and compare the methodologies used to study genome architecture, with an emphasis on recently developed key approaches including 3C and its derivatives. We discuss the crucial challenges facing current 3D studies based on 3C technologies and the direction of future technologies to address currently outstanding questions in the field.

The methodologies of 3C and 3C-derived technologies

The strategy of 3C to discover genomic architecture is based on quantifying the frequencies of contacts between distal DNA segments in cell populations [46]. In contrast to cytogenetic approaches, 3C-based genomics strategies yield incomparable information-rich data describing genome topology at the genome-wide level, enabling more systematic genome topology studies at a higher resolution and throughput and providing deep insights into genome architecture and its impact on genome function. Thus, 3C technologies are revolutionizing our ability to explore genome organization from specific loci up to the whole genome.

The principal steps of 3C and 3C-based experiments are theoretically similar and have following principal steps: crosslink chromatin using a fixative agent in solution, most often formaldehyde, to create covalent bonds between DNA fragments bridged by proteins; isolate and digest the chromatin using a restriction enzyme such as *Hind*III [46], *Bgl*II [47], *Eco*RI [48], *Aci*I [49], or *Dpn*II [50, 51] at a low concentration to create pairs of crosslinked DNA fragments that are distant in linear distance but close in space; re-ligate the sticky ends of crosslinked DNA fragments to form chimeric molecules; reverse the crosslinks to obtain 3C templates; and finally, interrogate the rearranged DNA fragments by PCR or sequencing technologies (Fig. 1). Eventually, 3D conformations at the regional, chromosome and whole-genome levels can be inferred by calculating the number of ligation junctions between genomic loci (Fig. 1). To describe in more detail and to facilitate comparisons among different methods, we describe current 3C and 3C-based approaches below.

Chromosome conformation capture (3C)

3C technology was developed to detect ligation junctions by PCR followed by gel electrophoresis (Fig. 1) [45]. The first 3C assay inferred the 3D conformation of yeast chromosome III and showed that it forms a contorted ring [46]. Next, this method was adapted for mammalian systems. 3C technology confirmed the existence of chromatin loops, which confer spatial contact between DNA fragments such as regulatory DNA elements and their

target genes [47, 52–57] or the start and end of a gene [58]. Remarkably, this chromatin loop is dynamic based on transcriptional state changes [48, 58], implying that this structure is associated with genomic function.

Although 3C provides a method for visualizing the genome at high resolution, some shortcomings remain, including the requirement for PCR primers designed to amplify regions of interest. For this reason, 3C can be used only to detect spatial relationships between known DNA sequences. Obviously, the "one versus one" (Fig. 2a) throughput of this method limits its application to genome-scale assays. In addition, it can detect contact only in a limited range (not exceeding a few hundred kilobases) [59]. To overcome these limitations, several 3C-derived methods have been developed to generate higher throughput chromatin interaction data.

Chromosome conformation capture-on-Chip (4C)

4C technology was developed by combining 3C with microarray [60, 61] or, more recently, next-generation sequencing (NGS) technologies [62, 63]. This method is able to assess chromatin interactions between one genomic locus of interest (referred to as bait or viewpoint) and all other genomic loci (one versus all) (Fig. 2b). In 4C experiments, small DNA circles are created by cleaving with a second restriction enzyme and re-ligating 3C DNA templates. Then, inverse PCR using bait-specific primers is applied to amplify any interacting fragments. Finally, the interacting fragments are evaluated using microarrays or NGS (Fig. 1).

4C was originally applied to elucidate the DNA contact maps of the β-globin and *Rad23a* genes [60], which showed that the housekeeping gene *Rad23a* tends to interact with other active regions on the chromosomes and that its contact maps were conserved in various tissues [60]. By contrast, the contact maps for the erythroid-specific gene β-globin changed depending on its expression status. More specifically, β-globin contacts other active regions in erythroid cells, whereas it contacts inactive regions in the fetal brain, where this gene is silent. Subsequently, a series of 4C experiments were carried out and have shown changes in gene regulation and interaction profiles during differentiation and development [64] and that chromosome conformation is relatively stable in a given cell type [65]. Furthermore, 4C has also been used to identify chromosomal rearrangements [66] and uncover disease mechanisms [67].

4C technology is an excellent strategy to survey the DNA contact profile of specific genomic sites. However, it is worth noting that the amplification of GC-rich fragments by inverse PCR during 4C library construction is inefficient, resulting in biases in the interaction profile [68]. In addition, it is not possible to differentiate PCR duplication in 4C data.

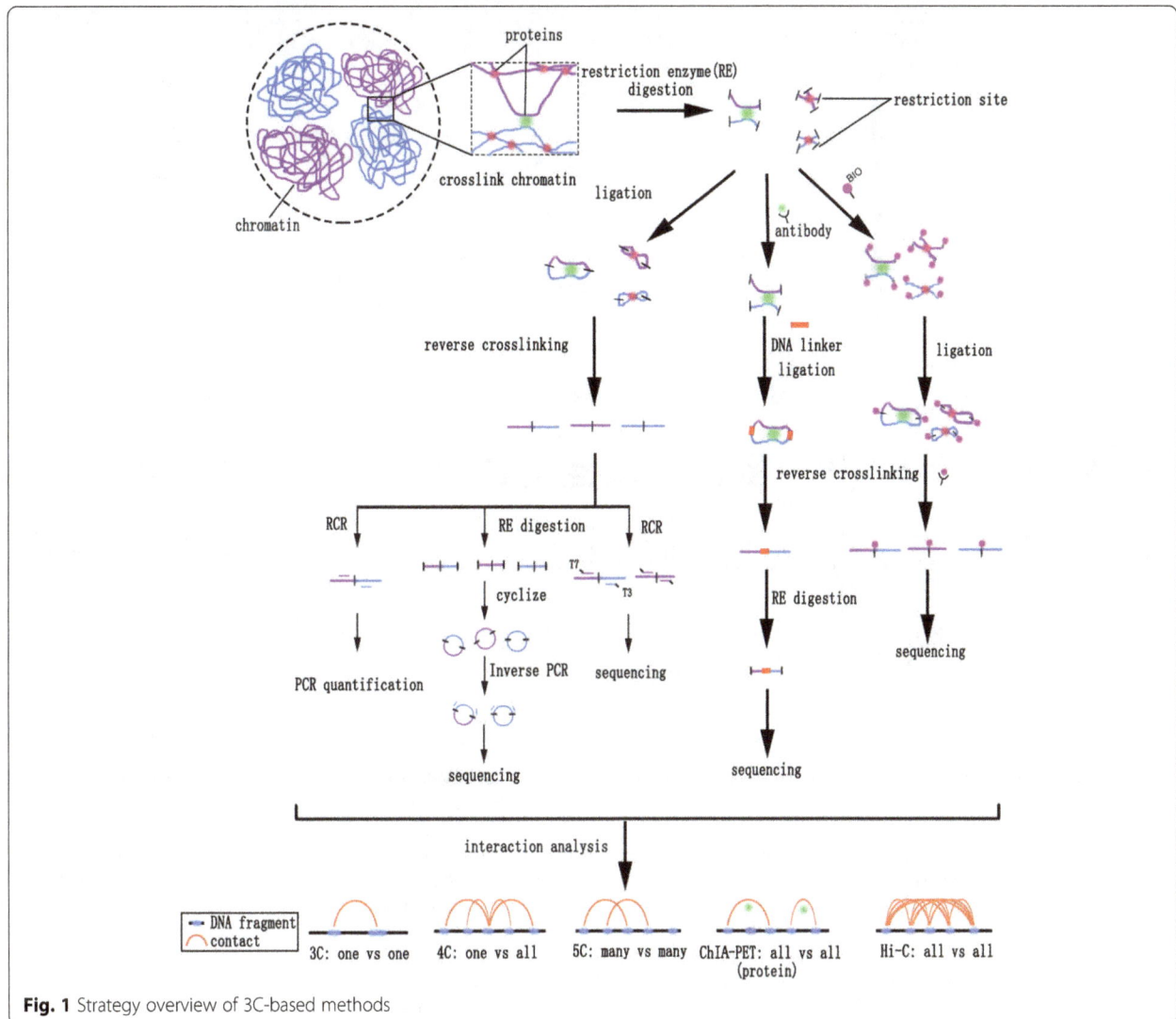

Fig. 1 Strategy overview of 3C-based methods

Chromosome conformation capture carbon copy (5C)

Another variant of 3C is 5C [69, 70]. It is analogous to 3C technology but is a "many versus many" method (Fig. 2c), allowing the simultaneous detection of millions of interactions through the use of thousands of primers in a single assay. The main difference between 3C and 5C is the strategy for primer design. 5C primers have a universal sequence (usually T7 and T3) appended to the 5′ ends. This change, combined with multiplex PCR amplification and sequencing, allows researchers to detect contact events within a particular locus (Fig. 1). Thus, in contrast to 3C, 5C has a higher throughput and a lower bias. The improvements due to this higher-throughput scale have been demonstrated by its application in the study of the human β-globin locus [69], human α-globin locus [71], and human HOXA–D gene clusters [72–74]. In addition, 5C provided the first evidence of the existence of topologically associating domains (TADs) by X chromosome analysis [75]. However, 5C is still limited in terms of the size of the genomic region that can be assayed because of the DNA sequence requirement of interested regions, as well as the quantitatively inestimable PCR duplication.

Chromatin interaction analysis by paired-end tag sequencing (ChIA-PET)

Another 3C-based technology is ChIA-PET, which combines chromatin immunoprecipitation (ChIP) with 3C-type analysis to study genome-wide long-range chromatin interactions bound by one specific protein [76–78]. The key features of ChIA-PET technology are that the interaction sites are enriched by ChIP using a specific antibody after chromatin digestion, as in a ChIP experiment. Then, DNA sequences tethered together and to the protein of interest are connected through proximity

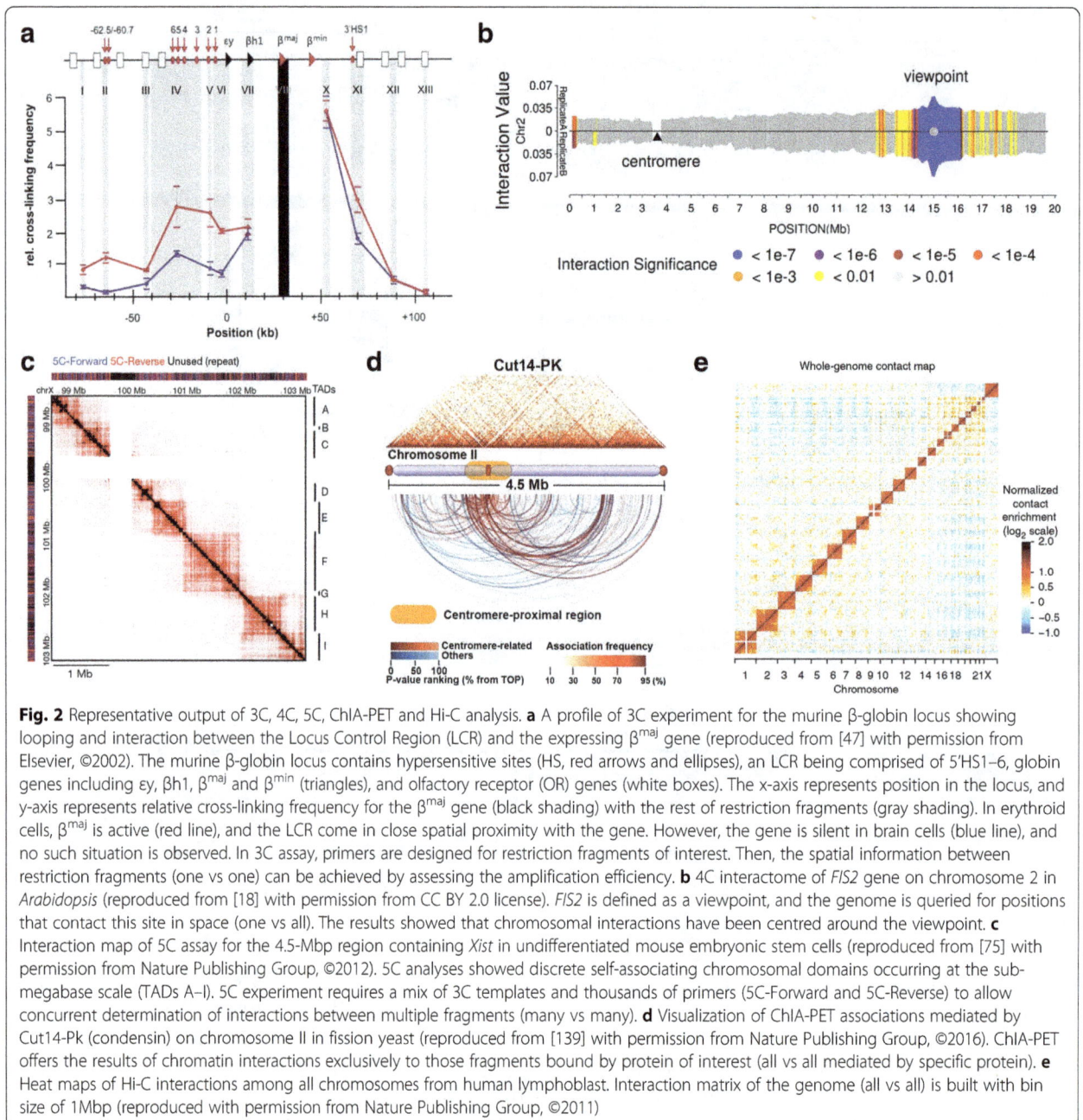

Fig. 2 Representative output of 3C, 4C, 5C, ChIA-PET and Hi-C analysis. **a** A profile of 3C experiment for the murine β-globin locus showing looping and interaction between the Locus Control Region (LCR) and the expressing β^{maj} gene (reproduced from [47] with permission from Elsevier, ©2002). The murine β-globin locus contains hypersensitive sites (HS, red arrows and ellipses), an LCR being comprised of 5'HS1–6, globin genes including εy, βh1, β^{maj} and β^{min} (triangles), and olfactory receptor (OR) genes (white boxes). The x-axis represents position in the locus, and y-axis represents relative cross-linking frequency for the β^{maj} gene (black shading) with the rest of restriction fragments (gray shading). In erythroid cells, β^{maj} is active (red line), and the LCR come in close spatial proximity with the gene. However, the gene is silent in brain cells (blue line), and no such situation is observed. In 3C assay, primers are designed for restriction fragments of interest. Then, the spatial information between restriction fragments (one vs one) can be achieved by assessing the amplification efficiency. **b** 4C interactome of *FIS2* gene on chromosome 2 in *Arabidopsis* (reproduced from [18] with permission from CC BY 2.0 license). *FIS2* is defined as a viewpoint, and the genome is queried for positions that contact this site in space (one vs all). The results showed that chromosomal interactions have been centred around the viewpoint. **c** Interaction map of 5C assay for the 4.5-Mbp region containing *Xist* in undifferentiated mouse embryonic stem cells (reproduced from [75] with permission from Nature Publishing Group, ©2012). 5C analyses showed discrete self-associating chromosomal domains occurring at the sub-megabase scale (TADs A–I). 5C experiment requires a mix of 3C templates and thousands of primers (5C-Forward and 5C-Reverse) to allow concurrent determination of interactions between multiple fragments (many vs many). **d** Visualization of ChIA-PET associations mediated by Cut14-Pk (condensin) on chromosome II in fission yeast (reproduced from [139] with permission from Nature Publishing Group, ©2016). ChIA-PET offers the results of chromatin interactions exclusively to those fragments bound by protein of interest (all vs all mediated by specific protein). **e** Heat maps of Hi-C interactions among all chromosomes from human lymphoblast. Interaction matrix of the genome (all vs all) is built with bin size of 1Mbp (reproduced with permission from Nature Publishing Group, ©2011)

ligation with oligonucleotide DNA linkers, the sequence of which contains restriction sites for digestion in the next step (Fig. 1). After high-throughput sequencing and bioinformatics analysis, an interactome map of the specific protein binding sites is achieved (Fig. 2d). Thus, ChIA-PET has been applied efficiently to study sites bound with specific transcription factors [76, 78, 79]. For example, some proteins, such as RAD21, SMC3, CTCF and ZNF143, that are important for the formation of a 3D chromatin structure were discovered with ChIA-PET analysis [80]. Another advantage is that ChIA-PET has relatively low levels of library complexity compared with other 3C techniques; therefore,

interactions that are identified with an extremely low number of reads are usually considered significant [76, 78]. Recently, an improved method, HiChIP was developed and it can improve over 10-fiold of the yield of chromatin interacting reads but with 100-fold lower requirement than that of ChIA-PET [81]. Results generated from HiChIP of cohesin achieved multiscale genome intact map with greater signal-to-background rations than that of in situ Hi-c [81]. More important is that the sustain high-confidence results are achieved from low cell number input, which will facilitate the investigation of chromatin conformation at cell- or tissue-specific aspects.

Hi-C

The development of high-throughput sequencing technology promoted the emergence of a series of "all versus all" methods (Fig. 2e). Of these, Hi-C was the first to be developed that does not depend on specific primers and generates genome-wide contact maps [82, 83]. In Hi-C experiments, the first step is to generate contact segments as with 3C, but the procedure is slightly different from that described above (Fig. 1). After restriction enzyme digestion, the sticky ends are filled in with biotin-labeled nucleotides followed by blunt-end ligation. The expected contacting DNAs are sheared and then purified in a biotin pull-down experiment using streptavidin beads to ensure that only biotinylated junctions are selected for further high-throughput sequencing and computational analysis (Fig. 1).

The strategy of Hi-C data analysis is thus different from above methods due to the massive parallel NGS data obtained. The basic data analysis typically involves the following aspects [84–86].

Read mapping

Paired-end reads are independently aligned to the corresponding reference genome. Given that effective sequence fragments used for sequencing are normally chimeras, which come from two or more chromatin loci, massive reads are discontinuous in the genome [87]. Considering this situation, various methods have been proposed to improve data-use efficiency during the mapping stage, including a pre-truncation process [88], iterative mapping [89], or allowing split alignments [87].

Read filtering

First, the mapping results are filtered at the level of reads and fragments, and only reads with information about chromatin conformation are included. Generally, valid reads are a limited distance from the nearest restriction site, and valid pairs will fall within distinct restriction fragments, which correspond to an interaction between DNA fragments. Then, the remaining read pairs are further filtered to discard PCR duplicates. Here, all uninformative reads are excluded.

Establishment of the contact matrix

For this step, the genome is divided into non-overlapping bins, each filtered read pair is assigned to a specific bin pair, the count of read pairs in the corresponding bin pair aggregated, and eventually, a contact matrix is created. Rows and columns of the contact matrix represent bins across the genome, and each entry contains the number of read pairs that reflects bin–bin interactions.

Normalization

Because of biases, such as GC content, the mappability, and the frequency of restriction sites, normalization (such as explicit-factor correction methods or matrix balancing-based methods) is essential to correct the raw contact matrix [89–91]. Once normalization is completed, one can generate a contact heatmap and infer genome-wide proximity information. Meanwhile, some tools have been developed to visualize Hi-C and other conformation capture data [92, 93]. These help researchers intuitively observe long-range genomic interactions.

In the original Hi-C study, two types of chromatin compartments (A and B) were identified, each of which has different functional and structural properties [82]. The former is enriched in genes and sites with active histone marks, such as H3K36me3, or DNase I hypersensitivity. By contrast, B compartments are enriched with inactive histone marks, such as H3K27me3, and contain few genes and DNase I hypersensitivity sites. Thereafter, other domain types (TAD and sub-TAD) were also identified [87, 94]. In addition, several polymer models have been showed by Hi-C data, including the fractal globule model [82], random loop model [95], dynamic loop model [96] and strings and binders switch model [97], to explain the underlying biophysical principles governing chromatin packing. For chromosome positioning, the previously observed Rabl configuration of chromosomes was confirmed once again, with the results showing clustering of the centromeres and clustering of the telomeres [98]. Due to its robust and powerful topology profiling at the genome scale, Hi-C has recently been applied extensively in genome conformation research [86, 99–102]. It is also important to mention that Hi-C can also assist in chromosomal rearrangements, genome assembly and haplotyping [16, 103–111].

Although Hi-C is a satisfactory technique for determining genome-wide chromatin interaction maps with relatively few biases compared with other existing C-methods, the acquisition of a reliable contact map with high-resolution still requires sufficient sequencing depth. Ordinarily, there is a direct relationship between mapping resolution and sequencing depth for Hi-C assay [82]. For example, generating contact profiles with resolution from 40 kbp to 1 kbp in the human genome requires hundreds of millions to multiple billion paired-end reads [112]. Thus, the cost and computational resources are certainly prohibitively expensive for most laboratories, which has seriously dampened the popularity of Hi-C.

Other 3C-based strategies

In addition to the above techniques, other seminal adaptations of 3C protocols have been developed for assessing proximity events between distal genomic elements. For example, UMI-4C uses a unique molecular identifier

(UMI) to derive quantitative and targeted chromosomal contact profiling [113]. In this approach, initial 3C ligation products are sonicated, and one end of each sonicated fragment is ligated to a sequencing adapter, generating a UMI. Using a bait-specific primer and a universal adaptor primer, physical linkage fragments can be amplified, sequenced and quantified. UMI-4C can eliminate PCR duplicates during data analysis based on the UMI and allows multiple baits (with a suggested number of 20–50 baits) to be selected [113].

Capture-C combines 3C, oligonucleotide capture technology and NGS to generate genome-wide contact profiles from hundreds of selected loci at a time [114]. In this method, 3C DNAs are sonicated, and paired-end sequencing adaptors are added. The resulting library is then enriched for junction fragments of interest by hybridization to biotinylated capture probes and streptavidin pull-down. Finally, the captured DNAs are amplified and sequenced, and the interaction maps are produced by corresponding bioinformatics methods. The Capture-C strategy can be used to enrich Hi-C libraries, and accordingly a new technique, known as Capture Hi-C (CHi-C), was developed [115]. This method enables deep sequencing of target fragments, excluding uninformative background [115, 116].

Subsequently, using an improved oligonucleotide capture strategy, Davies et al. re-designed the Capture-C protocol and developed another method, called next generation (NG) Capture-C [117]. NG Capture-C has higher assay sensitivity and resolution than Capture-C, and its sensitivity allows the analysis of weak long-range interactions. In addition, multiple 3C libraries from different cell types or different experimental conditions can be processed simultaneously in a single reaction by pooling differently indexed samples, which significantly increases throughput, removes experimental variation and allows the subtractive analysis of chromosome conformation from different samples.

Researchers have also developed DNase Hi-C technology [102]. Compared with Hi-C, the key difference is that DNase Hi-C uses DNase I rather than restriction enzymes for fragmenting crosslinked chromatin, leading to better genome coverage and resolution than Hi-C. Furthermore, the coupling of DNase Hi-C with DNA-capture technology, targeted DNase Hi-C has also been proposed and applied to characterize the 3D organization of large intergenic noncoding RNA promoters in different human cell lines [102]. Similarly, micro-C [118] and an updated micro-C XL version [119] uses micrococcal nuclease (MNase) to fragment chromatin, enabling the analysis of chromosome conformation at nucleosome resolution.

Further considerations for 3C technologies

Researchers have been working to improve the resolution of 3C technologies to clarify the specific relationship between genomic conformation and function. However, some challenges have been encountered in this process, indicating that resolution can be affected by many factors [120]. The most important limiting factor is the selection of the first restriction enzyme, which determines the maximum resolution of 3C experiments because contacts between DNA fragments can be detected only at restriction enzyme cut sites. If two restriction enzymes, four-cutter and six-cutter, are compared, the former will yield a 16-fold higher resolution library (256 bp vs. 4096 bp) in humans. However, we should also take into account that the distribution of restriction sites is not uniform in the genome, resulting in different resolutions at different genomic regions. A further increase in resolution can be achieved by substituting restriction enzymes with MNase [118] or DNase I [102], which can cut at any site along the genome and can theoretically generate single base pair resolution. After the restriction enzyme to be used in the 3C experiment is chosen, the resolution of the contact maps is further affected by sequencing depth. When it is insufficient to explore contacts at the level of individual restriction fragments, the resolution will be determined by an appropriate bin size. In addition, research on the 3D conformation of repeat regions in the genome is difficult and is mainly because sequence information in this region is often incomplete, and thus sequencing-based 3C methods cannot effectively handle data mapping in this area. Another experimental factor that may impact the output of 3C study is the bias caused potentially by the crosslinking agent. Because crosslinking treatment inappropriately will crosslink the fibers, which are in close physical proximity rather than directly interacting [121]. Therefore, the consideration that to isolate native nuclei in an isotonic buffer to retain the native chromosome loops will properly present the native chromosome conformation [121, 122]. Moreover, comparative study of 3C-type experiments with FISH indicated that 3C-type experiments or FISH alone must be interpreted with caution when studying chromatin architecture [39], thus cross-validation of Hi-C with FISH [123] or visible data achieved with super-resolution microscope [10, 124] still need to be considered. Resemble the concept of native chromosome loops, that joint assays will present crucial information for fully understanding chromatin organization.

Theoretically, 3C experiments can capture all DNA fragments that make contact in space. However, studies have showed that capture probability present an exponential decrease as the linear distance between DNA fragments increases [82, 125]. Thus, the ligation junctions between sites that are far apart on the chromosome will be difficult to detect. Moreover, the capacity for 3C-based methods to efficiently detect simultaneous contacts between multiple genomic loci is still overrated [126]. Most recently, Beagrie et al. [127] developed an all vs. all protocol described as Genome Architecture Mapping (GAM) to dissect the nuclear architecture [127]. Instead of a strong reliance on digestion and ligation as above 3C technologies, this method combines ultrathin cryosectioning, laser microdissection, DNA sequencing, and statistical inference of co-segregation to detect interacting DNA fragments, which significantly expands our ability to explore chromatin spatial organization. Using this tool, they have succeeded in constructing the 3D chromatin structures of mouse embryonic stem cells, and unequivocally found some triplet contacts between super-enhancers [127].

Due to the heterogeneity between cells [128], it cannot be overlooked for the impact on data statistical processing regarding these data derived from millions of cells. Therefore, the established 3D genome modeling can represent only an average state of whole cell populations. Thus, one promising challenge is the development of strategies that analyze genomic 3D structure in single- or low-cell samples. Benefiting from the progresses of single-cell sequencing technology [129–131], Hi-C assays based on single or low-cell samples have been fulfilled and presented the chromatin structure diversities cell versus cell [132–138]. A prospective idea is that, by combining with other single-cell data of chromatin states, including transcriptome, DNA methylome, and histone modification, single-cell Hi-C assay will be possible to build a comprehensive picture for the interplay between chromatin folding and its states inside of single cell.

Conclusions

C-technologies, especially Hi-C have heralded the advent of other methods that together offer tantalizing prospects for visualizing the abstract 3D structure of the genome. With the advent of other aspects such as high-throughput and long sequencing reads, single cell sequencing and other type of epigenomics data might provide us more insights on the 3D genome and reveal fundamental principles underlying genome structure and function.

Abbreviations

3C: Chromosome conformation capture; 4C: Chromosome Conformation Capture-on-Chip; 5C: Chromosome conformation capture carbon copy; ChIA-PET: Chromatin Interaction Analysis by Paired-End Tag Sequencing; cHi-C: Capture Hi-C; ChIP: Chromatin immunoprecipitation; CT: Chromosome territory; FISH: Fluorescence in situ hybridization; GAM: Genome architecture mapping; MNase: Micrococcal nuclease; NG: Next generation; NGS: Next-generation sequencing; TADs: Topologically associating domains; UMI: Unique molecular identifier

Acknowledgments
The authors apologize to all those authors whose work they were unable to describe owing to space constraints. The authors thank members of the laboratory for their input and feedback on the manuscript.

Funding
KW was funded by the National Natural Science Foundation of China (31771862, 31471170 and 31628013).

Author's contributions
JH and KW conceived the study and drafted the manuscript. ZZ commented and revised the manuscript. All authors read and approved the final manuscript.

Competing interests
The authors declare that they have no competing interests.

References
1. Cremer T, Cremer C. Chromosome territories, nuclear architecture and gene regulation in mammalian cells. Nat Rev Genet. 2001;2(4):292–301.
2. Parada L, Misteli T. Chromosome positioning in the interphase nucleus. Trends Cell Biol. 2002;12(9):425–32.
3. Meaburn KJ, Tom M. Cell biology: chromosome territories. Nature. 2007; 445(7126):379–81.
4. Grob S, Grossniklaus U. Chromosome conformation capture-based studies reveal novel features of plant nuclear architecture. Curr Opin Plant Biol. 2017;36:149–57.
5. Hakim O, Misteli T. SnapShot: chromosome confirmation capture. Cell. 2012; 148(5):1068. e1061–1062
6. Fraser J, Williamson I, Bickmore WA, Dostie J. An overview of genome organization and how we got there: from FISH to hi-C. Microbiol Mol Biol Rev. 2015;79(3):347–72.
7. Heard E. 3D solutions to complex gene regulation. Nat Rev Mol Cell Biol. 2016;17(12):739.
8. Krijger PH, de Laat W. Regulation of disease-associated gene expression in the 3D genome. Nat Rev Mol Cell Biol. 2016;17(12):771–82.
9. Schmitt AD, Hu M, Ren B. Genome-wide mapping and analysis of chromosome architecture. Nat Rev Mol Cell Biol. 2016;17(12):743–55.
10. Schmid VJ, Cremer M, Cremer T. Quantitative analyses of the 3D nuclear landscape recorded with super-resolved fluorescence microscopy. Methods. 2017;123:33–46.
11. Bonev B, Cavalli G. Organization and function of the 3D genome. Nat Rev Genet. 2016;17(11):661–78.
12. Feng S, Cokus SJ, Schubert V, Zhai J, Pellegrini M, Jacobsen SE. Genome-wide hi-C analyses in wild-type and mutants reveal high-resolution chromatin interactions in Arabidopsis. Mol Cell. 2014;55(5):694–707.
13. Bickmore W, Vansteensel B. Genome architecture: domain Organization of Interphase Chromosomes. Cell. 2013;152(6):1270–84.
14. Osorio J. Chromatin: moving a TAD closer to unravelling chromosome architecture. Nat Rev Genet. 2016;17(1):3–3.
15. Dekker J, Mirny L. The 3D genome as moderator of chromosomal communication. Cell. 2016;164(6):1110–21.
16. Makova KD, Hardison RC. The effects of chromatin organization on variation in mutation rates in the genome. Nat Rev Genet. 2015; 16(4):213–23.
17. Dixon JR, Jung I, Selvaraj S, Shen Y, Antosiewicz-Bourget JE, Lee AY, Ye Z, Kim A, Rajagopal N, Xie W, et al. Chromatin architecture reorganization during stem cell differentiation. Nature. 2015; 518(7539):331–6.
18. Grob S, Schmid MW, Luedtke NW, Wicker T, Grossniklaus U. Characterization of chromosomal architecture in Arabidopsis by chromosome conformation capture. Genome Biol. 2013;14(11):R129.

19. Shen Y, Yue F, McCleary DF, Ye Z, Edsall L, Kuan S, Wagner U, Dixon J, Lee L, Lobanenkov VV, et al. A map of the cis-regulatory sequences in the mouse genome. Nature. 2012;488(7409):116–20.

20. Francastel C, Schübeler D, Martin DI, Groudine M. Nuclear compartmentalization and gene activity. Nat Rev Mol Cell Biol. 2000;1(2):137–43.

21. Wasserman WW, Sandelin A. Applied bioinformatics for the identification of regulatory elements. Nat Rev Genet. 2004;5(4):276–87.

22. Branco MR, Pombo A. Chromosome organization: new facts, new models. Trends Cell Biol. 2007;17(3):127–34.

23. Won H, De la Torre-Ubieta L, Stein JL, Parikshak NN, Huang J, Opland CK, Gandal MJ, Sutton GJ, Hormozdiari F, Lu D, et al. Chromosome conformation elucidates regulatory relationships in developing human brain. Nature. 2016;538(7626):523–7.

24. Taberlay PC, Achinger-Kawecka J, Lun AT, Buske FA, Sabir K, Gould CM, Zotenko E, Bert SA, Giles KA, Bauer DC, et al. Three-dimensional disorganisation of the cancer genome occurs coincident with long range genetic and epigenetic alterations. Genome Res. 2016;26(6):719–31.

25. Dekker J. Mapping the 3D genome: aiming for consilience. Nat Rev Mol Cell Biol. 2016;17(12):741–2.

26. Moissiard G, Cokus SJ, Cary J, Feng S, Billi AC, Stroud H, Husmann D, Zhan Y, Lajoie BR, McCord RP, et al. MORC family ATPases required for heterochromatin condensation and gene silencing. Science. 2012; 336(6087):1448–51.

27. Cremer T, Cremer C. Rise, fall and resurrection of chromosome territories: a historical perspective. Part I. The rise of chromosome territories. Eur J Histochem. 2006;50(3):161–76.

28. Muller I, Boyle S, Singer RH, Bickmore WA, Chubb JR. Stable morphology, but dynamic internal reorganisation, of interphase human chromosomes in living cells. PLoS One. 2010;5(7):e11560.

29. Edelmann P, Bornfleth H, Zink D, Cremer T, Cremer C. Morphology and dynamics of chromosome territories in living cells. Biochim Biophys Acta. 2001;1551(1):M29–39.

30. Mahy NL, Perry PE, Bickmore WA. Gene density and transcription influence the localization of chromatin outside of chromosome territories detectable by FISH. J Cell Biol. 2002;159(5):753–63.

31. Chambeyron S, Bickmore WA. Chromatin decondensation and nuclear reorganization of the HoxB locus upon induction of transcription. Genes Dev. 2004;18(10):1119–30.

32. Boyle S, Rodesch MJ, Halvensleben HA, Jeddeloh JA, Bickmore WA. Fluorescence in situ hybridization with high-complexity repeat-free oligonucleotide probes generated by massively parallel synthesis. Chromosom Res. 2011;19(7):901–9.

33. Shopland LS, Lynch CR, Peterson KA, Thornton K, Kepper N, Hase J, Stein S, Vincent S, Molloy KR, Kreth G, et al. Folding and organization of a contiguous chromosome region according to the gene distribution pattern in primary genomic sequence. J Cell Biol. 2006;174(1):27–38.

34. Brown JM, Green J, das Neves RP, Wallace HAC, Smith AJH, Hughes J, Gray N, Taylor S, Wood WG, Higgs DR, et al. Association between active genes occurs at nuclear speckles and is modulated by chromatin environment. J Cell Biol. 2008;182(6):1083–97.

35. Cremer T, Cremer M, Dietzel S, Müller S, Solovei I, Fakan S. Chromosome territories–a functional nuclear landscape. Curr Opin Cell Biol. 2006;18(3):307–16.

36. van Steensel B, Dekker J. Genomics tools for unraveling chromosome architecture. Nat Biotechnol. 2010;28(10):1089–95.

37. Rego EH, Shao L, Macklin JJ, Winoto L, Johansson GA, Kamps-Hughes N, Davidson MW, Gustafsson MG. Nonlinear structured-illumination microscopy with a photoswitchable protein reveals cellular structures at 50-nm resolution. Proc Natl Acad Sci. 2011;109(3):E135–43.

38. Hu M, Deng K, Qin Z, Liu JS. Understanding spatial organizations of chromosomes via statistical analysis of hi-C data. Quant Biol. 2013;1(2):156–74.

39. Williamson I, Berlivet S, Eskeland R, Boyle S, Illingworth RS, Paquette D, Dostie J, Bickmore WA. Spatial genome organization: contrasting views from chromosome conformation capture and fluorescence in situ hybridization. Genes Dev. 2014;28(24):2778–91.

40. Sati S, Cavalli G. Chromosome conformation capture technologies and their impact in understanding genome function. Chromosoma. 2017;126(1):33–44.

41. Ramani V, Shendure J, Duan Z. Understanding spatial genome organization: methods and insights. Genomics Proteomics Bioinformatics. 2016;14(1):7–20.

42. Risca VI, Greenleaf WJ. Unraveling the 3D genome: genomics tools for multiscale exploration. Trends Genet. 2015;31(7):357–72.

43. Wang C, Liu C, Roqueiro D, Grimm D, Schwab R, Becker C, Lanz C, Weigel D. Genome-wide analysis of local chromatin packing in Arabidopsis thaliana. Genome Res. 2014;

44. Lesne A, Riposo J, Roger P, Cournac A, Mozziconacci J. 3D genome reconstruction from chromosomal contacts. Nat Meth. 2014;11(11):1141–3.

45. Louwers M, Splinter E, van Driel R, de Laat W, Stam M. Studying physical chromatin interactions in plants using chromosome conformation capture (3C). Nat Protoc. 2009;4(8):1216–29.

46. Dekker J, Rippe K, Dekker M, Kleckner N. Capturing chromosome conformation. Science. 2002;295(5558):1306–11.

47. Tolhuis B, Palstra RJ, Splinter E, Grosveld F, Laat WD. Looping and interaction between hypersensitive sites in the active beta-globin locus. Mol Cell. 2002;10(6):1453–65.

48. Robert-Jan P, Bas T, Erik S, Rian N, Frank G, Wouter DL. The ÄŸ-globin nuclear compartment in development and erythroid differentiation. Nat Genet. 2003;35(2):190–4.

49. Miele A, Bystricky K, Dekker J. Yeast silent mating type loci form heterochromatic clusters through silencer protein-dependent long-range interactions. PLoS Genet. 2009;5(5):e1000478.

50. Sue Mei TW, French JD, Proudfoot NJ, Brown MA. Dynamic interactions between the promoter and terminator regions of the mammalian BRCA1 gene. Proc Natl Acad Sci U S A. 2008;105(13):5160–5.

51. Comet I, Schuettengruber B, Sexton T, Cavalli G. A chromatin insulator driving three-dimensional Polycomb response element (PRE) contacts and Polycomb association with the chromatin fiber. Proc Natl Acad Sci U S A. 2011;108(6):2294–9.

52. Murrell A, Heeson S, Reik W. Interaction between differentially methylated regions partitions the imprinted genes Igf2 and H19 into parent-specific chromatin loops. Nat Genet. 2004;36(8):889–93.

53. Spilianakis CG, Lalioti MD, Town T, Lee GR, Flavell RA. Interchromosomal associations between alternatively expressed loci. Nature. 2005;435(7042):637–45.

54. Erik S, Helen H, Jurgen K, Robert-Jan P, Petra K, Frank G, Niels G, Wouter DL. CTCF mediates long-range chromatin looping and local histone modification in the beta-globin locus. Genes Dev. 2006;20(2):178.

55. Douglas V, De GM, Sloane-Stanley JA, Wood WG, Higgs DR. Long-range chromosomal interactions regulate the timing of the transition between poised and active gene expression. EMBO J. 2007;26(8):2041–51.

56. Nele G, Smith EM, Tabuchi TM, Koch CM, Ian D, Stamatoyannopoulos JA, Job D. Cell-type-specific long-range looping interactions identify distant regulatory elements of the CFTR gene. Nucleic Acids Res. 2010; 38(13):4325–36.

57. Dekker J, Marti-Renom MA, Mirny LA. Exploring the three-dimensional organization of genomes: interpreting chromatin interaction data. Nat Rev Genet. 2013;14(6):390–403.

58. O'Sullivan JM, Tan-Wong SM, Morillon A, Lee B, Coles J, Mellor J, Proudfoot NJ. Gene loops juxtapose promoters and terminators in yeast. Nat Genet. 2004;36(9):1014–8.

59. Simonis M, Kooren J, De LW. An evaluation of 3C-based methods to capture DNA interactions. Nat Methods. 2007;4(11):895–901.

60. Marieke S, Petra K, Erik S, Yuri M, Rob W, Elzo DW, Bas VS, Wouter DL. Nuclear organization of active and inactive chromatin domains uncovered by chromosome conformation capture-on-chip (4C). Nat Genet. 2006;38(11):1348–54.

61. Zhao Z, Tavoosidana G, Sjolinder M, Gondor A, Mariano P, Wang S, Kanduri C, Lezcano M, Sandhu KS, Singh U, et al. Circular chromosome conformation capture (4C) uncovers extensive networks of epigenetically regulated intra- and interchromosomal interactions. Nat Genet. 2006;38(11):1341–7.

62. Splinter E, Wit ED, Nora EP, Klous P, Werken HJGVD, Zhu Y, Kaaij LJT, Ijcken WV, Gribnau J, Heard E. The inactive X chromosome adopts a unique three-dimensional conformation that is dependent on Xist RNA. Genes Dev. 2011;25(13):1371–83.

63. van de Werken HJ, Landan G, Holwerda SJ, Hoichman M, Klous P, Chachik R, Splinter E, Valdes-Quezada C, Oz Y, Bouwman BA, et al. Robust 4C-seq data analysis to screen for regulatory DNA interactions. Nat Methods. 2012;9(10):969–72.

64. Andrey G, Montavon T, Mascrez B, Gonzalez F, Noordermeer D, Leleu M, Trono D, Spitz F, Duboule D. A switch between topological domains underlies HoxD genes collinearity in mouse limbs. Science. 2013; 340(6137):1234167.

65. Daan N, Elzo DW, Petra K, Harmen VDW, Marieke S, Melissa LJ, Bert E, Annelies DK, Singer RH, Wouter DL. Variegated gene expression caused by cell-specific long-range DNA interactions. Nat Cell Biol. 2011;13(8):944–51.

66. Simonis M, Klous P, Homminga I, Galjaard RJ, Rijkers EJ, Grosveld F, Meijerink JP, de Laat W. High-resolution identification of balanced and complex chromosomal rearrangements by 4C technology. Nat Methods. 2009;6(11):837–42.

67. Groschel S, Sanders MA, Hoogenboezem R, de Wit E, Bouwman BA, Erpelinck C, van der Velden VH, Havermans M, Avellino R, van Lom K, et al. A single oncogenic enhancer rearrangement causes concomitant EVI1 and GATA2 deregulation in leukemia. Cell. 2014;157(2):369–81.

68. Stadhouders R, Kolovos P, Brouwer R, Zuin J, van den Heuvel A, Kockx C, Palstra RJ, Wendt KS, Grosveld F, van Ijcken W, et al. Multiplexed chromosome conformation capture sequencing for rapid genome-scale high-resolution detection of long-range chromatin interactions. Nat Protoc. 2013;8(3):509–24.

69. Dostie J, Richmond TA, Arnaout RA, Selzer RR, Lee WL, Honan TA, Rubio ED, Krumm A, Lamb J, Nusbaum C, et al. Chromosome conformation capture carbon copy (5C): a massively parallel solution for mapping interactions between genomic elements. Genome Res. 2006;16(10):1299–309.

70. Dostie J, Dekker J. Mapping networks of physical interactions between genomic elements using 5C technology. Nat Protoc. 2007;2(4):988–1002.

71. Baù D, Sanyal A, Lajoie BR, Capriotti E, Byron M, Lawrence JB, Dekker J, Marti-Renom MA. The three-dimensional folding of the a-globin gene domain reveals formation of chromatin globules. Nat Struct Mol Biol. 2011; 18(1):107–14.

72. Fraser J, Rousseau M, Shenker S, Ferraiuolo MA, Hayashizaki Y, Blanchette M, Dostie J. Chromatin conformation signatures of cellular differentiation. Genome Biol. 2009;10(4):1–18.

73. Ferraiuolo MA, Mathieu R, Carol M, Solomon S, Wang XQD, Michelle N, Mathieu B, Josée D. The three-dimensional architecture of Hox cluster silencing. Nucleic Acids Res. 2010;38(21):7472–84.

74. Wang KC, Yang YW, Bo L, Amartya S, Ryan CZ, Yong C, Lajoie BR, Angeline P, Flynn RA, Gupta RA. A long noncoding RNA maintains active chromatin to coordinate homeotic gene expression. Nature. 2011; 472(7341):120–4.

75. Nora EP, Lajoie BR, Schulz EG, Giorgetti L, Okamoto I, Servant N, Piolot T, van Berkum NL, Meisig J, Sedat J, et al. Spatial partitioning of the regulatory landscape of the X-inactivation Centre. Nature. 2012; 485(7398):381–5.

76. Fullwood MJ, Liu MH, Pan YF, Liu J, Xu H, Mohamed YB, Orlov YL, Velkov S, Ho A, Mei PH, et al. An oestrogen-receptor-alpha-bound human chromatin interactome. Nature. 2009;462(7269):58–64.

77. Li G, Fullwood MJ, Han X, Mulawadi FH, Velkov S, Vega V, Ariyaratne PN, Mohamed YB, Ooi HS, Tennakoon C. ChIA-PET tool for comprehensive chromatin interaction analysis with paired-end tag sequencing. Genome Biol. 2010;11(2):1–13.

78. Li X, Luo OJ, Wang P, Zheng M, Wang D, Piecuch E, Zhu JJ, Tian SZ, Tang Z, Li G, et al. Long-read ChIA-PET for base-pair-resolution mapping of haplotype-specific chromatin interactions. Nat Protocols. 2017;12(5):899–915.

79. Handoko L, Xu H, Li G, Ngan CY, Chew E, Schnapp M, Lee CW, Ye C, Ping JL, Mulawadi F, et al. CTCF-mediated functional chromatin interactome in pluripotent cells. Nat Genet. 2011;43(7):630–8.

80. Heidari N, Phanstiel DH, He C, Grubert F, Jahanbani F, Kasowski M, Zhang MQ, Snyder MP. Genome-wide map of regulatory interactions in the human genome. Genome Res. 2014;24(12):1905–17.

81. Mumbach MR, Rubin AJ, Flynn RA, Dai C, Khavari PA, Greenleaf WJ, Chang HY. HiChIP: efficient and sensitive analysis of protein-directed genome architecture. Nat Methods. 2016;13(11):919–22.

82. Lieberman-Aiden E, Dekker J. Comprehensive mapping of long-range interactions reveals folding principles of the human genome. Science. 2009; 326(5950):289–93.

83. van Berkum NL, Lieberman-Aiden E, Williams L, Imakaev M, Gnirke A, Mirny LA, Dekker J, Lander ES. Hi-C: a method to study the three-dimensional architecture of genomes. J Vis Exp. 2010;39:e1869.

84. Ay F, Noble WS. Analysis methods for studying the 3D architecture of the genome. Genome Biol. 2015;16:183.

85. Lajoie BR, Dekker J, Kaplan N. The Hitchhiker's guide to hi-C analysis: practical guidelines. Methods (San Diego, Calif). 2015;72:65–75.

86. Forcato M, Nicoletti C, Pal K, Livi CM, Ferrari F, Bicciato S. Comparison of computational methods for hi-C data analysis. Nat Meth. 2017;14(7):679–85.

87. Rao SS, Huntley MH, Durand NC, Stamenova EK, Bochkov ID, Robinson JT, Sanborn AL, Machol I, Omer AD, Lander ES, et al. A 3D map of the human genome at Kilobase resolution reveals principles of chromatin looping. Cell. 2014;159(7):1665–80.

88. Wingett S, Ewels P, Furlan-Magaril M, Nagano T, Schoenfelder S, Fraser P, Andrews S. HiCUP: pipeline for mapping and processing hi-C data. F1000Res. 2015;4:1310.

89. Imakaev M, Fudenberg G, McCord RP, Naumova N, Goloborodko A, Lajoie BR, Dekker J, Mirny LA. Iterative correction of hi-C data reveals hallmarks of chromosome organization. Nat Methods. 2012;9(10):999–1003.

90. Yaffe E, Tanay A. Probabilistic modeling of hi-C contact maps eliminates systematic biases to characterize global chromosomal architecture. Nat Genet. 2011;43(11):1059–65.

91. Hu M, Deng K, Selvaraj S, Qin Z, Ren B, Liu JS. HiCNorm: removing biases in hi-C data via Poisson regression. Bioinformatics. 2012;28(23):3131–3.

92. Asbury TM, Mitman M, Tang J, Zheng WJ. Genome3D: a viewer-model framework for integrating and visualizing multi-scale epigenomic information within a three-dimensional genome. BMC Bioinformatics. 2010;11:444.

93. Zhou X, Lowdon RF, Li D, Lawson HA, Madden PA, Costello JF, Wang T. Exploring long-range genome interactions using the WashU epigenome browser. Nat Methods. 2013;10(5):375–6.

94. Dixon JR, Selvaraj S, Yue F, Kim A, Li Y, Shen Y, Hu M, Liu JS, Ren B. Topological domains in mammalian genomes identified by analysis of chromatin interactions. Nature. 2012;485(7398):376–80.

95. Mateos-Langerak J, Bohn M, de Leeuw W, Giromus O, Manders EM, Verschure PJ, Indemans MH, Gierman HJ, Heermann DW, van Driel R, et al. Spatially confined folding of chromatin in the interphase nucleus. Proc Natl Acad Sci U S A. 2009;106(10):3812–7.

96. Bohn M, Heermann DW. Diffusion-driven looping provides a consistent framework for chromatin organization. PLoS One. 2010;5(8):521–6.

97. Barbieri M, Chotalia M, Fraser J, Lavitas LM, Dostie J, Pombo A, Nicodemi M. Complexity of chromatin folding is captured by the strings and binders switch model. Proc Natl Acad Sci U S A. 2012; 109(40):16173–8.

98. Duan Z, Andronescu M, Schutz K, McIlwain S, Kim YJ, Lee C, Shendure J, Fields S, Blau CA, Noble WS. A three-dimensional model of the yeast genome. Nature. 2010;465(7296):363–7.

99. Le TB, Imakaev MV, Mirny LA, Laub MT. High-resolution mapping of the spatial organization of a bacterial chromosome. Science. 2013;342(6159):731–4.

100. Jin F, Li Y, Dixon JR, Selvaraj S, Ye Z, Lee AY, Yen CA, Schmitt AD, Espinoza CA, Ren B. A high-resolution map of the three-dimensional chromatin interactome in human cells. Nature. 2013;503(7475):290–4.

101. Ay F, Bunnik EM, Varoquaux N, Bol SM, Prudhomme J, Vert JP, Noble WS, Le Roch KG. Three-dimensional modeling of the P. Falciparum genome during the erythrocytic cycle reveals a strong connection between genome architecture and gene expression. Genome Res. 2014;24(6):974–88.

102. Ma W, Ay F, Lee C, Gulsoy G, Deng X, Cook S, Hesson J, Cavanaugh C, Ware CB, Krumm A, et al. Fine-scale chromatin interaction maps reveal the cis-regulatory landscape of human lincRNA genes. Nat Methods. 2015;12(1):71–8.

103. Burton JN, Adey A, Patwardhan RP, Qiu R, Kitzman JO, Shendure J. Chromosome-scale scaffolding of de novo genome assemblies based on chromatin interactions. Nat Biotechnol. 2013;31(12):1119–25.

104. Selvaraj S, RD J, Bansal V, Ren B. Whole-genome haplotype reconstruction using proximity-ligation and shotgun sequencing. Nat Biotechnol. 2013; 31(12):1111–8.

105. Dudchenko O, Batra SS, Omer AD, Nyquist SK, Hoeger M, Durand NC, Shamim MS, Machol I, Lander ES, Aiden AP, et al. De novo assembly of the Aedes aegypti genome using hi-C yields chromosome-length scaffolds. Science. 2017;356(6333):92–5.

106. Avni R, Nave M, Barad O. Wild emmer genome architecture and diversity elucidate wheat evolution and domestication. Science. 2017;357(6346):93–7.

107. Jarvis DE, Ho YS, Lightfoot DJ, Schmockel SM, Li B, Borm TJ, Ohyanagi H, Mineta K, Michell CT, Saber N, et al. The genome of Chenopodium quinoa. Nature. 2017;542(7641):307–12.

108. Mascher M, Gundlach H, Himmelbach A, et al. A chromosome conformation capture ordered sequence of the barley genome. Nature. 2017;544(7651): 427–433.

109. Wu P, Li T, Li R, Jia L, Zhu P, Liu Y, Chen Q, Tang D, Yu Y, Li C. 3D genome of multiple myeloma reveals spatial genome disorganization associated with copy number variations. Nat Commun. 2017;8:1937.

110. Harewood L, Kishore K, Eldridge MD, Wingett S, Pearson D, Schoenfelder S, Collins VP, Fraser P. Hi-C as a tool for precise detection and characterisation of chromosomal rearrangements and copy number variation in human tumours. Genome Biol. 2017;18(1):125.

111. Aymard F, Aguirrebengoa M, Guillou E, Javierre BM, Bugler B, Arnould C, Rocher V, Iacovoni JS, Biernacka A, Skrzypczak M, et al. Genome-wide mapping of long-range contacts unveils clustering of DNA double-strand breaks at damaged active genes. Nat Struct Mol Biol. 2017;24(4):353–61.

112. Servant N, Varoquaux N, Lajoie BR, Viara E, Chen CJ, Vert JP, Heard E, Dekker J, Barillot E. HiC-pro: an optimized and flexible pipeline for hi-C data processing. Genome Biol. 2015;16:259.

113. Schwartzman O, Mukamel Z, Oded-Elkayam N, Olivares-Chauvet P, Lubling Y, Landan G, Izraeli S, Tanay A. UMI-4C for quantitative and targeted chromosomal contact profiling. Nat Methods. 2016;13(8):685–91.

114. Hughes JR, Roberts N, McGowan S, Hay D, Giannoulatou E, Lynch M, De Gobbi M, Taylor S, Gibbons R, Higgs DR. Analysis of hundreds of cis-regulatory landscapes at high resolution in a single, high-throughput experiment. Nat Genet. 2014;46(2):205–12.

115. Mifsud B, Tavares-Cadete F, Young AN, Sugar R, Schoenfelder S, Ferreira L, Wingett SW, Andrews S, Grey W, Ewels PA, et al. Mapping long-range promoter contacts in human cells with high-resolution capture hi-C. Nat Genet. 2015;47(6):598–606.

116. Jager R, Migliorini G, Henrion M, Kandaswamy R, Speedy HE, Heindl A, Whiffin N, Carnicer MJ, Broome L, Dryden N, et al. Capture hi-C identifies the chromatin interactome of colorectal cancer risk loci. Nat Commun. 2015;6:6178.

117. Davies JO, Telenius JM, McGowan SJ, Roberts NA, Taylor S, Higgs DR, Hughes JR. Multiplexed analysis of chromosome conformation at vastly improved sensitivity. Nat Methods. 2016;13(1):74–80.

118. Hsieh TH, Weiner A, Lajoie B, Dekker J, Friedman N, Rando OJ. Mapping nucleosome resolution chromosome folding in yeast by micro-C. Cell. 2015;162(1):108–19.

119. Hsieh TS, Fudenberg G, Goloborodko A, Rando OJ. Micro-C XL: assaying chromosome conformation from the nucleosome to the entire genome. Nat Methods. 2016;13(12):1009–11.

120. Davies JO, Oudelaar AM, Higgs DR, Hughes JR. How best to identify chromosomal interactions: a comparison of approaches. Nat Methods. 2017;14(2):125–34.

121. Brant L, Georgomanolis T, Nikolic M, Brackley CA, Kolovos P, van Ijcken W, Grosveld FG, Marenduzzo D, Papantonis A. Exploiting native forces to capture chromosome conformation in mammalian cell nuclei. Mol Syst Biol. 2016;12(12):891.

122. Rusk N. Genomics: native chromosome conformation. Nat Meth. 2017;14(2):105.

123. Fudenberg G, Imakaev M. FISH-ing for captured contacts: towards reconciling FISH and 3C. Nat Meth. 2017;14(7):673–8. advance online publication

124. Ou HD, Phan S, Deerinck TJ, Thor A, Ellisman MH, O'Shea CC. ChromEMT: visualizing 3D chromatin structure and compaction in interphase and mitotic cells. Science. 2017;357(6349):eaag0025.

125. Wijchers PJ, de Laat W. Genome organization influences partner selection for chromosomal rearrangements. Trends Genet. 2011;27(2):63–71.

126. Ay F, Vu TH, Zeitz MJ, Varoquaux N, Carette JE, Vert JP, Hoffman AR, Noble WS. Identifying multi-locus chromatin contacts in human cells using tethered multiple 3C. BMC Genomics. 2015;16:121.

127. Beagrie RA, Scialdone A, Schueler M, Kraemer DC, Chotalia M, Xie SQ, Barbieri M, de Santiago I, Lavitas LM, Branco MR, et al. Complex multi-enhancer contacts captured by genome architecture mapping. Nature. 2017;543(7646):519–24.

128. Nitzan R, Young JW, Uri A, Swain PS, Elowitz MB. Gene regulation at the single-cell level. Science. 2005;307(5717):1962–5.

129. Navin N, Kendall J, Troge J, Andrews P, Rodgers L, McIndoo J, Cook K, Stepansky A, Levy D, Esposito D, et al. Tumour evolution inferred by single-cell sequencing. Nature. 2011;472(7341):90–4.

130. De Souza N. Single-cell methods. Nat Methods. 2011;9(1):35.

131. Chi KR. Singled out for sequencing. Nat Methods. 2014;11(1):13–7.

132. Nagano T, Lubling Y, Stevens TJ, Schoenfelder S, Yaffe E, Dean W, Laue ED, Tanay A, Fraser P. Single-cell hi-C reveals cell-to-cell variability in chromosome structure. Nature. 2013;502(7469):59–64.

133. Stevens TJ, Lando D, Basu S, Atkinson LP, Cao Y, Lee SF, Leeb M, Wohlfahrt KJ, Boucher W, O'Shaughnessykirwan A. 3D structures of individual mammalian genomes studied by single-cell hi-C. Nature. 2017;544(7648):59.

134. Flyamer IM, Gassler J, Imakaev M, Brandão HB, Ulianov SV, Abdennur N, Razin SV, Mirny LA, Tachibana-Konwalski K. Single-nucleus Hi-C reveals unique chromatin reorganization at oocyte-to-zygote transition. Nature. 2017;544(7648):110–4. advance online publication

135. Nagano T, Lubling Y, Várnai C, Dudley C, Leung W, Baran Y, Mendelson Cohen N, Wingett S, Fraser P, Tanay A. Cell-cycle dynamics of chromosomal organization at single-cell resolution. Nature. 2017;547(7661):61–7.

136. Du Z, Zheng H, Huang B, Ma R, Wu J, Zhang X, He J, Xiang Y, Wang Q, Li Y, et al. Allelic reprogramming of 3D chromatin architecture during early mammalian development. Nature. 2017;547(7662):232–5.

137. Nagano T, Lubling Y, Yaffe E, Wingett SW, Dean W, Tanay A, Fraser P. Single-cell hi-C for genome-wide detection of chromatin interactions that occur simultaneously in a single cell. Nat Protocols. 2015;10(12):1986–2003.

138. Ke Y, Xu Y, Chen X, Feng S, Liu Z, Sun Y, Yao X, Li F, Zhu W, Gao L, et al. 3D chromatin structures of mature gametes and structural reprogramming during mammalian embryogenesis. Cell. 2017;170(2):367–81. e320

139. Kim KD, Tanizawa H, Iwasaki O, Noma K. Transcription factors mediate condensin recruitment and global chromosomal organization in fission yeast. Nat Genet. 2016;48(10):1242–52.

2

MLPA analysis in a cohort of patients with autism

Sara Peixoto[1,2,3*], Joana B. Melo[1,4,5], José Ferrão[1], Luís M. Pires[1], Nuno Lavoura[1], Marta Pinto[1], Guiomar Oliveira[2,6†] and Isabel M. Carreira[1,4,5*†]

Abstract

Background: Autism is a global neurodevelopmental disorder which generally manifests during the first 2 years and continues throughout life, with a range of symptomatic variations. Epidemiological studies show an important role of genetic factors in autism and several susceptible regions and genes have been identified. The aim of our study was to validate a cost-effective set of commercial Multiplex Ligation dependent Probe Amplification (MLPA) and methylation specific multiplex ligation dependent probe amplification (MS-MLPA) test in autistic children refered by the neurodevelopmental center and autism unit of a Paediatric Hospital.

Results: In this study 150 unrelated children with autism spectrum disorders were analysed for copy number variation in specific regions of chromosomes 15, 16 and 22, using MLPA. All the patients had been previously studied by conventional karyotype and fluorescence in situ hybridization (FISH) analysis for 15(q11.2q13) and, with these techniques, four alterations were identified. The MLPA technique confirmed these four and identified further six alterations by the combined application of the two different panels.

Conclusions: Our data show that MLPA is a cost effective straightforward and rapid method for detection of imbalances in a clinically characterized population with autism. It contributes to strengthen the relationship between genotype and phenotype of children with autism, showing the clinical difference between deletions and duplications.

Keywords: Autism, Autism spectrum disorders, Copy number variants, Genotype, Multiplex Ligation-dependent Probe Amplification (MLPA), Methylation Specific Multiplex Ligation-dependent Probe Amplification (MS-MLPA), Phenotype

Background

Autism is a global neurodevelopment disorder which, in most cases, manifests during the first 2 years and prolongs throughout life, having clinical variances with aging. It belongs to a large family of disorders - autism spectrum disorder (ASD), clinically characterized by difficulties with communication and social interaction, verbal language deficiencies and by repetitive and stereotype behaviour [1]. Epidemiological studies revealed that the number of children with ASD has been increasing throughout the world. In Portugal, a published study in 2007, suggested a prevalence of 9,2/10 000 cases, in the main land, and 15,6/10 000 in the Azores Islands [2]. Several epidemiologic

studies identified the importance of genetic factors in autism, specifically the existence of a higher rate of similarities in monozygotic twins (60 to 90%) in contrast to only 3 to 10% in dizygotic twins [3–6]. Structural chromosomic imbalances - copy number variants (CNVs) – seams to be a key player in the disorder and a risk factor for autism especially in the sporadic forms [7–11]. CNVs associated with autism may be inherited or *de novo*, affecting preferentially the chromosomes regions: 1q21, 2p16.3, 3p25-26, 7q36.2, 15q11-13, 15q24, 16p11.2, 16p13.11, 17q12 and 22q11.2 [12–14]. A recent genome wide copy number variation analysis projected between 156 and 280 genomic intervals contributing to autism. Exome sequencing of over 900 individuals provided an estimate of nearly 1.000 contributing genes [15–18]. The most consistently reported submicroscopic chromosome abnormalities detected by chromosomal microarray (10–20%) are recurrent CNVs at 16p11.2, 15q11-13 and

* Correspondence: saraccpeixoto@gmail.com; icarreira@fmed.uc.pt
†Equal contributors
[1]Cytogenetics and Genomics Laboratory, Faculty of Medicine, University of Coimbra, Coimbra, Portugal
Full list of author information is available at the end of the article

22q11.2 [12, 19, 20]. Submicroscopic rearrangements as deletions or duplications in 15q11-13 region, and especially proximal 15q duplications containing the critical regions of Prader-Willi and Angelman Syndrome (PWS/AS), have been reported in various patients with autism representing the majority of chromosome alterations described in this population [12, 21].

Microdeletions of the short arm of chromosome 16p11.2 were also identified in up to 1% of patients with autism [22–25]. The microduplication of this region was also observed in a similar percentage of individuals, however the association with autism is less convincing due to the increased frequency observed in the control groups [25, 26]. Deletions and duplications in the region 22q13.3 also appear to be risk factors for ASD. Among the three genes (*ACR, RABL2B, SHANK3*) in 22q subtelomeric region, *SHANK3* is the candidate gene for neurobehavioral symptoms observed in affected individuals with 22q13 deletions. This gene has a mutation frequency of 0.5 to 1% in individuals with ASD [27–29].

It is well accepted that array comparative genomic hybridization (CGH) should be the first genetic test to be offered for detection of genomic imbalances in patients with intellectual disability and ASD [30, 31], however access to these costly methods and techniques can be difficult especially given the current economic and financial context in many countries and consequently the pressure from the hospital administrations to contain expense. Clinicians often are confronted with this economical and financial issues and have difficulties to respond to families request to find the cause of these children pathology. One of the aims of this study was to evaluate the detection rate of MLPA technique that could allow a rapid and cost-saving response in a large consultation of children with ASD.

We analysed the presence of CNVs in the most common described chromosomic regions associated with ASD (15q11-q13, 16p11.2 and 22q13) in 150 children using MLPA and MS-MLPA techniques. A clinical assessment of each case was also done to allow genotype-phenotype correlations in the cases with genetic alterations.

Methods
Clinical assessment
For this study, a pilot population of 150 children was analysed. They were clinically diagnosed with autism by the Unit of Neurodevelopment and Autism of the Paediatric Hospital, Coimbra Hospital and University Centre, Portugal. The diagnosis was based on a clinical observation by a multidisciplinary team coordinated by a neurodevelopmental paediatrician. ASD diagnosis was assigned on the basis of the gold standard instruments: parental or caregiver interview (Autism Diagnostic Interview-Revised, ADI-R [32]), direct structured proband assessment (Autism

Diagnostic Observation Schedule, ADOS [33]), both history and observation for rating (Childhood Autism Rating Scale, CARS [34]) and clinical examination performed by an experienced neurodevelopmental Paediatrician. The latter allows the classification of the degree of autism into mild to moderate (score between 30 and 37) and severe (38–60). The current diagnostic criteria for autism were revised according to the Diagnostic and Statistical Manual of Mental Disorders fifth edition, DSM-5 [1]. It was considered a diagnosis of autism (this term being used synonymously to ASD) any case where ADI-R and ADOS presented as positive scores and all patients met the criteria for ASD from the DSM-5.

An EDTA blood sample from each child was collected for the genetic evaluation by MLPA and MS-MLPA for chromosomes 15q11-13, 16p11 and 22q13. A more detailed clinical evaluation was done for the ten children that presented alterations in the MLPA study, proceeding to the analysis of the relative clinical relevant data to the current clinical history of autism, accordingly to Table 1. Whenever possible, laboratory studies were done on the parents of the children with chromosome alterations.

Conventional cytogenetic and fluorescence in situ hybridization
All 150 children participating in this study, had been previously evaluated by high resolution conventional

Table 1 Clinical data relevant to the clinical history of the cohort

Personal history: pre and perinatal
Parturition type
Gestational age
Apgar index
Somatometry birth (weight/height/head circumference)
Personal history: Acquisition of neurodevelopment
Walking age
First words
First sentences
Global developmental quotient (GDQ) - Griffiths scale (between 2 and 6 years of age)
Global intelligence quotient (GIQ) - WISC-III (between 6 and 16 years of age)
Pathological personal history
Visual or auditory deficits
Epilepsy (two or more critical episodes in apyrexia)
Family history
Physical exam
Dysmorphisms and signs of neurocutaneous syndromes
Collection of anthropometric measurements (actual growing)
Classical neurologic exam

cytogenetic using standard GTG-banding on pro-metaphases obtained from 72 h PHA stimulated peripheral blood lymphocyte cultures according to standard procedures [35].

FISH for the critical region 15q11.2 was performed using two commercially available DNA probes: LSI SNRPN/CEP15 (locus D15Z1)/LSI PML and LSI D15S10/CEP15 (locus D15Z1)/LSI PML (Vysis, Chicago, IL) according to standard procedures and manufacturer's instructions [35].

Multiplex Ligation-dependent Probe Amplification (MLPA)
MLPA (P343-B1) and MS-MLPA (ME028) (Fig. 1a) probe panels were applied as described in the protocols of the manufacturer (MRC – Holland). The P343-B1 panel, applied to all cases, has 54 MLPA probes for the three regions 15q11-13, 16p11 and 22q13, implicated in autism. The 12 most relevant genes studied in chromosome 15 were: *SNRPN-HB2-85, UBE3A, ATP10A, GABRB3, OCA2, APBA2, NDNL2, TJP1, TRPM1, KLF13, CHRNA7, SCG5*). The MS-MLPA ME028 PWS/AS panel, was applied to the patients without alterations detected with the P343-B1 panel. This panel has 25 specific probes for the critical regions of Prader-Willi and Angelman syndromes, as well as five probes to assess the state of methylation, allowing the study of more proximal genes that are not included in P343-B1 panel, like *NIPA1* and *TUBGCP5*. In the region of microdeletion 16p11 the nine studied genes were *LAT, SPN, MAS, MVP, SEZ6L2, HIRIP3, DOC2A, MAPK3, CD2BP2*. The gene *SHANK3* in 22q13 was the one studied in chromosome 22. The products of amplification were identified and quantified by capillary electrophoresis in an

ABI 3130 genetic analyser (Applied Biosystems, Japan) and the results were analysed using the GeneMapper v4.1 software (Applied Biosystems, Foster City, USA) and Coffalyser (MRC-Holland, Amsterdam, Holland). The linear ratios of deletion and duplication were fixed at 0.7 e 1.3 respectively.

Results
The study of the conventional karyotype, together with FISH analysis for 15(q11.2q13) detected duplication of this proximal region in three cases (I, IV, V) and triplication in one case (VI) (Table 2).

The application of the MLPA – Panel P343 confirmed two of the cases identified by cytogenetics (I, VI), redefined to a triplication a duplication previously diagnosed by FISH (case V) and identified alterations in three more cases - a duplication (15q11.2-q13.1) (case II) and a deletion (15q13.2-q13.3) (case IX) of the critical region of the chromosome 15 and a duplication in 22q13.33 (case X) (Table 2 and Fig. 1b).

The use of Panel ME028 confirmed one of the alterations, diagnosed by FISH as a mosaic, to be a maternal duplication of the proximal region of 15q11.2 (case IV) and identified three more cases, with normal result after application of MLPA Panel P343: two microdeletions (cases VII and VIII) and one duplication (case III) of the most proximal region of 15q11.2 (*NIPA1, TUBGCP5*) (Table 2 and Fig. 1b).

No alterations were observed in these 150 patients for the critical region 16p11.2.

The main clinical data from these ten patients with structural chromosome alterations are described in Table 3.

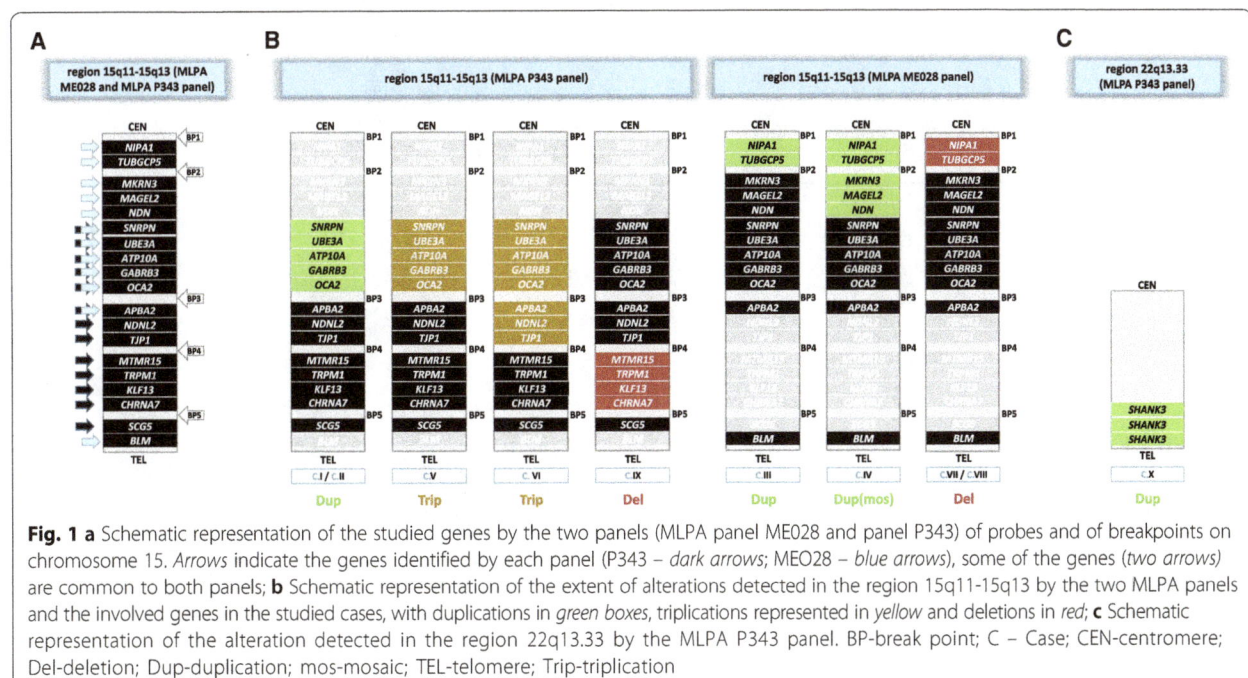

Fig. 1 a Schematic representation of the studied genes by the two panels (MLPA panel ME028 and panel P343) of probes and of breakpoints on chromosome 15. *Arrows* indicate the genes identified by each panel (P343 – *dark arrows*; MEO28 – *blue arrows*), some of the genes (*two arrows*) are common to both panels; **b** Schematic representation of the extent of alterations detected in the region 15q11-15q13 by the two MLPA panels and the involved genes in the studied cases, with duplications in *green boxes*, triplications represented in *yellow* and deletions in *red*; **c** Schematic representation of the alteration detected in the region 22q13.33 by the MLPA P343 panel. BP-break point; C – Case; CEN-centromere; Del-deletion; Dup-duplication; mos-mosaic; TEL-telomere; Trip-triplication

Table 2 Detailed clinical features of all ten probands with chromosomal abnormalities

Case/ Gender	Age (Y)	Diagnosis	Cognition	Family History	Karyotype and FISH (ISCN)	P343 MLPA panel (ISCN)	ME028 MLPA panel (ISCN)	Abnormality origin
I/M	17	ADI-R/ADOS + CARS: 44,5 Severe Autism	Severe/Profound Intellectual Disability (QIG:29)[a]	Brother has autism	46,XY.ish dup(15)(q11.2 q11.2)(SNRPN++,UBE3A++)	rsa15q11.2-q13.1(SNRPN, UBE3A,ATP10A,GABRB3, OCA2)x3	-	Mother normal Father unavailable
II/M	6	ADI-R/ADOS + CARS: 35 Severe Autism	Mild Intellectual Disability (QDG:54)[b]	Adopted Biological Mother has Depressive Disorder	46,XY	rsa 15q11.2-q13.1(SNRPN, UBE3A,ATP10A,GABRB3, OCA2)x3	-	unavailable
III/M	6	ADI-R/ADOS + CARS: 35 Mild Autism	No Intellectual Disability (QDG: 102)[b]	Father has drug addiction Brother has social disability	46,XY	rsa(P343)x2	rsa 15q11.2(NIPA1, TUBGCP5)x3mat	Mother
IV/M	12	ADI-R/ADOS + CARS: 30 Mild Autism	Mild Intellectual Disability (QDG:58)[b]	Paternal grandfather has schizophrenia Maternal grandmother is alcoholic Paternal Uncle has drug addiction	mos 47,XY,+r.ish r(15)(D15Z4 +,SNRPN-,UBE3A-)[69]/r(15)(D15Z4++,SNRPN-,UBE3A-)[2]/46,XY[105]	rsa(P343)x2	rsa 15q11.2(NIPA1, TUBGCP5,MKRN3, MAGEL2,NDN)X3mat	Mother
V/F	9	ADI-R/ADOS + CARS: 37 Moderate Autism	Mild/Moderate Intellectual Disability (QDG:39)[b]	Irrelevant	46,XX,dup(15)(q11.2q11.2)(SNRPN++,D15S10++)	rsa 15q11.2-q13.1(SNRPN, UBE3A,ATP10A,GABRB3, OCA2)x4	-	unavailable
VI/F	10	ADI-R/ADOS + CARS: 32 Mild Autism	Severe/profound Intellectual Disability (QDG:29)[b]	Irrelevant	46,XX,add(15)(q11.2).ish trp(15)(q11.2)(SNRPN, UBE3A)x4	rsa 15q11.2-q13.1(SNRPN, UBE3A,ATP10A,GABRB3, OCA2,APBA2,NDNL2,TJP1) x4dn	-	de novo
VII/M	7	ADI-R/ADOS + CARS: 30 Mild Autism	No intellectual Disability (QDG: 97)[b]	Irrelevant	46,XY	rsa(P343)x2	rsa 15q11.2(NIPA1, TUBGCP5)x1	unavailable
VIII/M	8	ADI-R/ADOS + CARS: 30 Mild Autism	Intellectual Disability (QDG:71)[b]	Mother has learning difficulties	46,XY	rsa(P343)x2	rsa 15q11.2(NIPA1, TUBGCP5)x1mat	Mother
IX/M	14	ADI-R/ADOS + CARS: 30 Mild Autism	Mild Intellectual Disability (QDG:61)[b]	Father has chromosomal abnormalities but no clinical issues Paternal grandmother has Depressive Disorder	46,XY	rsa 15q13.2-q13.3(MTMR15, TRPM, KLF13,CHRNA7)x1pat	-	Father
X/M	5	ADI-R/ADOS + CARS: 31 Mild Autism	No intellectual Disability (QDG:99)	Irrelevant	46,XY	rsa 22q13.33(SHANK3)x3mat	-	Mother

[a]WISC III; M-male, F-female

[b]Griffiths

ADI-R Autism Diagnostic Interview Revised

ADOS Autism Diagnostic Observation Schedule

ISCN International system for human cytogenetic nomenclature, 2016

Table 3 Prenatal and perinatal History and Neurodevelopment

Case	Prenatal History	Actual Growing	GPDD (1st year)	March (months)	1st Words (months)	1st sentences (months)	Epilepsy
I	Part/GA: Forceps/38w BW: 3350 g (P63); BL:52 cm (P90); BHC:35 cm (P72) AI :10	W: P75 H: P75 HC: >P50	No[a]	12	12	Doesn't build sentences	No
II	Part/GA: Eutocic/ ? BW: 3380 g (P?); AI:10	W: P95 H: P50 HC: P95	Yes	16	12	48	No
III	Part/GA: Ventouse/39w BW: 3450 g (P55); BL:50 cm (P47); BHC:35.5 cm (P69); AI :10	W: P90 H: P75 HC: >P50	No[a]	12	24	36	No
IV	Part/GA: CS/ 40w BW: 3460 g (P41); BL:50.5 cm (P39); BHC:35 cm (P45); AI:10	W: P75/90 H: P90 HC: P90	Yes	18	14	36	No
V	Part/GA: Ventouse/39w BW: 2485 g (P4); BL:47 cm (P8); BHC:32.5 cm (P11) AI :10	W: P25 H: P25 HC: P50	Yes	24	20	36	No
VI	Part/GA: Eutocic/? BW: 2840 g (P?); BL:50 cm (P?); IA:10	W: >P75 H: P50 HC: P50	Yes	24	60	Doesn't build sentences	Yes
VII	Part/GA: Eutocic/35w BW: 2510 g(P46); BL:45 cm (P31); BHC:33 cm (P72) AI:10	W: P50 H: P50 HC: P75	Yes	24	36	42	No
VIII	Part/GA: CS/ 38w High Risk in Pregnancy due to previous abortions (2) BW: 3470 g (P72); BL:49 cm (P47); BHC:36 cm (P88); AI:10	W: P95 H: P95 HC: > > P50	Yes	15	40	60	No
IX	Unknown	W: P50 H: P50 HC: >P95	Yes	19	30	42	No
X	Part: CS/ 41w BW: 4610 g (P94); BL:51 cm (P35); BHC:37 cm (P76); AI:10	W: P95 H: P90 HC: >P95	No[a]	12	12	36	No

[a]only identified at the age of 2 years old - followed by regression
Pre and perinatal history: *AI* Apgar Index at 5 min, *BHC* Birth head circumference, *BL* Birth length, *BW* Birth Weight, *CS* Caesarean Section, *GA* Gestational Age, *Part* Parturition type, *P* percentile according Fenton growth chart
Actual Growing: *HC* head circumference, *H* Height, *W* – Weight
GPDD Global psychomotor developmental delay, *w* pregnancy weeks, *g* grams, *cm* centimeters

The study of the patient's parents was possible in only six of the ten individuals with alterations: in four of them, the alteration is maternally inherited (cases III, IV, VIII and X), one has a paternal origin (case IX) and in case VI the alteration is *de novo*. For the remaining four cases, it was not possible to ascertain the parental origin because either child was adopted or because some parents rejected to be studied.

Cases I and II, are carriers of the same duplication on chromosome 15 [15q11.2q13.1(SNRPN,UBE3A,ATP10A, GABRB3,OCA2) x3] (Fig. 1b), both have severe autism but with different levels of cognition. Case II is an adopted boy with a global psychomotor developmental delay from the first year of age and currently with mild intellectual disability.

Cases III and IV, evaluated by the second MLPA probe panel have more proximal duplications of chromosome 15 (Fig. 1b). Both children have mild autism. Case III which has the more proximal duplication shows a normal global intelligence quotient (GIQ) and a normal motor and language development. Case IV has a mild intellectual deficit.

Cases V and VI (Fig. 1b), both presented mild to moderate autism but with distinct levels of intellectual disability, varying from mild in case V to severe in case VI, which is coincident with the extent of the triplicated region that includes a greater number of genes. In both patients, strabismus is present as well as motor

development delay, not found in previously described patients, carriers of duplications. This strongly suggests a gene dosage effect.

Cases VII and VIII (Fig. 1b) both have microdeletions of the proximal genes, both have similar levels of neurodevelopment features, presenting mild autism and mild (case VIII) or absent (case VII) intellectual disability. In case VIII, the alteration is of maternal origin and the progenitor is reported as having learning difficulties.

In case IX (Fig. 1b), the deleted region is distal to the previous two cases reported and involves a greater number of genes, however the clinical presentation is similar between the three cases (VII, VIII and IX). In this case the deletion was inherited from the father, but was not possible to ascertain his phenotype.

Lastly, from the 150 individual evaluated there was one case (X) identified with duplication of the SHANK3 gene on 22q13.33, associated with mild autism and average intellectual quotient and without other significant neurodevelopmental alterations except for clumsiness. The duplication was inherited from an asymptomatic mother.

Concerning to the prenatal history, most cases did not reveal any anomalies, being born from gestations of term, without prenatal incidents. As for the early development markers, half of the children walked after 18 months, which suggests an early alteration in neurodevelopment. However, the growth with regards to stature, weight and head circumference, did not reveal alterations (Table 3).

Discussion

Of the 150 children evaluated in this pilot study, only four (3%) had revealed alterations detected by conventional cytogenetics and FISH. This number increased after MLPA and MS-MLPA analysis with the identification of 6 more imbalances. Being a technique with higher resolution, MLPA also allowed the redefinition of a duplication, initially reported by conventional cytogenetics as a triplication (case V - Fig. 2) and allowed the identification of imbalances of six new cases (Table 2).

Of these ten patients, only one presented duplication on the *SHANK3* gene on 22q13.33, which is in accordance with the reported frequency in the population (1% of patients with ASD) [13, 28]. All the others showed imbalances on chromosome 15 (four duplications, two triplications and three deletions) [9, 36, 37]. No cases of deletion nor duplication on 16p11.2 were found in our sample, possibly due to the relative low frequency of up to 1% mentioned in other studies. Walsh and

Bracken in 2011 made a review of literature and a meta-analysis of 3613 ASD patients from seven studies redefining a prevalence of 16p11.2 microdeletion CNVs in 0.5% (0.31–0.82%, 95% CI) and 16p11.2 microdeletion CNVs in 0.28% (0.14–0.56%, 95% CI) not in disagreement with our results [25, 38].

CNVs in 15q11-15q13 region

In cases I, II, III and IV we found duplications of specific regions of chromosome 15 that involve several break points (Fig. 1b).

Two of the patients (case I and II) presented a duplication that affects BP2-BP3 (Fig. 1b). This alteration involves the critical region for Prader-Willi and Angelman Syndrome which is subjected to genomic imprinting and referred as the imbalance more frequently found in individuals with ASD [37, 39]. Numerous studies support that the majority of cases with this alteration are associated to maternal transmission or appear *de novo*, while the paternal inheritance leads to a normal phenotype [37, 40, 41]. It was not possible to ascertain the parental origin in these two patients (cases I and II), however the family history is

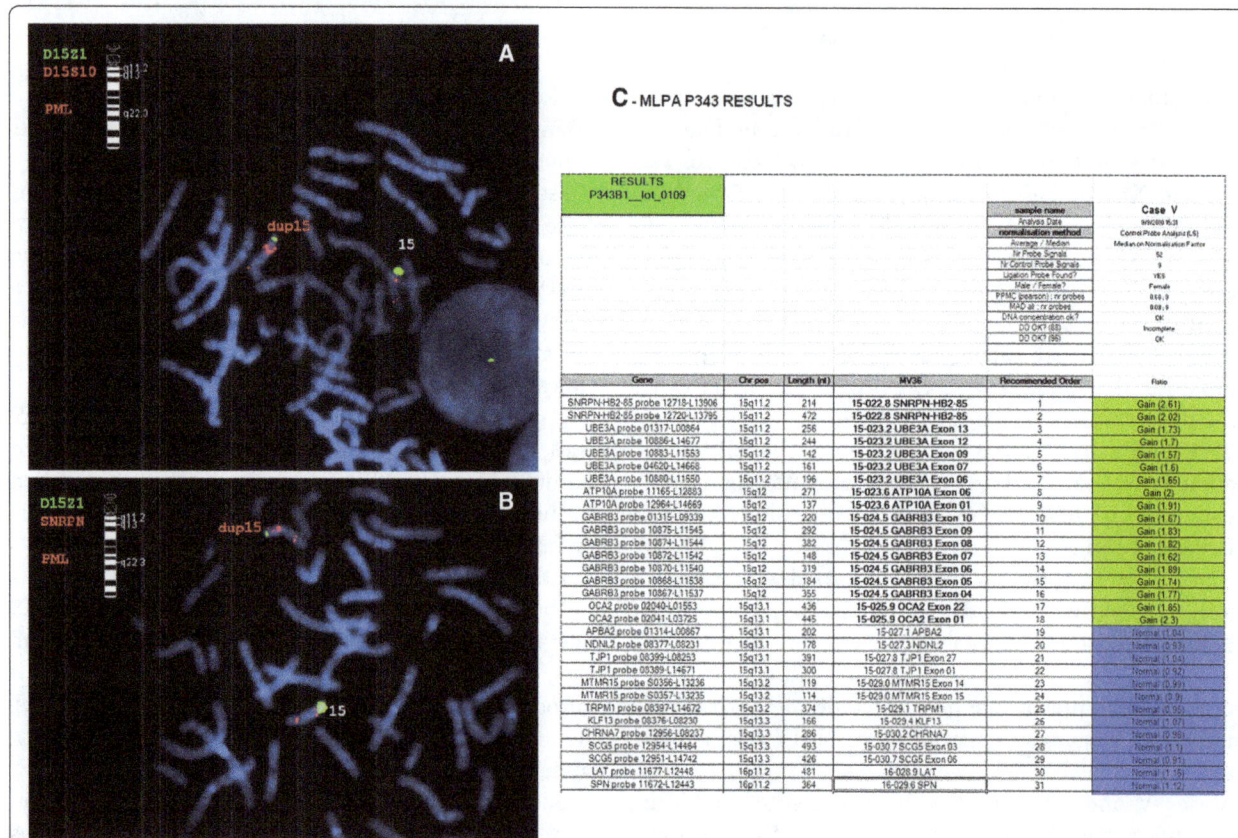

Fig. 2 FISH and MLPA results for patient V. **a** Metaphase hybridization showing a gain in 15q11.2 (D15S10 probe in *red*) interpreted as a duplication. **b** Metaphase hybridization showing a gain in 15q11.2 (SNRPN probe in *red*) interpreted as a duplication. **c** Overview of MLPA P343 result using CoffalyserV7 software (MRC Holland, Amsterdam, Netherland) revealing the presence of 4 copies and not 3 of region 15q11.2q12 in patient V compatible with a triplication and not a duplication

suggestive of neurodevelopmental delays, with a brother with autism (case I) and neuropsychiatric disorders, with mother with depressive disorder (case II), indicating a possible inheritance of the mentioned alterations (Table 2). These two cases (I and II) with the same genetic imbalances, both have severe autism although with different intellectual levels. According to Bolton PF et al. (2001) and Depienne C et al. (2009) the patients with duplication of the critical region (BP2-BP3), as occurs in these two cases, have frequently an abnormal phenotype that includes development delay, especially in speech and language, different degrees of intellectual disability, motor coordination difficulties and mild dysmorphisms (which are absent in our cases) [34, 40].

Case III, is a case of a more proximal duplication (between BP1-BP2) (Fig. 1b). The patient has mild autism, without intellectual impairment and with normal motor and language development. The common phenotype found in this alteration is highly variable, even between members of the same family [40, 42]. It can vary between autism, other neurodevelopmental disorders, mild socialization problems or learning difficulties, neuropsychiatric manifestations or even a normal phenotype, which is corroborated by other authors [37, 41]. The genetic alteration in this patient is also present in his mother who is phenotypically normal. One of the patient's brother, presents a serious socialization problem nevertheless he was not available for study.

Case IV also presents a duplication of the proximal region involving more genes than the previous one (case III) (Fig. 1b). It corresponds to a mosaicism with three cell lines. This patient presents mild intellectual disability and mild autism, as in case III. In this case IV, a milder phenotype could be expected since this aberration is present in a mosaic state. In the blood lymphocytes, the normal cellular lineage is the most representative. The ring chromosome was inherited from the mother that is not a mosaic in the blood and does not present with any type of clinical alteration. Other tissues were not evaluated for the detection of the mosaic state.

Regarding the two cases with triplication (V and VI), both have mild to moderate autism with distinct levels of intellectual disabilities which is, mild in case V but severe in case VI. The latter have a greater number of triplicated genes, being the distal breakpoint correspondent to BP4 (Fig. 1b). Genes APBA2, NDNL2 and TJP1 that are triplicated in case VI may be responsible for the more severe intellectual disability. Both patients had delay motor developmental skills (age of walking 24 months), which was not seen in the cases with duplication in our cohort, suggesting that a greater number of copies may be related to a more severe motor development delay. Both present vision deficit and one of them (case VI) also has epilepsy, which has been frequently associated with autism [43, 44].

Cases VII and VIII present microdeletion of proximal genes (NIPA1, TUBGCP5) and show similar levels of motor and cognitive development, both have mild autism with normal intelligence quotient and motor and language development delay, noted from the first year. These discrete phenotypes, as it happens in cases III and IV, that involve duplications of the same region, suggests that alterations involving this region, that not include the critical region of PWS and AS may not have any significant clinical effects. These alterations may also manifest as a milder form, like the mother in case VIII that, despite having the exact same deletion as her son, only had learning difficulties in her childhood which did not affect her adult independent life. Cases like this had been described repeatedly with significant phenotypic variability [39, 45]. Copy numbers losses and gains in this region have been identified with a frequency of 1% in the normal population, proving to be a challenge for genetic counselling [37, 39].

Case IX also corresponds to a microdeletion that is different from the previous ones since there are other breakpoints involved (BP4-BP5) (Fig. 1b) with a greater number of genes involved (MTMR15, TRPM1, KLF13, CHRNA7). The clinical condition is however similar to the two previous cases, contrary to what would be expected, based on the genetic differences. In this case, the deletion was inherited from an apparently normal father. This situation has already been reported in other cases, supporting the evidence of a higher frequency of deletions inherited from healthy parents, comparing to those that occur de novo [46, 47]. There are a great variety and heterogeneity of the phenotypic expression for this deletion of 1.6 Mb size. It ranges from normal phenotype (as it happens in the father), to intellectual disability with borderline intellectual quotient and autism (present in the patient), epilepsy, bipolar disorder, schizophrenia and other neuropsychiatric disorders [47, 48]. Depression that are frequently associated with this deletion, has been refered in the patient paternal grandmother but she was unavailable for study. In our sample, no cases of duplication of BP4-BP5 were found, which is in agreement with other reports [48–50]. If duplications involving this region cause phenotypical anomalies, its penetrance seems to be lower than it is in deletions which therefore may explain its minor frequency.

The structural alterations presented in this study involving various regions of chromosome 15, have a significant role in the pathogenesis of other different conditions. They affect predominantly the brain function like in ASD and intellectual disability (that varies from mild to severe), epilepsy and neuropsychiatric disorders like schizophrenia and bipolar disease. This phenotypic variability suggests that other events may contribute for the manifestation of those conditions.

Various factors have been proposed to explain this variability in phenotype. Besides from incomplete penetrance and the contribution of adjacent genes, the presence of a masked recessive mutation or functional polymorphism on one of the genes may be another factor, environmental and perinatal factors, maternal conditions [51, 52]. The possibility of different phenotypic expressions between diverse members of the family with a deletion, caused by defects of imprinting, would be another hypothesis to explain this variability, however it seems unlikely on the alterations that affect BP1-BP2 and BP4-BP5, as none of the genes in these regions have been described as imprinted (Genomic Imprinting Website: www.geneimprint.com/site/genes-by-species, September 2008).

Another hypothesis is the possible capability that some individuals may have to overcome one or more deficiencies caused by haploinsufficiency of specific genes during pre or postnatal development [53]. This supports the fact that some carriers have normal development from birth, while others have learning difficulties during their childhood that cause no impact in the adult life. This is enforced by the fact that some parents who present the same alterations as their children, have no problem related to social integration. In addition to all these possible explanations, one cannot exclude the presence of other CNVs not detected with this approach, neither the environmental factors that may also play a vital role in the child's development.

CNVs in SHANK3 at 22q13.33 region

A single duplication was found on gene *SHANK3* at 22q13.33 which is associated to mild autism with normal intellectual quotient. Microdeletions and point mutation involving *SHANK3* region have been reported as cause of a spectrum of neuropsychiatric disorders including "22q13 deletion syndrome" (also known as Phelan-Mcdermid syndrome) and ASD [28, 29]. In the same way, 22q13 duplications involving *SHANK3* were reported in patients with Asperger syndrome, attention deficit-hyperactivity disorder (ADHD) or schizophrenia, suggesting that an overexpression of this gene could be also pathogenic [27]. In our sample, case X is a patient with a *SHANK3* duplication that was inherited from a healthy mother which leads us to question of its pathogenicity. A situation of incomplete penetrance or expression variability cannot be ruled out in the same way as in 22q11.2 duplication syndrome [54], neither can be excluded the presence of other CNVs not detected with this approach.

Conclusion

In this study, it was also possible to establish some correlations between certain genotypes and corresponding phenotypes, despite of some variability.

The study of autism is a challenge due to the great variety of behavioural and neurodevelopmental manifestations with variable severity and many co-morbidities. With the development of new technologies that allow an approach to the whole genome, certainly there will be a greater contribution for a better comprehension of its aetiology. It is vital that children with ASD are followed-up by specialized professionals in the neurodevelopment area, so that clinical details can be well accurate to allow strong genotype-phenotype correlations.

Our study indicates that MLPA can be a cost-effective method for detection of microdeletions and microduplications in ASD population. In patients with relevant phenotypic characteristics, this approach could replace other expensive and laborious techniques in clinical diagnosis. Additionally, in some cases karyotype and/or FISH analysis should be considered, mainly for the detection of supernumerary marker chromosomes. For example, the invdup(15) is a well documented cause of ASD with distinct phenotype and prognosis.

It is well established that array-CGH should be the first-tier test for neurodevelopmental disorders, MLPA, although with some limitations, since it is a target method, can be considered as a test in large populations where the costs and economic pressures limits a more expensive method for diagnosis.

Abbreviations
ADHD: Attention deficit-hyperactivity disorder; ADIR: Autism Diagnostic Interview – Revised; ADOS: Autism Diagnostic Observation Schedule; AS: Angelman Syndrome; ASD: Autism spectrum disorder; BP: Break point; CARS: Childhood Autism Rating Scale; CGH: Comparative genomic hybridization; CNV: Copy number variants; DSM-5: Diagnostic and Statistical Manual of Mental Disorders; EDTA: Ethylenediaminetetraacetic acid; FISH: Fluorescence *in situ* hybridization; GIQ: Global intelligence quotient; MLPA: Multiplex ligation dependent probe amplification; MS-MLPA: Methylation specific multiplex ligation dependent probe amplification; PWS: Prader Willi Syndrome

Acknowledgements
The authors wish to thank the patients and their families.

Funding
Not applicable' for that section.

Authors' contributions

IMC, GO have designed the study and drafted the manuscript; SP have clinically evaluated the patients and their families, provided clinical information for the interpretation of results, partial participation in MLPA analysis and interpretation and drafted the manuscript; JBM data acquisition and drafted the manuscript; LMP, JF have been involved in MLPA data acquisition and analysis and drafted the manuscript. MP, NL have performed conventional cytogenetics procedures, including karyotype and FISH analysis and helped to draft the manuscript. All authors read and approved the final manuscript.

Competing interests

The authors declare that they have no competing interests.

Author details

[1]Cytogenetics and Genomics Laboratory, Faculty of Medicine, University of Coimbra, Coimbra, Portugal. [2]Neurodevelopmental and Autism Unit from Child Developmental Center and Centro de Investigação e Formação Clinica, Hospital Pediátrico, Centro Hospitalar e Universitário de Coimbra, Coimbra, Portugal. [3]Department of Paediatrics of the Centro Hospitalar de Trás-os-Montes e Alto Douro, EPE, Vila Real, Portugal. [4]CNC.IBILI, University of Coimbra, Coimbra, Portugal. [5]CIMAGO - Centro Investigação em Meio Ambiente, Genética e Oncobiologia, Faculty of Medicine, University of Coimbra, Coimbra, Portugal. [6]University Clinic of Pediatrics and Institute for Biomedical Imaging and Life Science, Faculty of Medicine, University of Coimbra, Coimbra, Portugal.

References

1. Association, A.P. Autism spectrum disorder. In: Diagnostic and Statistical Manual of Mental Disorders (DSM-5). 2013. p. 50.
2. Oliveira G, et al. Epidemiology of autism spectrum disorder in Portugal: prevalence, clinical characterization, and medical conditions. Dev Med Child Neurol. 2007;49(10):726–33.
3. Colvert E, et al. Heritability of Autism Spectrum Disorder in a UK Population-Based Twin Sample. JAMA Psychiatry. 2015;72(5):415–23.
4. Faras H, Al Ateeqi N, Tidmarsh L. Autism spectrum disorders. Ann Saudi Med. 2010;30(4):295–300.
5. Kumar RA, Christian SL. Genetics of autism spectrum disorders. Curr Neurol Neurosci Rep. 2009;9(3):188–97.
6. Sandin S, et al. The familial risk of autism. JAMA. 2014;311(17):1770–7.
7. Abrahams BS, Geschwind DH. Advances in autism genetics: on the threshold of a new neurobiology. Nat Rev Genet. 2008;9(5):341–55.
8. Autism Genome Project, C, et al. Mapping autism risk loci using genetic linkage and chromosomal rearrangements. Nat Genet. 2007;39(3):319–28.
9. Pinto D, et al. Convergence of genes and cellular pathways dysregulated in autism spectrum disorders. Am J Hum Genet. 2014;94(5):677–94.
10. Prasad A, et al. A discovery resource of rare copy number variations in individuals with autism spectrum disorder. G3 (Bethesda). 2012;2(12):1665–85.
11. Sebat J, et al. Strong association of de novo copy number mutations with autism. Science. 2007;316(5823):445–9.
12. Carter MT, Scherer SW. Autism spectrum disorder in the genetics clinic: a review. Clin Genet. 2013;83(5):399–407.
13. Freitag CM, et al. Genetics of autistic disorders: review and clinical implications. Eur Child Adolesc Psychiatry. 2010;19(3):169–78.
14. Mefford HC, Batshaw ML, Hoffman EP. Genomics, intellectual disability, and autism. N Engl J Med. 2012;366(8):733–43.
15. Iossifov I, et al. De novo gene disruptions in children on the autistic spectrum. Neuron. 2012;74(2):285–99.
16. Neale BM, et al. Patterns and rates of exonic de novo mutations in autism spectrum disorders. Nature. 2012;485(7397):242–5.
17. O'Roak BJ, et al. Exome sequencing in sporadic autism spectrum disorders identifies severe de novo mutations. Nat Genet. 2011;43(6):585–9.
18. Sanders SJ, et al. De novo mutations revealed by whole-exome sequencing are strongly associated with autism. Nature. 2012;485(7397):237–41.
19. Carreira IM, et al. Copy number variants prioritization after array-CGH analysis - a cohort of 1000 patients. Mol Cytogenet. 2015;8:103.
20. Moreira DP, et al. Investigation of 15q11-q13, 16p11.2 and 22q13 CNVs in autism spectrum disorder Brazilian individuals with and without epilepsy. PLoS One. 2014;9(9):e107705.
21. Schaaf CP, et al. Truncating mutations of MAGEL2 cause Prader-Willi phenotypes and autism. Nat Genet. 2013;45(11):1405–8.
22. Marshall CR, et al. Structural variation of chromosomes in autism spectrum disorder. Am J Hum Genet. 2008;82(2):477–88.
23. Tabet AC, et al. Autism multiplex family with 16p11.2p12.2 microduplication syndrome in monozygotic twins and distal 16p11.2 deletion in their brother. Eur J Hum Genet. 2012;20(5):540–6.
24. Weiss LA, et al. Association between microdeletion and microduplication at 16p11.2 and autism. N Engl J Med. 2008;358(7):667–75.
25. Walsh KM, Bracken MB. Copy number variation in the dosage-sensitive 16p11.2 interval accounts for only a small proportion of autism incidence: a systematic review and meta-analysis. Genet Med. 2011;13(5):377–84.
26. Lord C, Rutter M, Le Couteur A. Autism Diagnostic Interview-Revised: a revised version of a diagnostic interview for caregivers of individuals with possible pervasive developmental disorders. J Autism Dev Disord. 1994;24(5):659–85.
27. Han K, et al. SHANK3 overexpression causes manic-like behaviour with unique pharmacogenetic properties. Nature. 2013;503(7474):72–7.
28. Leblond CS, et al. Meta-analysis of SHANK Mutations in Autism Spectrum Disorders: a gradient of severity in cognitive impairments. PLoS Genet. 2014;10(9):e1004580.
29. Uchino S, Waga C. SHANK3 as an autism spectrum disorder-associated gene. Brain Dev. 2013;35(2):106–10.
30. Friedman JM, et al. Oligonucleotide microarray analysis of genomic imbalance in children with mental retardation. Am J Hum Genet. 2006;79(3):500–13.
31. Miller DT, et al. Consensus statement: chromosomal microarray is a first-tier clinical diagnostic test for individuals with developmental disabilities or congenital anomalies. Am J Hum Genet. 2010;86(5):749–64.
32. Lord C, et al. Autism diagnostic observation schedule: a standardized observation of communicative and social behavior. J Autism Dev Disord. 1989;19(2):185–212.
33. Rellini E, et al. Childhood Autism Rating Scale (CARS) and Autism Behavior Checklist (ABC) correspondence and conflicts with DSM-IV criteria in diagnosis of autism. J Autism Dev Disord. 2004;34(6):703–8.
34. Depienne C, et al. Screening for genomic rearrangements and methylation abnormalities of the 15q11-q13 region in autism spectrum disorders. Biol Psychiatry. 2009;66(4):349–59.
35. Melo JB, et al. Chromosome 5 derived small supernumerary marker: towards a genotype/phenotype correlation of proximal chromosome 5 imbalances. J Appl Genet. 2011;52(2):193–200.
36. Bijlsma EK, et al. Extending the phenotype of recurrent rearrangements of 16p11.2: deletions in mentally retarded patients without autism and in normal individuals. Eur J Med Genet. 2009;52(2–3):77–87.
37. Pujana MA, et al. Human chromosome 15q11-q14 regions of rearrangements contain clusters of LCR15 duplicons. Eur J Hum Genet. 2002;10(1):26–35.
38. Browne CE, et al. Inherited interstitial duplications of proximal 15q: genotype-phenotype correlations. Am J Hum Genet. 1997;61(6):1342–52.
39. Burnside RD, et al. Microdeletion/microduplication of proximal 15q11. 2 between BP1 and BP2: a susceptibility region for neurological dysfunction including developmental and language delay. Hum Genet. 2011;130(4):517–28.
40. Bolton PF, et al. The phenotypic manifestations of interstitial duplications of proximal 15q with special reference to the autistic spectrum disorders. Am J Med Genet. 2001;105(8):675–85.
41. Piard J, et al. Clinical and molecular characterization of a large family with an interstitial 15q11q13 duplication. Am J Med Genet A. 2010;152A(8):1933–41.
42. Combi R, et al. Clinical and genetic evaluation of a family showing both autism and epilepsy. Brain Res Bull. 2010;82(1–2):25–8.
43. De Wolf V, et al. Genetic counseling for susceptibility loci and neurodevelopmental disorders: the del15q11.2 as an example. Am J Med Genet A. 2013;161A(11):2846–54.
44. Tuchman R, Hirtz D, Mamounas LA. NINDS epilepsy and autism spectrum disorders workshop report. Neurology. 2013;81(18):1630–6.
45. Cox DM, Butler MG. The 15q11.2 BP1-BP2 microdeletion syndrome: a review. Int J Mol Sci. 2015;16(2):4068–82.
46. Sharp AJ, et al. A recurrent 15q13.3 microdeletion syndrome associated with mental retardation and seizures. Nat Genet. 2008;40(3):322–8.
47. van Bon BW, et al. Further delineation of the 15q13 microdeletion and duplication syndromes: a clinical spectrum varying from non-pathogenic to a severe outcome. J Med Genet. 2009;46(8):511–23.

48. Miller DT, et al. Microdeletion/duplication at 15q13.2q13.3 among individuals with features of autism and other neuropsychiatric disorders. J Med Genet. 2009;46(4):242–8.

49. Helbig I, et al. 15q13.3 microdeletions increase risk of idiopathic generalized epilepsy. Nat Genet. 2009;41(2):160–2.

50. Kolevzon A, et al. Analysis of a purported SHANK3 mutation in a boy with autism: clinical impact of rare variant research in neurodevelopmental disabilities. Brain Res. 2011;1380:98–105.

51. Lopez-Rangel E, Lewis ME. Loud and clear evidence for gene silencing by epigenetic mechanisms in autism spectrum and related neurodevelopmental disorders. Clin Genet. 2006;69(1):21–2.

52. Krakowiak P, et al. Maternal metabolic conditions and risk for autism and other neurodevelopmental disorders. Pediatrics. 2012;129(5):e1121–8.

53. Seidman JG, Seidman C. Transcription factor haploinsufficiency: when half a loaf is not enough. J Clin Invest. 2002;109(4):451–5.

54. Courtens W, Schramme I, Laridon A. Microduplication 22q11.2: a benign polymorphism or a syndrome with a very large clinical variability and reduced penetrance?–Report of two families. Am J Med Genet A. 2008; 146A(6):758–63.

3

Molecular cytogenetic characterization of *Dasypyrum breviaristatum* chromosomes in wheat background revealing the genomic divergence between *Dasypyrum* species

Guangrong Li, Dan Gao, Hongjun Zhang, Jianbo Li, Hongjin Wang, Shixiao La, jiwei Ma and Zujun Yang[*] ⓘ

Abstract

Background: The uncultivated species *Dasypyrum breviaristatum* carries novel diseases resistance and agronomically important genes of potential use for wheat improvement. The development of new wheat-*D. breviaristatum* derivatives lines with disease resistance provides an opportunity for the identification and localization of resistance genes on specific *Dasypyrum* chromosomes. The comparison of wheat-*D. breviaristatum* derivatives to the wheat-*D. villosum* derivatives enables to reveal the genomic divergence between *D. breviaristatum* and *D. villosum*.

Results: The mitotic metaphase of the wheat- *D. breviaristatum* partial amphiploid TDH-2 and durum wheat -*D. villosum* amphiploid TDV-1 were studied using multicolor fluorescent *in situ* hybridization (FISH). We found that the distribution of FISH signals of telomeric, subtelomeric and centromeric regions on the *D. breviaristatum* chromosomes was different from those of *D. villosum* chromosomes by the probes of Oligo-pSc119.2, Oligo-pTa535, Oligo-(GAA)$_7$ and Oligo-pHv62-1. A wheat line D2139, selected from a cross between wheat lines MY11 and TDH-2, was characterized by FISH and PCR-based molecular markers. FISH analysis demonstrated that D2139 contained 44 chromosomes including a pair of *D. breviaristatum* chromosomes which had originated from the partial amphiploid TDH-2. Molecular markers confirmed that the introduced *D. breviaristatum* chromosomes belonged to homoeologous group 7, indicating that D2139 was a 7V^b disomic addition line. The D2139 displayed high resistance to wheat stripe rust races at adult stage plant, which may be inherited from, *D. breviaristatum* chromosome 7V^b.

Conclusion: The study present here revealed that the large divergence between *D. breviaristatum* and *D. villosum* with respected to the organization of different repetitive sequences. The identified wheat- *D. breviaristatum* chromosome addition line D2139 will be used to produce agronomically desirable germplasm for wheat breeding.

Keywords: *Dasypyrum breviaristatum*, Fluorescence *in situ* hybridization, Molecular marker, Wheat

Background

The genus *Dasypyrum* (or *Haynaldia*) consists of only two diploid species, the annual *Dasypyrum villosum* and perennial *D. breviaristatum* [1]. The genomes of diploid *D. villosum* and *D. breviaristatum* were assigned the symbols V and V^b, respectively [2, 3]. Based on the sequences comparison of nr5S DNA multigene family, Baum et al. [4] suggested that the genome constitution of 4x *D. breviaristatum* should be considered as an allotetraploid VVV^{b}V^b. *Dasypyrum* species possess agronomically important genes such as disease resistance, high protein quality and drought tolerance, all of which represent valuable resources for global wheat breeding [3]. The species *D. villosum* has been extensively hybridized with wheat for at least 6 decades, and several disease resistance genes have been successfully transferred to wheat [5–7]. Above all, over 20 elite cultivars carrying the wheat- *D. villosum* chromosome T6AL·6VS translocation with powdery mildew resistance gene *Pm21* have been released into agricultural production in China [8, 9]. Given the widespread success of this introgression from *D. villosum*, researches

* Correspondence: yangzujun@uestc.edu.cn
School of Life Science and Technology, University of Electronic Science and Technology of China, Chengdu 610054, China

have been conducted with a similar aim to transfer useful genes from *D. breviaristatum* into wheat. Subsequently, the wheat- *D. breviaristatum* partial amphiploid [10] and wheat- *D. breviaristatum* introgression lines with multiply disease resistances have developed [11, 12].

Molecular and cytogenetic methods have been previously employed to assess the level of chromosomal divergence of these two *Dasypyrum* species [13, 14]. A large number of interspecific and intraspecific chromosome variations and significant genomic diversification were observed among different *Dasypyrum* accessions, probably due to the out-crossing characteristic of these two *Dasypyrum* species [2]. Each pair of *Dasypyrum* chromosomes were transferred into a wheat background after intergeneric hybridizations. The wheat- *Dasypyrum* chromosome addition lines with different *Dasypyrum* species or accession origins allow comparison of the different *Dasypyrum* genomes in wheat backgrounds. In the present study, fluorescent *in situ* hybridization (FISH) was carried out to characterize differences between *D. breviaristatum* and *D. villosum* chromosomes by comparing karyotypes between the wheat- *D. breviaristatum* partial amphiploid TDH-2 and *Triticum turgidum - D. villosum* amphiploid TDV-1, The FISH and molecular markers were applied to identify new wheat- *D. breviaristatum* addition line with stripe rust resistance, which will be a useful germplasm for wheat genetics and breeding.

Results

Comparative FISH karyotype of TDH-2 and TDV-1

The mitotic metaphase chromosomes of the wheat- *D. breviaristatum* partial amphiploid TDH-2, were hybridized with probes Oligo-pSc119.2, Oligo-pTa535, Oligo-(GAA)$_7$ by sequential multicolor-FISH (Fig. 1). As shown in Fig. 1a, the FISH hybridization signals of the probes Oligo-pSc119.2 and Oligo-pTa535 can easily identify the 28 wheat chromosomes from 1A-7A and 1B-7B based on the standard FISH karyotype of wheat chromosomes using the same probes described by Tang et al. [15]. Yang et al. [10] reported that the partial amphiploid TDH-2 was produced by the elimination of some chromosomes from the wheat Chinese Spring (CS)- *D. breviaristatum* decaploid amphiploid. It is likely that the A and B chromosomes of TDH-2 originated from CS. By comparing the FISH patterns of Oligo-pSc119.2 and Oligo-pTa535 probes of TDH-2 to those of CS by Tang et al. [15], we found additional signals corresponding to probe Oligo-pSc119.2 on the terminal regions of 1BS and 2BL in TDH-2 (Fig. 1b). After comparing the (GAA)n signal distribution on TDH-2 chromosomes with those of CS reported by Danilova et al. [16], we observed that the (GAA)n signals on chromosome 7A of CS were absent in TDH-2. The results suggest that at least three wheat chromosomes have undergone structural change(s) which may

be related to the presence of *D. breviaristatum* chromosomes. Each of the seven pairs of *D. breviaristatum* chromosomes were also distinguished using probes Oligo-pSc119.2, Oligo-pTa535 in TDH-2 (Fig. 1b). These chromosomes were temporarily named Vb1-Vb7 (Fig. 1b).

FISH using probes Oligo-pSc119.2, Oligo-pTa535, Oligo-(GAA)$_7$ were also carried out on the chromosomes of the *Triticum turgidum* cv. Jorc-69- *D. villosum* amphiploid TDV-1 (Fig. 1c and d). We found that the signals of probe Oligo-pSc119.2 were mainly located on terminal sites, while the hybridization signals of Oligo-pTa535 were distributed along the chromosome arms of *D. villosum*. The probe Oligo- (GAA)$_7$ hybridized to 2V-7V of *D. villosum* chromosomes at their centromeric or sub-terminal regions. Moreover, we produced a high tandem repeat sequences probe Oligo-pHv62-1 as reported by Li et al. [17]. FISH revealed that Oligo-pHv62-1 present in terminal or sub-terminal heterochromatic C-banding regions of *D. villosum* chromosomes in TDV-1, but was absent in *D. breviaristatum* chromosomes of TDH-2 (Fig. 1e and f). The comparative FISH karyotypes of the *D. breviaristatum* and *D. villosum* chromosomes allows easily to distinguish each individual *Dasypyrum* chromosome in wheat background.

FISH of wheat- D. breviaristatum addition line D2139

Sequential multi-color ND-FISH by probes Oligo-pSc119.2, Oligo-pTa535, Oligo-(GAA)$_7$ was conducted to characterize the mitotic metaphase cells of D2139 (Fig. 2). The chromosome number of D2139 is 2n = 44, including all the 42 wheat chromosomes and two alien chromosomes added in the wheat background. The probes Oligo-pSc119.2, Oligo-pTa535, showed a pair of chromosomes with faint Oligo-pSc119.2 hybridization signals at the telomeric region of long arm, and strong hybridization signals of Oligo-pTa535 along the long and short arm in D2139 (Fig. 2). The FISH hybridization pattern of the chromosomes was identical to *D. breviaristatum* chromosomes Vb7 (Fig. 1). Therefore, we concluded that the line D2139 was a chromosome Vb7 addition line. Comparing the FISH patterns of D2139 parents MY11 [15] and TDH-2 (Fig. 1), it appeared that the D2139 line inherited the A and B- genome chromosomes from MY11 and/or TDH-2. Based on the FISH patterns, D2139 inherited chromosomes 5A, 7A, 1B, and 7B which were identical to the TDH-2 parent, while 6B, 2B appeared to be from MY11. Since there is no D-genome in the partial amphiploid TDH-2, D2139 would have inherited D-chromosomes from MY11. As shown in Fig. 2c, chromosomes 1D and 3D revealed clear differences in the distribution of Oligo-pSc119.2 signals compared to previously published FISH patterns of D-genome chromosomes of MY11 [15]. The terminal region of 1DL showed strong Oligo-pSc119.2 signals, while the Oligo-pSc119.2 signals were absent from the 3DS terminal

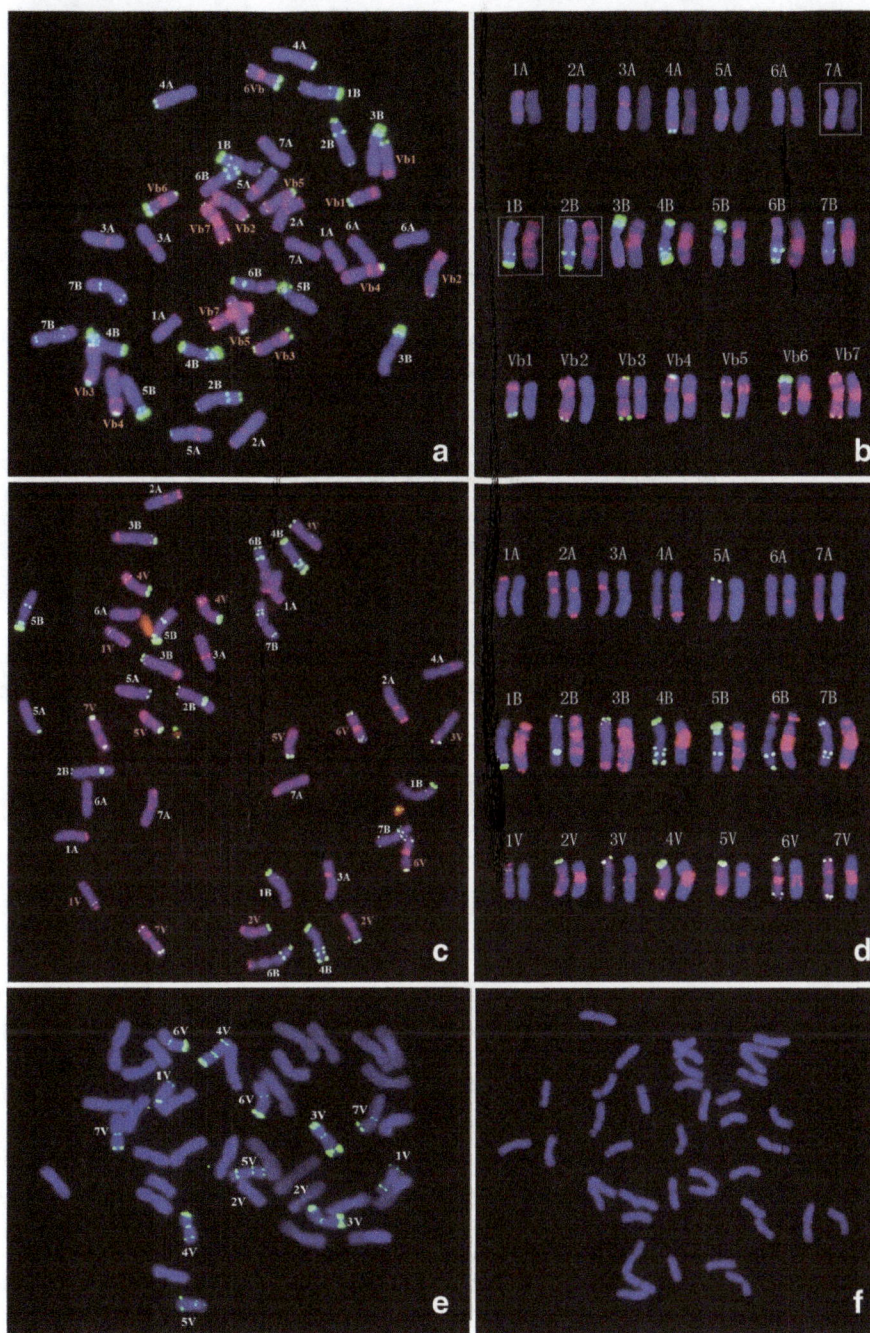

Fig. 1 FISH and karyotypes of TDH-2 (**a**, **b**, **f**) and TDV-1(**c**, **d**, **e**). The mitotic metaphase chromosomes (**a**, **c**) after hybridization with probes Oligo-pTa535 (red) and Oligo-pSc119.2 (green), or (**b**, **d**) hybridized with Oligo-(GAA)₇ (red) The boxes shows the modified chromosomes compared to its parents. Figures **e** and **f** are hybridized by probe of pHv62-3 (green)

region. The observation implies that the transmission of the *D. breviaristatum* chromosomes may be associated with structural changes in wheat chromosomes.

Molecular markers analysis

PLUG primers were designed from rice genomic DNA sequences specific for the syntenic regions, in the expectation

that they would presumably amplify fragments from the corresponding linkage group(s) of wheat genomes [18]. Our previous studies showed that the PLUG markers were useful for producing alien chromosome-specific markers [19, 20]. A total of 21 PLUG markers from wheat homoeologous group 7 were tested on D2139 compared to its parents MY11 and TDH-2 (Table 1). Based on the

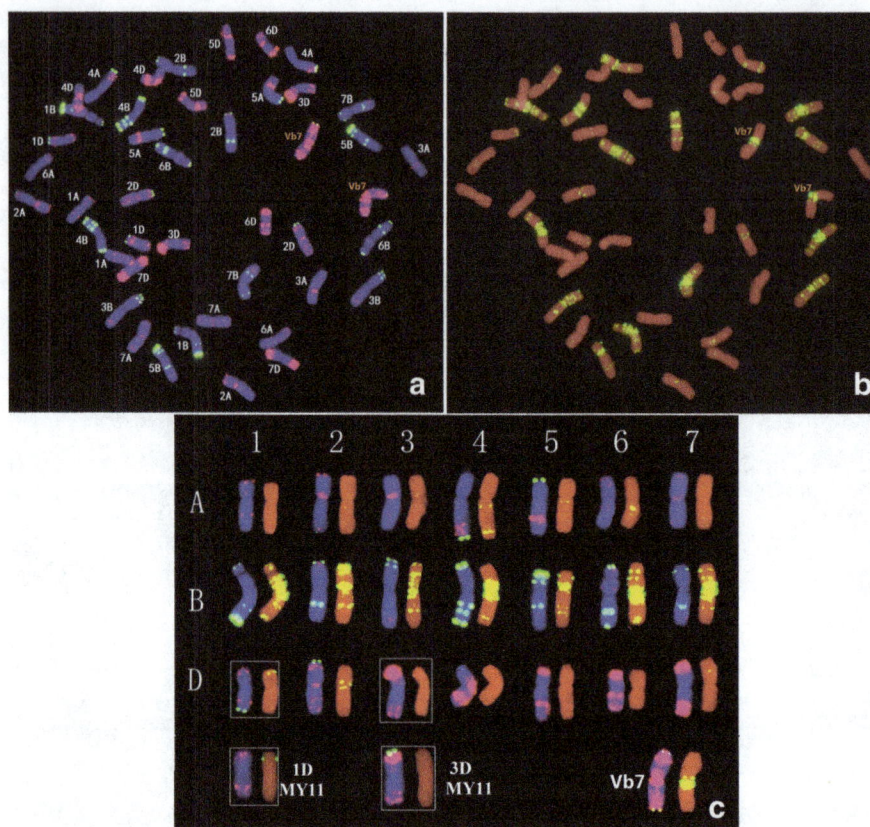

Fig. 2 Sequential FISH karyotypes of D2139. Left figure (**a**) was stained with DAPI (blue), Oligo-pTa535 (red) and Oligo-pSc119.2 (green), while the right figure (**b**) chromosomes were stained by PI (red) and Oligo-GAA (green). The box shows the modified chromosomes compared to the parent line MY11 (**c**)

amplification of nulli-tetrasomic lines of Chinese Spring, the PLUG markers give rise to the 7A, 7B and 7D specific bands, respectively (Fig. 3). A total of 13 pairs of primers generated the identical bands from *D. breviaristatum* V^{b}V^b and TDH-2 to those from the disomic addition line D2139. These results suggested that the *D. breviaristatum* chromosome in D2139 belonged to homoeologous group 7. Five markers out of the 13 had previously been mapped onto the short arms and eight mapped onto the long arms of group 7 (Table 1). After combining these PCR results with the FISH patterns, we concluded that the D2139 was a 7V^b addition line, and the Vb7 was chromosome 7V^b. The wheat CS - *D. villosum* 7V addition line TA7683 was also used to test the PLUG markers. We found that seven of 13 primer pairs showed polymorphic amplification differences between the *D. breviaristatum* 7V^b and *D. villosum* 7V chromosomes (Table 1). The results suggested that sequence divergence may have occurred among *Dasypyrum* species during their evolution.

Agronomic traits and rust resistance analysis

The spike phenotype and stripe rust resistance of lines D2139, TDH-2, CS and MY11 were observed. As shown in Fig. 4a, the spike length of D2139 was 11–12 cm, which was longer than the wheat parents (9–10 cm), while the D2139 had 22–22 spikelets per spike, closely resembling MY11. When inoculated with *P. striiformis* f. sp. *tritici* (PST) races CYR32 and CYR33 at adult plant stage, the TDH-2 and D2139 lines were highly resistance to the isolates, whereas wheat MY11 and CS were highly susceptible (Fig. 4b). These results indicated that the stripe rust resistance in D2139 was from the TDH-2 parent, and originates from *D. breviaristatum*.

Discussion

With respect to the genomic relationship between two *Dasypyrum* species, *D. breviaristatum* and *D. villosum*, cytogenetic and molecular evidence has revealed the huge genetic divergence between the two species. Friebe et al. [21] established the C-banded patterns of *D. villosum*, and then Linde-Laursen and Frederiksen [22] observed extensive C-band karyotype differences between the two genomes. De Pace et al. [23] isolated a repeat sequence that was mapped further distally on *D. villosum* chromosomes using FISH compared to wheat chromosomes. Galasso et al. [13] found that the differentiated GISH

Table 1 The primers used to localize the Vb7 specific amplification in D2139

No.	Primers name	Primer sequences (5′–3′)	Wheat bin map	Restriction enzyme	Length of Vb7 bands
1	TNAC1776	F: ATCATCCTGCTGCTACTGTGC	7AS2-0.73–0.83	–	
		R: CCTTCTCAGCTTAGCGATGTG	4AL2-0.75–0.80		
			7DS4-0.73–1.00		
2	TNAC1782	F: TCACTGAACAGCCTAGACATGG	7AS2-0.73–0.83	HaeIII	690 bp
		R: ATTCGCAGACCGCATCTATC	7BS2-0.27–1.00		
			7DS4-0.73–1.00		
3	TNAC1803	F: TGCGACCAGTCTCTTTGAAAT	C-7AL1-0.39	HaeIII	800 bp*
		R: GTCGGAGCCTGGATCTCTAGT	7BL2-0.38–0.63		
			7DL5-0.30–0.61		
4	TNAC1806	F: ATTCCTCGTGAATTGCTGGAT	7AS8-0.45–0.59	TaqI	350 bp*
		R: TCTGCAGTTAGGGACTTGAAA	7BS2-0.27–1.00		
			7DS2-0.61–0.73		
5	TNAC1811	F: CTGCTCAACGAGTTCATCGAC	7AL1-0.39–0.63	TaqI	740 bp
		R: TTGGAGTGGACGTTGCATT	7BL2-0.38–0.63		
			7DL5-0.30–0.61		
6	TNAC1812	F: ACTTCGCTTGGTCTCCTCAAT	7AL5-0.63–0.71	TaqI	860 bp
		R: GAGAAGTGTGCCAATTCCAAA	7BL7-0.63–0.78		
			7DL5-0.30–0.61		
7	TNAC1815	F: AGCAGACATCAGCAAGTTTGAG	7AL1-0.39–0.63	TaqI	600 bp*
		R: ACTGACAAGCCCATGATTGAC	7BL2-0.38–0.63		
			7DL5-0.30–0.61		
8	TNAC1822	F: CCCTCCGTCCGTGCAAAT	7AL5-0.63–0.71	TaqI	730 bp*
		R: GGCTGATGATGGAGACGTG	7BL2-0.38–0.63		
			7DL2-0.61–0.82		
9	TNAC1867	F: GCCTTTCCTTTGGTAGTCTGG	C-7AL1-0.39	–	840 bp
		R: CGATCCAAATGATCCTGAAGA	7BL2-0.38–0.63		
			7DL1-0.14–0.30		
10	TNAC1903	F: TCGCTTCTTCTGCTTGTTCTT	C-7AL1–0.39	TaqI	920 bp*
		R: CTGCTACTAGGCCACCCAAA	C-7BL2–0.38		
			7DL1-0.14–0.30		
11	TNAC1926	F: CGTCAGCTACAGCGACATCTA	C-7AS8–0.45	TaqI	700 bp*
		R: AACTTGAGCAGCGTGGTGTT	7BS2-0.27–1.00		
			7DS3-0.15–0.36		
12	TNAC1943	F: GCTGCTATGGTCCACGAATTA	7AS5-0.59–0.73	HaeIII	600 bp*
		R: AGAGTATCGTATCCGGGCAAT	7BS2-0.27–1.00		
			7DS4-0.73–1.00		
13	TNAC1957	F: TCAACATTTGCAGGATTGTCA	7AL21-0.74–0.86	–	730 bp
		R: TTTCACAGGAACCTCTGCATC	7BL10-0.78–0.84		
			7DL2-0.61–0.82		

The primers and the location in wheat bin map were referred to Ishikawa et al. [18]. The star indicated the Vb7 specific bands were polymorphic to 7V band

patterns reflected the large genomic divergence between the *D. villosum* and *D. breviaristatum* chromosomes. Liu et al. [14] used FISH probed by a ribosomal DNA sequence and proposed a hypothesis that the diploid *D. villosum* and tetraploid *D. breviaristatum* evolved in parallel from an ancestral species. Recently, we used the pDbC2 probe to hybridize to tetraploid *D. breviaristatum* and diploid *D. villosum* chromosomes, and found more

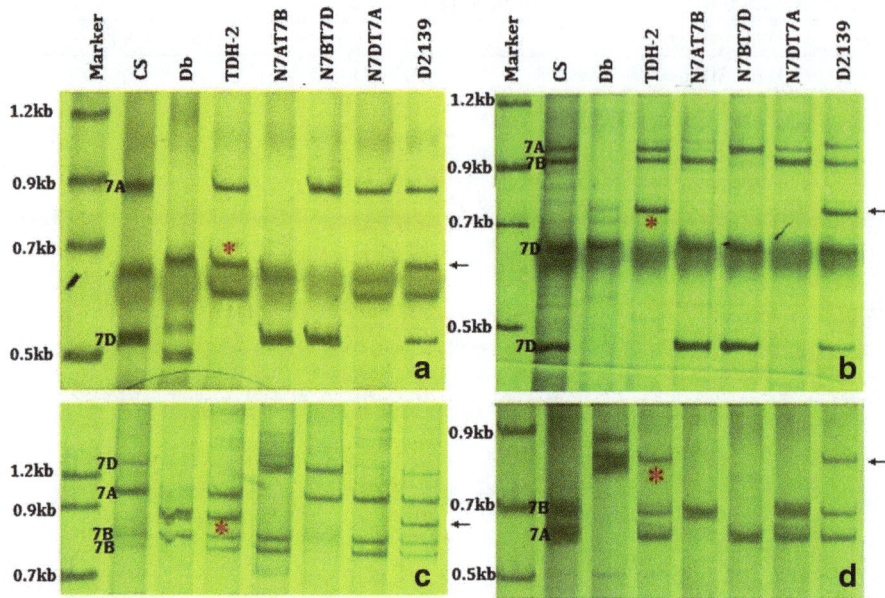

Fig. 3 PCR using PLUG primers TNAC1782/HaeIII (**a**), TNAC1811/TaqI (**b**), TNAC1812/TaqI (**c**) and TNAC1867 (**d**). The stars and arrows indicate the *D. breviaristatum* specific bands in TDH-2 and D2139, respectively

Ty3-gypsy retrotransposon copy numbers in centromeric regions of *D. villosum* than those in *D. breviaristatum* [24]. In the present study, we compared *D. breviaristatum* and diploid *D. villosum* chromosomes through the distribution of FISH signals of Oligo-pSc119.2, Oligo-pTa535, Oligo-(GAA)₇ by sequential multicolor-FISH (Fig. 1) and the molecular markers (Table 1) by PCR. The results suggested that strong evolutionary divergence involving copy number of repeated sequences and nucleotide sequence rearrangement may have occurred among *Dasypyrum* species during species evolution. Moreover, the Oligo-

pHv62-1 can hybridize *D. villosum* chromosomes in TDV-1 (Fig. 1e). It confirmed that the high tandem repeat sequences present largely in telomeric heterochromatin regions of *D. villosum* as reported by Li et al. [17]. However, FISH revealed that Oligo-pHv62-1 was absent in *D. breviaristatum* chromosomes of TDH-2 (Fig. 1f). This significant amplification of different types of repetitive sequences between the *D. villosum* and *D. breviaristatum* chromosomes may be related to adaptation of the plant species to their environments [3]. The cytogenetic and molecular markers which are species-specific can be used

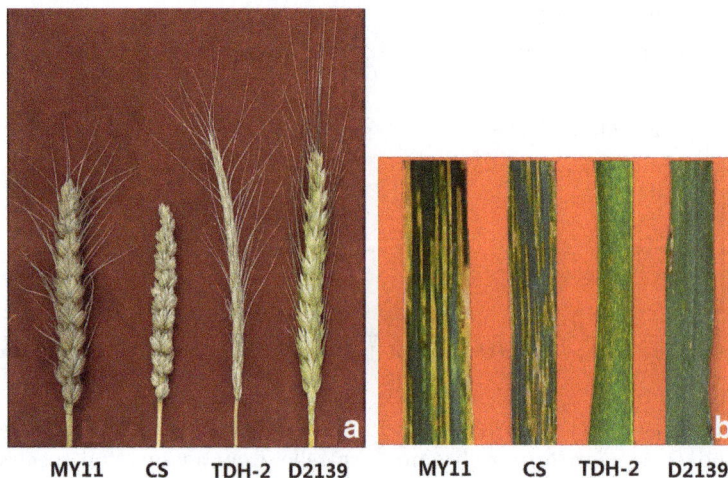

Fig. 4 The spikes morphology (**a**) and leaf response to stripe rust (**b**) of the lines

to identify and characterize the introgression of *D. villosum* and *D. breviaristatum* chromosome segments into a wheat background.

Rapid genomic and epigenomic changes have been commonly found in some newly synthesized wheat-alien amphiploids [25, 26]. Alterations of alien chromosomal structure in wheat background have also been described especially wheat-rye chromosome addition, substitution and translocation lines [27, 28]. However, the variations in the karyotype of wheat chromosomes have been less reported. Recently, Fu et al. [29] reported that pSc119.2 FISH signals could be observed at the telomeric regions of 3DS arms which was not observed in the current material, and structural variation and abnormal mitotic behavior of the 3D chromosome were detected in the selfed progeny of wheat "MY11"-rye 6R monosomic addition line. Furthermore, Fu et al. [30] reported the occurrence of 14 chromosomal rearrangements in wheat -rye hybrids. Our studies found that chromosomes 1B, 2B and 7A of the wheat- *D. breviaristatum* partial amphiploid TDH-2 (Fig. 1), and chromosomes 1D and 3D of the $7V^b$ addition lines D2139 (Fig. 2) showed apparent structural changes revealed by FISH patterns compared to the parental lines. Patokar et al. [31] characterized several novel wheat-*Thinopyrum bessarabicum* recombinant lines carrying intercalary translocations and did not report any observable wheat chromosomal rearrangements using FISH. It is likely that the distant species of genera *Secale* and *Dasypyrum* may induce such structural changes while present in a wheat background, while chromosomes derived from *Thinopyrum* species may not have the same effect due to their close relationship to wheat [32]. Thus, we suggest that the introgression of chromosomes from closely related species may not lead to the significant structural changes of wheat chromosomes, although the introduction of closely related *Aegilops* chromosomes causes massive deletions of wheat chromosomes [33], which were mainly useful for physical mapping of genes. There is the other possibility that the recipient wheat genotype may also increase the chromosomal rearrangement with visible changes of representative repeats. Taking advantage of fast multicolor FISH methods [15], we recently identified some chromosomal changes in high yielding elite cultivars originating from wheat distant hybridization. The association between the visibly rearranged wheat chromosomes and the yield or disease resistances are being verified for breeding purpose.

D. villosum chromosomes are known to contain genetic variability of value for incorporation into wheat. At least three sets of *D. villosum* chromosomes addition lines in wheat background have been developed [34–36]. Novel genes including disease resistance and quality-related characters have been found in different wheat- *D. villosum* derived lines [7]. With the aim to transfer novel genes

from *D. breviaristatum* to wheat, we identified the two *D. breviaristatum* chromosomes addition lines Y93-1-A6-4 and Y93-1-6-6, which showed novel resistance to powdery mildew isolates and stem rust Ug99 (pathotype TTKSK) [11]. Molecular marker and GISH analysis revealed that those introduced *D. breviaristatum* chromosomes were rearranged chromosomes involved groups 2, 6 and 7. Recently, Li et al. [12] reported a wheat - *D. breviaristatum* substitution line D11-5 possessing a pair of $2V^b$ chromosomes which had replaced wheat 2D. Based on the FISH analysis, we found that the $2V^b$ chromosome in line D11-5 was identical to chromosome Vb2 of TDH-2 (Fig. 1). We thus suggest that chromosome Vb2 can be provisionally assigned to linkage group 2, subject to confirmation using other genetic markers.

In the present study, we identified line D2139 which contained a pair of *D. breviaristatum* chromosomes confirmed herein to be "$7V^b$". This disomic substitution line D2139 may be potentially useful germplasm for agronomic traits including enhance spike length and the stripe rust resistance from the *D. breviaristatum* $7V^b$ into the wheat genome using marker-assisted chromosome engineering [37]. The divergence between the individual *D. villosum* 7V and *D. breviaristatum* $7V^b$ chromosomes was revealed by FISH and molecular markers in wheat background, which will provide the basis for future detailed comparative genomics analysis. Guo et al. [38] compared chromosomes $7el_1$, $7el_2$, 7E(e), and $7E^i$ derived from different *Thinopyrum* species by molecular and cytological methods. In a similar manner, we intend to create hybrid populations between wheat- *Dasypyrum* 7 V and $7V^b$ addition lines for further and direct localization of genes on these alien chromosomes.

Conclusions

In summary, the different FISH patterns between *D. breviaristatum* and *D. villosum* chromosomes were observed clearly by using different repetitive sequences as probes, which allows to identify the individual *Dasypyrum* chromosomes in wheat background. The changes of FISH patterns of wheat chromosomes were induced by the induction of *D. breviaristatum* to wheat. The *D. breviaristatum* specific molecular markers can be used to assign the homologous group of *D. breviaristatum* to wheat. We identified wheat- *D. breviaristatum* chromosome $7V^b$ addition line with novel stripe rust resistances will be potential useful for wheat breeding. The molecular and cytogenetic markers will assist to trace the *D. breviaristatum* chromatin in wheat background.

Methods
Plant materials
D. breviaristatum accession PI 546317 was obtained from the National Small Grains Collection at Aberdeen,

Idaho, USA. The wheat– *D. breviaristatum* partial amphiploid TDH-2 (genome AABBV^{b}V^b) was as described by Yang et al. [10]. The accession of *Dasypyrum villosum* TA10220 and the Chinese Spring- *D. villosum* chromosome 7 V addition line TA7683 [39] were obtained from Dr. Bernd Friebe of Wheat Genetic and Genomic Resources Center at Kansas State University, Manhattan, KS, USA. The *T. turgidum* cv. Jorc-69- *D. villosum* amphiploid TDV-1 (genome AABBVV) was developed and provided by Prof. Hua-Ren Jiang at Sichuan Agricultural University, China [40]. Line D2139 was obtained from a BC$_1$F$_5$ generation of the crosses between wheat cultivar 'Mianyang 11' (MY11) and TDH-2.

Fluorescence *in situ* hybridization (FISH)

Seedling root tips were collected and then treated with nitrous oxide followed by enzyme digestion, using the procedure of Han et al. [41]. The synthesized oligonucleotide probes Oligo-pSc119.2, Oligo-pTa535, Oligo-(GAA)$_7$ were used for identifying the wheat chromosomes according to the description of Tang et al. [15]. A new probe, Oligo-pHv62-1 (5' CGAAGGATTG AAAAAAGG AA CAATTTCGCA CTTACAGCTC AAAAATATA TG GGACA 3') was synthesized and labeled at 5' 6-carboxyfluorescein (FAM) based on high tandem repeat sequences pHv62 in *D. villosum* as reported by Li et al. [17]. The protocol of non-denaturing FISH by the synthesized probes was described by Fu et al. [30]. Photomicrographs of FISH chromosomes were taken with an Olympus BX-51 microscope equipped with a DP-70 CCD camera.

Molecular marker analysis

DNA was extracted from young leaves of *D. breviaristatum*, TDH-2, TDV-1, lines D11-5 and CS [42]. PCR-based Landmark Unique Gene (PLUG) primers were designed according to Ishikawa et al. [18]. Polymerase chain reaction (PCR) was performed in an Icycler thermalcycler (Bio-RAD Laboratories, Emeryville, CA) in a 25 μl reaction, containing 10 mmol Tris–HCl (pH 8.3), 2.5 mmol MgCl$_2$, 200 μmol of each dNTP, 100 ng template DNA, 0.2 U Taq polymerase (Takara, Japan) and 400 nmol of each primer. The cycling parameters were 94 °C for 3 min for denaturation; followed by 35 cycles at 94 °C for 1 min, 55 °C for 1 min, 72 °C for 2 min; and a final extension at 72 °C for 10 min. The amplified products were separated by 8 % PAGE gel as described by Hu et al. [43].

Disease resistance screening

Wheat- *D. breviaristatum* derivative lines were evaluated for adult-plant resistance to *Pst* strains CYR32 and CYR33 during the 2013 and 2015 cropping seasons as described by Li et al. [12].

Competing interests

The authors declare that they have no competing interests.

Authors' contributions

GL and ZY designed the study. GL, DG, HZ, JL conducted the experiments. HW, SL and JM helped to conduct experiment and data analysis. GL and ZY participated in paper writing. All authors read and approved the final manuscript.

Acknowledgement

We particularly thank Dr. I. Dundas at University of Adelaide, Australia, for reviewing the manuscript. We thank the National Natural Science Foundation of China (No. 31171542), and Sichuan wheat breeding community for the financial support.

References

1. Frederiksen S. Taxonomic studies in *Dasypyrum* (Poaceae). Nord J Bot. 1991;11:135–42.
2. Gradzielewska A. The genus *Dasypyrum*–part 1. The taxonomy and relationships within Dasypyrum and with Triticeae species. Euphytica. 2006;152:429–40.
3. De Pace C, Vaccino P, Cionini PG, Pasquini M, Bizzarri M, Qualset CO. *Dasypyrum*. In: Kole C, editor. Wild Crop Relatives, Genomic and Breeding Resources, Cereals, vol. 4. Heidelberg: Springer; 2011. p. 185–292.
4. Baum BR, Edwards T, Johnson DA. What does the nr5S DNA multigene family tell us about the genomic relationship between *Dasypyrum breviaristatum* and *D. villosum* (Triticeae: Poaceae)? Mol Genet Genomics. 2014;289:553–65.
5. Chen PD, Qi LL, Zhang SZ, Liu DJ. Development and molecular cytogenetic analysis of wheat-*Haynaldia* 6VS/6AL translocation lines specifying resistance to powdery mildew. Theor Appl Genet. 1995;91:1125–8.
6. Yildirim A, Jones SS, Murray TD. Mapping a gene conferring resistance to *Pseudocercosporella herpotrichoides* on chromosome 4 V of *Dasypyrum villosum* in a wheat background. Genome. 1998;41:1–6.
7. Qi LL, Pumphrey MO, Friebe B, Zhang P, Qian C, Bowden RL, et al. A novel Robertsonian translocation event leads to transfer of a stem rust resistance gene (*Sr52*) effective against race Ug99 from *Dasypyrum villosum* into bread wheat. Theor Appl Genet. 2011;123:159–67.
8. He ZH, Xia XC, Chen XM, Zhuang QS. Progress of wheat breeding in China and the future perspective. Acta Agron Sin. 2011;37:202–15.
9. Bie T, Zhao R, Zhu S, Chen S, Cen B, Zhang B, et al. Efficient marker-assisted screening of structural changes involving *Haynaldia villosa* chromosome 6V using a double-distal-marker strategy. Mol Breeding. 2015;35:34.
10. Yang ZJ, Li GR, Feng J, Jiang HR, Ren ZL. Molecular cytogenetic characterization and disease resistance observation of wheat - *Dasypyrum breviaristatum* partial amphiploid and its derivatives. Hereditas. 2005;142:80–5.
11. Liu C, Li G, Yan H, Zhou J, Hu L, Lei M, et al. Molecular and cytogenetic identification of new wheat- *D. breviaristatum* additions conferring resistance to stem rust and powdery mildew. Breeding Sci. 2011;61:366–72.
12. Li GR, Zhao JM, Li DH, Yang EN, Huang YF, Liu C, et al. A novel wheat–*Dasypyrum breviaristatum* substitution line with stripe rust resistance. Cytogenet Genome Res. 2014;143:280–7.
13. Galasso I, Blanco A, Katsiotis A, Pignone D, Heslop-Harrison HS. Genomic organization and phylogenetic relationships in the genus *Dasypyrum* analysed by Southern and *in situ* hybridization of total genomic and cloned DNA probes. Chromosoma. 1997;106:53–61.
14. Liu C, Li GR, Sunish S, Jia JQ, Yang ZJ, Friebe B, et al. Genome relationships in the genus *Dasypyrum*: evidence from molecular phylogenetic analysis and *in situ* hybridization. Plant Syst Evol. 2010;288:149–56.
15. Tang ZX, Yang ZJ, Fu SL. Oligonucleotides replacing the roles of repetitive sequences pAs1, pSc119.2, pTa-535, pTa71, CCS1, and pAWRC.1 for FISH analysis. J Appl Genet. 2014;55:313–8.
16. Danilova TV, Friebe B, Gill BS. Single-copy gene fluorescence *in situ* hybridization and genome analysis: Acc-2 loci mark evolutionary chromosomal rearrangements in wheat. Chromosoma. 2012;121:597–611.
17. Li WL, Chen PD, Qi LL, Liu DJ. Isolation, characterization and application of a species-specific repeated sequence from *Haynaldia villosa*. Theor Appl Genet. 1995;90:526–33.
18. Ishikawa G, Nakamura T, Ashida T, Saito M, Nasuda S, Endo T, et al. Localization of anchor loci representing five hundred annotated rice genes to wheat chromosomes using PLUG markers. Theor Appl Genet. 2009;118:499–514.

19. Jia J, Li G, Liu C, Zhou J, Yang Z. Sequence variations of PDHA1 gene in Triticeae species allow for identifying wheat-alien introgression lines. Frontiers Agric China. 2010;4:137–44.

20. Hu LJ, Liu C, Zeng ZX, Li GR, Song XJ, Yang ZJ. Genomic rearrangement between wheat and *Thinopyrum elongatum* revealed by mapped functional molecular markers. Genes Genomics. 2012;34:67–75.

21. Friebe B, Cermeno MC, Zeller FJ. C-banding polymorphism and the analysis of nucleolar activity in *Dasypyrum villosum* (L.) Candargy, its added chromosomes to hexaploid wheat and the amphiploid *Triticum dicoccum-D. villosum*. Theor Appl Genet. 1987;73:337–42.

22. Linde Laursen IB, Frederiksen S. Comparison of the Giemsa C-banded karyotypes of *Dasypyrum villosum* (2×) and *D. breviaristatum* (4×) from Greece. Hereditas. 1991;114:237–44.

23. De Pace C, Delre V, Scarascia Mugnozza GT, Qualset CO, Cremonini R, Frediani M, et al. Molecular and chromosomal characterization of repeated and single copy DNA sequences in the genome of *Dasypyrum villosum*. Hereditas. 1992;116:55–65.

24. Li GR, Liu C, Wei P, Song XJ, Yang ZJ. Chromosomal distribution of a new centromeric Ty3-gypsy retrotransposon sequence in *Dasypyrum* and related Triticeae species. J Genet. 2012;91:343–8.

25. Gustafson JP, Lukaszewski AJ, Bennett MD. Somatic deletion and redistribution of telomeric heterochromatin in the genus *Secale* and in Triticale. Chromosoma. 1983;88:293–8.

26. Dou QW, Tanaka H, Nakata N, Tsujimoto H. Molecular cytogenetic analyses of hexaploid lines spontaneously appearing in octoploid Triticale. Theor Appl Genet. 2006;114:41–7.

27. Alkhimova AG, Heslop-Harrison JS, Shchapova AI, Vershinin AV. Rye chromosome variability in wheat-rye addition and substitution lines. Chromosome Res. 1999;7:205–12.

28. Bento M, Gustafson P, Viegas W, Silva M. Genome merger: from sequence rearrangements in triticale to their elimination in wheat-rye addition lines. Theor Appl Genet. 2010;121:489–97.

29. Fu S, Yang M, Fei Y, Tan F, Ren Z, Yan B, et al. Alterations and abnormal mitosis of wheat chromosomes induced by wheat-rye monosomic addition lines. PLoS One. 2013;8:e70483.

30. Fu S, Chen L, Wang Y, Li M, Yang Z, Qiu L, et al. Oligonucleotide probes for ND-FISH analysis to identify rye and wheat chromosomes. Sci Rep. 2015;5:10552.

31. Patokar C, Sepsi A, Schwarzacher T, Kishii M, Heslop-Harrison JS: Molecular cytogenetic characterization of novel wheat-*Thinopyrum bessarabicum* recombinant lines carrying intercalary translocations. Chromosoma 2015. DOI: 10.1007/s00412-015-0537-6.

32. Dvořák J. Homology between *Agropyron elongatum* chromosomes and *Triticum aestivum* chromosomes. Can J Genet Cytol. 1980;22:237–59.

33. Endo TR, Gill BS. The deletion stocks of common wheat. J Heredity. 1996;87: 295–307.

34. Sears ER. Addition of the genome of *H. villosa* to *T. aestivum*. Am J Bot. 1953;40:168–74.

35. Lukaszewski AJ. A comparison of several approaches in the development of disomic alien addition lines of wheat. In: Miller TE, Koebner RMD, editors. Proceedings of the 7th international wheat genetics symposium, vol. 1. Cambridge, UK: Institute of Plant Sciences Research; 1988. p. 363–7.

36. Chen PD, Liu DJ. Identification of *H. villosa* chromosomes in alien wheat addition of *T. aestivum-H. villosa*. In: Li ZS, editor. Proceedings of the 1st international symposium on chromosome engineering in plants. Xian, China: BookPublisher; 1986. p. 31–3.

37. Niu Z, Klindworth DL, Friesen TL, Chao S, Jin Y, Cai X, et al. Targeted introgression of a wheat stem rust resistance gene by DNA marker-assisted chromosome engineering. Genetics. 2011;187:1011–21.

38. Guo J, He F, Cai JJ, Wang HW, Li AF, Wang HG, et al. Molecular and Cytological Comparisons of Chromosomes 7el$_1$, 7el$_2$, 7E(e), and 7E^l Derived from *Thinopyrum*. Cytogenet Genome Res. 2015;145:68–74.

39. Liu C, Qi L, Liu W, Zhao W, Wilson J, Friebe B, et al. Development of a set of compensating *Triticum aestivum-Dasypyrum villosum* Robertsonian translocation lines. Genome. 2011;54:836–44.

40. Jiang HR, Dai DQ, Sun DF, Xiao SH. New artificial genetic resources of wheat: several polyploids of *Triticum-Dasypyrum*. Sci Agric Sin. 1992;25:89.

41. Han FP, Lamb JC, Birchler JA. High frequency of centromere inactivation resulting in stable dicentric chromosomes of maize. Proc Natl Acad Sci U S A. 2006;103:3238–43.

42. Yang ZJ, Liu C, Feng J, Li GR, Deng KJ, Zhou JP, et al. Studies on genome relationship and species-specific PCR marker for *Dasypyrum breviaristatum* in Triticeae. Hereditas. 2006;143:47–54.

43. Hu LJ, Li GR, Zeng ZX, Chang ZJ, Liu C, Zhou JP, et al. Molecular cytogenetic identification of a new wheat-*Thinopyrum* substitution line with stripe rust resistance. Euphytica. 2011;177:169–77.

4

Dissection of partial 21q monosomy in different phenotypes: clinical and molecular characterization of five cases

Edoardo Errichiello[1*†], Francesca Novara[1†], Anna Cremante[2], Annapia Verri[2], Jessica Galli[3], Elisa Fazzi[3], Daniela Bellotti[4], Laura Losa[5], Mariangela Cisternino[5] and Orsetta Zuffardi[1]

Abstract

Background: Partial deletion of chromosome 21q is a very rare chromosomal abnormality associated with highly variable phenotypes, such as facial dysmorphic features, heart defects, seizures, psychomotor delay, and severe to mild intellectual disability, depending on the location and size of deletions. So far, three broad deletion regions of 21q have been correlated with the clinical phenotype.

Results: We described the clinical and genetic features of three family members (father and two siblings) and other two unrelated patients with very wide range in age of diagnosis. All of them showed intellectual disability with very variable symptoms, from mild to severe, and carried 21q interstitial deletions with different sizes and position, as detected by conventional karyotype and array-CGH.

Conclusions: Our study provided additional cases of partial 21q deletions, allowing to better delineate the genotype-phenotype correlations. In contrast to previous observations, we showed that deletions of the 21q proximal region are not necessarily associated with severe phenotypes and, therefore, that mild phenotypes are not exclusively related to distal deletions. To the best of our knowledge, this is the first report showing 21q deletions in adult patients associated with mild phenotypes, mainly consisting of neurobehavioral abnormalities, such as obsessive-compulsive disorders, poor social interactions and vulnerability to psychosis.

Keywords: Array Comparative Genomic Hybridization (array-CGH), Behavioral disorders, BTG3 (BTG family, Member 3), DNA Copy Number Variations (CNVs), GRIK1 (glutamate receptor, Ionotropic, Kainate 1), Intellectual Disability (ID), Partial 21q monosomy, RBM11 (RNA binding motif protein 11)

Background

Partial deletion of chromosome 21q (ORPHA574) is a very rare condition (<1/1,000,000) associated with highly variable phenotypes, which include facial dysmorphic features, heart defects, seizures, psychomotor delay, and severe to mild intellectual disability, depending on the size and position of the deletion [1].

In one of the most complete studies to date, Lyle et al. [2] reported 11 cases of partial monosomy 21 and outlined three deletion regions with the associated phenotypic severity ranging from mild to severe to lethal. Deletions in the first region, ranging from the centromere to approximately 31.2 Mb (21q21.3), are associated with a severe phenotype. Deletions in the second region (31.2–36 Mb), corresponding to the 21q22.11 band with a higher gene density, produce a severe phenotype not compatible with survival. On the other hand, deletions in the third region, from 36 to 37.5 Mb to the telomere (21q22.12-qter, approximately 10 Mb), result in a relatively mild phenotype. However, other studies reported patients with proximal deletions of chromosome 21 and mild or even normal phenotypes [3–5].

* Correspondence: edoardo.errichiello01@universitadipavia.it
†Equal contributors
[1]Department of Molecular Medicine, University of Pavia, Via Forlanini 14, 27100 Pavia, Italy
Full list of author information is available at the end of the article

In this study, we investigated five patients from three unrelated Italian families with deletions of chromosome 21q by conventional and molecular karyotyping (array-CGH), in order to underline new insights on genotype-phenotype correlations. In addition, previously published cases with chromosome 21q monosomies and similar deletions have been reviewed. Altogether, our data provide a further dissection of the complex 21q monosomy phenotype.

Results

Clinical reports

Patient 1

Patient 1 was a 53 years old male, father of cases 2 and 3. The patient was born full-term. He achieved the middle school graduation and then experienced different jobs (gardener, bricklayer, crane worker), being frequently fired after short periods. His mother (79 years old) was affected by hypertension and the father (80 years old) by insulin dependent diabetes mellitus and stroke. The patient had a 55 years old brother who was also affected by diabetes. He was first evaluated at the age of 53 years, after that chromosome 21 deletion had been ascertained in his children.

The clinical evaluation documented mild facial dysmorphisms, such as deep set eyes, large ears and prominent nose (Fig. 1a). The neurological evaluation revealed mild head tremor and postural hand tremor. The Nuclear Magnetic Resonance (NMR) documented a periventricular white matter hyperintensity and enlarged cisterna magna. The electromyography (EMG) showed bilateral entrapment of median nerve at the wrist. The patient was scarcely collaborating and quite anxious. He frequently showed the tendency to give a very positive image of himself. The language was rather simple. The evaluation by DSM-IV (Diagnostic and Statistical Manual of Mental Disorders, Fourth Edition) documented a psychotic disorder with persecutory delusion. High levels of aggressiveness and impairment in behavioural control were well documented as well as alcohol abuse. Total IQ was 87, without any important discrepancy among verbal subtests (Verbal IQ = 88,) and the performance ones (Performance IQ = 88). Poor attentive skills, short-term memory and limited funds of knowledge acquired through school and cultural experience were documented by verbal subtests. Abstract thinking and understanding were very simple, with limited ability to synthesize verbal relationships and

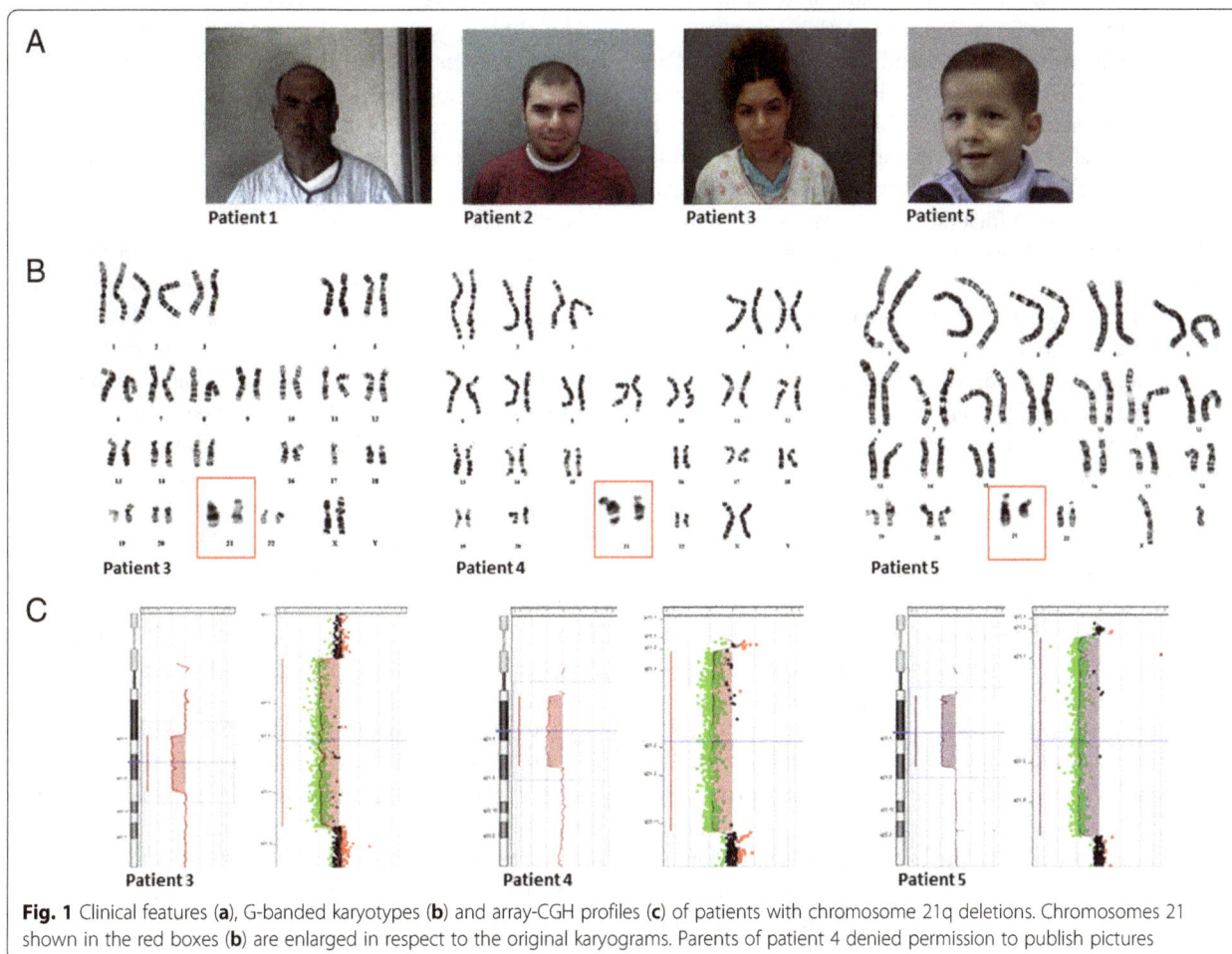

Fig. 1 Clinical features (**a**), G-banded karyotypes (**b**) and array-CGH profiles (**c**) of patients with chromosome 21q deletions. Chromosomes 21 shown in the red boxes (**b**) are enlarged in respect to the original karyograms. Parents of patient 4 denied permission to publish pictures

social knowledge. The computational skills were also very limited, as well as the logical-deductive and abstract reasoning.

Patient 2

Patient 2 was the oldest child of patient 1. He was born at term by caesarean section (weight 2,900 g). He started walking at 18 months and pronounced the first comprehensible words at 14 months. He attended 3 years of pre-school and started the primary school at 7 years. Then he attended a professional school care for mentally-disabled people. He was first evaluated at the age of 20 years because of mild intellectual disability, requiring a dedicated teacher at school, and autistic-like features.

The clinical examination revealed a coarse facies with nuchal low set hair, frontal alopecia, prominent forehead, small palpebral fissures, prominent nose, prognathism and large ears (Fig. 1a). The neurological evaluation revealed mild postural hand tremor and altered saccadic eye movements. The Magnetic Resonance Imaging (MRI), performed at the age of 18 years, showed mild periventricular white matter hyperintensity and enlarged cisterna magna. The EMG revealed mild sensorimotor axonal neuropathy and autonomic dysfunction. During examination, the patient showed adequate levels of attention and concentration. The evaluation by DSM-IV criteria for ID diagnosis documented the presence of a compulsive-obsessive disorder. The patient referred binge eating episodes, occurring during the night, and compulsive smoking (60 cigarettes/day). He was sufficiently autonomous and able to work. His global IQ was 79 (borderline level), without discrepancy among the verbal subtests (Verbal IQ = 79) and the performance ones (Performance IQ = 82). He demonstrated good comprehension skills, but low attitudes in numerical reasoning and a poor vocabulary. Selective and focused attention, mental control and response flexibility, as assessed by the Stroop Test, resulted inadequate.

Patient 3

Patient 3 was a 22 years old female, the younger child of patient 1. She was born at term with caesarean section (weight 2,600 g). She pronounced the first words at 18 months of age. She was first evaluated at the age of 18 years because of mild intellectual disability requiring a dedicated teacher at school.

The clinical evaluation revealed coarse facies with nuchal low set hair, small palpebral fissures, prominent nose, large ears and large flat mouth (Fig. 1a), as documented in cases 1 and 2. The neurological evaluation revealed mild postural hand tremor and normal saccadic eye movements. Visual and BAEP (Brainstem Auditory Evoked Potentials) evoked potentials were normal. The

audiometric examination documented mild neurosensory hypoacusia. The EMG showed no sign of peripheral neuropathy and mild autonomic dysfunction. The MRI showed mega cisterna magna. At the cognitive and behavioural assessment, the patient was generally collaborating and cooperative. During the talks, she often showed propensity to give fast and impulsive answers. The evaluation by DSM-IV criteria revealed – as in patients 1 and 2 – the presence of impulsivity (compulsive buying disorder). Cognitive evaluation documented a borderline IQ of 78, with a light discrepancy among the verbal subtests and the performance ones (Verbal IQ = 81; Performance IQ = 76). As documented in the brother, she had good comprehension skills, but low attitudes in numerical reasoning and poor vocabulary. In addition, social insight, spatial perception, problem solving, logical and sequential reasoning appeared limited.

Patient 4

Patient 4 was a 16 years old girl, daughter of two non-consanguineous healthy parents. She was born at term after uneventful pregnancy (birth weight: 3,400 g, birth length: 50 cm). The mother had a spontaneous miscarriage during a previous pregnancy.

The clinical evaluation documented some dysmorphic features, such as low hair line and widely spaced nipples. In primary school she was noted to have learning difficulties associated with dyslexia and dyscalculia. She was diagnosed with a visual-praxis difficulty and a full-scale IQ at the lower end of normal range (77), with significant discrepancies between verbal (IQ = 100) and performance (IQ = 59) scores. At the neuropsychological evaluation the patient revealed low self-esteem, strong insecurity and poor social adaptation skills. Major depressive episodes, together with anxiety and distress, and behavioral disorganization were also well documented. Written communication skills were deeply impaired due to deficient visuospatial organization and global movement impairment. She started gaining weight progressively at the age of 6, and developed primary amenorrhoea at the age of 15. She presented thelarche and pubarche at the age of 13 and familial history of delayed puberty was reported in the paternal pedigree. Although GnRH stimulation test showed a pubertal response of LH and FSH (LH peak of 12.7 mU/ml, FSH peak of 11 mU/ml), with a concentration of oestradiol (E2) of 40 pg/ml (normal pubertal values >15 pg/ml), FSH and LH peaks were lower than the expected for age, according to functional immaturity of the hypothalamus-pituitary-gonadal axis. The brain MRI showed normal signal of both anterior and posterior pituitary gland, with a normal pituitary stalk. The MRI with contrast highlighted the presence of a microadenoma (35 mm) at the centre of the hypophysis.

Patient 5

Patient 5 was a 6 years old boy, son of two non-consanguineous healthy parents. His father suffered from idiopathic focal epilepsy of infancy and childhood, and the mother was healthy. He was born at term after an uneventful pregnancy (birth weight: 3,070 g, birth length: 50 cm). The proband also had a heterozygotic twin brother with normal neurological assessment, normal IQ score (88), and obesity.

A mild psychomotor delay was reported since the proband was only 5 months old. A delay of the expressive language was revealed at 2 years of life, with speech very poor and simple. Personal autonomy skills (e.g. toilet training, routine clothing, and use of cutlery) were also deeply impaired. At the present age the patient had bilateral iris and choroidal coloboma, Duane syndrome type 3 of the left eye (Fig. 1a), hypotonia of both arms and legs, and developmental coordination disorder (DCD), as confirmed by the Movement Assessment Battery for Children (MABC), with a score below the 5th percentile. The patient presented a borderline IQ [total IQ = 74, without discrepancy between verbal (IQ = 80) and performance (IQ = 82) scores] and required the support of a dedicated teacher. He also lacked proactivity in the relationship game and in accessing language expression, characterized by simple speech with a reduced vocabulary. The instrumental examination by Nuclear Magnetic Resonance (NMR) revealed hypoplasia of corpus callosum, inferior vermis and pons, as well as bilateral anomalies of the course of the sixth cranial nerve.

Conventional and molecular karyotyping

In the three affected family members (patients 1–3), the karyotyping and the array-CGH analysis revealed a chromosome 21q interstitial deletion of approximately 10.6 Mb (chr21:21,754,822-32,380,347, hg38), and excluded the presence of any other genomic imbalance (Table 1, Fig. 1b and c). In patient 4, both karyotype and array-CGH detected a larger deletion, spanning approximately 14.5 Mb (chr21:13,048,294-27,532,614, hg38; Table 1, Fig. 1b and c). No other significant chromosomal rearrangements were revealed in the proband and the parental GTG-banded karyotypes showed a normal chromosomal asset. In case 5, the array-CGH demonstrated two genomic rearrangements: arr[hg38] 21q11.2q21.3 (14,000,146-27,785,985)x1 (Table 1, Fig. 1b and c), and the typical 220-kb deletion on chromosome 16p11.2 (OMIM 613444), arr[hg38] 16p11.2 (28,813,473-29,030,738)x1. The parental GTG-banded karyotypes were normal and the array-CGH analysis confirmed that the large 21q deletion appeared *de novo* in their child. On the contrary, the rearrangement on chromosome 16 was also detected in the mother and the proband's heterozygotic twin. The molecular and clinical details of

our cases have been referenced in the ClinVar database (http://www.ncbi.nlm.nih.gov/clinvar): Patients 1–3 (#SCV000239859), Patient 4 (#SCV000239860), Patient 5 (#SCV000239861).

Discussion

Partial deletions of chromosome 21q are commonly associated with highly heterogeneous phenotypes. In this study we characterized five patients with partial 21q monosomies by array-CGH and conventional karyotyping. The three family members (patients 1–3) showed mild clinical features, such as facial dysmorphisms and behavioral abnormalities, mainly consisting of obsessive-compulsive features, poor social interactions and vulnerability to psychosis, fully expressed in the father. High levels of impulsivity, repeatedly identified as a major problem in schizophrenia, were present in all the family members: alcohol abuse (father), compulsive smoking (son) and shopping/spending addiction (daughter). The phenotypic intrafamilial variability might be due to additive genetic and environmental factors that potentially have accumulated in the oldest member of the family. A deletion comprising 21q21.2 and the proximal segment of 21q22.1 has been previously associated with schizophrenia susceptibility [6], although a recent multi-stage genome-wide association study failed to detect schizophrenia-associated genetic locus on chromosome 21 [7]. Interestingly, all family members presented postural hand tremor, a symptom never described in association with chromosome 21q deletions. In agreement with our observations, it has been reported that *Sod1-/-* mice presented tremors along with gait disturbances and skeletal muscle atrophy [8, 9]. However, according to Decipher, no cases of *SOD-1* deletions (chr21:31659622-31668930, hg38) have been associated with tremor until now and the unique family with *SOD-1* null mutation manifested an atypical form of familial amyotrophic lateral sclerosis [10].

Compared to patients 4 and 5, the three family members carried the deletion of *GRIK1* mapping to the 21q21.3 region (Fig. 2). This gene (OMIM 138245) might be considered a plausible candidate for autism and other neurobehavioral disorders, since it codifies for a protein belonging to the kainate family of excitatory glutamate receptors that are activated in a variety of neurophysiologic processes. Moreover, *GRIK1* alterations were shown to be associated with various neurobehavioral phenotypes in humans, such as anxiety disorders, schizophrenia, bipolar disorder, epilepsy and PDD-NOS (pervasive developmental disorder not otherwise specified) [11–13], as well as with anxiety-like behaviors in *GRIK1* knockout mice – due to its regulation of inhibitory circuits in the amygdala [14]. Accordingly, the behavioral disorders observed in our family suggest that

Table 1 Summary of patients harboring 21q deletions overlapping with patients 1–5 and corresponding clinical features

Patient	Age at diagnosis (yr)	Phenotype (main features)	Chromosomal coordinates of deletion (hg38)	Size (Mb)	Genes (protein coding)	Inheritance	Pathogenicity
Patients 1-2-3 (present study)	53 (#1), 20 (#2), 18 (#3)	Obsessive-compulsive disorders, impaired social interactions, aggressiveness, delayed speech and language development, mild facial dismorphisms	chr21:21754822-32380347	10.63	112 (52)	Paternal	Pathogenic
Patient 4 (present study)	6	Intellectual disability, global movement impairment, dysmorphic features, dyslexia, dyscalculia, primary amenorrhoea, obesity, pituitary microadenoma	chr21:13048294-27532614	14.48	117 (21)	De novo	Pathogenic
Patient 5 (present study)	4	Intellectual disability, mild psychomotor delay, speech delay, hypotonia, DCD[a], Duane syndrome type 3, bilateral iris/choroidal coloboma	chr21:14000146-27785985	13.79	112 (23)	De novo	Pathogenic
			chr16:28813473-29030738	0.22	35 (24)	Maternal	Pathogenic
Case 1 (Petit et al., 2015) [24] Decipher#276325	7	Behavioural/psychiatric abnormality, attention deficit, impaired social interactions, frustration, aggressiveness, delayed speech and language development	chr21:21062316-24943120	3.88	16 (1)	Maternal	Unknown
Case 2 (Petit et al., 2015) [24] Decipher#254181	9	Global developmental delay, speech delay, hyperactivity, impairment of social interactions	chr21:15619936-23525918	7.91	50 (9)	Paternal (mosaicism)	Unknown
Case 3 (Petit et al., 2015) [24] Decipher#274603	5	Global developmental delay, hypotonia, constipation, impaired social interactions	chr21:16079383-24575840	8.50	48 (7)	Unknown	Unknown
KKI patient 3 - cohort A (Roberson et al., 2011)	6	Speech delay, mild/moderate mental retardation, dysmorfic features, hypotonia, GERD[b], eczema, dermatographism	chr21:16814345-33232252	16.42	159 (69)	De novo	Unknown
			chr4:65863868-66006319	0.14	0	Maternal	Unlikely pathogenic
			chr14:22625231-22795061[c]	0.17[c]	2 (2)	Paternal	Unlikely pathogenic
GM00137 - cohort B (Roberson et al., 2011) [1]	6	Severe psychomotor retardation, microcephaly, dysmorphic features, bilateral iris coloboma	chr21:13403408-28392024	14.99	124 (23)	Unknown	Unknown
			chr4:68917-11238519	11.17	229 (122)	Unknown	Unknown
GM06918 - cohort B (Roberson et al., 2011) [1]	9	Mental retardation, dysmorphic features	chr21:14981488-32298829	17.32	156 (61)	De novo	Unknown
Haldeman-Englert et al., 2010 [13]	2	Poor social interactions, speech delay, mild dysmorphic features, PDD-NOS[d]	chr21:21085454-29813876	8.73	62 (18)	De novo	Pathogenic
Case 31 (Lyle et al., 2009) [2]	Unknown	Dysmorphic features, short stature, mental retardation, synbrachydactily	chr21:12965809-30890916	17.93	180 (56)	Unknown	Unknown
Case 32 (Lyle et al., 2009) [2]	Unknown	Dysmorphic features, short stature, mental retardation, microcephaly, clinodactily, hypotonia	chr21:12965809-30218169	17.26	145 (31)	Unknown	Unknown
Case 33 (Lyle et al., 2009) [2]	Unknown	Mental retardation	chr21:12965809-26199556	13.23	108 (15)	Unknown	Unknown
Hannachi et al., 2011 [20]	26	Moderate mental retardation, minor brain malformations, craniofacial dysmorphic features, azoospermia, diffuse cerebral atrophy	chr21:3603505-29194209	15.59	130 (23)	Maternal	Likely pathogenic

Table 1 Summary of patients harboring 21q deletions overlapping with patients 1–5 and corresponding clinical features (*Continued*)

Decipher#285024	2	Ataxia, intellectual disability, poor speech, lower limb spasticity, speech articulation difficulties	chr21:13224687-27912651	14.69	124 (23)	Unknown	Pathogenic
Decipher#285691	10	Cognitive impairment, generalized myoclonic seizures, microcephaly, asymmetry of the ears	chr21:13045202-33522318	20.48	217 (76)	Unknown	Pathogenic
ECARUCA#4777	16	Mental retardation, seizures/abnormal EEG [e], short stature, prominent maxilla, dislocation of hip, atrial septum defect	chr21:14166659-20412272	6.25	66 (13)	De novo	Unknown
			chr21:43013575-46699983	3.69	116 (67)	De novo	Unknown
ECARUCA#4841	9	Mental retardation, seizures/abnormal EEG [e], facial dysmorphisms	chr21:15292766-19704615	4.41	31 (6)	De novo	Unknown

[a]*DCD* developmental coordination disorder [b]*GERD* gastroesophageal reflux disease [c]duplication [d]*PDD-NOS* pervasive developmental disorder not otherwise specified [e]*EEG* Electroencephalogram

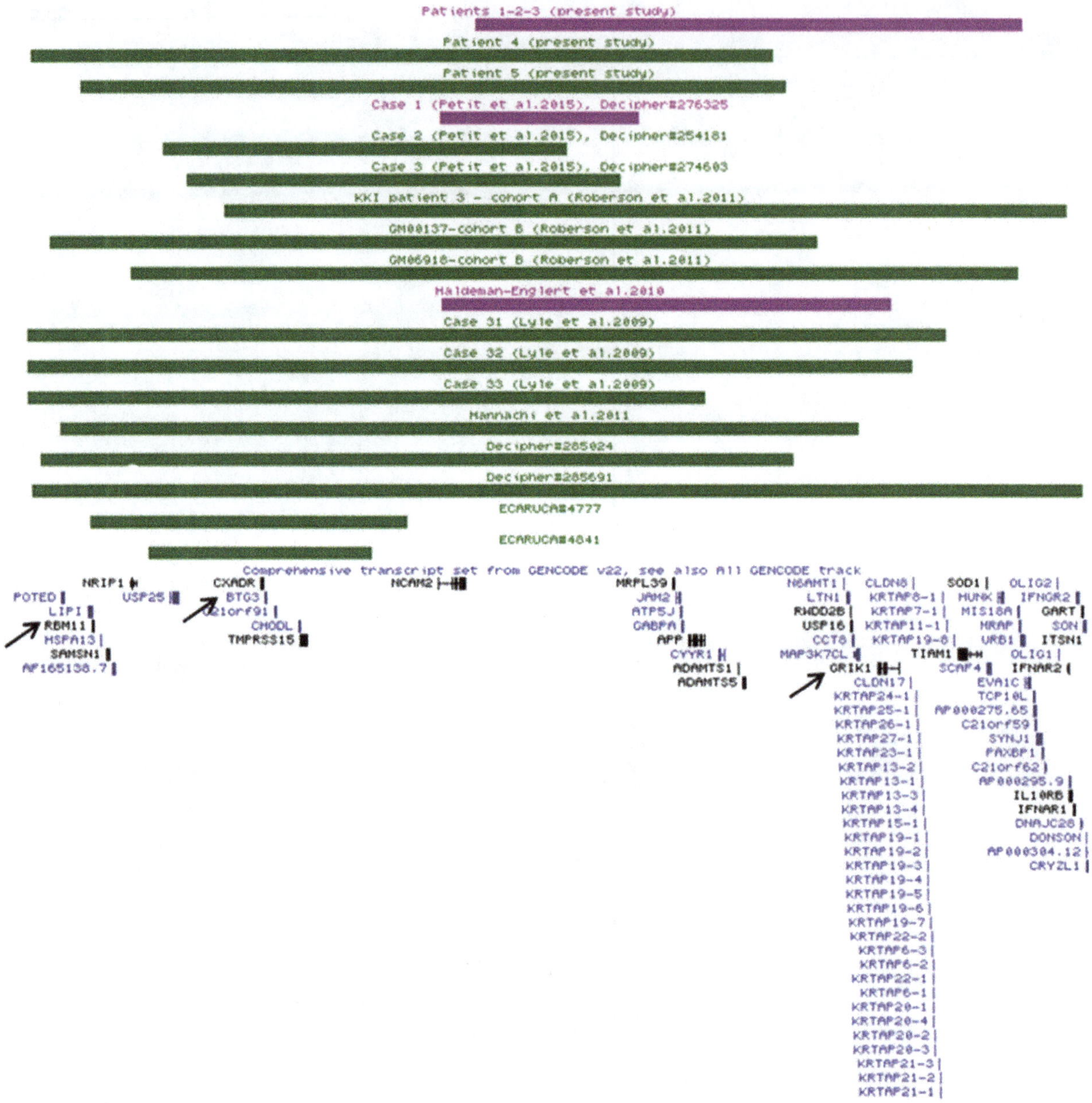

Fig. 2 Comparison of 21q deletion cases with mild (purple) and moderate/severe (green) phenotypes (behavioral disorders and intellectual disability, respectively). The protein-coding genes of 21q region are mainly grouped into two main clusters. The proximal cluster includes genes more likely involved in intellectual disability (*BTG3* and *RBM11*), whereas the distal cluster mainly contains genes related to behavioral disorders, such as *GRIK1* (almost completely deleted in the case reported by Haldeman-Englert et al., [13]). KKI-3, GM00137, and ECARUCA#4777 cases also had rearrangements involving chromosomes other than 21 (as reported in Table 1) that might contribute to the clinical severity

GRIK1 might be considered the most favorable candidate gene.

Patients 4 and 5, with similar proximal 21q deletions, showed the most severe clinical features, mainly consisting in intellectual disability (Table 1). Moreover, case 5 also harbored an additional deletion at 16p11.2, inherited from the clinically normal mother. Since this deletion has been previously linked to developmental delay, autism spectrum disorder and epilepsy [15–17], its additive effect on our patient's phenotype might also be considered. In addition, the 220-kb 16p11.2 deletion has also been widely associated with susceptibility to isolated severe early-onset obesity (OMIM 613444) [18]. Interestingly, the proband and his mother were normal weight, whereas the proband's heterozygotic twin harboring the same deletion was obese, thus supporting the incomplete penetrance and the clinical variability of this chromosomal alteration [19].

The findings that patients 4 and 5 presented more severe clinical features than patients 1–3 are in agreement with previously reported cases (Table 1 and Fig. 2) [1, 2, 20], where the proximal 21q deletions encompassed two genes expressed in the central nervous system, *RBM11* (21q11.2) and *BTG3* (21q21.1), that might play a role in intellectual disability. *RBM11* was deleted in 10 out of 15 cases with the most severe phenotype (intellectual disability), whereas *BTG3* in all of these cases (Fig. 2). *RBM11* is a tissue-specific splicing factor that mediates the alternative splicing process during neuronal differentiation [21]. *BTG3* (OMIM 605674) is involved in the neurogenesis of the developing central nervous system, where it acts as a regulator of cell proliferation and apoptosis [22]. Deletions of *BTG3* have been reported in a subset of patients with autism characterized by developmental regression [23] and in patients with neurodevelopmental delay [24] (Decipher 285691, 285987, 288573, 291626, and 300775). Moreover, *BTG3* deletions have also been associated with delayed speech (Decipher 249224, 277597, and 285024), as observed in our patient 5.

Conclusions

Although further investigations of other cases are needed, our preliminary results provide new insights on the traditional model firstly proposed by Lyle and colleagues in 2009 [2], making it possible to tentatively subset their original great region 1 (21qcen-21q21.3) into two smaller subregions. Deletions in the subregion 1, spanning from the centromere to approximately 21 Mb (21q21.1), are mainly associated with intellectual disability, whereas deletions of subregion 2, until approximately 32 Mb (21q22.11), are more tightly associated with neurobehavioral disorders, such as obsessive-compulsive disorders, poor social interactions and vulnerability to psychosis (Fig. 3). Interestingly, the subregion 2 also includes a portion of the 21q22.11 band,

whose deletion was traditionally considered associated with severe and even lethal phenotypes. This finding may be due to the fact that most of the disease-related genes, such as *SYNJ1*, *ITSN1*, *SLC5A3/SMIT1* and *KCNE2* [25–29], are clustered in the distal part of the band with the highest gene density.

According to the literature, very few cases of behavioral disorders with 21q deletions have been described until now [13, 24]. Indeed, attenuated phenotypes, such as poor social interactions, may be easily neglected and further genetic analyses are undertaken only when a suggestive familiar history is clearly ascertained. The spreading of genetic tests along with increasing evidences that copy number variations are linked to complex neuropsychiatric disorders [30, 31] will certainly unveil new cases in the near future.

Methods
Conventional karyotyping
Phytohaemagglutinin (PHA)-stimulated lymphocyte cultures were set up from peripheral blood samples and the chromosomal analysis was carried out on GTG banded metaphases, according to standard procedures.

Molecular karyotyping
Molecular karyotyping (array-CGH) was performed on DNA samples, extracted from patient's peripheral blood according to standard methods, by using a whole-genome 180 K Agilent array (Human Genome CGH Microarray, Agilent Technologies, Santa Clara, CA, USA), according to manufacturer's protocol. Data were analyzed by using the Agilent Genomic Workbench Standard Edition 6.5.0.58. All genomic positions were reported according to the latest human genome assembly (GRCh38/hg38).

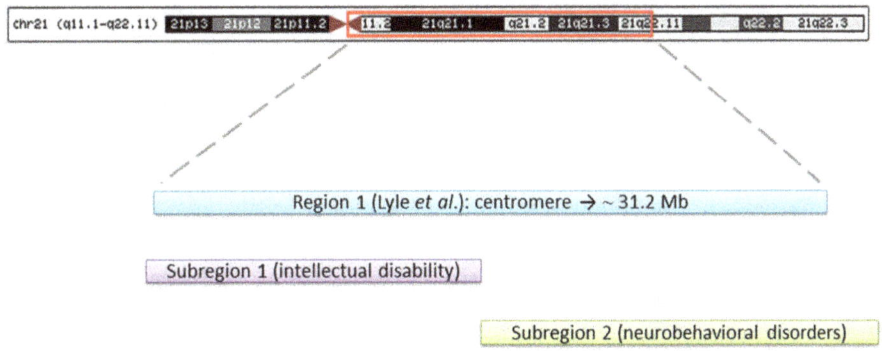

Fig. 3 Subsetting of the great 21q region 1 described by Lyle and colleagues in 2009 into two smaller subregions. Deletions in the subregion 1, from the centromere to ~ 21 Mb (including *BTG3* and *RBM11*), are mainly associated with severe intellectual disability, whereas deletions of the subregion 2, until approximately 32 Mb (including *GRIK1*), are more tightly associated with milder neurobehavioral disorders, such as poor social interactions. Patients with a deletion overpassing the two subregions clinically manifested the most severe phenotype

Abbreviations

Array-CGH: array comparative genomic hybridization; BAEP: Brainstem Auditory Evoked Potentials; DCD: developmental coordination disorder; DSM-IV: diagnostic and statistical manual of mental disorders, fourth edition; EEG: electroencephalogram; EMG: electromyography; GERD: gastroesophageal reflux disease; IQ: intelligence quotient; MABC: movement assessment battery for children; MRI: magnetic resonance imaging; NMR: nuclear magnetic resonance; PDD-NOS: pervasive developmental disorder not otherwise specified.

Competing interests

The authors declare that they have no competing interests.

Authors' contributions

EE and FN analyzed and interpreted the cytogenetic data, and drafted the manuscript. AC, AV, JG, EF and MC collected clinical data and revised the manuscript. DB carried out the karyotype analysis of patient 5. LL contributed to the final revision of the article. OZ conceived the work, participated in its design and finally revised the manuscript. All authors read and approved the final manuscript.

Acknowledgements

We would like to thank the patients and their family members who participated in this study. We also thank Professor Adriano Chiò (ALS Center,'Rita Levi Montalcini' Department of Neuroscience, University of Torino, Torino, Italy) for the fruitful discussion about ALS symptomatology. OZ is supported by Telethon Italy Grant GGP13060; FN is supported by Progetto Cariplo IMPROVE 2015.

Author details

[1]Department of Molecular Medicine, University of Pavia, Via Forlanini 14, 27100 Pavia, Italy. [2]National Neurological Institute IRCCS C, Mondino, Pavia, Italy. [3]Mother-Child Department, Child Neurology and Psychiatry Unit, Spedali Civili, Brescia, Italy. [4]Department of Molecular and Translational Medicine, University of Brescia, Brescia, Italy. [5]Department of Pediatrics, IRCCS Policlinico San Matteo, University of Pavia, Pavia, Italy.

References

1. Roberson ED, Wohler ES, Hoover-Fong JE, Lisi E, Stevens EL, Thomas GH, et al. Genomic analysis of partial 21q monosomies with variable phenotypes. Eur J Hum Genet. 2011;19(2):235–8.
2. Lyle R, Béna F, Gagos S, Gehrig C, Lopez G, Schinzel A, et al. Genotype-phenotype correlations in Down syndrome identified by array CGH in 30 cases of partial trisomy and partial monosomy chromosome 21. Eur J Hum Genet. 2009;17(4):454–66.
3. Korenberg JR, Kalousek DK, Anneren G, Pulst SM, Hall JG, Epstein CJ, et al. Deletion of chromosome 21 and normal intelligence: molecular definition of the lesion. Hum Genet. 1991;87(2):112–8.
4. Tinkel-Vernon H, Finkernagel S, Desposito F, Pittore C, Reynolds K, Sciorra L. Patient with a deletion of chromosome 21q and minimal phenotype. Am J Med Genet A. 2003;120A(1):142–3.
5. Lindstrand A, Malmgren H, Sahlén S, Schoumans J, Nordgren A, Ergander U, et al. Detailed molecular and clinical characterization of three patients with 21q deletions. Clin Genet. 2010;77(2):145–54.
6. Murtagh A, McTigue O, Ramsay L, Hegarty AM, Green AJ, Stallings RL, et al. Interstitial deletion of chromosome 21q and schizophrenia susceptibility. Schizophr Res. 2005;78(2–3):353–6.
7. Ripke S, Neale BM, Corvin A, Walters JT, Farh KH, Holmans PA, et al. Biological insights from 108 schizophrenia-associated genetic loci. Nature. 2014;511(7510):421–7.
8. Saccon RA, Bunton-Stasyshyn RK, Fisher EM, Fratta P. Is SOD1 loss of function involved in amyotrophic lateral sclerosis? Brain. 2013;136:2342–58.
9. Muller FL, Song W, Liu Y, Chaudhuri A, Pieke-Dahl S, Strong R, et al. Absence of CuZn superoxide dismutase leads to elevated oxidative stress and acceleration of age-dependent skeletal muscle atrophy. Free Radic Biol Med. 2006;40(11):1993–2004.
10. Hu J, Chen K, Ni B, Li L, Chen G, Shi S. A novel SOD1 mutation in amyotrophic lateral sclerosis with a distinct clinical phenotype. Amyotroph Lateral Scler. 2012;13(1):149–54.
11. Lucarini N, Verotti A, Napolioni V, Bosco G, Curatolo P. Genetic polymorphisms and idiopathic generalized epilepsies. Pediatr Neurol. 2007;37:157–64.
12. Woo TU, Shrestha K, Amstrong C, Minns MM, Walsh JP, Benes FM. Differential alterations of kainite receptor subunits in inhibitory interneurons in the anterior cingulated cortex in schizophrenia and bipolar disorder. Schizophr Res. 2007;96:46–61.
13. Haldeman-Englert CR, Chapman KA, Kruger H, Geiger EA, McDonald-McGinn DM, Rappaport E, et al. A de novo 8.8-Mb deletion of 21q21.1-q21.3 in an autistic male with a complex rearrangement involving chromosomes 6, 10, and 21. Am J Med Genet A. 2010;152A(1):196–202.
14. Wu LJ, Ko SW, Toyoda H, Zhao MG, Xu H, Vadakkan KI, et al. Increased anxiety-like behavior and enhanced synaptic efficacy in the amygdala of GluR5 knockout mice. PLoS One. 2007;2:e167.
15. Bassuk AG, Geraghty E, Wu S, Mullen SA, Berkovic SF, Scheffer IE, et al. Deletions of 16p11.2 and 19p13.2 in a family with intellectual disability and generalized epilepsy. Am J Med Genet A. 2013;161A(7):1722–5.
16. Gerundino F, Marseglia G, Pescucci C, Pelo E, Benelli M, Giachini C, et al. 16p11.2 de novo microdeletion encompassing SRCAP gene in a patient with speech impairment, global developmental delay and behavioural problems. Eur J Med Genet. 2014;57(11–12):649–53.
17. Ciuladaitė Z, Kasnauskienė J, Cimbalistienė L, Preikšaitienė E, Patsalis PC, Kučinskas V. Mental retardation and autism associated with recurrent 16p11. 2 microdeletion: incomplete penetrance and variable expressivity. J Appl Genet. 2011;52(4):443–9.
18. Bochukova EG, Huang N, Keogh J, Henning E, Purmann C, Blaszczyk K, et al. Large, rare chromosomal deletions associated with severe early-onset obesity. Nature. 2010;463(7281):666–70.
19. Sampson MG, Coughlin CR, Kaplan P, Conlin LK, Meyers KE, Zackai EH, et al. Evidence for a recurrent microdeletion at chromosome 16p11.2 associated with congenital anomalies of the kidney and urinary tract (CAKUT) and Hirschsprung disease. Am J Med Genet A. 2010;152A(10):2618–22.
20. Hannachi H, Mougou-Zerelli S, BenAbdallah I, Mama N, Hamdi I, Labalme A, et al. Clinical and molecular characterization of a combined 17p13.3 microdeletion with partial monosomy 21q21.3 in a 26-year-old man. Cytogenet Genome Res. 2011;135(2):102–10.
21. Pedrotti S, Busà R, Compagnucci C, Sette C. The RNA recognition motif protein RBM11 is a novel tissue-specific splicing regulator. Nucleic Acids Res. 2012;40(3):1021–32.
22. Ren XL, Zhu XH, Li XM, Li YL, Wang JM, Wu PX, et al. Down-regulation of BTG3 promotes cell proliferation, migration and invasion and predicts survival in gastric cancer. J Cancer Res Clin Oncol. 2015;141(3):397–405.
23. Molloy CA, Keddache M, Martin LJ. Evidence for linkage on 21q and 7q in a subset of autism characterized by developmental regression. Mol Psichiatry. 2005;10(8):741–6.
24. Petit F, Plessis G, Decamp M, Cuisset JM, Blyth M, Pendlebury M, et al. 21q21 deletion involving NCAM2: report of 3 cases with neurodevelopmental disorders. Eur J Med Genet. 2015;58(1):44–6.
25. Dyment DA, Smith AC, Humphreys P, Schwartzentruber J, Beaulieu CL, Bulman DE, et al. Homozygous nonsense mutation in SYNJ1 associated with intractable epilepsy and tau pathology. Neurobiol Aging. 2015;36(2):1222. e1-5.
26. Fukai R, Hiraki Y, Nishimura G, Nakashima M, Tsurusaki Y, Saitsu H, et al. A de novo 1.4-Mb deletion at 21q22.11 in a boy with developmental delay. Am J Med Genet A. 2014;164A(4):1021–8.
27. Dai Z, Chung SK, Miao D, Lau KS, Chan AW, Kung AW. Sodium/myo-inositol cotransporter 1 and myo-inositol are essential for osteogenesis and bone formation. J Bone Miner Res. 2011;26(3):582–90.
28. Roepke TK, King EC, Reyna-Neyra A, Paroder M, Purtell K, Koba W, et al. Kcne2 deletion uncovers its crucial role in thyroid hormone biosynthesis. Nat Med. 2009;15(10):1186–94.
29. Ying SW, Kanda VA, Hu Z, Purtell K, King EC, Abbott GW, et al. Targeted deletion of Kcne2 impairs HCN channel function in mouse thalamocortical circuits. PLoS One. 2012;7(8):e42756.

5

First molecular-cytogenetic characterization of Fanconi anemia fragile sites in primary lymphocytes of FA-D2 patients in different stages of the disease

Jelena Filipović[1], Gordana Joksić[1*], Dragana Vujić[2], Ivana Joksić[1], Kristin Mrasek[3], Anja Weise[3] and Thomas Liehr[3]

Abstract

Background: Fanconi anemia (FA) is a chromosomal instability syndrome characterized by increased frequency of chromosomal breakages, chromosomal radial figures and accelerated telomere shortening. In this work we performed detailed molecular-cytogenetic characterization of breakpoints in primary lymphocytes of FA-D2 patients in different stages of the disease using fluorescent in situ hybridization.

Results: We found that chromosomal breakpoints co-localize on the molecular level with common fragile sites, whereas their distribution pattern depends on the severity of the disease. Telomere quantitative fluorescent in situ hybridization revealed that telomere fusions and radial figures, especially radials which involve telomere sequences are the consequence of critically shortened telomeres that increase with the disease progression and could be considered as a predictive parameter during the course of the disease. Sex chromosomes in FA cells are also involved in radial formation indicating that specific X chromosome regions share homology with autosomes and also could serve as repair templates in resolving DNA damage.

Conclusions: FA-D2 chromosomal breakpoints co-localize with common fragile sites, but their distribution pattern depends on the disease stage. Telomere fusions and radials figures which involve telomere sequences are the consequence of shortened telomeres, increase with disease progression and could be of predictive value.

Keywords: Fanconi anemia, Fragile sites, Telomere fusions, Radial figures, X chromosome

Background

Fanconi anemia (FA) is a rare, inherited, genetically heterogeneous chromosomal instability syndrome. To date, 19 different complementation groups, which correspond to distinct DNA repair genes have been identified, FA-A, FA-B, FA-C, FA-D1 (*BRCA2*), FA-D2, FA-E, FA-F, FA-G, FA-I, FA-J (*BRIP1*), FA-M, FA-N (*PALB2*), FA-O (*RAD51C*), FA-P (*SLX4*), FA-Q (*ERCC4*), FA-S (*BRCA1*), FA-R (*RAD51*) and FA-T (*UBE2T*) [1]. The genes that correspond to different FA complementation groups are involved in the FA/BRCA DNA damage repair pathway having an essential function in the cellular response to stress induced by DNA alkylating agents [2]. The most frequent complementation group in Serbia is FA-D2 [3], which is in contrast to the FA-D2 frequency in the general population where it accounts for approximately 4 % of all complementation groups [4]. FA-D2 patients are characterized by a broad spectrum of congenital abnormalities and, unlike most of the other FA complementation groups, an early onset of hematological manifestations including acute myelogenous leukemia and bone marrow failure [5]. One of the most significant FA cellular characteristics is an increase of chromosomal aberrations induced by interstrand cross-linking (ICL) agents [6]. When exposed to these agents, FA cells show an increased frequency of chromosomal breakages and chromosomal radial figures, prolonged cell-cycle arrest in G2/M phase, reduced cellular survival and accelerated telomere shortening [7]. With respect to chromosomal

* Correspondence: gjoksic@vinca.rs
[1]Vinca Institute of Nuclear Sciences, University of Belgrade, Mike Petrovica Alasa 12-14, Belgrade 11001, Serbia
Full list of author information is available at the end of the article

breakages, Schoder and coworkers [8] reported that chromosomal breakpoints in cells derived from FA-A and FA-C patients co-localize with the chromosomal regions that are constitutionally prone to breakage in each individual, known as common fragile sites (CFSs). In addition to standard FS classification, it was shown that cells exposed to replication stress also display breakages in telomeric regions; therefore they were attributed to CFSs [9]. Recent studies of telomere maintenance in FA cells showed that telomere fusions arise either as a consequence of their critical shortening or altered capping function. High percentage of dysfunctional telomeres and marked telomere fragility was found to be typical for FA-D2 cellular phenotype [10]. However, the role of telomeres in formation of induced chromosomal aberrations such as radial figures has not been determined, yet.

The aim of this study was to provide the first molecular-cytogenetic characterization of breakpoint distribution and co-localization with FSs, formation of radial figures and involvement of telomeres in formation of chromosomal aberrations in FA-D2 primary lymphocytes originated from patients in different stages of the disease, severe and mild bone marrow failure stage.

Methods
Patients and sampling
A total of six patients (five females, one male) previously diagnosed with FA-D2 [3, 10] were included in our study. Mean age of children at the time of study was 8 ± 5 years. Routine control of those children was undertaken at the Mother and Child Health Care Institute of Serbia, Hematooncology department. Disease stage was determined based on complete blood count (CBC) and bone marrow examination using standard criteria. Children were divided into two groups accordingly: severe (group A) or mild (group B) bone marrow failure (BMF). Informed consents from the families were obtained and peripheral blood was collected in Li-heparin vaccutainers for additional testing. The study was approved by The Ethical Committee of Mother and Child Health Care Institute of Serbia.

Whole blood cultures
Aliquots of heparinized whole blood (0.5 ml) were set up in cultures containing PBmax-karyotyping medium (Invitrogen-Gibco, Paisley, UK) and treated with diepoxibuthan (DEB, Sigma Chemicals Co., Germany) (final concentration 0.1 µg/ml) 48 h after culture initiation and further harvested 72 h after initiation. Colchicine (Sigma-Aldrich, Munich, Germany) was added during the last 3 h (final concentration 2.5 µg/ml). Cells were collected by centrifugation and treated with hypotonic solution (0.56 % KCl). Cell suspensions were fixed in

methanol/acetic acid (3:1), washed three times with fixative and dropped onto clean slides.

DAPI banding
Slides were incubated overnight at room temperature, dehydrated in series of ethanol (70, 95 and 100 %, respectively), 5 min each, and counterstained with 4′,6′-diamidino-2-phenylindole (DAPI)-containing Vectashield solution (Vector Laboratories Ltd, Peterborough, UK). DAPI selectively binds to heterochromatin regions, which produces a banding pattern known as inverse DAPI banding. According to the unique pattern of differentially stained regions each chromosome can be identified. Analysis was performed with a Zeiss-Axioimager A1 microscope and the ISIS imaging software package (MetaSystems, Altlussheim, Germany).

Locus-specific fluorescent in situ hybridization (Locus-specific FISH, BAC-FISH)
After determination of the most frequent chromosomal breakpoints by inverse DAPI staining, molecular characterization was performed by hybridization with appropriate bacterial artificial chromosome probes (BAC-probes) as described by Mrasek et al. [11]. In short, after removing DAPI, slides were incubated in pepsin solution for 5 min, washed in 1xPBS and fixed in 1 % formalin buffer solution. Prior to applying the BAC-probe, slides were dehydrated in series of ethanol (70, 90, 100 %, 5 min each), denatured in 70 % formamide solution for 2–3 min on a hot plate at 75 °C and immediately placed in 70 % ethanol (4 °C) to conserve target DNA single-stranded. Dehydration in 90 and 100 % ethanol followed. The probe mixture (the probe in hybridization buffer and COT1 Human DNA) was denatured in a thermocycler at 75 °C for 5 min, pre-annealed at 37 °C for 30 min and cooled down to 4 °C. Prepared denatured probes were applied to the slides and hybridized overnight in a dark humid chamber at 37 °C. After hybridization, the slides were washed in 4xSSC/0.2 % Tween20 at the room temperature and 1xSSC-solution (62–65 °C), dehydrated in series of ethanol, counterstained with DAPI solution and observed under the fluorescence microscope. The results were analyzed using ISIS software (MetaSystems, Germany). The chromosomal regions and associated BAC-probes used for hybridization are shown in Table 1.

Telomere quantitative fluorescent in situ hybridization (Q-FISH)
After metaphase analysis DAPI was removed, slides hybridized with telomere cPNA oligonucleotide probe (TTAGGG) as described by Slijepcevic [12]. Briefly, hybridization was performed with the Cy-3 labeled telomeric PNA probe (CCCTAA) 3′ supplemented with PNA

Table 1 BAC-probes used for fluorescence in situ hybridization for the most breakpoint-affected chromosomal regions

Chromosomal region	Fragile site (FS)	FS type[a]	BAC-probe	Co-localization of FA breakpoints and FS
1p13.3	FRA1N	Aphidicolin[b]	RP11-242D10	+
1q21.2	FRA1F	Aphidicolin	RP11-301 M17	+
1q42.2	Near FRA1H	Azacytidin	RP11-109G24	−
2q35	FRA2U	Aphidicolin	RP11-316O14	+
3p14.2	FRA3B	Aphidicolin	RP11-129 K20	+
3p21.31	FRA3H	New nomenclature[c]	RP11-787O14 RP11-159A17	+
3q27.1	FRA3C	Aphidicolin	RP11-110C15	+
5q13.2	FRA5K	New nomenclature[d]	RP11-497H16	+
5q33.2	FRA5O	New nomenclature[d]	RP11-265I24 RP11-494C5	+
7q22.3	FRA7F	Aphidicolin	CTB-20D2	+
7q32.3	FRA7H	Aphidicolin	RP11-138A9 RP11-36B6	+
11q13	FRA11H	Aphidicolin	RP11-449G14	+
14q24.3	FRA14G	Aphidicolin[b]	RP3-414A15	+
16q22.1	FRA16C, FRA16B	Aphidicolin	RP11-106 J23	+
16q23	FRA16D	Aphidicolin	RP11-358 L22	+
18q21.3	FRA18B	Aphidicolin	RP11-15C15	+

BAC-probes for the appropriate FSs were selected according to the literature data:
[a]Nomenclature according to Lukusa et al. [33]
[b]New extended nomenclature according to Mrasek et al. [34]
[c]Common according to the nomenclature by Borgaonkar [35]
[d]Common according to the nomenclature by Simonic and Gericke [36]

centromeric probe for chromosome 2 (DAKO, Glostrup, Denmark) in final concentration 2 ng/ml. The PNA probe for centromere 2 was added in ready to use telomere probe. After hybridization slides were left in a dark humidified chamber for 2 h. The slides were then washed in 70 % formamide and stained with 4′,6′-diamidino-2-phenylindole (DAPI)-containing mounting medium (Vector Laboratories, UK). Analysis was performed using the ISIS software, MetaSystems (Altlussheim, Germany). Measurements were reported as arbitrary relative telomere length units (RTLU), which are defined as the ratio of signal intensity between telomeres and a centromere chromosome 2 reference signals.

Metaphase analysis

Metaphase spreads were analyzed according to the International System for Human Cytogenetic Nomenclature (ISCN, 2013). For each sample at least 1000 metaphases were analyzed for the breakpoint characterization, whereas at least 500 metaphases were scored for fusions and radial formation with regard to the chromosomes involved in their formation, and involvement of telomeres in arising of those aberrations.

Statistical analysis

FA breakpoints were expressed as the percentage of total number of breaks per patient. Telomere fusions and radial figures were presented as percentage of total number of metaphases analyzed and were statistically analyzed using nonparametric Mann-Whitney U test in the program SPSS 10 for Windows. Differences at $p < 0.05$ were considered as significant.

Results

FA breakpoints and assignment to FSs

Results of molecular cytogenetic characterization concerning chromosomal breakages, telomere fusions and radial figures in DEB treated peripheral blood derived from three FA-D2 patients in the severe stage of diseases (group A), and three patients in the mild stage of the disease (group B) are presented in Table 2.

The FA breakpoint analysis showed that frequency of breakages, and breakpoint distribution pattern depend on the stage of the disease: most of the breakpoints in both groups of patients corresponded to CFSs, except for patient 1 in group A where one of the most frequent breaks was 1q42.2 (Fig. 1). In the group A patients, breakpoints were dispersed throughout the genome with a much lower frequency of breakage at the particular

Table 2 FA-D2 patients' karyotypes and molecular cytogenetic findings

	FA-D2 patient	Age (years)	Karyotype	Most frequent breakpoints	Fragile site (FS)	Breakpoint frequency (%)	Telomere fusion frequency (%)	Average telomere length (RTLU[a] ± SD)	Radial figures frequency (%)
Group A	1	8	46,XX	1q42.2	distal to FRA1H	1.72	1.95	14.76 ± 3.23	7.06
				14q24.3	FRA14G	3.09			
				18q21.3	FRA18B	1.72			
	2	6	46,XX	2q35	FRA2U	2.4	1.54	23.02 ± 12.73	1.78
				3p14.2	FRA3B	2.4			
				5q33.2	FRA5O	2			
				7q32.3	FRA7H	1.6			
	3	17	46,XX	3q27.1	FRA3C	2.75	1.62	35.72 ± 7.00	1.88
				5q13.2	FRA5K	2.75			
				5q33.2	FRA5O	3.29			
Group B	4	3	46,XX	3p14.2	FRA3B	11.07	0.08	20.48 ± 12.24	0.78
				3p21.31	FRA3H	3.95			
				7q32.3	FRA7H	1.19			
	5	3	46,XX,der(21)t(15;21)(q15;p11.1)[5]/ 46,XX [15]	1p13	FRA1N	1.76	0.72	21.01 ± 10.33	0.715
				1q21	FRA1F	1.32			
				3p21.31	FRA3H	1.32			
				11q13	FRA11H	0.88			
	6	11	46, XY, der(16)t(1;16)(q42;p11.2)del(1)(q42)[1]/46,XY[31]	3p14.2	FRA3B	1.88	0.23	23.91 ± 6.92	0.23
				3p21.31	FRA3H	0.63			
				16q22.1	FRA16C	1.88			
				16q23	FRA16D	6.88			

[a]RTLU–relative telomere length units

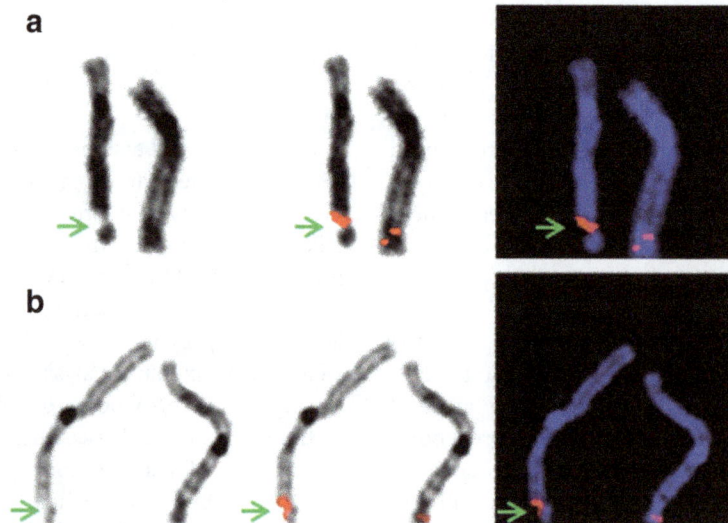

Fig. 1 Representative images of BAC-FISH in FA-D2 metaphases, inverted DAPI and DAPI staining. Arrows indicate breakpoints and hybridized BAC-probes; RP11-265I24 located within FRA5O (**a**), and RP11-109G24 located within 1q42.2, near FRA1H (**b**)

chromosomal locus, i.e. the most frequent breakpoints within this group did not exceed 3.297 % of the total number of breaks.

In contrast, chromosomes in patients of B group tended to break with the higher frequency in the chromosomal regions where the most CFSs are reported (Table 2). Inter-individual variability in frequency of the most common breakages was significant in this group, but the breakage pattern in two patients from this group was similar: in patients 4 and 6 the highest frequency of breakage was observed in regions that correspond to FRA3B (11.07 %) and FRA16D (6.87 %), respectively. However, patient 5 had a different breakage pattern compared to other two patients within this group, where low frequencies of the common breakages were found. However, this patient also shows an unbalanced karyotype, mos 46,XX,der(21)t(15;21)(q15;p 11.1)[5]/46,XX[15].

Telomeres and radial figures
Frequency of telomere fusions and radial figures, with special regard to their structure and telomere involvement in radial figures formation, are presented in Table 2 and Figs. 2, 3 and 6.

The results showed significantly higher frequency of telomere fusions in patients from group A versus group B ($p = 0.05$, Fig. 2). Within A group of patients, telomere fusions occurred most frequently between chromosomes 2p, 2q, 5q and 18q, whereas in group B fusions mostly occurred between 6q, 7q, 9p, 10q, 18q (Fig. 4). Relative quantification of telomere length revealed that the average telomere length (RTLU) was not significantly different between two groups ($p = 0.442$). However, quantification of telomere length at single chromosomes showed that p/q ratio ranged from 0.41 to 2.18 and that

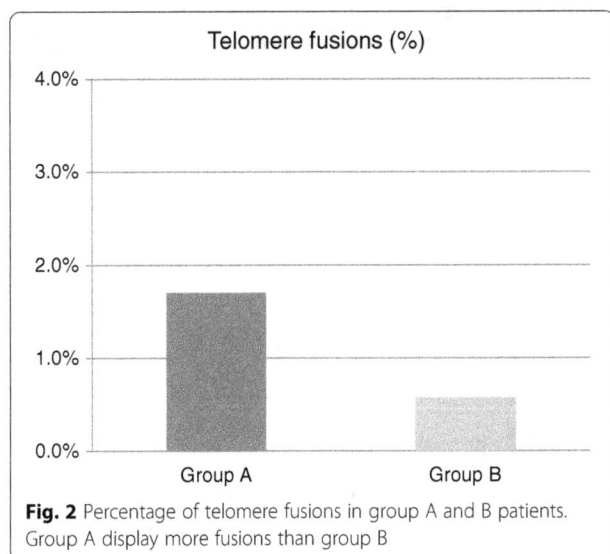

Fig. 3 Percentage of radial figures in group A and B patients. In Group A incidence of radials was six fold higher compared to group B

chromosomes with the shortest telomeres constituted telomere end-to-end fusions.

The percentage of radial figures was low in group B (below 1 %), whereas in group A the percentage was on average six times higher than in group B ($p = 0.05$, Fig. 3). Regarding radial figure structure, great percentage of radials found in group A was a consequence of exchange between telomeres of one and non-telomeric, interstitial regions of other chromosomes, 25.49 % (50 % of all radials in patient 1, and 22.7 % for patients 2 and 3, each). Only two radials between telomeres and interstitial chromosomal sequences were observed in patient 4 and 5, and neither one was observed in patient 6. Although radials always arose between non-homologous chromosomes, distribution of involved chromosomes was heterogeneous—chromosomes 1, 2, 9, 10 and 14 were frequently present in radial figures in group A patients, and chromosome 1 was most frequent in group B. Chromosome X was found to be involved in radial figures in all group A patients and one group B patient (Fig. 5). Representative images of telomere fusions, radials and X chromosome in radial formation are presented in the Fig. 6.

Discussion
The results of our study revealed that chromosomes are not equally prone to breakages in FA-D2 cells exposed to DEB. Matching the data of DAPI banding and BAC-FISH pointed out that regions with increased frequency of breakages co-localize with the CFSs, indicating that frequency of breakpoints as well as their distribution pattern is different among patients and is related to the disease stage.

Assignment of breakpoints to FS in FA-D2 cells is in accordance to previously reported data for FA-A and

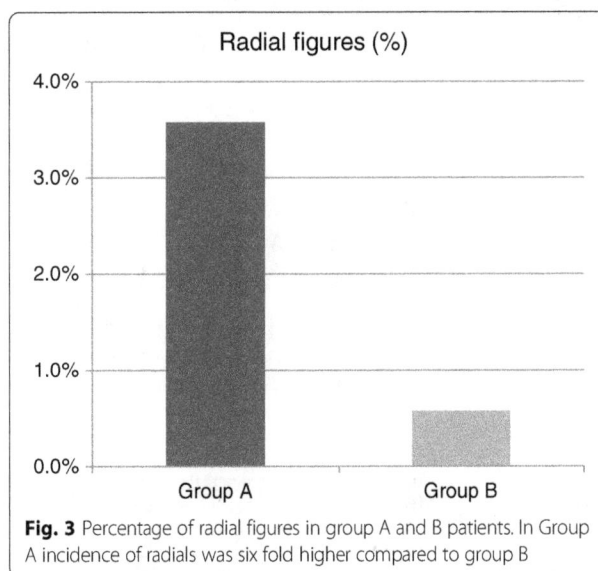

Fig. 2 Percentage of telomere fusions in group A and B patients. Group A display more fusions than group B

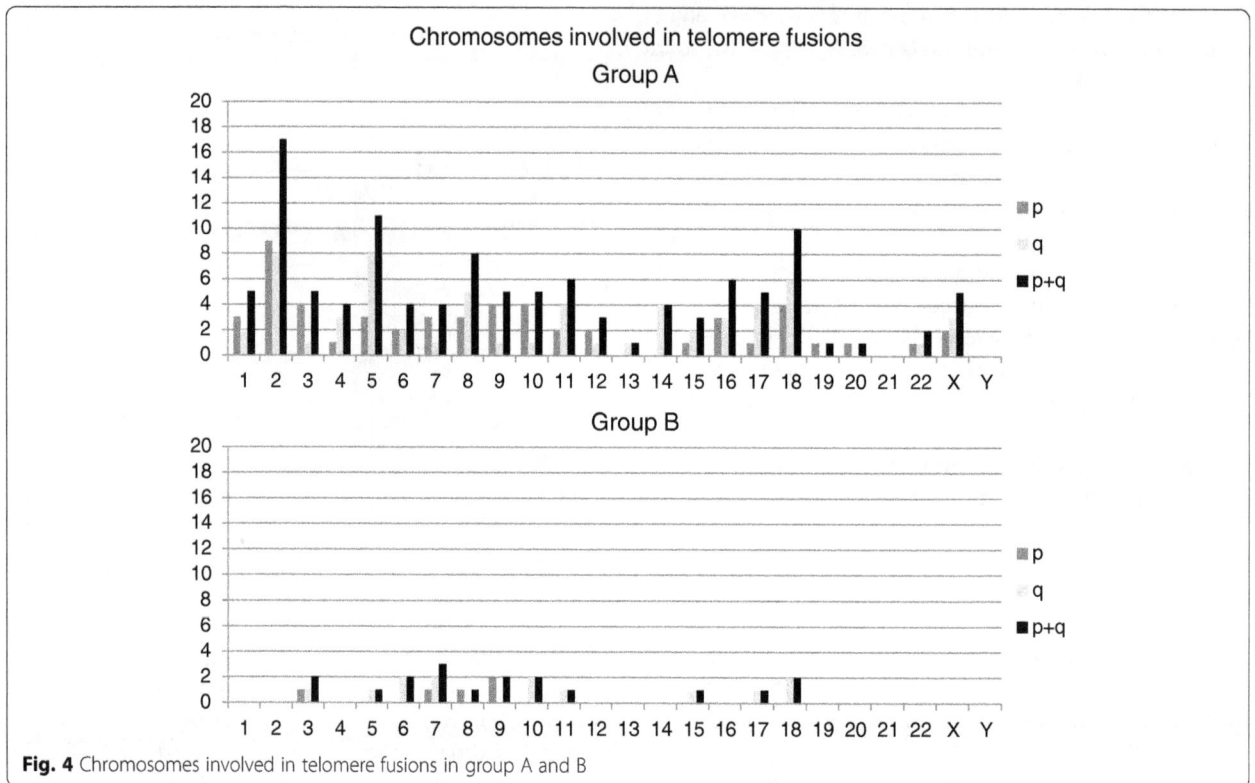

Fig. 4 Chromosomes involved in telomere fusions in group A and B

FA-C cell lines, although the disease stage for the patients in this study was not determined [8]. In FA-D2 patients in the severe stage of the disease (group A) the most frequent breakpoints were present within the CFSs regions (FRA14G, FRA5O, FRA5K and FRA3C, Table 2) except for patient 1 in group A where one of the most frequent breaks was 1q42.2 which is near the FRA1H [13]. However, previously it was not attributed as FS. Their distribution pattern was similar to that found in FA-A and FA-C patients, although different breakpoints were observed in these groups (FRA1A, FRA1D, FRA1E and FRA1J) [8]. The average incidence of chromosomal breaks didn't increase with the disease progression, but the breakpoint distribution pattern was quite different.

Mild stage patients (group B) displayed higher frequencies of breakpoints within the most common FSs, FRA3B and FRA16D except for the patient with unbalanced karyotype (Table 2).

FA pathway plays an essential role in regulation of maintenance and stability of CFSs [14]. Howlett et al. [15], was the first who establishes that disrupted FA pathway leads to increased chromosomal instability at CFSs underlying that their stability depends on the ATR-FANCD2 signaling pathway, i.e. following DNA replication stress, ATR kinase phosphorylates FANCD2 promoting its monoubiquqtination, which activates homologous recombination (HR). Replication stress leads to accumulation of FANCD2 protein in the chromosomal

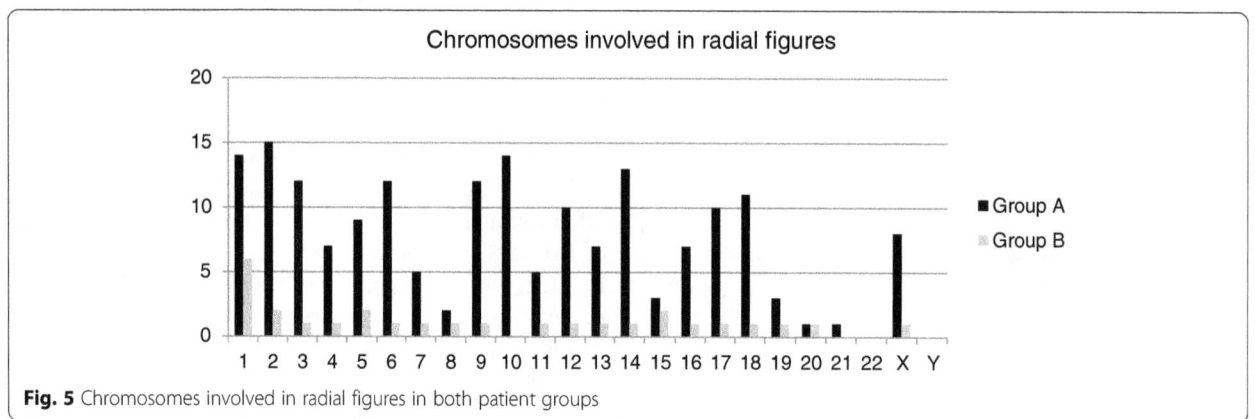

Fig. 5 Chromosomes involved in radial figures in both patient groups

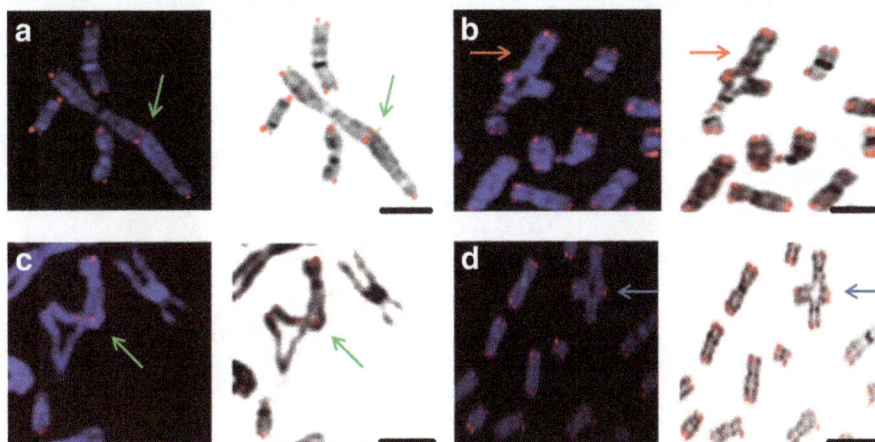

Fig. 6 Representative images of telomere FISH in FA-D2 metaphases. Telomere signals at the fusion points are indicated by *green arrow*: telomere end-to-end fusion, three signals are present between two chromosomes (**a**), radial figure between chromosomes X and 13, *red arrow* indicates X chromosome in radial figure (**b**), *green arrow* indicates radial figure between telomere of one and interstitial region of another chromosome (**c**), *blue arrow* indicates simple radial figure (**d**). Scale bars = 10 µm

regions prone to breakage, whether they are broken or not [16]; however altered FANCD2 protein in FA-D2 cells couldn't maintain stability of existing FSs which in turn activates alternative mechanisms of repair. Apart from HR the CFSs are maintained by non-homologous end-joining (NHEJ) mechanisms, as well as with specialized polymerases that perform by-pass function in DNA synthesis [17, 18].

On the other hand, CFSs are AT-rich sequences prone to form DNA secondary structures which can lead to the replication fork collapse [19]. In addition, replication timing is delayed along CFSs, whereas exposure to DNA polymerase inhibitors intensifies the deceleration of the fork progression, so the CFSs enter G2 phase unreplicated [20]. Both give rise for chromosomal breaks.

Increasing body of evidence now show that large genes constitute the pool of CFSs [21] indicating relationship between instability and transcription of these genes. Since more than one cell cycle is required for their transcription, transcription and replication machineries collide and CFSs expression may occur [22]. Although different FS distribution pattern with the disease progression remains unclear, it is possible that with the progression of the disease different genes could be expressed as a cellular attempt to compensate progressive genomic instability, leading to different CFSs expression.

Up to now, 19 CFSs have been molecularly characterized [23]. Among them are the most common FSs (FRA3B and FRA16D, Table 3) which both contain very large genes (>1 Mbp) important for tumor suppression. These FSs are, along with FRA7H, most frequently expressed in mild stage. In severe stage of the disease different FSs appear as the most common. These

chromosomal regions are also very large, extending from 2 to 6 Mbp, but are comprised by a great number of genes (Table 3); many of those are included in control of cell cycle and tumor suppression. For example, *BCL2* gene (spans approximately 200 kbp), which is the first discovered anti-apoptotic gene, is located within FRA18B, whereas it is known that breakpoints and translocations within this region disrupt its function and lead to myeloproliferative diseases [24]. Similarly, proto-oncogene *C-FOS*, located within FRA14G, also has important role in regulation of cell proliferation and differentiation [25].

Patients in the severe stage of the disease have significantly higher percentage of telomere fusions compared to the patients in the mild stage. Interestingly, there was no significant difference in average telomere length between two groups of patients, but measurement of telomere length at each individual chromosome revealed that the chromosomes with the shortest telomeres were most frequently involved in telomere fusions. Our previous research showed that lymphocyte telomeres in FA-D2 patients are shortened when compared to the age-matched control [10]. Taking into account that FA cells are breakage prone, increased breakages at telomeres and complexity of their function could be the cause of their shortening. Recent review of Holohan et al. [26] pointed out that impaired telomere maintenance and attrition is a hallmark of FA-D2 group, not FA in general. Our previous study showed that FA-D2 cells displayed heterogeneous telomere length and high frequency of double-strand breaks in telomere regions (telomere dysfunction–induced foci - TIFs) which lead to telomere fragility [10]. Altered FANCD2 protein is not capable to maintain telomeres,

Table 3 Genes located within common fragile sites according to the literature data[a, b, c, d]

Fragile site	Chromosomal region	Start	End	Gene	Gene length
Molecularly characterized fragile sites					
FRA3B	3p14.2	58 600 001	63 800 000	FHIT[a]	>1.5 Mbp
FRA7H	7q32.3	130 800 001	132 900 000	/[b]	/
FRA16D	16q23.2	79 200 001	81 600 000	WWOX[c]	1.1 Mbp
Not-characterized fragile sites[d]					
FRA1F	1q21.2	147 500 001	150 600 000	33 genes	/
FRA1N	1p13.3	106 700 001	111 200 000	52 genes	/
FRA2U	2q35	214 500 001	220 700 000	70 genes	/
FRA3C	3q27.1	183 000 001	184 800 000	20 genes	/
FRA3H	3p21.31	44 200 001	50 600 000	78 genes	/
FRA5K	5q13.2	69 100 001	74 000 000	25 genes	/
FRA5O	5q33.2	153 300 001	156 300 000	8 genes	/
FRA7F	7q22.3	104 900 001	107 800 000	14 genes	/
FRA11H	11q13.4	70 500 001	75 500 000	48 genes	/
FRA14G	14q24.3	73 300 001	78 800 000	69 genes	/
FRA16C	16q22.1	66 600 001	70 800 000	95 genes	/
FRA18B	18q21.3	61 300 001	63 900 000	10 genes	/

[a]According to Zimonjic et al. [37].
[b]According to Mishmar et al. [38].
[c]According to Ried et al. [39].
[d]According to National Center for Biotechnology Information [40]

leaving the telomeres unprotected and prone to increased fragility and attrition.

FA-D2 patients in the severe stage had significantly more radials than the patients in the mild phase of the disease, particularly radials formed between telomeres of one and interstitial chromosomal regions of other chromosomes, which was rarely observed in group B. This is unreported finding. Since shortened and fragile telomeres act as double strand breaks (DSB) interchromosomal recombination with other impaired chromosomal regions in attempt to repair the damage is not surprising. Additionally, two patients in severe stage developed bone marrow failure several months after cytogenetic examination and became candidates for bone marrow transplantation.

In both groups of patients, radials were composed of non-homologous chromosomes, which is consistent with the previously reported results [27, 28]. Distribution of involved chromosomes was heterogeneous and not specific for the disease stage. However, X chromosome was found in radials in both groups of patients, which is opposite to the report of Newell and colleagues [27], who found that sex chromosomes are not involved in FA-A and FA-G cells and suggested that alternative mechanisms of ICL repair, which avoid recombination between sex and autosome chromosomes, play the main repair role in FA cells. Involvement of Y chromosome was not observed, but only one male patient in the mild stage and with very low number of radials was part of the study. The presence of sex chromosomes in radial figures in FA patients was not previously reported.

Although radials are described in many genomic instability syndromes, only a few studies clarified the mechanism of their formation. Kuhn and Therman [29] and Scully et al. [30], suggested that they arise as an attempt of cellular repair machinery to resolve DSBs, especially when cells with hampered repair machinery are exposed to ICLs employing homologous recombination [31, 32]. Radials formation in FA cells between non-homologous chromosomes, as well as between autosomes and sex chromosomes indicate that short dispersed chromosomal regions that share homology could act as repair templates in resolving the DNA damage. In FA-D2 cells the X chromosome is not spared from such recombination.

Conclusions

Overall, our results indicate that regions with increased frequency of breakage co-localize with CFSs, whereas their distribution pattern relates to the severity of the disease.

Telomere fusions, as well as interchromosomal recombination and radials formation which involve telomere sequences are the consequence of critically shortened telomeres, increase with disease progression and could be of predictive value.

Acknowledgement
The authors are thankful to patient, parents and medical staff of the Institute of mother and Child Health Care of Serbia. This work is financially supported by Ministry of Education, Science and Technological Development of the Republic of Serbia ON173046 and DAAD project No 57127754.

Funding
This study was funded by Ministry of Education, Science and Technological Development of the Republic of Serbia ON173046 and DAAD project No 57127754.

Authors' contributions
JF and IJ performed experiments and analytical procedures, and drafted the manuscript. GJ, DV, KM, AW and TL supervised the experiments, edited and approved the manuscript.

Competing interests
The authors declare that they have no competing interests.

Author details
[1]Vinca Institute of Nuclear Sciences, University of Belgrade, Mike Petrovica Alasa 12-14, Belgrade 11001, Serbia. [2]Mother and Child Health Care Institute of Serbia, "Dr Vukan Cupic", Radoja Dakica 6, Belgrade 11070, Serbia. [3]Institute of Human Genetics, Jena University Hospital, Friedrich Schiller University, Kollegiengasse 10, Jena D-07743, Germany.

References
1. Dong H, Nebert DW, Bruford EA, Thompson DC, Joenje H, Vasiliou V. Update of the human and mouse Fanconi anemia genes. Hum Genomics. 2015;9:32.
2. Kee Y, D'Andrea AD. Expanded roles of the Fanconi anemia pathway in preserving genomic stability. Gene Dev. 2010;24:1680–94.
3. Vujic D, Petrovic S, Lazic E, Kuzmanovic M, Leskovac A, Joksic I, Micic D, Jovanovic A, Zecevic Z, Guc-Scekic M, Cirkovic S, Joksic G. Prevalence of FA-D2 Rare Complementation Group of Fanconi Anemia in Serbia. Indian J Pediatr. 2014;81:260–5.
4. Whitney M, Thayer M, Reifsteck C, Olson S, Smith L, Jakobs P, Leach R, Naylor S, Joenje H, Grompe M. Microcell mediated chromosome transfer maps the Fanconi anaemia group D gene to chromosome 3p. Nat Genet. 1995;11:341–3.
5. Kalb R, Neveling K, Hoehn H, Schneider H, Linka Y, Batish SD, Hunt C, Berwick M, Callen E, Surralles J, Casado JA, Bueren J, Dasi A, Soulier J, Gluckman E, Zwaan CM, van Spaendonk R, Pals G, de Winter JP, Joenje H, Grompe M, Auerbach AD, Hanenberg H, Schindler D. Hypomorphic mutations in the gene encoding a key Fanconi anemia protein, FANCD2, sustain a significant group of FA-D2 patients with severe phenotype. Am J Hum Genet. 2007;80:895–910.
6. Auerbach AD. Fanconi anemia and its diagnosis. Mutat Res. 2009;668:4–10.
7. Adelfalk C, Lorenz M, Serra V, von Zglinicki T, Hirsch-Kauffmann M, Schweiger M. Accelerated telomere shortening in Fanconi anemia fibroblasts–a longitudinal study. FEBS Lett. 2001;506:22–6.
8. Schoder C, Liehr T, Velleuer E, Wilhelm K, Blaurock N, Weise A, Mrasek K. New aspects on chromosomal instability: Chromosomal break-points in Fanconi anemia patients co-localize on the molecular level with fragile sites. Int J Oncol. 2010;36:307–12.
9. Sfeir A, Kosiyatrakul ST, Hockemeyer D, MacRae SL, Karlseder J, Schildkraut CL, de Lange T. Mammalian telomeres resemble fragile sites and require TRF1 for efficient replication. Cell. 2009;138:90–103.
10. Joksic I, Vujic D, Guc-Scekic M, Leskovac A, Petrovic S, Ojani M, Trujillo JP, Surralles J, Zivkovic M, Stankovic A, Slijepcevic P, Joksic G. Dysfunctional telomeres in primary cells from Fanconi anemia FANCD2 patients. Genome Integr. 2012;3:6.
11. Mrasek K, Wilhelm K, Quintana LG, Theuss L, Liehr T, Leskovac A, Filipovic J, Joksic G, Joksic I, Weise A. BAC-probes applied for characterization of fragile sites (FS). Methods Mol Biol. 2015;1227:289–98.
12. Slijepcevic P. Telomere length measurement by Q-FISH. Methods Cell Sci. 2001;23:17–22.
13. Curatolo A, Limongi ZM, Pelliccia F, Rocchi A. Molecular Characterization of the Human Common Fragile Site FRA1H. Genes Chromosomes Cancer. 2007;46:487–93.
14. Durkin SG, Glover TW. Chromosome fragile sites. Annu Rev Genet. 2007; 41:169–92.
15. Howlett NG, Taniguchi T, Durkin SG, D'Andrea AD, Glover TW. The Fanconi anemia pathway is required for the DNA replication stress response and for the regulation of common fragile site stability. Hum Mol Genet. 2005;14:693–701.
16. Chan KL, Palmai-Pallag T, Ying S, Hickson ID. Replication stress induces sister-chromatid bridging at fragile site loci in mitosis. Nat Cell Biol. 2009;11:753–60.
17. Schwartz M, Zlotorynski E, Goldberg M, Ozeri E, Rahat A, Sage C, Chen BP, Chen DJ, Agami R, Kerem B. Homologous recombination and nonhomologous end-joining repair pathways regulate fragile site stability. Gene Dev. 2005;19:2715–26.
18. Bergoglio V, Boyer AS, Walsh E, Naim V, Legube G, Lee MY, Rey L, Rosselli F, Cazaux C, Eckert KA, Hoffmann JS. DNA synthesis by Pol eta promotes fragile site stability by preventing under-replicated DNA in mitosis. J Cell Biol. 2013;201:395–408.
19. Shah SN, Opresko PL, Meng X, Lee MY, Eckert KA. DNA structure and the Werner protein modulate human DNA polymerase δ-dependent replication dynamics within the common fragile site FRA16D. Nucleic Acids Res. 2010; 38:1149–62.
20. Zlotorynski E, Rahat A, Skaug J, Ben-Porat N, Ozeri E, Hershberg R, Levi A, Scherer SW, Margalit H, Kerem B. Molecular basis for expression of common and rare fragile sites. Mol Cell Biol. 2003;23:7143–51.
21. Le Tallec B, Koundrioukoff S, Wilhelm T, Letessier A, Brison O, Debatisse M. Updating the mechanisms of common fragile site instability: how to reconcile the different views? Cell Mol Life Sci. 2014;71:4489–94.
22. Helmrich A, Ballarino M, Tora L. Collisions between replication and transcription complexes cause common fragile site instability at the longest human genes. Mol Cell. 2011;44:966–77.
23. Ma K, Qiu L, Mrasek K, Zhang J, Liehr T, Quintana LG, Li Z. Common fragile sites: genomic hotspots of DNA damage and carcinogenesis. Int J Mol Sci. 2012;13:11974–99.
24. Yip KW, Reed JC. Bcl-2 family proteins and cancer. Oncogene. 2008;27:6398–406.
25. Milde-Langosch K. The Fos family of transcription factors and their role in tumourigenesis. Eur J Cancer. 2005;41:2449–61.
26. Holohan B, Wright WE, Shay JW. Telomeropathies: An emerging spectrum disorder. J Cell Biol. 2014;205:289–99.
27. Newell AE, Akkari YM, Torimaru Y, Rosenthal A, Reifsteck CA, Cox B, Grompe M, Olson SB. Interstrand crosslink-induced radials form between non-homologous chromosomes, but are absent in sex chromosomes. DNA Repair (Amst). 2004;3:535–42.
28. Owen N, Hejna J, Rennie S, Mitchell A, Hanlon Newell A, Ziaie N, Moses RE, Olson SB. Bloom syndrome radials are predominantly non-homologous and are suppressed by phosphorylated BLM. Cytogenet Genome Res. 2014;144:255–63.
29. Kuhn EM, Therman E. Origin of symmetrical triradial chromosomes in human cells. Chromosoma. 1982;86:673–81.
30. Scully R, Puget N, Vlasakova K. DNA polymerase stalling, sister chromatid recombination and the BRCA genes. Oncogene. 2000;19:6176–83.
31. Joksic I, Petrovic S, Leskovac A, Filipovic J, Guc-Scekic M, Vujic D, Joksic G. Enhanced frequency of sister chromatid exchanges induced by diepoxybutane is specific characteristic of Fanconi anemia cellular phenotype. Genetika. 2013;45:393–403.

32. Thyagarajan B, Campbell C. Elevated homologous recombination activity in Fanconi anemia fibroblasts. J Biol Chem. 1997;272:23328–33.
33. Lukusa T, Fryns JP. Human chromosome fragility. Biochim Biophys Acta. 2008;1779:3–16.
34. Mrasek K, Schoder C, Teichmann AC, Behr K, Franze B, Wilhelm K, Blaurock N, Claussen U, Liehr T, Weise A. Global screening and extended nomenclature for 230 aphidicolin-inducible fragile sites, including 61 yet unreported ones. Int J Oncol. 2010;36:929–40.
35. Borgaonkar DS. Chromosomal Variation in Man. 7th ed. New York: Wiley-Liss; 1994.
36. Simonic I, Gericke GS. The enigma of common fragile sites. Hum Genet. 1996;97:524–31.
37. Zimonjic DB, Druck T, Ohta M, Kastury K, Croce CM, Popescu NC, Huebner K. Positions of Chromosome 3p14.2 Fragile Sites (FRA3B) within the FHIT Gene. Cancer Res. 1997;57:1166–70.
38. Mishmar D, Rahat A, Scherer SW, Nyakatura G, Hinzmann B, Kohwi Y, Mandel-Gutfroind Y, Lee JR, Drescher B, Sas DE, Margalit H, Platzer M, Weiss A, Tsui LC, Rosenthal A, Kerem B. Molecular characterization of a common fragile site (FRA7H) on human chromosome 7 by the cloning of a simian virus 40 integration site. Proc Natl Acad Sci U S A. 1998;95:8141–6.
39. Ried K, Finnis M, Hobson L, Mangelsdorf M, Dayan S, Nancarrow JK, Woollatt E, Kremmidiotis G, Gardner A, Venter D, Baker E, Richards RI. Common chromosomal fragile site FRA16D sequence: identification of the FOR gene spanning FRA16D and homozygous deletions and translocation breakpoints in cancer cells. Hum Mol Genet. 2000;9:1651–63.
40. National Center for Biotechnology Information. http://www.ncbi.nlm.nih.gov. Accessed 10 Jun 2016.

6

Segmental paleotetraploidy revealed in sterlet (*Acipenser ruthenus*) genome by chromosome painting

Svetlana A. Romanenko[1,2*], Larisa S. Biltueva[1], Natalya A. Serdyukova[1], Anastasia I. Kulemzina[1], Violetta R. Beklemisheva[1], Olga L. Gladkikh[1], Natalia A. Lemskaya[1], Elena A. Interesova[3,4], Marina A. Korentovich[5], Nadezhda V. Vorobieva[1,2], Alexander S. Graphodatsky[1,2] and Vladimir A. Trifonov[1]

Abstract

Background: Acipenseriformes take a basal position among Actinopteri and demonstrate a striking ploidy variation among species. The sterlet (*Acipenser ruthenus*, Linnaeus, 1758; ARUT) is a diploid 120-chromosomal sturgeon distributed in Eurasian rivers from Danube to Enisey. Despite a high commercial value and a rapid population decline in the wild, many genomic characteristics of sterlet (as well as many other sturgeon species) have not been studied.

Results: Cell lines from different tissues of 12 sterlet specimens from Siberian populations were established following an optimized protocol. Conventional cytogenetic studies supplemented with molecular cytogenetic investigations on obtained fibroblast cell lines allowed a detailed description of sterlet karyotype and a precise localization of 18S/28S and 5S ribosomal clusters. Localization of sturgeon specific HindIII repetitive elements revealed an increased concentration in the pericentromeric region of the acrocentric ARUT14, while the total sterlet repetitive DNA fraction (C_0t30) produced bright signals on subtelomeric segments of small chromosomal elements. Chromosome and region specific probes ARUT1p, 5, 6, 7, 8 as well as 14 anonymous small sized chromosomes (probes A-N) generated by microdissection were applied in chromosome painting experiments. According to hybridization patterns all painting probes were classified into two major groups: the first group (ARUT5, 6, 8 as well as microchromosome specific probes C, E, F, G, H, and I) painted only a single region each on sterlet metaphases, while probes of the second group (ARUT1p, 7 as well as microchromosome derived probes A, B, D, J, K, M, and N) marked two genomic segments each on different chromosomes. Similar results were obtained on male and female metaphases.

Conclusions: The sterlet genome represents a complex mosaic structure and consists of diploid and tetraploid chromosome segments. This may be regarded as a transition stage from paleotetraploid (functional diploid) to diploid genome condition. Molecular cytogenetic and genomic studies of other 120- and 240-chromosomal sturgeons are needed to reconstruct genome evolution of this vertebrate group.

Keywords: Acipenseriformes, Fish cell line, Banding, Satellite DNA, Telomeric repeat, rRNA, FISH, Microdissection

* Correspondence: rosa@mcb.nsc.ru
[1]Institute of Molecular and Cellular Biology SB RAS, Novosibirsk, Russia
[2]Novosibirsk State University, Novosibirsk, Russia
Full list of author information is available at the end of the article

Background

A great interest in the study of the sturgeon genomes (Acipenseridae, Acipenseriformes) is primarily connected with a high commercial value of the representatives of the family and a necessity in conservation measures due to a rapid population decline in the wild. At present, most of sturgeons became commercially valuable and popular objects of industrial farming. A detailed investigation of sturgeon biology including molecular characterization of chromosomal complement and understanding of genetic mechanisms of sex determination are essential for improvement of aquaculture and development of a viable conservation strategy. The group of Aciperseriformes also draws attention due to a basal position within Actinopteri on the evolutionary tree of ray-finned fishes. Deep investigation of sturgeon's genomes is critical for eliciting information about genetic composition through comparative approach.

Despite a high interest in sturgeon biology, the phylogenetic relationships between species, the number of chromosomes and other important biological characteristics remained controversial for a long time. Recent work on sturgeon phylogeny finally resolved many questions [1–3]. However, the cytogenetic investigation of sturgeons was particularly complicated because of the high number of chromosomes in acipenserid karyotypes (a minimal diploid number is about 120). The average diploid number chromosomes in Acipenseriformes considerably exceeds that in other vertebrate groups due to presumed ancient polyploidization event with no diploid ancestral forms survived [4]. Sturgeons' karyotypes were investigated only by conventional cytogenetics and no molecular chromosome probes were developed for in-depth study of sturgeons' chromosome structure. The same reasons resulted in the lack of accurate knowledge about the system of sex determination of all members of Acipenseriformes.

However, through pioneering cytogenetic studies of sturgeons karyotypes some essential information about composition and molecular structure of sturgeon chromosomal complements is available [5]. A considerable amount of work on conventional cytogenetics was carried out on other acipenserid species, as well as the study of distribution of telomeric sequences, 5S, 18S, and 28S ribosomal RNA genes, different satellite DNA sequences by fluorescent in situ hybridization (FISH) [6–8]. Up to now the description of some chromosome rearrangements was obtained for only one sturgeon species – *Acipenser gueldenstaedtii* [7].

The sterlet (*Acipenser ruthenus*) is one of the well-known representatives of Acipenseridae family with a relatively wide distribution (from Danube to Enisey) and small body size (in comparison to other sturgeons). The species is considered as vulnerable by the IUCN but it was successfully bred in captivity and sterlet fishing is currently allowed in some Russian regions. The mechanism of sex determination is not established in acipenseriformes, while some existing data suggest genetic sex determination with females being heterogametic in certain species [9–11]. Cell cultures were obtained for sterlet previously which advanced the species cytogenetics [12]. The data on sterlet karyotype description obtained up to 1999 are summarized in [5]. The most recent data show that even the question about precise diploid chromosome number remains open; with 2n reported to vary between 118 ± 2 and 118 ± 4 (see [13]). It was proposed that the sterlet genome, along with other acipenserid genomes with $2n \approx 120$, was formed by duplication of the ancestral 60-chromosomal genome [13]. Other cytogenetic data for *A. ruthenus* include information about C-banding [14], NORs visualization by Ag-staining [4, 15], localization of telomeric repeats [7], detection and mapping of 18S/28S and 5S rRNA [8, 16], and distribution of HindIII satellite [17]. GTG (G-banding by trypsin using Giemsa) differential staining as well as comparison of different markers localization between males and females has not been reported. The comparative information about distinguishing features of male and female karyotypes is also missing. Most cytogenetic works have been accomplished on captive individuals or involved European sterlet populations, no karyotypes of wild sterlet from Siberian rivers were reported so far.

Although chromosome painting using chromosome specific probes was found to be a method of choice for contemporary cytogenetic studies of mammals [18], birds [19], reptiles [20] and even some teleosts [21], no such studies have been performed so far within the group of sturgeons.

Generation of detailed cytogenetic maps saturated with molecular and cytogenetic markers is a prerequisite for a profound study of any genome. However quality metaphases and high-resolution chromosomes are required for reliable localization of molecular probes and for distinguishing of individual chromosome pairs. Here we established an array of sterlet primary cell lines and present a molecular cytogenetic study of sterlet karyotype from Siberian populations using C- and G-banding, localization of variety of repetitive sequences (telomeric repeats, 18S/28S and 5S rDNAs, repetitive DNA fraction (C_0t 30), and HindIII satellite). Besides, through microdissection we created molecular markers for some of the sterlet chromosomes and applied chromosome painting to male and female metaphases to estimate to copy numbers of homologous regions. We explore and discuss ploidy phenomenon in the sterlet.

Results

Optimization of cell culture conditions for primary cell lines of sterlet

To optimize conditions for sterlet cell lines establishment, fin tissues from 5 specimens from the wild population of

Ob river (Middle Ob, Tomsk region) (ARUT"1-5") (Table 1) were used. Cell proliferation was observed in all culturing conditions but growth rates varied. We compared cell growth from explants that undergone collagenase/hyaluronidase proteolytic treatment and those simply plated onto culturing surface. New cell growth was observed after one to three days following seeding of tissue explants regardless of whether proteolytic treatment of explants was performed or not. The cells demonstrated rapid growth and formed a monolayer after seven-ten days of culturing. In all cases fin-derived cells appeared to look better and grew faster if the cultures were established without tissue treatment with proteolytic enzymes. We also compared an array of media: αMEM, DMEM, RPMI, L-15, and 199. The worst results of growing were shown with L-15 medium, the best results was achieved using 199 medium or αMEM supplemented with 15 % FBS. This optimal media combination was validated on fin tissues from ARUT"6-9" individuals and was applied in all subsequent experiments. Moreover, we revealed that sterlet cells are sensitive to standard trypsin/EDTA treatment, therefore we used scrapers to dissociate cells. Post-recovery survival of cells frozen in plain FBS with 10 % DMSO was much higher than for cells frozen in medium with 40 % FBS + 10 % DMSO. In primary sterlet cultures we observed a high viscosity of the post-culture media that decreased with subsequent passaging. This phenomenon is worth additional investigation and could possibly be caused by changes in hyaluronic pathway in sterlet cells similar to that described for the naked mole rat cells [22].

In another experiment besides fins we took three different kinds of tissues from ARUT"10-12": notochord, swim bladder, and barbels and observed similar pattern of growth despite variation in cell morphology (Table 2, Fig. 1). While the cells originated from swim bladder and notochord showed typical fibroblast-like morphology, other cell lines were heterogeneous. We postulate

that seeding without enzyme treatment can be more efficient in the case of fin tissues, while notochord tissues demonstrate better growth after preliminary treatment with collagenase and hyaluronidase in comparison to seeding without any treatment. Both methods of swim bladder seeding gave similar results. The establishment of sterlet cell cultures from barbel tissues looked unpromising because of the high risk of contamination and a poor survival of cells after passaging.

Conventional cytogenetics

Routine Giemsa staining was used to count chromosomes. It appears that 2n in sterlet karyotype is seemingly 120 (Fig. 2). GTG-banding allowed us to further rank chromosome pairs. All pairs of autosomes were placed in order of decreasing size. No distinct G-blocks were identified on large chromosomes (Fig. 3). Heterochromatic blocks were identified in the pericentromeric regions of some sterlet chromosomes (Fig. 4). The largest eight pairs of chromosomes exhibit only interstitial heterochromatin blocks with almost no detectable C-blocks in the centromeric regions of chromosomes.

Distribution pattern of telomeric repeats and ribosomal DNA

We localized the 18S/28S-rDNA probe in dual-color FISH with 5S-rDNA probe both on sterlet male and female (Fig. 5a, b). The 5S-rDNA probe marked a pericentromeric region of one of the small pairs of chromosomes in both sexes (ARUT41-50). The pair was DAPI-positive. The 18S/28S-rDNA probe gave 3 pairs of signals on male karyotype: in the p-arms of one pair of chromosomes (ARUT21-30), on the pericentromeric region of a small pair (ARUT31-40) and on the long arm of a small pair of chromosomes (ARUT31-40) (Fig. 5a). Moreover in the female karyotype we detected some additional weak signals produced by 18S/28S-rDNA probe (Fig. 5b). On average

Table 1 List of *Acipenser ruthenus* specimens

Abbreviation	Sex	Age	Origin
ARUT"1f"	♀	3–4 years	Shegarsky district, Ob river, N 56°34'45", E 84 °10'46", Tomsk oblast, Russia
ARUT"2m"	♂	3–4 years	Shegarsky district, Ob river, N 56°34'45", E 84 °10'46", Tomsk oblast, Russia
ARUT"3m"	♂	3–4 years	Shegarsky district, Ob river, N 56°34'45", E 84 °10'46", Tomsk oblast, Russia
ARUT"4f"	♀	3–4 years	Shegarsky district, Ob river, N 56°34'45", E 84 °10'46", Tomsk oblast, Russia
ARUT"5f"	♀	3–4 years	Shegarsky district, Ob river, N 56°34'45", E 84 °10'46", Tomsk oblast, Russia
ARUT"6f"	♀	4 years	Kostylevo, Sturgeon Hatchery Farm of State Scientific-and-Production Centre for Fisheries, Tyumen, Russia
ARUT"7m"	♂	4 years	Kostylevo, Sturgeon Hatchery Farm of State Scientific-and-Production Centre for Fisheries, Tyumen, Russia
ARUT"8f"	♀	4 years	Kostylevo, Sturgeon Hatchery Farm of State Scientific-and-Production Centre for Fisheries, Tyumen, Russia
ARUT"9m"	♂	4 years	Kostylevo, Sturgeon Hatchery Farm of State Scientific-and-Production Centre for Fisheries, Tyumen, Russia
ARUT"10m"	♂	unknown	Fish Farm, Seversk, Tomsk oblast, Russia
ARUT"11f"	♀	unknown	Fish Farm, Seversk, Tomsk oblast, Russia
ARUT"12f"	♀	unknown	Fish Farm, Seversk, Tomsk oblast, Russia

Table 2 Types of seeding and culture media used for ARUT″10-12″ cultivation

Tissues	Without enzymes	With collagenase and hyaluronidase
Barbels	αMEM	-
	199	-
Notochord	αMEM	αMEM
	199	199
Swim bladder	αMEM	αMEM
	199	199
Fin	αMEM	-
	199	-

The optimal condition for each sample is underlined

we identified from two to four additional signals on different homologs (usually only on a single homolog from the pair). Telomeric repeats were localized in the terminal regions of all chromosomes. Although no interstitial blocks of telomeric repeats were visualized, some small chromosome had increased subtelomeric signals (Fig. 5e, f).

Distribution pattern of C_0t30 DNA and HindIII repeat

In all metaphases of both male and female of *A. ruthenus* the hybridization signals with the HindIII satellite DNA probe were weak but clearly visible (Fig. 5c, d). In both sexes the satellite DNA was localized in the pericentromeric region of the large acrocentric pair (ARUT14). No clear signals were detected on other chromosomes.

C_0t30 DNA probe has highlighted pericentromeric regions of all chromosomes as well as some interstitial

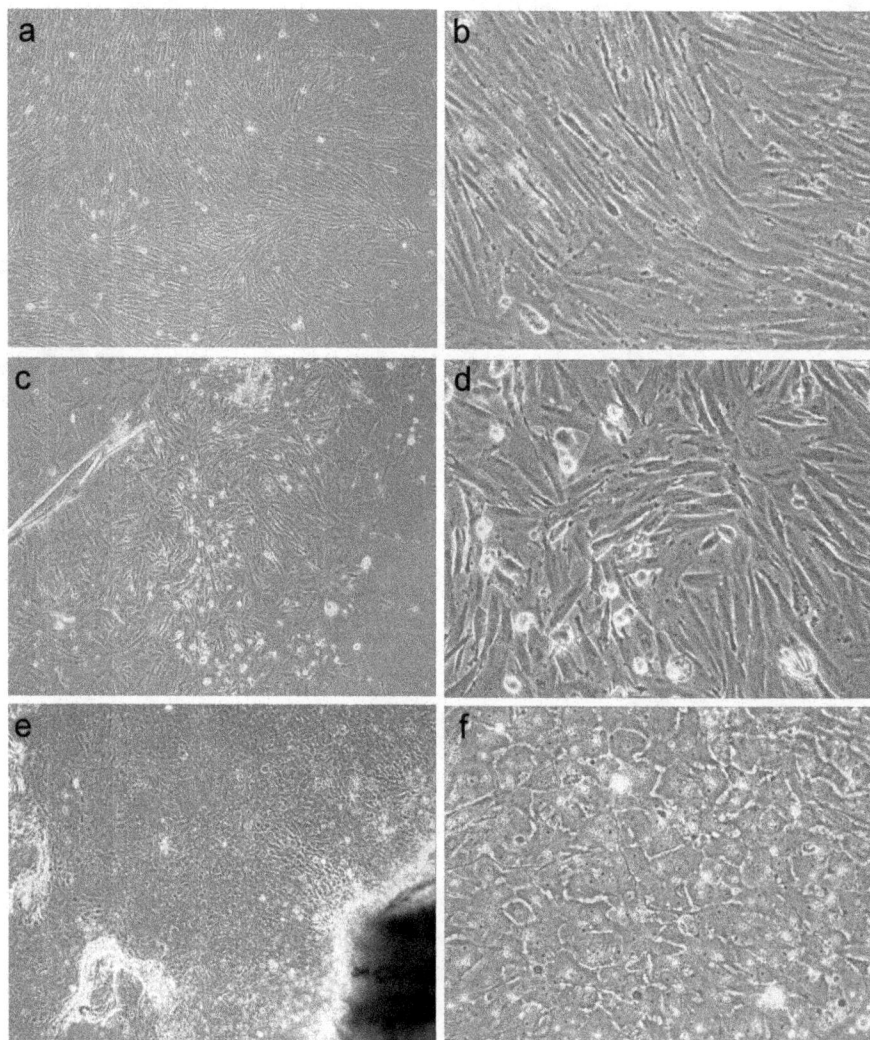

Fig. 1 The variety of cell types in primary cultures of sterlet. Left column – 100-fold magnification, right column – the same area at 400-fold magnification. **a**, **b** – cell cultures established from notochord of the male sterlet (ARUT″10m″); **c**, **d** – cell cultures established from swim bladder of the female sterlet (ARUT″11f″); **e**, **f** – cell cultures established from fin of the female sterlet (ARUT″12f″)

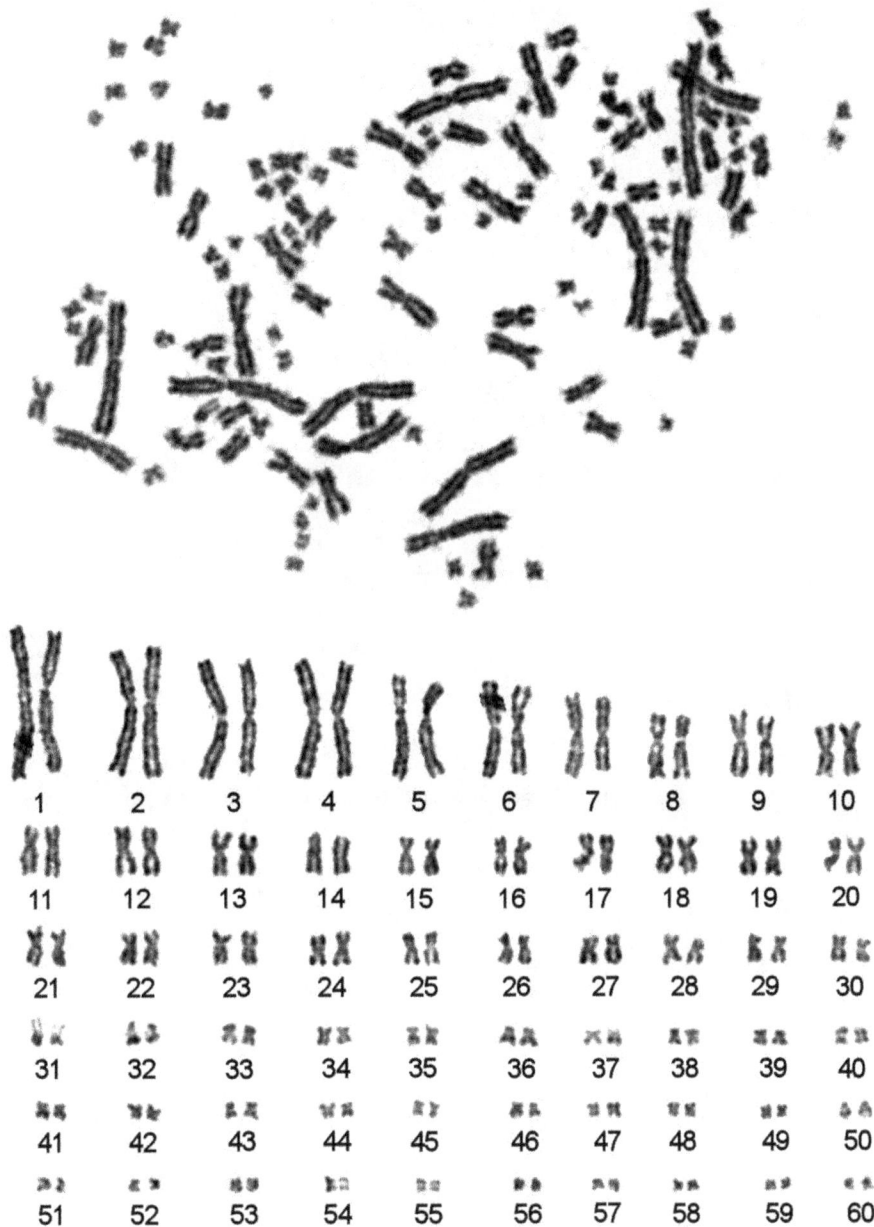

Fig. 2 A metaphase plate and karyotype of the male sterlet (ARUT"2m", 2n = 120) after routine Giemsa staining

regions and p- and q-arms of most small metacentrics (Fig. 5g, h). Signal intensity was higher on small chromosomes suggesting uneven distribution of repetitive DNAs across genome.

Chromosome painting of microdissection-derived painting probes

We obtained painting probes from single chromosomes (regions) ARUT1p, 5, 6, 7, 8 as well as for 14 small sized chromosomes (probes A-N: we used letters to designate the probes of microchromosomes as no precise chromosome assignment had been accomplished yet). All probes

obtained can be classified into two major groups: the first group (ARUT5, 6, 8 as well as microchromosome specific probes C, E, F, G, H, and I) painted only a single region each in sterlet genome (Fig. 6a (green signals), c (green signals), d), while probes of the second group (ARUT1p, 7 as well as microchromosome derived probes A, B, D, J, K, M, and N) marked two genomic segments each on different chromosomes (Fig. 6a (red signals), b, c (red signals)). Similar results were obtained on male and female metaphases, revealing no sex specific localization pattern.

It is interesting to note that the most tetraploid segments were localized on chromosomes of similar size

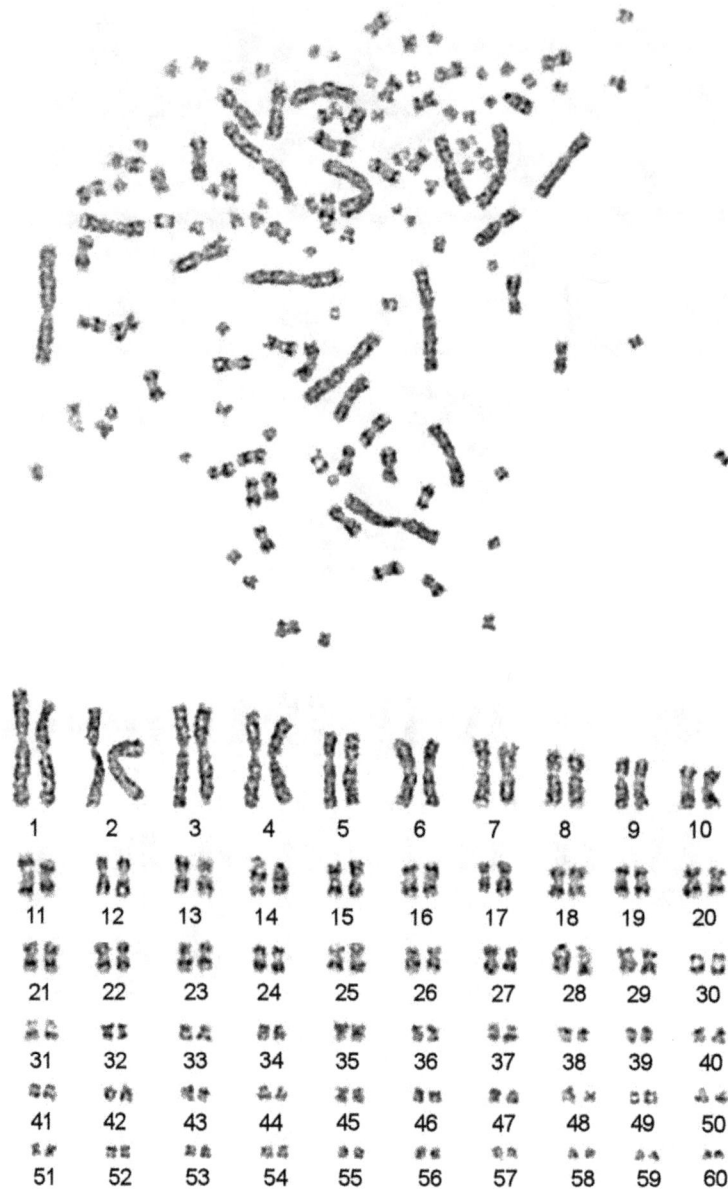

Fig. 3 GTG-banded chromosomes of the male sterlet (ARUT"2m"): metaphase plate and karyotype

(i.e., ARUT1p and ARUT2p), but the probe ARUT7 additionally painted much smaller and different in morphology chromosome ARUT14. We assume that some material of ARUT7 is present in diploid and some in tetraploid state.

Discussion

Features of sterlet cell culture

Cell cultures of different sturgeon species have been established since 1985 [23]. Previously published data showed that fish cell cultures can be grown using variety of culture media [24–27]. Fin tissues are the most commonly used material for establishing primary cell line in fishes. However, we show that primary cell line could be established successfully from variety of sterlet tissues types (notochord, bladder). In present work we used the established growth temperature and FBS concentration shown to be optimal for other sturgeon species [26, 27]. We varied several parameters of culturing and show that proteolytic treatment is very efficient for establishment of primary cell lines from notochord, but not useful for fins [28, 29]. We demonstrated that 199 and alphaMEM media are suitable for prolific cell growth in sterlet cell lines, while L-15 media is not (Table 2). Sterlet cells from all tissues are sensitive to trypsin and freezing, so extra measures should be taken to not damage the cells

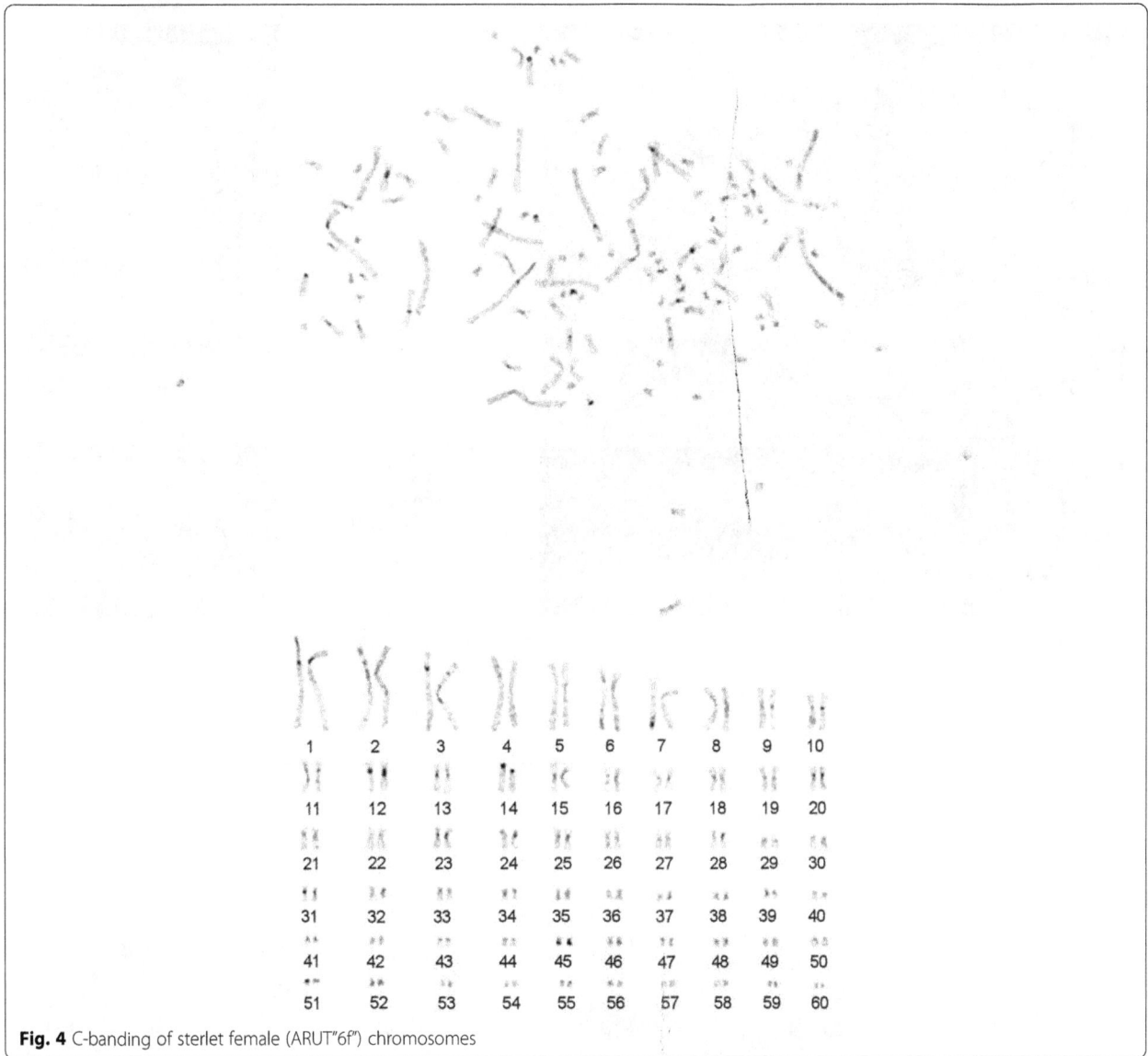

Fig. 4 C-banding of sterlet female (ARUT"6f") chromosomes

by harsh handling. Scrapers and mild composition of cryopreservation media (90 % FBS + 10%DMSO) should be used to keep cells alive through standard cell line procedures. Successful application of this protocol for another sturgeon species (*A. baerii*) (unpublished data) indicates that this method can be used for tissue culture establishment from variety of sturgeon species.

Karyotype of the sterlet
Cytogenetic description of the sterlet karyotype have been published previously (e.g., [5, 14, 30]).

The karyotype of *A. ruthenus* is very similar to karyotypes of other 120-chromosomal acipenserids. Most of the chromosomes are bi-armed, whereas two pairs (ARUT14 and ARUT50) are acrocentric. Previously, the presence of at least two pairs of acrocentric chromosomes was described by Rab [30]. At the same time, on

the basis of routine staining authors could not establish unambiguously morphology of small pairs of chromosomes (ARUT32-60). Establishment of cell cultures and optimization of harvesting protocol allowed us to obtain metaphase chromosomes with a high resolution and to characterize the morphology of small chromosome pairs as bi-armed.

As it was previously shown the largest eight pairs of chromosomes contain only interstitial heterochromatin blocks with almost no visible C-blocks in the pericentromeric regions (Fig. 4, [14]). Precise pair-by-pair comparison of data obtained here with published previously is complicated by the lack of standard nomenclature. Many microchromosomes of *A. ruthenus* were previously described as almost or totally heterochromatic [14, 31], while here we show that most of these chromosomes contain euchromatic regions. Based on present data,

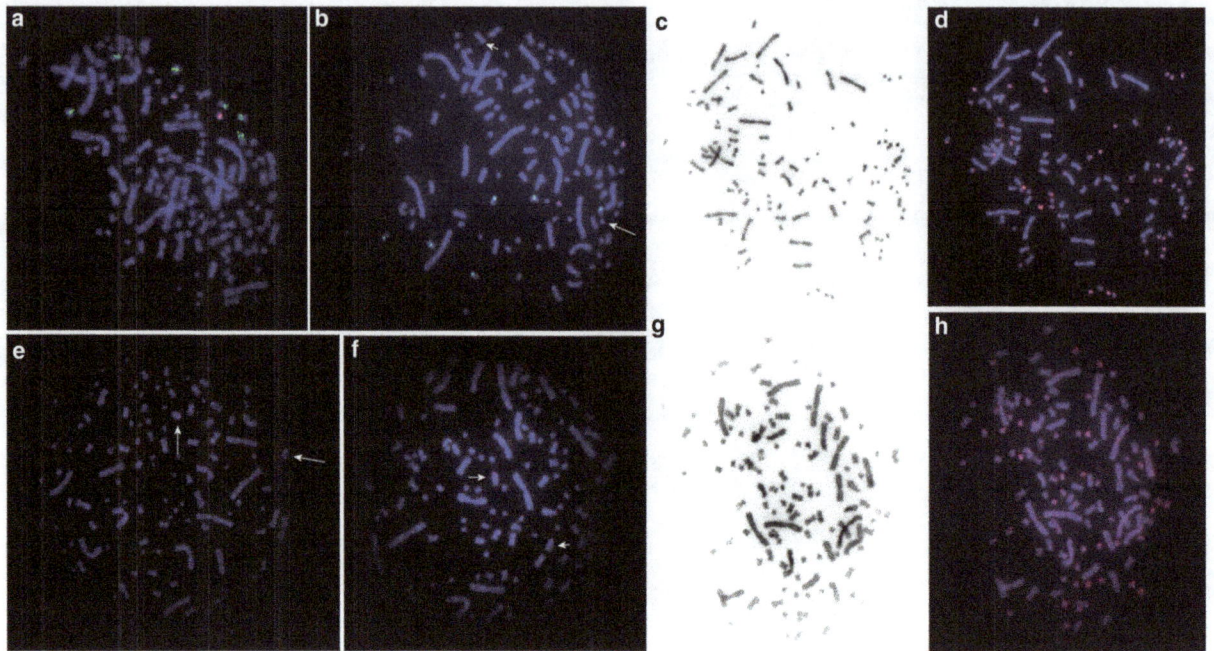

Fig. 5 Fluorescent in situ hybridization (FISH) of repetitive DNA probes: **a**, **b** – dual-color FISH with 18S/28S-rDNA probe (*green*) and 5S-rDNA probe (*red*) onto sterlet male and female, respectively; arrows mark some weak additional signals on female chromosomes; **c** – inverted-DAPI image of a male chromosome metaphase spread; **d** – localization of telomeric DNA probe (*red*) onto the same metaphase; **e**, **f** – HindIII satellite onto male and female, respectively; **g** – inverted-DAPI image of a female chromosome metaphase spread, **h** – localization of labeled C_0t30 DNA (*red*) onto the same metaphase

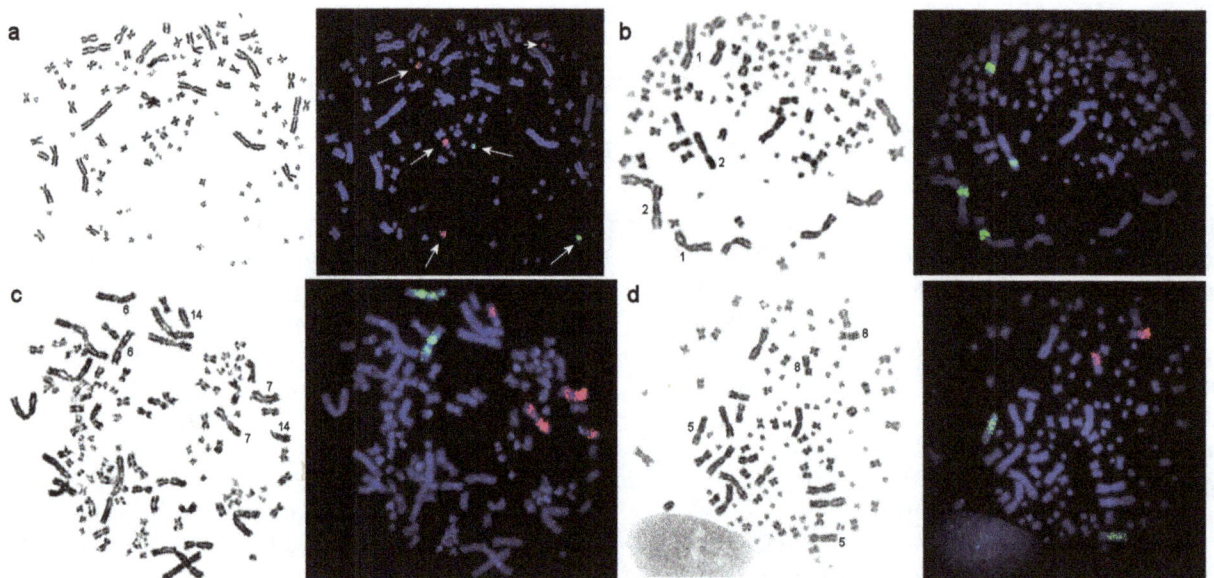

Fig. 6 FISH of microdissection-derived painting probes: **a** – painting probes ARUT"A" (*red*) and ARUT"G" (*green*) mark 4 and 2 chromosomes, respectively, on metaphase plate of sterlet female; **b** – painting ARUT1p marks p-arms of chromosomes ARUT1 and ARUT2 in sterlet female; **c** – painting probes ARUT6 (*green*) and ARUT7 (*red*) mark 2 and 4 homologous regions, respectively, in sterlet female; **d** – painting probes ARUT5q (*green*) and ARUT8q (*red*) paint a single chromosome pair each in sterlet male

clearly visible C-bands were detected at pericentromeric regions of chromosomes ARUT9-10, 12–14, 20, 23, 25, 31 and 51. Only two microchromosomes ARUT45 and 59 contained large stretches of heterochromatin and no visible euchromatic components.

It is noteworthy that no distinct and reproducible G-block pattern was detected in the sterlet karyotype, which is usually observed in the karyotypes of warm-blooded vertebrates and some fishes [32]. Previously a parallelism between chromosome banding and compositional compartmentalization of fishes genome was supported [32]. We suggest that the absence of reproducible G-banding pattern in sterlet might also be result of a compositional homogeneity of its genome.

Distribution pattern of telomeric repeats and ribosomal RNA genes

The telomeric repeated sequence $(TTAGGG)_n$ is highly conserved in structure and function among eukaryotes [33]. At the moment the sequence has been localized in over 100 vertebrate species, including fishes. In *A. ruthenus* karyotype the telomere signals were detected by FISH as definite spots at both ends of each chromosome, although the signal intensity varied between chromosomes [7]. Rather large blocks of repeats have been found on some small metacentrics. We could not find any variation in telomeric repeats distribution between male and female specimens. In general telomeric blocks distribution in studied here sterlet individuals is similar to previously published for wild and captive populations [7].

Different cytogenetic approaches reveal specific features of nucleolar organizing regions (NORs). Interesting that sturgeon NORs were not stained by GC specific fluorochromes as in other groups fishes studied [31]. While conventional Ag-staining reveals only active NORs, FISH with rDNA probes detects all clusters of rDNA, regardless of their activity. Using Ag-staining NORs were detected at the terminal ends of two chromosome pairs in sterlet [4, 15]. Localization of rRNA genes in *A. ruthenus* by FISH with the 28S and 5S probes yielded signals at 3 and 1 pairs of chromosomes, respectively [16]. Later studies revealed from 6 to 8 chromosomes (3–4 pairs) as NOR-bearing using FISH with the 18S/28S probe [8]. Moreover, the authors mentioned that all 5S rDNA signals overlapped with some of the 18S/28S rDNA signals [8]. In the present study we revealed unusual features in 18S/28S-rDNA probe distribution in two studied individuals (ARUT"9m" (male) and ARUT"12f" (female)) (Fig. 5a, b). In the female specimen three pairs of intense signal were detected (common with male), but additionally, we observed some weak signals on different chromosomes (Fig. 5b). The number of the additional signals varied from 2 to 4. Moreover in some cases we could clearly identify only

one of the homologs bearing NOR. As for now only one individual of each sex was investigated and most likely that such pattern of 18S/28S-rDNA probe localization points out at individual variation, although it also could result from heteromorphism of some *A. ruthenus* chromosomes. Additional investigation of NOR localization in more male and female individuals is needed. The amount of signals revealed using 5S-rDNA probe in the male and female was the same as published previously [16]. Dual-color FISH did not show any overlapping between 5S and 18S/28S-rDNA probes localizations (Fig. 5a). The discrepancy between the results obtained here and previously published could be attributed to variation between sterlet populations.

Distribution patterns of C_0t30 DNA and HindIII repeat

Satellite DNA is an important component of eukaryotic genome, mostly composed of tandemly repeated nucleotide sequences. The satellite DNA does not encode proteins and is localized in the regions of constitutive heterochromatin, preferentially in pericentromeric and subtelomeric areas of chromosomes [34]. The pattern of distribution of different kinds of satellite DNA sequences is one of the distinguishing features of species karyotype. Previous studies of satellite DNA sequence distribution in sturgeons included description of HindIII and PstI enriched heterochromatic blocks in some acipenserid species [17, 35].

In earlier studies the HindIII satellite DNA probe revealed minimum 8 signals on chromosomes of sterlet [17]. In our samples HindIII repetitive DNA was localized in the pericentromeric region of only one chromosome pair (the large acrocentric ARUT14) in both sexes and we did not detect any clear signals on other chromosomes (Fig. 5c, d). Such variation in the amount of signals obtained here and in the previous work could point out at a variation of HindIII satellite DNA content and chromosomal distribution between populations. The amount and the size of HindIII specific blocks indicate that it is not the major component of sterlet heterochromatin.

C_0t DNA fraction is rich in numerous types of repetitive sequences and isolation of the repetitive DNAs was proved to be useful for genome characterization in many animal and plant species [36–39]. Depending on the fraction C_0t DNA contains various amounts of satellite DNAs, DNA transposons, and retrotransposons. In some species localization of C_0t DNA onto metaphase chromosomes could produce a banding pattern, useful for chromosome identification [38]. We isolated C_0t30 fraction of DNA that includes wide range of repetitive elements. Physical mapping of the C_0t30 probe in *A. ruthenus* karyotypes revealed repeat-rich blocks on both arms of all small chromosomes except for their pericentromeric regions (Fig. 5g, h). On the contrary, a higher intensity of signals was detected in pericentromeric regions of large chromosomes, but signals were diffused. Generally, the variation in the pattern of C_0t30 DNA distribution between small and large chromosomes revealed here could indicate the repeat homogeneity of chromosomes inside these two groups and will help in future development of chromosome specific markers.

Partial tetraploidization of sterlet genome

In his classical work S. Onho has proposed that genome evolution might have been accompanied by polyploidization events [40]. Modern genomic studies largely confirm this hypothesis and provide evidence that whole genome duplication events were quite common in the past and are characteristic for different eukaryotic taxa [41]. Interestingly some animal groups (such as mammals and birds) seem to be highly intolerant to genome duplications (or even to partial chromosome segment duplication). Although it was proposed that the 102-chromosomal genome of the South American red vizcacha rat (*Tympanoctomys barrerae*) resulted from tetraploidization [42], subsequent chromosome painting data clearly demonstrated that all chromosomal segments are present in diploid state [43]. On the other hand, chromosome painting turned out to be very useful in confirmation of triploidy in some lizards [44]. As most fish genomes have not been involved yet in chromosome painting experiments, future molecular cytogenetic works may shed light onto the level of ploidy in their genomes.

It was proposed that all modern 120-chromosomal acipenserids represent functional diploids, originated over 200 million years ago by a whole genome duplication of a 60-chromosomal ancestor [13, 45, 46]. The transition between 120-chromosomal tetraploid to modern functional diploid might have been accompanied by a functional reduction [2, 7, 15, 47]. Here using chromosome painting we present a direct evidence of partial genome tetraploidy combined with partial diploidy in the same species genome for the first time. It is noteworthy that most chromosomes and chromosomal regions were found to be in either diploid or in tetraploid state. However it is notable that chromosome 7 seems to consist of two blocks – tetrapoid (which also paints chromosome 14) and diploid (paints only a part of chromosome 7) (Fig. 6c). Of course we cannot exclude that the sterlet genome may contain additional highly divergent copies of regions revealed as diploid in FISH experiments. It is interesting, that tetraploidy of 120-chromosomal paddlefish was first proposed by Dingerkus and Howell on the basis on karyotype analysis [48], but later the accumulation of data on molecular markers [15] provided evidence for a diploid state of 120-chromosomal sturgeons and paddlefish. Here we demonstrate that both these hypotheses are partly correct and the genomes of sturgeons

might be more complex than it was proposed earlier. Whole genome sequencing is urgently needed to resolve multiple questions regarding the structure and origin of sterlet genome.

Conclusion

Genome evolution of Acipenseriformes is characterized by many independent polyploidization events on the one hand and by relatively low rates of molecular evolution the other hand [49]. Still very little is known about fundamental issues of sturgeon biology related to genetic mechanism of sex determination, predisposition to polyploidization and interspecific hybridization, genome composition and evolution. The establishment of sterlet cell cultures allowed us to obtain high quality chromosome preparations for molecular cytogenetic experiments including FISH, chromosome microdissection and chromosome specific painting probe generation. Chromosome painting revealed a complex structure of sturgeon genome comprising regions with different ploidy levels and indicated that further work is necessary to estimate precisely the ratio between diploid and tetraploid genomic components. Besides, we did not find any sex specific hybridization patterns among probes obtained here assuming that the search for sex chromosomes should be continued by means of the construction of more chromosome specific markers and comparative genome sequencing.

Methods
Ethics statement

The protocol was approved by the Committee on the Ethics of Animal Experiments of the Institute of Molecular and Cellular Biology SB RAS. Sterlet individuals were incubated in the water with 10^{-4} (v/v) Eugenol for about 5 min for euthanasia. All efforts were made to minimize suffering.

Samples origin

In total 12 sterlet specimens (6 males and 6 females) originating from Ob (ARUT"1-5"), Irtysh (ARUT"6-9") and Enisey (ARUT"10-12") rivers were provided for study by State Science-and-Production Centre for Fisheries (Table 1).

Optimization of sterlet cell culture conditions

To find optimal conditions for sterlet cell lines establishment, tissues from 5 specimens from the wild population of Ob river (Middle Ob, Tomsk region) (ARUT"1-5") were used.

Before dissecting fish was patted with dry paper towel to remove mucus. Abdominal and pectoral fins were additionally wiped with 70 % ethanol. Fins and surrounding tissue were cut and incubated in 70 % ethanol for 3 min. Subsequent manipulations were made in a sterile environment. Fins were rinsed out twice in 199 medium with penicillin ($5*10^5$ U/L), streptomycin (500 mg/L) and amphotericin B (12.5 mg/L) and incubated overnight in a fresh portion of the same medium. All samples were cultivated in CO_2 controlled incubator (5 % CO_2) at 25 °C, in each case growth medium contained 15 % of FBS, penicillin ($1*10^5$ U/L), streptomycin (100 mg/L) and amphotericin B (2.5 mg/L).

We used two protocols for cell culture establishment. Some samples were digested by proteolytic enzymes (collagenase and hyaluronidase) to dissociate tissue and release individual cells, other samples were attached to flask surface without preliminary treatments. The modified protocol of tissue culture establishment without enzymes was described earlier [50]. In both variants all five types of culture media (αMEM, DMEM, RPMI, L-15 and 199) were used for cells cultivation.

Establishment of cell cultures using collagenase/hyaluronidase treatment of tissues
We used the protocol suggested by Stanyon and Galleny [28] for mammalian tissues with some modification. The tissue pieces were finely minced and placed in a tube with 1–2 ml collagenase/hyaluronidase mixture: 1 mg/ml collagenase, 1 mg/ml hyaluronidase, 15 % fetal bovine serum in the growth medium. Dispersed tissues were incubated in CO_2 controlled incubator for 24 h at 25 °C. After that the pelleted cells were placed in culture flask with the growth medium.

Cell line passaging
For sequential passages the cells were dissociated with 0.25 % tripsin, 0.2 % EDTA or taken off by scrapers.

Application of the optimal conditions for establishment of cell cultures from notochord, swim bladder and barbels
The optimized conditions were applied for establishment of additional cell lines from 7 specimens (ARUT"6-12") from fishery farms of Tyumen Oblast and Tomsk Oblast. We took some other tissues (notochord, swim bladder and barbels) for cultivation (Table 2). Notochord and swim bladder tissue were aseptically removed for culturing. Barbles were cleaned and immersed as fins in 70 % ethanol for 3 min.

Cryopreservation and thawing of cells
We applied two different protocols for freezing cells. In the first protocol we used 199 medium with 40 % FBS and 10 % DMSO, in the second we used plain FBS with 10 % DMSO for freezing. The cryovials were placed in CoolCell (BioCision) freezing container and stored at –72 °C overnight. Cryovials were then transferred into cryotank with liquid nitrogen (–196 °C) for a prolonged storage.

For recovery, vials were thawed in the water at 30 °C, cells were then resuspended in 5X volume of 199 medium with 15 % FBS and centrifuged at 0,6× g for 5 min. After removing the supernatant, the cells were resuspended in the 199 medium with 15 % FBS, then counted in Goryaev's chamber using trypan blue stain (most cells appeared alive upon staining) and seeded into cell culture flasks to estimate the number of survived cells.

Chromosome preparation
Cells were split at a ratio 1:2 in a medium with 5-10 % of AmnioMax (Gibco). After two days of culturing colcemid (KaryoMAX, Gibco) was added to a final concentration of 0.1 μg/ml for overnight incubation. Three hours before cell harvesting ethidium bromide was added to a final concentration of 1.5 μg/ml. Cells were dissociated mechanically by scraping and centrifuged for 5 min at 0.6× g. Cell pellet was gently resuspended in hypotonic solution (33.5 mM KCl, 7.75 mM sodium citrate) and incubated for 2 h at 25 °C. For prefixation treatment 1/20 volume of fresh ice-cold fixative (methanol: acetic acid - 3:1) was added, mixed carefully and incubated for 12 min at 4 °C. Then cells were centrifuged for 5 min at 0.6× g and supernatant was discarded. For cell fixation, the pellet was covered by ice-cold fixative (–20 °C) and kept for 30 min at –20 °C without mixing. Cells were then centrifuged for 5 min at 0.6× g and resuspended in ice-cold fixative. The chromosome suspensions were stored long-term at –20 °C.

Chromosome staining
Routine Giemsa staining, C- and G-banding were performed as described previously [51].

Telomeric and ribosomal DNA probes
The telomeric DNA probe was generated by PCR using the oligonucleotides (TTAGGG)₅ and (CCCTAA)₅ [52]. Clones of human ribosomal DNA containing the complete 18S-rRNA and 28S-rRNA genes were obtained as described [53] and labeled by nick translation following the manufacturer's protocol (Nick Translation System, Life Technologies). 5S-rDNA probe was amplified by PCR using following primers: 5′-TACAGCACTTGA TATTCCCA-3′ and 5′-GTCATGAAAGCAGAAATG CA-3′. 5S-rDNA PCR amplification was performed in a 100 μl reaction mixture, containing 65 mM Tris–HCl (pH 8.9), 16 mM $(NH_4)_2SO_4$, 2.5 mM $MgCl_2$, 0.05 % tween-20, 0.25 mM 3dNTP, 0.1 mM TTP, 0.1 mM dig-dUTP, 400 ng of sterlet genomic DNA, 2 U of Taq DNA-polymerase, 1 μM of each primer. The PCR protocol included denaturing at 94 °C for 2 min, 30 cycles of denaturing at 94 °C for 30 s, annealing at 58 °C for 30 s and extension at 72 °C for 1 min 20 s. Agarose gel electrophoresis was performed to estimate the size of the PCR product (~100 bp).

HindIII satellite probe

The probe of HindIII satellite previously described by De la Herrán et al. [49] was obtained by PCR using primers: 5′-TTGATCTTCAGAACTACCAA-3′ and 5′-GGAACGAACCTGTAAGCTT-3′. PCR amplification was performed in 100 µl reaction mixture, containing 65 mM Tris–HCl (pH 8.9), 16 mM $(NH_4)_2SO_4$, 2.5 mM $MgCl_2$, 0.05 % tween-20, 0.25 mM 4dNTP, 0.08 mM dig-dUTP, 400 ng of sterlet genomic DNA, 2 U Taq DNA-polymerase, 1 µM of each primer. PCR protocol included denaturation at 94 °C for 2 min, 35 cycles of denaturing at 94 °C for 20 s, annealing at 58 °C for 50 s and extension at 72 °C for 1 min 20 s.

C_0t fraction of repeated DNA

C_0t30 DNA was obtained as described previously [54]. Labeling was carried out using Nick Translation Kit (Sigma). Labeled C_0t30 DNA was used as a probe for fluorescent in situ hybridization (FISH).

Painting probe generation by chromosome microdissection

Microdissection was performed as described earlier [55]. DNA from a single copy of each microdissected chromosome was amplified and labelled using WGA kits (Sigma). In total we obtained painting probes from following chromosomes (regions): ARUT1p, 5, 6, 7, 8 as well as for 14 small sized chromosomes.

Fluorescent in situ hybridization

FISH was performed on freshly made chromosome preparations not subject to any proteinase or RNAse treatment. Hybridization mixture contained 12 µl of 50 % formamide, 2 × SSC, 0.2 % Tween 20, and 0.2 µg of probe. Probes were denatured at 95 °C for 5 min. Slides were incubated in PBS with 0.05M $MgCl_2$ for 5 min and then in 2xSSC for 5 min. Chromosome denaturation was done in 70 % formamide with 2xSSC at 67 °C for 30–40 s. FISH protocol was described previously [56]. The slides were analyzed with fluorescence microscopes Olympus BX53 and Axioskop 2 plus (Zeiss) using VideoTesT-Karyo and VideoTesT-FISH (VideoTesT, Saint-Petersburg, Russia) digital imaging systems.

Competing interests
The authors declare that they have no competing interests.

Authors' contributions
SAR established all cell lines, made chromosome suspensions, carried out microdissection, FISH, microscopy analysis and wrote the manuscript. LSB made chromosome suspensions, carried out the routine staining, C- and G-banding, performed karyotype and chromosome painting analyses. NAS extracted C_0t DNA, prepared probes for FISH, optimized and carried out FISH experiments. AIK performed microdissection of macrochromosomes, prepared probes and analyzed FISH data. VRB performed comparative painting with microdissected probes and was involved in data analysis. OLG and NAL established cell cultures, prepared suspensions of chromosomes, carried out FISH experiments and helped to draft the manuscript. EAI and MAK presented samples and helped to draft the manuscript. NVV prepared probes for FISH,

provided conceptual advice and helped to draft the manuscript. ASG discussed the results and revised the manuscript. VAT conceived and supervised the project, analyzed data, and wrote the manuscript. All authors read and approved the final manuscript.

Acknowledgements
This study was funded by RSF № 14-14-00275.

Author details
[1]Institute of Molecular and Cellular Biology SB RAS, Novosibirsk, Russia. [2]Novosibirsk State University, Novosibirsk, Russia. [3]Novosibirsk Branch of the Federal State Budgetary Scientific Institution "State Scientific-and-Production Centre for Fisheries (Gosrybcenter)", Novosibirsk, Russia. [4]Tomsk State University, Tomsk, Russia. [5]Federal State Budgetary Scientific Institution "State Scientific-and-Production Centre for Fisheries (Gosrybcenter)", Tyumen, Russia.

References
1. Birstein VJ, DeSalle R. Molecular phylogeny of Acipenserinae. Mol Phylogenet Evol. 1998;9(1):141–55. doi:10.1006/mpev.1997.0443.
2. Ludwig A, Belfiore NM, Pitra C, Svirsky V, Jenneckens I. Genome duplication events and functional reduction of ploidy levels in sturgeon (Acipenser, Huso and Scaphirhynchus). Genetics. 2001;158(3):1203–15.
3. Sallan LC. Major issues in the origins of ray-finned fish (Actinopterygii) biodiversity. Biol Rev. 2014;89(4):950–71. doi:10.1111/brv.12086.
4. Birstein VJ, Vasiliev VP. Tetraploid-octoploid relationships and karyological evolution in the order acipenseriformes (Pisces) - karyotypes, nucleoli, and nucleolus-organizer regions in 4 Acipenserid species. Genetica. 1987;72(1):3–12. doi:10.1007/Bf00126973.
5. Acipenser ruthenus. http://sveb.unife.it/it/ricerca-1/laboratori/geneweb/acipenser-ruthenus. Accessed 13 Nov 2015.
6. Fontana F, Congiu L, Mudrak VA, Quattro JM, Smith TI, Ware K, et al. Evidence of hexaploid karyotype in shortnose sturgeon. Genome. 2008; 51(2):113–9. doi:10.1139/g07-112.
7. Fontana F, Lanfredi M, Chicca M, Aiello V, Rossi R. Localization of the repetitive telomeric sequence (TTAGGG)n in four sturgeon species. Chromosome Res. 1998;6(4):303–6.
8. Fontana F, Lanfredi M, Congiu L, Leis M, Chicca M, Rossi R. Chromosomal mapping of 18S-28S and 5S rRNA genes by two-colour fluorescent in situ hybridization in six sturgeon species. Genome. 2003;46(3):473–7. doi:10.1139/g03-007.
9. Flynn SR, Matsuoka M, Reith M, Martin-Robichaud DJ, Benfey TJ. Gynogenesis and sex determination in shortnose sturgeon, Acipenser brevirostrum Lesuere. Aquaculture. 2006;253(1–4):721–7. doi:10.1016/j.aquaculture.2005.09.016.
10. Saber MH, Hallajian A. Study of sex determination system in ship sturgeon, Acipenser nudiventris using meiotic gynogenesis. Aquac Int. 2014;22(1):273–9. doi:10.1007/s10499-013-9676-z.
11. Shelton WL, Mims SD. Evidence for female heterogametic sex determination in paddlefish Polyodon spathula based on gynogenesis. Aquaculture. 2012;356: 116–8. doi:10.1016/j.aquaculture.2012.05.029.
12. Fontana F, Lanfredi M, Rossi R, Bronzi P, Arlati G. Established cell lines from three sturgeon species. Sturgeon Q. 1995;3(4):6–7.
13. Havelka M, Kaspar V, Hulak M, Flajshans M. Sturgeon genetics and cytogenetics: a review related to ploidy levels and interspecific hybridization. Folia Zool. 2011;60(2):93–103.
14. Ráb P, Arefjev VA. M. R. C-banded karyotype of the sterlet, Acipenser ruthenus, from the Danube River. Sturgeon Q. 1996;4(4):10–2.
15. Fontana F. Chromosomal nucleolar organizer regions in 4 sturgeon species as markers of karyotype evolution in Acipenseriformes (Pisces). Genome. 1994;37(5):888–92.
16. Fontana F, Lanfredi M, Chicca M, Congiu L, Tagliavini J, Rossi R. Fluorescent in situ hybridization with rDNA probes on chromosomes of Acipenser ruthenus and Acipenser naccarii (Osteichthyes Acipenseriformes). Genome. 1999;42(5):1008–12. doi:10.1139/gen-42-5-1008.
17. Lanfredi M, Congiu L, Garrido-Ramos MA, de la Herran R, Leis M, Chicca M, et al. Chromosomal location and evolution of a satellite DNA family in

seven sturgeon species. Chromosome Res. 2001;9(1):47–52. doi:10.1023/A:1026739616749.

18. Graphodatsky AS, Trifonov VA, Stanyon R. The genome diversity and karyotype evolution of mammals. Mol Cytogenet. 2011;4:22. doi:10.1186/1755-8166-4-22.

19. Guttenbach M, Nanda I, Feichtinger W, Masabanda JS, Griffin DK, Schmid M. Comparative chromosome painting of chicken autosomal paints 1–9 in nine different bird species. Cytogenet Genome Res. 2003;103(1–2):173–84. doi:10.1159/000076309.

20. Pokorna M, Giovannotti M, Kratochvil L, Kasai F, Trifonov VA, O'Brien PCM, et al. Strong conservation of the bird Z chromosome in reptilian genomes is revealed by comparative painting despite 275 million years divergence. Chromosoma. 2011;120(5):455–68. doi:10.1007/s00412-011-0322-0.

21. Cioffi MD, Sanchez A, Marchal JA, Kosyakova N, Liehr T, Trifonov V, et al. Whole chromosome painting reveals independent origin of sex chromosomes in closely related forms of a fish species. Genetica. 2011;139(8):1065–72. doi:10.1007/s10709-011-9610-0.

22. Tian X, Azpurua J, Hine C, Vaidya A, Myakishev-Rempel M, Ablaeva J, et al. High-molecular-mass hyaluronan mediates the cancer resistance of the naked mole rat. Nature. 2013;499(7458):346–U122. doi:10.1038/nature12234.

23. Li MF, Marrayatt V, Annand C, Odense P. Fish cell-culture - 2 newly developed cell-lines from Atlantic sturgeon (Acipenser-Oxyrhynchus) and guppy (Poecilia-Reticulata). Can J Zool. 1985;63(12):2867–74.

24. Fontana F, Rossi R, Lanfredi M, Arlati G, Bronzi P. Cytogenetic characterization of cell lines from three sturgeon species. Caryologia. 1997;50(1):91–5.

25. Hedrick RP, Mcdowell TS, Rosemark R, Aronstein D, Lannan CN. 2 cell-lines from white sturgeon. T Am Fish Soc. 1991;120(4):528–34. doi:10.1577/1548-8659(1991)120<0528:Tclfws>2.3.Co;2.

26. Wang G, LaPatra S, Zeng L, Zhao Z, Lu Y. Establishment, growth, cryopreservation and species of origin identification of three cell lines from white sturgeon, Acipenser transmontanus. Methods Cell Sci. 2003;25(3–4):211–20.

27. Fontana F. Establishment of sturgeon primary cell lines. In: Ozouf-Costaz C, Pisano E, Foresti F, Foresti L, Foresti de Almeida Toledo L, editors. Fish cytogenetic techniques (Chondrichthyans and Teleosts). Enfield: CRC Press Inc; 2015. p. 49–57.

28. Stanyon R, Galleni L. A rapid fibroblast-culture technique for high-resolution karyotypes. B Zool. 1991;58(1):81–3.

29. Wolf K, Ahne W. Fish cell culture. In: Maramorosch K, editor. Advances in cell culture. New York: Academic Press, Inc; 1982. p. 305–28.

30. Rab P. A note on the karyotype on the sterlet, Acipenser ruthenus (Pisces, Acipenseridae). Folia Zool. 1986;35(1):73–8.

31. Fontana F, Rossi R, Lanfredi M, Arlati G, Bronzi P. Chromosome banding in sturgeons. J Appl Ichthyol. 1999;15:9–11.

32. Medrano L, Bernardi G, Couturier J, Dutrillaux B, Bernardi G. Chromosome-banding and genome compartmentalization in fishes. Chromosoma. 1988;96(2):178–83. doi:10.1007/Bf00331050.

33. Meyne J, Baker RJ, Hobart HH, Hsu TC, Ryder OA, Ward OG, et al. Distribution of non-telomeric sites of the (TTAGGG)n telomeric sequence in vertebrate chromosomes. Chromosoma. 1990;99(1):3–10.

34. Charlesworth B, Sniegowski P, Stephan W. The evolutionary dynamics of repetitive DNA in eukaryotes. Nature. 1994;371(6494):215–20. doi:10.1038/371215a0.

35. Fontana F, Lanfredi M, Kirschbaum F, Garrido-Ramos MA, Robles F, Forlani A, et al. Comparison of karyotypes of Acipenser oxyrinchus and A. sturio by chromosome banding and fluorescent in situ hybridization. Genetica. 2008;132(3):281–6. doi:10.1007/s10709-007-9171-4.

36. Cioffi MB, Martins C, Vicari MR, Rebordinos L, Bertollo LAC. Differentiation of the XY sex chromosomes in the fish hoplias malabaricus (Characiformes, Erythrinidae): unusual accumulation of repetitive sequences on the X chromosome. Sex Dev. 2010;4(3):176–85. doi:10.1159/000309726.

37. Schemberger MO, Oliveira JI, Nogaroto V, Almeida MC, Artoni RF, Cestari MM, et al. Construction and characterization of a repetitive DNA library in Parodontidae (Atinopterygii:Characiformes): a genomic and evolutionary approach to the degeneration of the w sex cromosome. Zebrafish. 2014;11(6):518–27. doi:10.1089/zeb.2014.1013.

38. Wang YM, Minoshima S, Shimizu N. Cot-1 banding of human-chromosomes using fluorescence in-situ hybridization with Cy3 labeling. Jpn J Hum Genet. 1995;40(3):243–52. doi:10.1007/Bf01876182.

39. Zhang L, Xu C, Yu W. Cloning and characterization of chromosomal markers from a Cot-1 library of peanut (Arachis hypogaea L.). Cytogenet Genome Res. 2012;137(1):31–41. doi:10.1159/000339455.

40. Ohno S. Evolution by gene duplication. Berlin Heidelberg: Springer; 1970.

41. Furlong RF, Holland PWH. Polyploidy in vertebrate ancestry: Ohno and beyond. Biol J Linn Soc. 2004;82(4):425–30. doi:10.1111/j.1095-8312.2004.00329.x.

42. Gallardo MH, Bickham JW, Honeycutt RL, Ojeda RA, Kohler N. Discovery of tetraploidy in a mammal. Nature. 1999;401(6751):341. doi:10.1038/43815.

43. Svartman M, Stone G, Stanyon R. Molecular cytogenetics discards polyploidy in mammals. Genomics. 2005;85(4):425–30. doi:10.1016/j.ygeno.2004.12.004.

44. Trifonov VA, Paoletti A, Caputo Barucchi V, Kalinina T, O'Brien PC, Ferguson-Smith MA, et al. Comparative chromosome painting and NOR distribution suggest a complex hybrid origin of triploid lepidodactylus lugubris (Gekkonidae). PLoS One. 2015;10(7):e0132380. doi:10.1371/journal.pone.0132380.

45. Birstein VJ, Hanner R, DeSalle R. Phylogeny of the Acipenseriformes: cytogenetic and molecular approaches. Environ Biol Fish. 1997;48(1–4):127–56. doi:10.1023/A:1007366100353.

46. Fontana F, Tagliavini J, Congiu L. Sturgeon genetics and cytogenetics: recent advancements and perspectives. Genetica. 2001;111(1–3):359–73. doi:10.1023/A:1013711919443.

47. Tagliavini J, Conterio F, Gandolfi G, Fontana F. Mitochondrial DNA sequences of six sturgeon species and phylogenetic relationships within Acipenseridae. J Appl Ichthyol. 1999;15(4–5):17–22. doi:10.1111/J.1439-0426.1999.tb00198.x.

48. Dingerkus G, Howell WM. Karyotypic analysis and evidence of tetraploidy in the North American paddlefish, Polyodon spathula. Science. 1976;194(4267):842–4.

49. de la Herran R, Fontana F, Lanfredi M, Congiu L, Leis M, Rossi R, et al. Slow rates of evolution and sequence homogenization in an ancient satellite DNA family of sturgeons. Mol Biol Evol. 2001;18(3):432–6.

50. Lemskaya NA, Romanenko SA, Golenishchev FN, Rubtsova NV, Sablina OV, Serdukova NA, et al. Chromosomal evolution of Arvicolinae (Cricetidae, Rodentia). III. Karyotype relationships of ten Microtus species. Chromosome Res. 2010;18(4):459–71. doi:10.1007/s10577-010-9124-0.

51. Graphodatsky AS, Radjabli SI. Chromosomes of agricultural and laboratory mammals. Novosibirsk: Nauka; 1988.

52. Ijdo JW, Wells RA, Baldini A, Reeders ST. Improved telomere detection using a telomere repeat probe (TTAGGG)n generated by PCR. Nucleic Acids Res. 1991;19(17):4780.

53. Maden BE, Dent CL, Farrell TE, Garde J, McCallum FS, Wakeman JA. Clones of human ribosomal DNA containing the complete 18 S-rRNA and 28 S-rRNA genes. Characterization, a detailed map of the human ribosomal transcription unit and diversity among clones. Biochem J. 1987;246(2):519–27.

54. Trifonov VA, Vorobieva NV, Rens W. FISH with and without COT1 DNA. In: Liehr T, editor. Fluorescence in situ hybridization (FISH) – application guide. 2009. p. 99–112.

55. Kosyakova N, Hamid AB, Chaveerach A, Pinthong K, Siripiyasing P, Supiwong W, et al. Generation of multicolor banding probes for chromosomes of different species. Mol Cytogenet. 2013;6:6. doi:10.1186/1755-8166-6-6.

56. Yang F, Graphodatsky AS. Animal probes and ZOO-FISH fluorescence in situ hybridization (FISH). In: Liehr T, editor. Fluorescence in situ hybridization (FISH) – application guide. Berlin: Springer; 2009. p. 323–47.

7

Meiotic outcome in two carriers of Y autosome reciprocal translocations: selective elimination of certain segregants

Harita Ghevaria[1]* ⓘ, Roy Naja[1], Sioban SenGupta[1], Paul Serhal[2] and Joy Delhanty[1]

Abstract

Background: Reciprocal Y autosome translocations are rare but frequently associated with male infertility. We report on the meiotic outcome in embryos fathered by two males with the karyotypes 46,X,t(Y;4)(q12;p15.32) and 46,X,t(Y;16)(q12;q13). The two couples underwent preimplantation genetic diagnosis (PGD) enabling determination of the segregation types that were compatible with fertilization and preimplantation embryo development. Both PGD and follow up analysis were carried out via fluorescence in situ hybridization (FISH) or array comparative genomic hybridization (aCGH) allowing the meiotic segregation types to be determined in a total of 27 embryos.

Results: Interestingly, it was seen that the number of female embryos resulting from alternate segregation with the chromosome combination of X and the autosome from the carrier gamete differed from the corresponding balanced males with derivative Y and the derivative autosome by a ratio of 7:1 in each case ($P = 0.003$) while from the adjacent-1 mode of segregation, the unbalanced male embryos with the combination of der Y and the autosome were seen in all embryos from couple A and in couple B with the exception of one embryo only that had the other chromosome combination of X and derivative autosome ($P = 0.011$). In both cases the deficit groups have in common the der autosome chromosome that includes the segment Yq12 to qter.

Conclusion: The most likely explanation may be that this chromosome is associated with the X chromosome at PAR2 (pseudoautosomal region 2) in the sex-body leading to inactivation of genes on the autosomal segment that are required for the meiotic process and that this has led to degeneration of this class of spermatocytes during meiosis.

Keywords: Y-autosome Translocation, Meiosis, Segregation, Infertility

Background

Reciprocal translocations between the Y chromosome and an autosome are rare and highly associated with male infertility. From a review of 22 cases of balanced Y-autosome translocations, it became clear that if the break occurs within the Yq critical segment (AZF) or near the primary pseudoautosomal segment (PAR1) and hence the SRY gene, germ cell maturation may be severely damaged, resulting in azoospermia or severe oligozoospermia in the carrier males [1, 2].

However, translocations involving breaks in the Yq12 heterochromatic region also frequently lead to infertility. During normal male meiosis, recombination normally takes place between the X and Y chromosomes at PAR 1 located at the tips of both the Xp and Yp and the remainder of the chromosome remains unsynapsed. However, synapsis may also occur at PAR 2, located at the terminal region of the long arms of X & Y. Thus in the first meiotic metaphase the two sex chromosomes form the XY-body or the sex-body, which is genetically inactivated during the pachytene stage of meiosis. The formation of the sex-body enables normal meiotic progression even in the presence of unsynapsed regions [3]. In the case of a Y-autosome translocation, if a translocated chromosome is associated with the sex-body, inactivation may extend to the autosomal segment. If this segment houses pachytene critical genes the consequence may be degeneration of most of the spermatocytes after the pachytene stage [4].

A few clinical investigations involving Y-autosome translocations with familial histories have been reported

* Correspondence: h.ghevaria@ucl.ac.uk
[1]Preimplantation Genetics Group, Institute for Women's Health, University College London, 86-96 Chenies Mews, London WC1E 6HX, UK
Full list of author information is available at the end of the article

previously in the literature. An infertile man with severe oligoasthenospermia was found to have the karyotype 46,X,t(1;Y) (q11;q11). His father who was proved to have the same translocation, also had two daughters and one other son [5]. The report of the family investigated by (Sklower Brooks et al. in 1998), describes a couple where the male had the abnormal karyotype 46,X,t(Y;8)(q12;p21.3) and the woman had reported a third miscarriage involving the t(Y;8) translocation. This couple also had a normal daughter. The man had four brothers and two sisters. The investigation revealed that their deceased father must have carried the abnormal karyotype which was passed on to four of his sons in a balanced state and in an unbalanced state to the remaining one [6]

We present here the meiotic outcome for two carriers of reciprocal Y-autosome translocations ascertained after a total of six cycles of preimplantation genetic diagnosis (PGD). The data provide evidence for the selective elimination of certain gametic segregants.

Methods
Patient Details
Two couples, where the male patient was a carrier of a reciprocal Y-autosome translocation, underwent six cycles of PGD between the years 2014–2015. The necessary IVF (in vitro fertilization) treatment took place at the Centre for Reproductive and Genetic Health (CRGH). All genetic diagnoses were carried out at UCL Centre for PGD with the exception of those for one cycle of treatment for couple B. The karyotype of the carrier patients along with their reproductive histories is shown in Table 1.

IVF and PGD
For both couples, fresh semen was retrieved on the day of the egg collection. Routine semen analysis revealed sub-optimal semen parameters and both male carriers presented with severe oligozoospermia. Hence during the IVF treatment, intracytoplasmic sperm injection (ICSI) was the chosen method of insemination (Table 1).

Three PGD cycles were carried out for each of the two couples. For couple A, all three cycles were performed using Fluorescence In Situ Hybridisation (FISH) at cleavage stage (day 3 of embryo development) where one or two blastomeres were biopsied for diagnosis. For couple

B, one cycle was performed using FISH at cleavage stage and the remaining two using array comparative genomic hybridisation (aCGH) at the blastocyst stage (day 5 or 6 of embryo development) where diagnosis was performed on a few trophectoderm (TE) cells.

Analysis by FISH
For cycles where PGD was performed by FISH, a patient specific protocol was developed and optimized on lymphocytes from peripheral blood prior to the clinical application of PGD on single blastomeres. Ideograms were constructed in order to choose the appropriate probes based on the position of the breakpoint for each translocation. The details of probes used for both the diagnosis and follow up analyses are given in Table 2. In these two cases, the probe strategies selected could distinguish normal female embryos from males chromosomally balanced for the translocation.

Fluorescence In Situ Hybridisation was performed in two rounds of hybridisation (Table 2). The FISH protocol was carried out as described previously with slight modifications [7]. Microscopic analysis and scoring of FISH signals were carried out using an epifluorescence Olympus microscope (Olympus BX 40, London, UK). FISH signals were scored according to [8]

Analysis by array-CGH
For both diagnosis and follow up cells were subjected to aCGH using 24Sure + arrays (BlueGnome Ltd., Fulbourn, Cambridge UK, now Illumina). Prior to the aCGH, whole genome amplification was carried out using the Sureplex™ amplification kit (BlueGnome Ltd., Fulbourn, Cambridge UK, now Illumina). Amplification efficiency was assessed by gel electrophoresis. Array-CGH was carried out according to the manufacturer's protocol with slight modifications. Images were scanned and analysed using BlueFuse Multi software (BlueGnome Ltd, now Illumina). Details for both the protocol and analysis has been described elsewhere [9].

Follow up analysis in embryos obtained on day 5–7 post-fertilisation
After transfer of embryos diagnosed as unaffected, the untransferred embryos were available for confirmation of diagnosis and follow up. Where diagnosis was by FISH, embryos were either subjected to follow up using

Table 1 Reproductive histories and karyotypes of the two carriers of reciprocal Y-autosome translocations

	Type of ART used	Male Karyotype	Sperm Parameters	Reproductive History
Couple A	ICSI	46,X,t(Y;4)(q12;p15.32)	Severe oligozoospermia	Primary infertility No previous pregnancies
Couple B	ICSI	46,X,t(Y;16)(q12;q13)	Severe oligozoospermia	Primary infertility No previous pregnancies

ART Assisted Reproductive Technology, *ICSI* Intracytoplasmic Sperm Injection

Table 2 Probes used in FISH analysis for couples A and B.

	Male karyotype	Probes used for FISH
Couple A	46,X,t(Y;4)(q12;p15.32)	1st Round: CEP 4 (SA); Tel 4p (SG); CEP X (SO) 2nd Round: [a]CEP Y (DYZ1) (SA); Tel Xq/Yq (SO)
Couple B	46,X,t(Y;16)(q12;q13)	1st Round: Tel Xq/Yq (SO), CEP 16 (SA); [b]Tel 16q (SG) 2nd Round: [c]CEP Y (DYZ3) (SO), CEP X (SG).

SA Spectrum Aqua, *SG* Spectrum Green, *SO* Spectrum Orange
All probes were from Abbott Molecular, UK unless stated
[a]CEP Y (DYZ1) : Cytogenetic Location Yq12, Satellite III DNA
[b] = Kreatech FISH Probes, Leica Biosystems, UK
[c]CEP Y (DYZ3) : Cytogenetic Location Yp11.1-q11.1, Alpha Satellite DNA

the same strategy or via aCGH. If PGD was carried out using aCGH, then follow up was also via aCGH. The diagnostic and follow up result using aCGH also revealed aneuploidies of other unrelated chromosomes; these are not reported here.

Meiotic segregation analysis

The segregation mode at meiosis was recorded for each embryo after follow up analysis. If no follow up information was available, or if the embryo had been transferred, then the segregation mode was deduced from the PGD results obtained on the biopsied cells (day 3 or 5). This was done in order to determine the contributions of the

Table 3 Summary of the follow up results of embryos from three PGD cycles performed for couple A with a male karyotype 46,X,t(Y;4)(q12;p15.32)

PGD cycle no. / Embryo no.	Follow up method	Day 5–7 Follow up result (Diagnostic result where follow up result not available)	Meiotic segregation (stage determined)	Chromosomes contributed by carrier parent	Embryo grade on follow up
C1 E2	aCGH	Female embryo with additional aneuploidies	Alternate (follow up)	X and 4	cavitating morula
C1 E3	aCGH	Female embryo with multiple chromosome abnormalities	Alternate (follow up)	X and 4	pre-morula
C1 E4	n/a	Embryo transferred (normal female embryo)	Alternate (diagnosis)	X and 4	7 cells 2+
C1 E6	FISH	Male unbalanced for translocation	Adjacent-1 (follow up)	der Y and 4	blastocyst
C1 E9	FISH	Male unbalanced for translocation	Adjacent-1 (follow up)	der Y and 4	degenerating embryo
C1 E10	FISH	Male unbalanced for translocation	Adjacent-1 (follow up)	der Y and 4	hatched blastocyst
C1 E12	FISH	Male unbalanced for translocation	Adjacent-1 (follow up)	der Y and 4	morula
C2 E1	n/a	Embryo transferred (normal female embryo)	Alternate (diagnosis)	X and 4	pre-morula
C2 E2	FISH	No result (Female unbalanced for translocation)	Unknown segregation (diagnosis)	-	blastocyst
C2 E3	FISH	No result (Male unbalanced for translocation)	3:1 (diagnosis)	der Y	blastocyst
C2 E4	FISH	No result (Male; mosaic)	Unknown segregation (diagnosis)	-	blastocyst
C3 E1	n/a	Embryo cryopreserved ([a]aCGH – Male embryo with no gains or losses detected)	Alternate (diagnosis)	der Y and der 4	blastocyst
C3 E2	n/a	Embryo cryopreserved ([a]aCGH result – normal female embryo with no gains or losses detected)	Alternate (diagnosis)	X and 4	blastocyst
C3 E3	aCGH	Male embryo unbalanced for the translocation, with additional aneuploidies	Adjacent-1 (follow up)	der Y and 4	morula
C3 E4	n/a	Embryo transferred (normal female embryo)	Alternate (diagnosis)	X and 4	pre-morula
C3 E5	n/a	Embryo cryopreserved- ([a]aCGH result – normal female embryo with no gains or losses detected)	Alternate (diagnosis)	X and 4	blastocyst

C PGD cycle no, *E* Embryo no
[a]Diagnostic aCGH result using 24Sure + arrays after a re-biopsy at blastocyst stage on day 6 of embryo development

chromosomes involved in the translocation by the different male gametes.

Statistical Analysis

The relative frequencies of combinations of chromosomal constitutions for the alternate and the adjacent-1 segregation products deduced from the embryos were analysed using the Chi-Square for Goodness of Fit test. $P < 0.05$ was considered significant. $P < 0.01$ was considered highly significant.

Results

Results from the follow up analysis of untransferred embryos

For couple A, follow up analysis on day 5–7 was carried out on a total of 10 untransferred embryos of which 7 gave conclusive results (Table 3). Four embryos (C1E6, C1E9, C1E10, C1E12) diagnosed as unbalanced for the translocation on day 3 were confirmed as so after follow up by FISH. Follow up of the remaining three embryos by aCGH gave results showing two embryos (C1E2, C1E3) (that had no result with PGD), to be female but with additional aneuploidies unrelated to the chromosomes involved in the translocation and confirmed one (C3E3) as an unbalanced male embryo with additional aneuploidy (Table 3). In addition, results from PGD were used for nine embryos, making a total of 16 for which segregation analysis could be attempted. Figure 1 shows the FISH result of the follow up analysis of an untransferred embryo from couple A.

For couple B, follow up analysis was carried out on a total of 11 embryos of which 10 gave conclusive results (Table 4). Of the embryos followed up by FISH from cycle 1, four (C1E4, C1E5, C1E6, C1E8) were confirmed as unbalanced for the translocation. The remaining two embryos were characterised as a normal female (C1E1) and a balanced

male (C1E3). In addition, follow up of four embryos from cycle 3 (initially diagnosed and followed up by aCGH) confirmed three embryos as females (C3E1, C3E3, C3E5) and one as male, unbalanced for the translocation (C3E4). For four embryos use was made of the diagnostic results giving segregation analysis results for a total of 14 embryos. One embryo gave no result (C1E2) either diagnostically or on follow up (Table 4).

Meiotic segregation analysis

Analysis of meiotic segregation was performed for 30 embryos in total. Overall, the analysis performed on all the embryos for rearrangements involving t(Y;4) and t(Y;16) revealed alternate segregation (53%) as the most frequent mode followed by adjacent-1 (33%) and 3:1 (3%). In three embryos (10%) a segregation pattern could not be determined. For both rearrangements no embryos resulting from adjacent-2 segregation were found.

Meiotic segregation outcomes obtained for the 16 embryos belonging to couple A showed eight embryos resulting from alternate segregation; five from adjacent-1 segregation and one from 3:1 segregation (analysis based on day 3 biopsy result). A segregation pattern could not be determined for two embryos. Similarly for couple B, meiotic segregation analysis for 14 embryos was carried out. Eight embryos resulted from alternate segregation and five from adjacent-1 segregation. In this case, the segregation pattern could not be determined for one embryo. An example of the presumed pachytene quadrivalent of a Y-autosome translocation carrier is shown (Fig. 2).

Detailed analysis of the chromosome contributions from the carrier gamete in both the reciprocal Y-autosome translocation carriers showed interesting outcomes. Firstly, it was seen that the number of female embryos resulting from alternate segregation with the chromosome combination of X and the autosome (4 or 16) from the carrier gamete, was

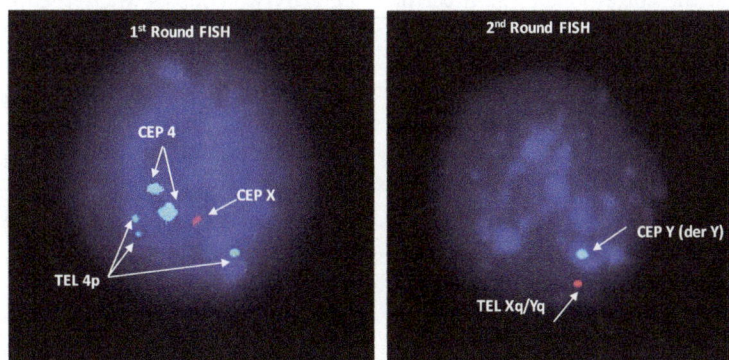

Fig. 1 FISH image of an embryonic blastomere from the untransferred embryo no. 10 (Table 3) belonging to couple A with karyotype 46,X,t(Y;4)(q12;p15.32). The FISH signal pattern is of an unbalanced male embryo consistent with 2 × CEP 4 (SA), 3 × Tel 4p(SG), 1 × CEP X(SO) in the 1st round and 1 × CEP Y (der Y) (SA), 1 × Tel Xq/Yq (SO) in the second round of hybridisation. The expected FISH signals pattern for an embryo to be a balanced male would be 2 × CEP 4 (SA), 2 × Tel 4p(SG), 1 × CEP X(SO) in the 1st round of hybridisation and 1 × CEP Y(der Y)(SA), 2 × Tel Xq/Yq (SO) in the 2nd round. Meiotic segregation analysis revealed that chromosomes der Y and 4 was the contribution from the male gamete

Table 4 Summary of the follow up results of embryos from three PGD cycles performed for couple B with a male karyotype 46,X,t(Y;16)(q12;q13)

PGD cycle no./ Embryo no.	Follow up method	Day 6 Follow up result (Diagnostic result where follow up result not available)	Meiotic segregation (stage determined)	Chromosomes contributed by carrier parent	Embryo grade on follow up
C1 E1	FISH	Normal female	Alternate (follow up)	X and 16	cavitating morula
C1 E2	FISH	No result	No result	No result	pre-morula
C1 E3	FISH	Male balanced for the translocation	Alternate (follow up)	der Y and der 16	blastocyst
C1 E4	FISH	Abnormal	Unknown (follow up)	-	blastocyst
C1 E5	FISH	Male unbalanced for the translocation	Adjacent-1 (follow up)	der Y and 16	blastocyst
C1 E6	FISH	Female unbalanced for the translocation	Adjacent-1 (follow up)	X and der 16	blastocyst
C1 E7	n/a	Embryo transferred (normal female embryo)	Alternate (diagnosis)	X and 16	blastocyst
C1 E8	FISH	Male unbalanced for the translocation	Adjacent-1 (follow up)	der Y and 16	blastocyst
C2 E1	n/a	Embryo transferred (normal female embryo)	Alternate (diagnosis)	X and 16	blastocyst
C2 E2	n/a	No result (Male unbalanced for the translocation)	Adjacent-1 (diagnosis)	der Y and 16	blastocyst
C3 E1	aCGH	Normal Female	Alternate (follow up)	X and 16	blastocyst
C3 E2	n/a	Embryo transferred (normal female embryo)	Alternate (diagnosis)	X and 16	blastocyst
C3 E3	aCGH	Female embryo with additional aneuploidy	Alternate (follow up)	X and 16	blastocyst
C3 E4	aCGH	Male unbalanced for the translocation with additional aneuploidy	Adjacent-1 (assumed) (follow up)	der Y and 16	blastocyst
C3 E5	aCGH	Female embryo with additional aneuploidy	Alternate (follow up)	X and 16	blastocyst

n/a – embryo not available for follow up. The diagnostic results of cycle 3 were available from Reprogenetics,UK

found to be far higher than the corresponding number of embryos characterised as balanced males with derivative Y and the derivative autosome, a ratio of 7:1 in each case. This observed outcome of alternate segregation deviated highly significantly ($P = 0.003$) from the expected 1:1 ratio (Table 5). Secondly, from the adjacent-1 mode of meiotic segregation, the unbalanced male embryos with the combination of der Y and the autosome were seen in all embryos from couple A and in couple B with the exception of one embryo only that had the other chromosome combination of X and derivative autosome. Again this observed outcome of adjacent-1 segregation deviated significantly ($P = 0.011$) from the expected 1:1 ratio (Table 5).

Discussion

We have reported the detailed analysis of the translocated chromosome constitution of the embryos generated by

PGD in two couples where the male partner has a Y- autosome translocation. This information has provided a rare opportunity to assess the translocation segregation types that led to successful fertilisation and early embryogenesis. As the analysis of the embryonic samples took place between days 3 and 6 of development this was prior to any post-implantation selection with regard to embryo viability.

In such carriers of Y autosome translocations, like any typical balanced autosomal reciprocal translocation, a formation of closed ring or open chain type of quadrivalent is expected at meiosis I. Gametes with 2:2 alternate, 2:2 adjacent 1 or 2, or 3:1 or 4:0 modes of segregation may be expected. In the two cases investigated the segregation mode of the male gamete was determined in a total of 27 embryos of which alternate segregation was the most common (53%) followed by adjacent-1 (33%) with a single example of the 3:1 type and no instances of

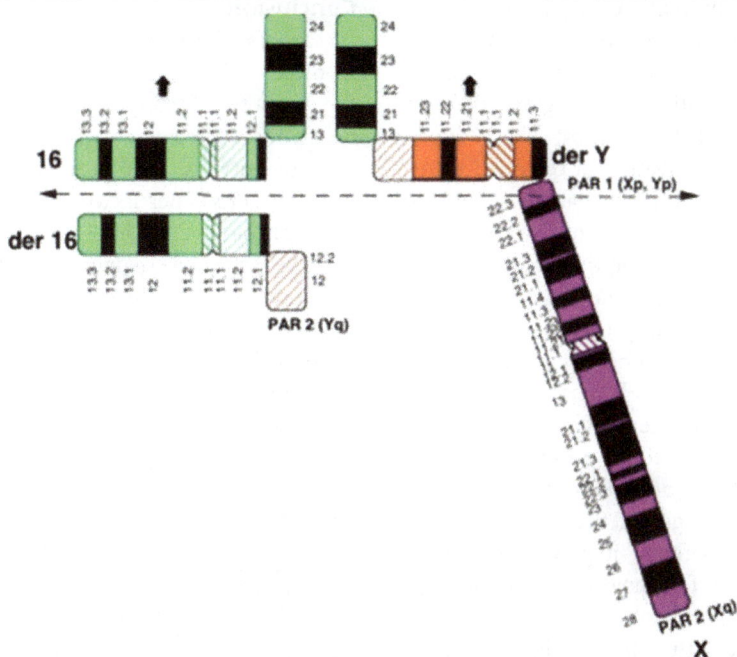

Fig. 2 Presumed configuration of the pachytene quadrivalent at meiosis I in the gametes of the male carrier of 46,X,t(Y;16)(q12;q13), couple B. The dotted line is the adjacent-1 segregation line. Black arrows indicate the two chromosomes (der Y and 16) that were passed on to the majority of the unbalanced embryos observed after PGD in couple B

adjacent-2. As is clear from the information in Table 5, there is a significant deficit of certain types of gametes for both the alternate and adjacent-1 modes. The deficit types are the der Y and der autosome combination from the alternate segregation and the X and der autosome combination from adjacent-1. In both translocation cases the deficit groups have in common the der autosome chromosome that includes the segment Yq12 to qter (Fig. 2).

A similar meiotic segregation analysis was performed on spermatozoa from a carrier of 46,X,t(Y;16)(q11.21;q24) translocation. The aim of this analysis was to estimate the risk of using a chromosomally unbalanced spermatozoan during ICSI. Using four-colour FISH, meiotic segregation analysis of 500 sperm revealed that the risk of the combination of chromosomes yielding an unbalanced sperm cell

is close to 50%. The most frequent mode of segregation seen in sperm cells was alternate segregation with normal or balanced sperm cells (51%) followed by adjacent-1 (36%) and 3:1 segregation (12%) [10].

Oliver-Bonet and colleagues studied the meiotic behaviour in spermatogenesis of two balanced reciprocal translocation carriers, t(10;14) with normal sperm parameters and t(13;20) with azoospermia. Increased pairing abnormalities, association of the quadrivalent with the sex-body and decreased recombination was seen in the t(13;20) azoospermic carrier whereas in the t(10;14) normozoospermic carrier fewer pairing abnormalities, no association of the quadrivalent with the sex body and a normal frequency of recombination were seen. These observations indicated that pairing abnormalities, association of the quadrivalent with the sex-

Table 5 Details of meiotic segregation patterns of embryos from the two reciprocal Y-autosome translocation carriers following alternate or adjacent- 1 separation

Mode of segregation	Embryo characterization with respect to the translocation	Combination of chromosomes	Embryos possessing the combination of the segregation mode for the chromosomal abnormality		Observed no. of embryos	Expected no. of embryos	Statistical Significance
			t (Y;4)	t (Y;16)			
Alternate segregation	Normal Female	X and 4/16	7 embryos	7 embryos	14	8	Deviation from 1:1 ratio, $P = 0.003$
	Balanced Male	der Y and der 4/16	1 embryo	1 embryo	2	8	
Adjacent −1	Unbalanced Male	der Y and 4/16	5 embryos	4 embryos	9	5	Deviation from 1:1 ratio, $P = 0.011$
	Unbalanced Male	X and der 4/16	0	1 embryo	1	5	

body and decreased recombination frequency were the possible mechanisms leading to spermatogenic arrest [11]. Similarly, in carriers of Y-autosome translocations involving the heterochromatic Yq12 region, defective spermatogenesis is thought to be most likely due to pairing abnormalities and association of the quadrivalent with sex-body formed during male meiosis [4, 12, 13].

In spermatocytes from Y-autosomal translocation carriers, it was observed that, during the pachytene stage of meiosis I, if a segment of autosome is associated with the sex-body, there is a possibility of it being unpaired or unsynapsed and therefore silenced genetically. It is also thought likely that the sex-body derived inactivation extends to the autosomal segment affecting (silencing) any genes required for the meiotic progression of the spermatocyte, thus leading to degeneration of spermatocytes after the pachytene stage via the pachytene stage checkpoint [12, 13]. Alternatively, it may be that if the autosomal genes required for meiotic progression are not inactivated then the sperm cell will progress through the meiotic prophase but at the time of alignment of the quadrivalent, the presence of asynapsed segments attached to the sex-body will trigger the meiotic spindle checkpoint leading to apoptosis of the sperm cell [14]. Therefore either one of the two mechanisms may be responsible for the arrested spermatogenesis.

Delobel and colleagues studied meiotic configurations at the pachytene stage in testicular biopsies from a carrier with karyotype 46,X,t(Y;6)(q12;p11.1). They clearly observed that in more than three quarters of the cells at pachytene the heterochromatic segment of Y (Yq12 to qter) translocated to the autosome 6 (i.e., der 6) is paired with Xqter, at the PAR2 and is associated with the sex body. In these cells the translocated segment of chromosome 6 is condensed in a similar fashion to the X chromosome. Although they do not comment upon it, critically for the interpretation of our data, close examination of their figures reveals that the translocated segment of the autosome that is attached to the derivative Y is not associated with the sex body and does not appear condensed [12].

To return to the present study, where there is a statistically significant deficit of embryos derived from sperm with the derivative autosome chromosome that includes the segment Yq12 to qter, the most likely explanation may be that this chromosome is associated with the X chromosome at PAR2 in the sex-body leading to inactivation of genes on the autosomal segment that are required for the meiotic process and that this has led to degeneration of this class of spermatocytes during meiosis. Whereas the spermatocytes with the derivative Y chromosome survive because the autosomal segment is not inactivated and genes essential for meiosis are active.

Conclusion

In carriers of reciprocal translocations the chromosomes involved and position of the breakpoints greatly influence the geometry of the quadrivalent formed at pachytene and hence the segregation types produced. In the particular case of carriers of more rarely occurring Y-autosome translocations other factors such as the association of the heterochromatic region of the chromosome Y (Yqh), bearing the attached segment of the autosome, with the chromosome X via the sex-body during meiosis may affect the expression of genes that are vital for the completion of meiosis (12). This in turn would play an important role in determining the final meiotic outcome and the types of gametes produced.

Abbreviations
aCGH: Array comparative genomic hybridization; ART: Assisted Reproductive Technology; AZF: Azoospermia factor; FISH: Fluorescence in situ hybridization; ICSI: Intracytoplasmic sperm injection; IVF: In vitro fertilization; PAR: Pseudoautosomal region, PGD. Preimplantation Genetic Diagnosis; SRY: Sex-determining region Y; TE: Trophectoderm; Yqh: Heterochromatic region of the chromosome Y

Acknowledgements
We thank Carleen Heath of The Centre for Reproductive and Genetic Health for much help in obtaining patient samples.

Funding
This work was supported for consumables by the Leverhulme Trust in the form of an Emeritus Fellowship for J.D. (reference EM/2/EM/2008/0061).

Authors' contributions
HG: collected samples, involved in conducting the experiments, data analysis, data interpretation, preparation of manuscript. RN: involved in acquisition of data, data analysis, reviewing of the manuscript, statistical analysis. SS: involved in critical reading of the manuscript. PS: Clinical responsibility for, and consent to the use of embryonic material. JD: contributed to the study design and conception, preparation of the manuscript, data analysis and interpretation, revised it critically for important intellectual content, final approval of the version to be published. All authors read and approved the final manuscript.

Competing interests
The authors declare that they have no competing interests.

Author details
[1]Preimplantation Genetics Group, Institute for Women's Health, University College London, 86-96 Chenies Mews, London WC1E 6HX, UK. [2]The Centre for Reproductive and Genetic Health, 230-232 Great Portland Street, London W1W 5QS, UK.

References

1. Rivera H, Diaz-Castanos L. Is Yq11 the main critical segment in balanced Y; autosome translocations? Ann Genet. 1992;35(4):224–6.

2. Van Assche E, Bonduelle M, Tournaye H, Joris H, Verheyen G, Devroey P, Van Steirteghem A, Liebaers I. Cytogenetics of infertile men. Hum Reprod. 1996; 11 Suppl 4:1–24. discussion 25–26.

3. Turner JM. Meiotic sex chromosome inactivation. Development. 2007; 134(10):1823–31.

4. Alves C, Carvalho F, Cremades N, Sousa M, Barros A. Unique (Y;13) translocation in a male with oligozoospermia. cytogenetic and molecular studies. European journal of human genetics. EJHG. 2002;10(8):467–74.

5. Teyssier M, Rafat A, Pugeat M. Case of (Y;1) familial translocation. Am J Med Genet. 1993;46(3):339–40.

6. Sklower Brooks SS, Genovese M, Gu H, Duncan CJ, Shanske A, Jenkins EC. Normal adaptive function with learning disability in duplication 8p including band p22. Am J Med Genet. 1998;78(2):114–7.

7. Harper JC, Coonen E, Ramaekers FC, Delhanty JD, Handyside AH, Winston RM, Hopman AH. Identification of the sex of human preimplantation embryos in two hours using an improved spreading method and fluorescent in-situ hybridization (FISH) using directly labelled probes. Hum Reprod. 1994;9(4):721–4.

8. Mantzouratou A, Mania A, Fragouli E, Xanthopoulou L, Tashkandi S, Fordham K, Ranieri DM, Doshi A, Nuttall S, Harper JC, et al. Variable aneuploidy mechanisms in embryos from couples with poor reproductive histories undergoing preimplantation genetic screening. Hum Reprod. 2007;22(7):1844–53.

9. Ghevaria H, SenGupta S, Shmitova N, Serhal P, Delhanty J. The origin and significance of additional aneuploidy events in couples undergoing preimplantation genetic diagnosis for translocations by array comparative genomic hybridization. Reprod Biomed Online. 2016;32(2):178–89.

10. Giltay JC, Kastrop PM, Tiemessen CH, van Inzen WG, Scheres JM, Pearson PL. Sperm analysis in a subfertile male with a Y;16 translocation, using four-color FISH. Cytogenet Cell Genet. 1999;84(1–2):67–72.

11. Oliver-Bonet M, Benet J, Sun F, Navarro J, Abad C, Liehr T, Starke H, Greene C, Ko E, Martin RH. Meiotic studies in two human reciprocal translocations and their association with spermatogenic failure. Hum Reprod. 2005;20(3):683–8.

12. Delobel B, Djlelati R, Gabriel-Robez O, Croquette MF, Rousseaux-Prevost R, Rousseaux J, Rigot JM, Rumpler Y. Y-autosome translocation and infertility. usefulness of molecular, cytogenetic and meiotic studies. Hum Genet. 1998; 102(1):98–102.

13. Sun F, Oliver-Bonet M, Turek PJ, Ko E, Martin RH. Meiotic studies in an azoospermic human translocation (Y;1) carrier. Mol Hum Reprod. 2005; 11(5):361–4.

14. Oliver-Bonet M, Ko E, Martin RH. Male infertility in reciprocal translocation carriers: the sex body affair. Cytogenet Genome Res. 2005;111(3–4):343–6.

8

Identification of small marker chromosomes using microarray comparative genomic hybridization and multicolor fluorescent *in situ* hybridization

Woori Jang[1,2], Hyojin Chae[1,2,5*], Jiyeon Kim[2], Jung-Ok Son[2], Seok Chan Kim[2], Bo Kyung Koo[2], Myungshin Kim[1,2], Yonggoo Kim[1,2], In Yang Park[3] and In Kyung Sung[4]

Abstract

Background: Marker chromosomes are small supernumerary chromosomes that cannot be unambiguously identified by chromosome banding techniques alone. However, the precise characterization of marker chromosomes is important for prenatal diagnosis and proper genetic counseling. In this study, we evaluated the chromosomal origin of marker chromosomes using a combination of banding cytogenetics and molecular cytogenetic techniques including diverse fluorescence *in situ* hybridization (FISH) assays and array comparative genomic hybridization (array CGH).

Results: In a series of 2871 patients for whom cytogenetic analysis was requested, 14 cases with small supernumerary marker chromosomes (sSMCs) were identified. Nine sSMCs were mosaic, and five nonmosaic. Of the nine cases with known parental origins, four were identified as de novo, and four and one were maternally and paternally inherited, respectively. Six sSMCs were identified by FISH using centromeric probes; three sSMCs were derived from chromosome 15, including two heterochromatic sSMC(15)s and a large sSMC(15) spanning 15q11.1q13.1, and three sSMCs originated from chromosome 14 or 22. Array CGH revealed two cases with derivatives of chromosome 2 and whole chromosome painting multicolor-FISH (M-FISH) identified three cases with derivatives of chromosome 6, 16, and 19, respectively. One maker chromosome in Turner syndrome was characterized as sSMC(X) by preferential application of a centromeric probe for X-chromosome. In addition, one sSMC composed of genomic materials from chromosomes 12 and 18 was identified in parallel with parental karyotype analysis that revealed the reciprocal balanced translocation.

Conclusions: This report is the largest study on sSMCs in Korea and expands the spectrum of sSMCs that are molecularly characterized.

Keywords: Marker chromosome, Array comparative genomic hybridization, Fluorescence *in situ* hybridization

Background

Marker chromosomes, also known as small supernumerary marker chromosomes (sSMCs), are structurally abnormal chromosomes that cannot be unambiguously identified or characterized by conventional banding cytogenetics (ISCN 2013) [1]. They are generally equal or smaller in size than a chromosome 20 of the same metaphase spread [2], and the small size of markers precludes the identification of their chromosomal origin by conventional banding techniques, and molecular cytogenetic techniques are necessary for their characterization.

According to a recent, comprehensive review [3], marker chromosomes are found in 0.075 % of unselected prenatal cases, and in 0.044 % of consecutive postnatal cases, but frequencies are elevated to 0.125 % in infertile subjects and to 0.255 % in developmentally retarded patients [3]. In terms of the parental origin of marker chromosomes, approximately 30 % of markers are familial, while 70 % are *de novo*. The clinical phenotypes

* Correspondence: chez@catholic.ac.kr
[1]Department of Laboratory Medicine, College of Medicine, The Catholic University of Korea, Seoul, Korea
[2]Catholic Genetic Laboratory Center, Seoul St. Mary's Hospital, College of Medicine, The Catholic University of Korea, Seoul, Korea
Full list of author information is available at the end of the article

associated with marker chromosomes are also highly variable, from normal to severely abnormal [4], and this renders marker chromosomes a particularly difficult problem in genetic counseling, especially in prenatal *de novo* cases. There has been a previous report on marker chromosomes identified in Korean patients [5] investigated with fluorescence *in situ* hybridization (FISH) analysis, but with advancements in molecular cytogenetic diagnostics, tools including whole-chromosome painting FISH and array comparative genomic hybridization (array CGH) have been applied in characterization of marker chromosomes.

Therefore, in this study, we aimed to characterize consecutive marker chromosomes identified from a single genetic center in Korea, with multiple molecular cytogenetic methods in combination with banding cytogenetics, to accurately characterize the chromosomal origin and the genetic content of marker chromosomes.

Methods

Chromosomal analysis, referred for constitutional abnormality, was performed on 2871 patients (1974 peripheral blood specimens, 897 amniotic fluid specimens) from January 2010 to December 2013 at Seoul St. Mary's Hospital. Written informed consent was obtained from the patients and/or their family members. Whenever available, the familial occurrence of markers was evaluated through parental studies. Information on the phenotypic features of the patients was obtained by a review of medical records. This study was conducted in accordance with the ethical guidelines of the Declaration of Helsinki and was approved by the Institutional Review Board (IRB)/Ethics Committee of Seoul St. Mary's Hospital (IRB No.KC11TISI0277).

Banding cytogenetics

Banding cytogenetics was performed on G-banded metaphase chromosomes of cultured peripheral blood lymphocytes and/or amniotic fluid cells using routine techniques. Karyotypes were interpreted according to the ISCN 2013.

FISH studies

If the size of the marker chromosome is similar to a chromosome 20 of the same metaphase spread, FISH analysis using centromeric probes for chromosomes 15, 18, and 12 was performed. If the size of the marker is smaller than a chromosome 20, FISH analysis using centromeric probes for all acrocentric chromosomes 15, 13/21, and 14/22 was performed. In Turner syndrome (TS) patients with a marker chromosome (45,X/46,X,+mar), FISH studies using X centromeric probe as well as SRY were performed. And in all patients with marker chromosomes, parental study was performed in parallel, whenever possible. The

FISH probes used in this study are summarized in Additional file 1: Table S1.

If the origin of the marker chromosome was not clarified by the above strategies, we then performed whole chromosome painting multicolor-FISH (M-FISH) and/or array CGH, based on the level of mosaicism, and the amount of specimen available. M-FISH was performed using the 24 *X*Cyte Human Multicolor FISH Probe kit (MetaSystems, Altlussheim, Germany) according to the manufacturer's instructions. Fluorescent images were captured and analysed using an Axio Imager 2 fluorescence microscope (Zeiss, Jena, Germany) and Isis image analysis software (MetaSystems).

Array CGH

Array CGH analysis was performed using a SurePrint G3 Human CGH Microarray 8 X 60 K kit (Agilent Technologies, Santa Clara, CA, USA), which consisted of 62,976 oligonucleotide probes spaced at 41 kbp intervals (median probe spacing) throughout the genome. Control DNA (Promega Corp., Nepean, Canada) was used as the reference DNA. DNA digestion, labeling and hybridization were performed following the manufacturer's instructions. Scanned images were quantified using Agilent Feature Extraction software (v10.0), and the resulting data were imported into Agilent Genomic Workbench 7.0.4.0 software for visualization, and copy number variations were detected using the Aberration Detection Method-2 (ADM-2) algorithm. All genomic coordinates were based on human genome build hg19/GRCh37.

Results

Of 2871 patients referred for chromosomal analysis, marker chromosomes were identified in 14 patients. Parental study was performed in nine patients, and five marker chromosomes (55.6 %) were inherited from one of the parents, while four markers (44.4 %) were *de novo*. Of the five inherited markers, four (80 %) were maternally inherited and only one (20 %) was paternally inherited. Mosaicism was detected in nine patients (64 %), whereas a single cell line was observed in the remaining five patients (36 %). Three marker chromosomes (21 %) were equal in size to a chromosome 20, whereas the other 11 (79 %) were smaller than a chromosome 20 of the same metaphase spread. Although the depth of clinical information available differed among the subjects, most postnatal cases (10/11, 91 %) showed abnormal phenotypes of variable severity (Table 1). All three prenatal cases were referred for advanced maternal age, and in two cases parental study was available, and one was maternally inherited and one *de novo*, and the outcome of the pregnancies could not be followed up.

In the present study, chromosomal origins were identified in 13 of 14 identified marker chromosomes, and in

Table 1 Summary of fourteen cases showing marker chromosomes

Case No.	Gender	Age at testing	Karyotype	Chr. Origin	Size	Inheritance	Phenotype	Molecular cytogenetic method	Molecular cytogenetic method results	Fig
1	female	19 y	mos 45,X[25]/46,X,+mar[5]	X	<20	NE	Short stature, Primary amenorrhea	Centromeric FISH	nuc ish(DXZ1x1)[340/400]/nuc ish(DXZ1x2) [60/400]	Fig. 1
2	female	1 m	47,XX,+der(12;18)(p10p10)	der(12;18)(p10p10)	<20	paternal	Incomplete cleft palate, Developmental coordination disorder, Developmental delay	M-FISH	ish der(12;18)(wcp12+wcp18+) pat	Fig. 2
3	female	25 m	mos 47,XX,+mar[24]/ 46,XX[6]	15	~20	NE	Developmental delay, Failure to thrive	Centromeric FISH	ish idic(15)(D15Z1++, D15S11-)	Fig. 3a, 3b
4	male	prenatal	47,XY,+mar	15	~20	maternal	NA	Centromeric FISH, M-FISH	ish idic(15)(wcp15+, D15Z1++, D15S11-) mat	Fig. 3c, 3d
5	female	32 m	47,XX,+mar	15	~20	maternal	Developmental delay	Centromeric FISH, Array CGH	ish der(15)(D15Z1+),arr[hg19]15q11.1q13.1 (20,102,541-28,525,460)x3 mat	Fig. 3e
6	male	prenatal	mos 47,XY,+mar[14]/ 46,XY[26]	14	<20	NE	NA	Centromeric FISH, M-FISH	ish der(14)(D14Z1+wcp14+)	Fig. 4a
7	NA	NA	NA	22	<20	NE	NA	Centromeric FISH, M-FISH	ish idic(22)(D22Z1++, wcp22+)	Fig. 4b
8	female	11 y	mos 47,XX,+mar[45]/ 46,XX[5]	14 or 22	<20	maternal	Short stature	Centromeric FISH, M-FISH	ish der(14/22)(D14Z1/D22Z1+) mat	Fig. 4c
9	female	prenatal	mos 46,XX,min[4]/ 46,XX[11]	6	<20	de novo	NA	Centromeric FISH, M-FISH	ish der(6)(wcp6+) de novo	NA
10	female	8 y	mos 47,XX,+mar[5]/ 46,XY[45]	16	<20	NE	Short stature, Elevated TSH level	M-FISH	ish der(16)(wcp16+)	Fig. 7a
11	male	18 m	mos 47,XY,+mar[14]/ 46,XY[26]	19	<20	de novo	Developmental delay	M-FISH	ish der(19)(wcp19+) de novo	Fig. 7b
12	female	10 y	47,XX,+mar	2	<20	maternal	Short stature, Developmental delay	Array CGH	arr[hg19]2q11.1q12.3(95,529,039-108,083,956)x3 mat,18p11.32p11.31(142,096-5,853,122)x1 dn	Fig. 5a
13	male	2 m	mos 47,XY,+mar[8]/ 46,XY[42]	2	<20	de novo	Prematurity, Developmental delay, ASD	Array CGH, FISH	arr[hg19]2q11.1q12.1(95,529,039-105,358,887)x3 dn,7q11.23(72,726,578-74,139,390)x3 mat	Fig. 5c, Fig. 6
14	male	20 m	mos 48,XY,+2mar[16]/ 47,XY,+mar[9]/46,XY[5]	NE	<20	de novo	Developmental delay	NE	NE	NE

Chr chromosomal, *CGH* comparative genomic hybridization, *M-FISH* whole chromosome painting multicolor- fluorescence *in situ* hybridization, *NA* not available, *NE* not established

one case, further characterization was not possible because there was not enough material. These marker chromosomes originated from various chromosomes and consisted of three cases (23 %) with derivatives of chromosome 15, two cases (15 %) with derivatives of chromosome 2, and one case (8 %) each with derivatives of chromosome 6, 14, 16, 19, 22, 14/22 and der(12;18)(p10;p10). Also, in a patient with TS (45,X/46,X,+mar), the marker chromosome originated from the X chromosome.

In accordance with the presented approach for marker chromosome characterization, preferential application of a centromeric probe specific for X- and Y-chromosome identified the marker as mar(X) in a TS patient (Fig. 1). And for an inherited marker chromosome (case 2), the identification of a balanced translocation in one of the parents led to a straightforward characterization of the marker chromosome as 47,XX,+der(12;18)(p10;p10) (Fig. 2).

The three marker chromosomes equal in size to a chromosome 20 (cases 3, 4 and 5) were all derived from chromosome 15, and this was readily identified by FISH analysis using centromeric probes for chromosome 15. FISH with centromeric probes for chromosome 12, and 18 was also performed to identify i(12p) associated with Pallister-Killian (OMIM 601803) syndrome and i(18p) syndrome, respectively, but no i(12p) nor i(18p) was found in this study. For both sSMC(15)s of case 3 and 4, FISH analysis using probe D15S11(15q11.2) lacked a positive hybridization signal and were therefore considered as heterochromatic (Fig. 3a-d). However, in sSMC(15) of case 5, array CGH showed a 8.4 Mb gain of chromosome 15q11.1q13.1 (chr15:20,102,541-28,525,460) encompassing *ATP10A*, *CYFIP1*, *GABRA5*, *GABRB3*, *GABRG3*, *HERC2*, *MAGEL2*, *MKRN3*, *NDN*, *NIPA1*, *NIPA2*, *OCA2*, *POTEB*, *SNRPN*, *TUBGCP5*, and *UBE3A* genes, with a $\log_2$ ratio of 1.0409, inherited from a phenotypically normal mother

(Fig. 3e). For the marker chromosomes smaller than that of a chromosome 20, FISH analysis using centromeric probes for all acrocentric chromosomes was performed sequentially according to their reported frequency in the literature, starting with chromosome 15, followed by 14/22 and 13/21. This led to the characterization of three cases that originated from chromosome 14 and/or 22 (Fig. 4). Therefore, in a total of six cases, the chromosomal origin of the marker chromosome was ascertained by FISH probes targeting the centromere.

For the remaining five marker chromosomes, M-FISH and/or array CGH identified the chromosomal origin. Two cases with a marker originating from chromosome 2 were characterized by array CGH. Array CGH detected a maternally inherited gain of 12.6 Mb derived from chromosome 2q11.1q12.3 (chr2: 95,529,039-108,083,956) with a $\log_2$ratio of 0.4890 and a de novo 5.7 Mb loss of chromosome 18p11.32p11.31 (chr18: 142,096-5,853,122) with a $\log_2$ ratio of -0.8833 in case 12 (Fig. 5a-b). A de novo 9.8 Mb gain of chromosome 2q11.1q12.1 (chr2: 95,529,039-105,358,887) with a $\log_2$ ratio of 0.3365 and maternally inherited 1.4 Mb gain of chromosome 7q11.23 (chr7: 72,726,578-74,139,390) with a $\log_2$ ratio of 0.4710 were identified in case 13 (Fig. 5c-e). Further FISH analysis confirmed that the 2q-amplified region, detected by array CGH, was localized to the marker chromosomes (Fig. 6). Three cases with low-level mosaicism were evaluated with M-FISH and the origin of the sSMCs was chromosome 6, 16 and 19, respectively (cases 9, 10 and 11) (Fig. 7).

On the basis of our experience, the present knowledge of sSMC frequency [5] and the previously suggested characterization schemes [6–8], we have followed a modified algorithm that allowed the determination of the chromosomal origin of the marker chromosome in an effective manner using diverse techniques including banding cytogenetics, M-FISH and array CGH (Fig. 8).

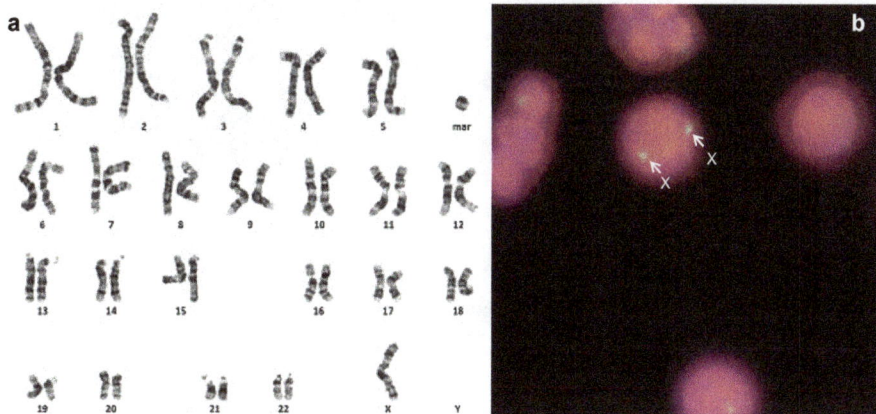

Fig. 1 a Karyotype of the patient with Turner syndrome; **b** Interphase FISH analysis using the probes of DXZ (Xp11.1-q11.1; spectrum green) and SRY (Yp11.31; spectrum red) probes shows two copies of green and absence of red signals

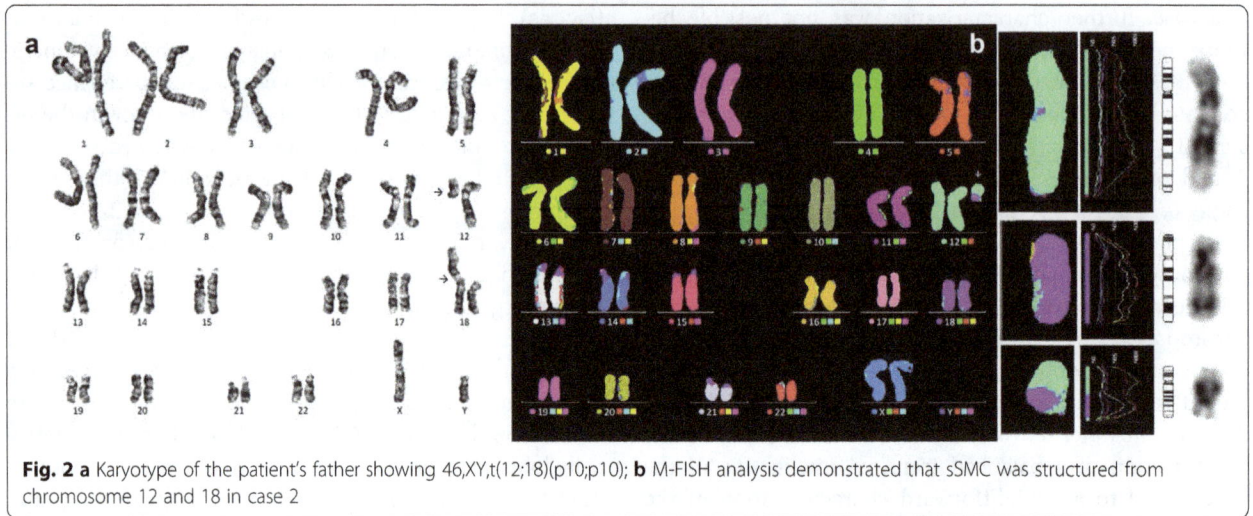

Fig. 2 a Karyotype of the patient's father showing 46,XY,t(12;18)(p10;p10); **b** M-FISH analysis demonstrated that sSMC was structured from chromosome 12 and 18 in case 2

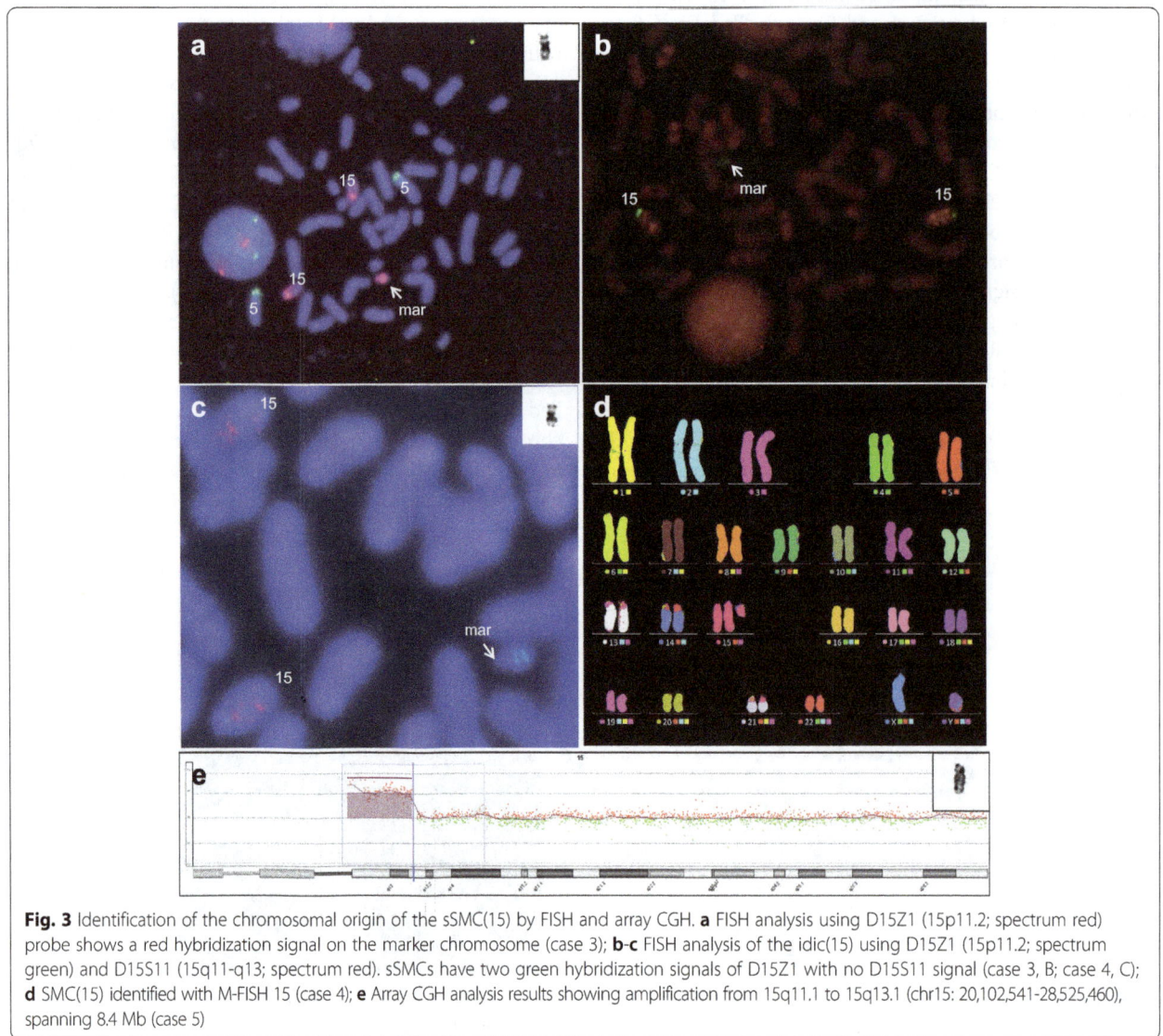

Fig. 3 Identification of the chromosomal origin of the sSMC(15) by FISH and array CGH. **a** FISH analysis using D15Z1 (15p11.2; spectrum red) probe shows a red hybridization signal on the marker chromosome (case 3); **b-c** FISH analysis of the idic(15) using D15Z1 (15p11.2; spectrum green) and D15S11 (15q11-q13; spectrum red). sSMCs have two green hybridization signals of D15Z1 with no D15S11 signal (case 3, B; case 4, C); **d** SMC(15) identified with M-FISH 15 (case 4); **e** Array CGH analysis results showing amplification from 15q11.1 to 15q13.1 (chr15: 20,102,541-28,525,460), spanning 8.4 Mb (case 5)

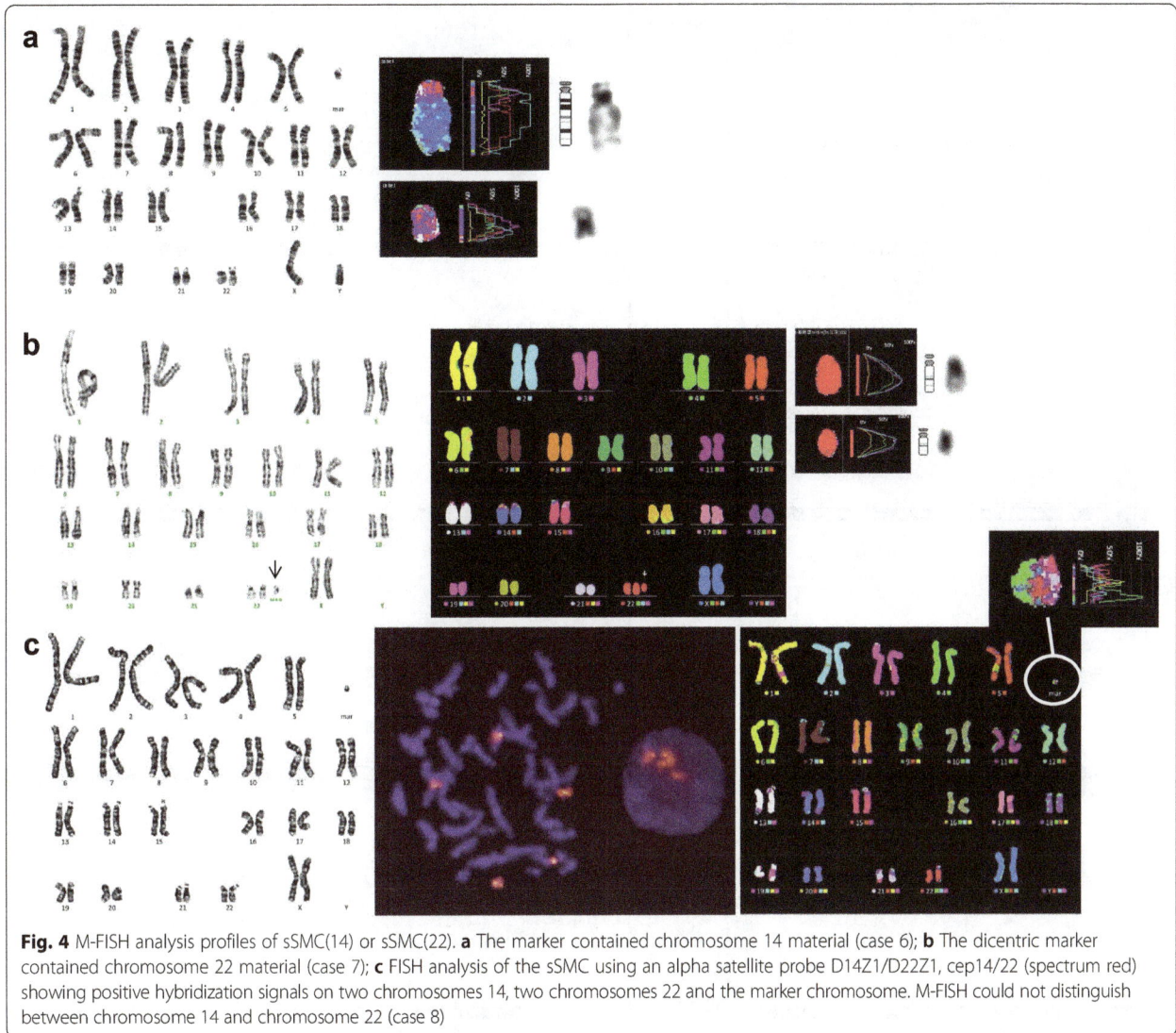

Fig. 4 M-FISH analysis profiles of sSMC(14) or sSMC(22). **a** The marker contained chromosome 14 material (case 6); **b** The dicentric marker contained chromosome 22 material (case 7); **c** FISH analysis of the sSMC using an alpha satellite probe D14Z1/D22Z1, cep14/22 (spectrum red) showing positive hybridization signals on two chromosomes 14, two chromosomes 22 and the marker chromosome. M-FISH could not distinguish between chromosome 14 and chromosome 22 (case 8)

Discussion

In our study population, six (6/12, 50 %) marker chromosomes were derived from acrocentric autosomes, six were derived from non-acrocentric autosomes and one from the X chromosome. Marker chromosome derived from chromosome 15 was the most frequent sSMC identified in individuals with karyotype 47,XN,+mar (3/12, 25 %), similar to the reported frequency of 30 % in the literature [8]. In the present study, 2 sSMC(15)s were without euchromatin, but 1 sSMC(15) showed a maternally inherited euchromatic sSMC(15) spanning 15q11.1 to 15q13.1. Larger sSMC(15) with euchromatic content has been associated with a wide spectrum of clinical features from normal to full phenotype of the 15q11-q13 duplication syndrome (OMIM #608636) including autism, mental retardation, ataxia, seizures, developmental delays, and behavioral problems [9, 10], and generally, sSMC(15) spanning 15pter to 15q12 tend to have less

severe phenotype than larger ones including 15pter to 15q14. While the identical large sSMC(15) was also identified in her phenotypically normal mother, the mother had a mosaic sSMC(15) (mos 47,XX,+mar[37]/ 46,XX[3]) while the proband had a single cell line, suggesting that the lack of mosaicism may be associated with the abnormal phenotype seen in the proband.

FISH analysis using centromeric probes for 14/22, confirmed three sSMCs as derived from chromosome 14 or 22. Following M-FISH analysis, two cases were identified as sSMC(14) and sSMC(22), respectively. However, the sSMC of case 8 was not resolved by M-FISH. This may be due to an underrepresentation of the region in M-FISH probes or a "flaring effect" of the fluorescence-intense centromeric signal [11]. The presence of a sSMC(14) is very rare [12] and among sSMC(14) cases with clinical signs, dysmorphic features and mental retardation are most often reported [8]. Regarding sSMC(22), 70 % of

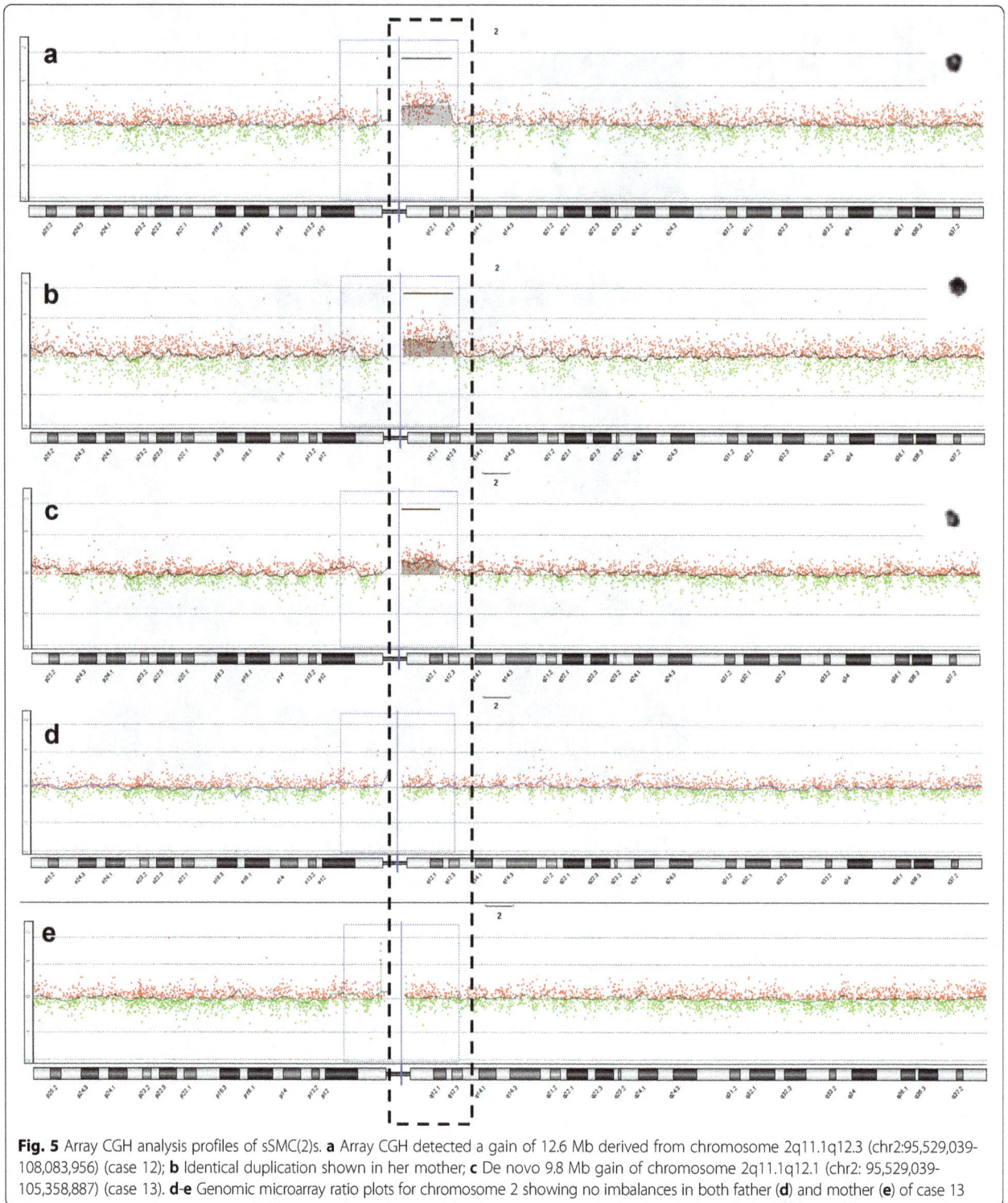

Fig. 5 Array CGH analysis profiles of sSMC(2)s. **a** Array CGH detected a gain of 12.6 Mb derived from chromosome 2q11.1q12.3 (chr2:95,529,039-108,083,956) (case 12); **b** Identical duplication shown in her mother; **c** De novo 9.8 Mb gain of chromosome 2q11.1q12.1 (chr2: 95,529,039-105,358,887) (case 13). **d-e** Genomic microarray ratio plots for chromosome 2 showing no imbalances in both father (**d**) and mother (**e**) of case 13

carriers are clinically normal [13] but distinct pathologic phenotypes, including CES (cat-eye syndrome, OMIM #115470) and ES (Emanuel syndrome, OMIM #609029) are associated with sSMC(22). The majority of CES is caused by bisatellited isodicentric marker chromosome containing CES critical region located in the most proximal 2-2.5 Mb of 22q11 [14] and ES is most often caused by a balanced translocation, t(11;22)(q23;q11.2), in one of the parents. Case 7 had an extra dicentric chromosome 22, however, analysis for CES critical region could not be done due to the insufficient amount of specimen. Furthermore, we were unable to obtain detailed clinical

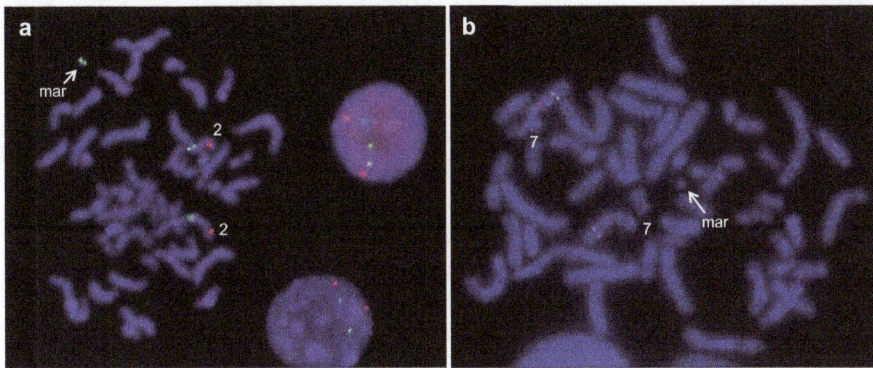

Fig. 6 Identification of the chromosomal origin of the sSMC(2) by FISH in case 13. FISH analysis with MYCN (2p24,3; spectrum red) probe and LAF4 (2q11.2; spectrum green) probe shows a green hybridization signal on the marker chromosome, indicating that it is a derivative of chromosome 2 (**a**). No red signal was observable on any structure other than normal homologues of chromosome 7 using FISH analysis with the probes of ELN (7q11.23; spectrum red) and D7S485/D7S522 (7q31; spectrum green) (**b**)

information regarding the presence or absence of major CES phenotypes including ocular coloboma, anal atresia, and renal malformations.

Marker chromosomes derived from non-acrocentric autosomes comprise about 40 % of all markers among individuals with karyotype 47,XN,+mar, and the risk of an abnormal phenotype associated with non-acrocentric autosomes is approximately 28 % [8, 15, 16]. In our study, five cases (5/12, 42 %) were derived from non-acrocentric

autosomes and had clinical features of developmental delay or short stature, with the exception of case 9 for whom phenotypic information was not available. Two ring-shaped marker chromosomes were characterized by array CGH as originating from chromosome 2q. The majority of previously reported sSMC(2)s are ring-shaped sSMCs, as in this study, and a correlation of 2p11.2 with the presence of clinical abnormalities, and 2q11.2 with an absence of clinical signs have been suggested [17]. For

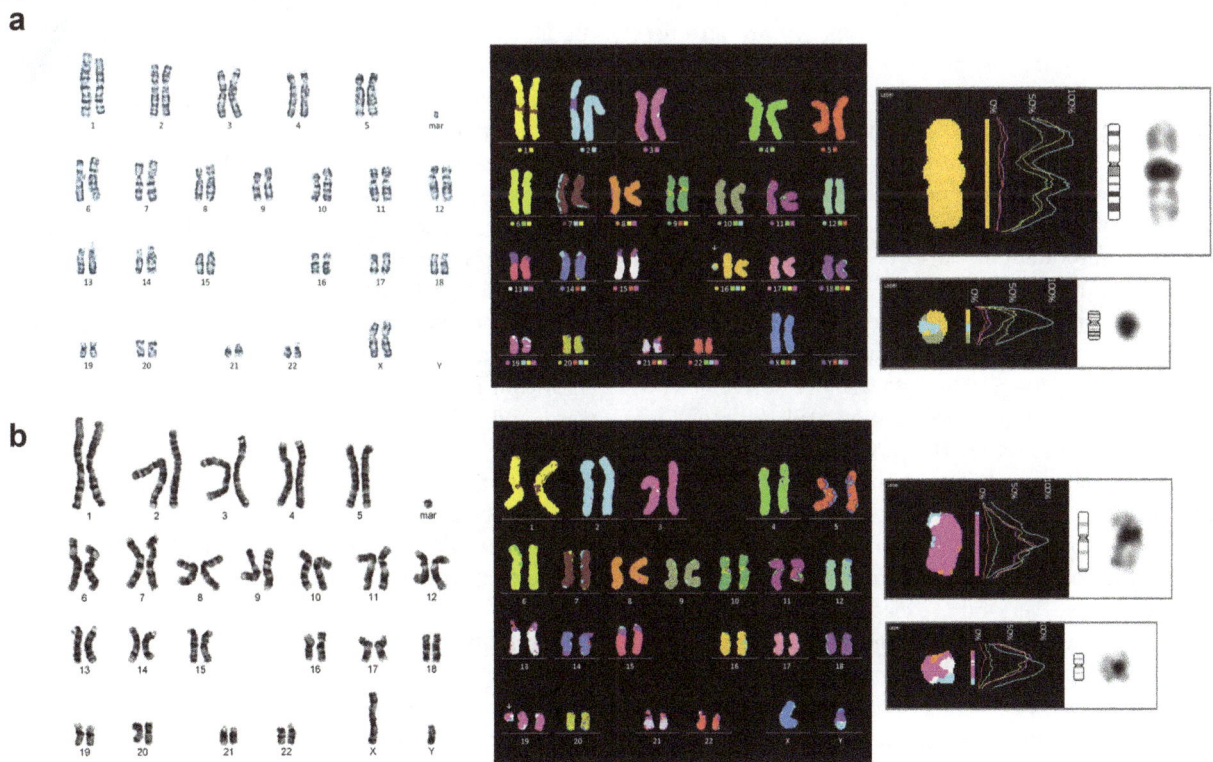

Fig. 7 Two sSMCs were characterized using multicolor FISH (M-FISH), which demonstrated the presence of additional material that originated from chromosome 16 (**a**, case 10) and 19 (**b**, case 11)

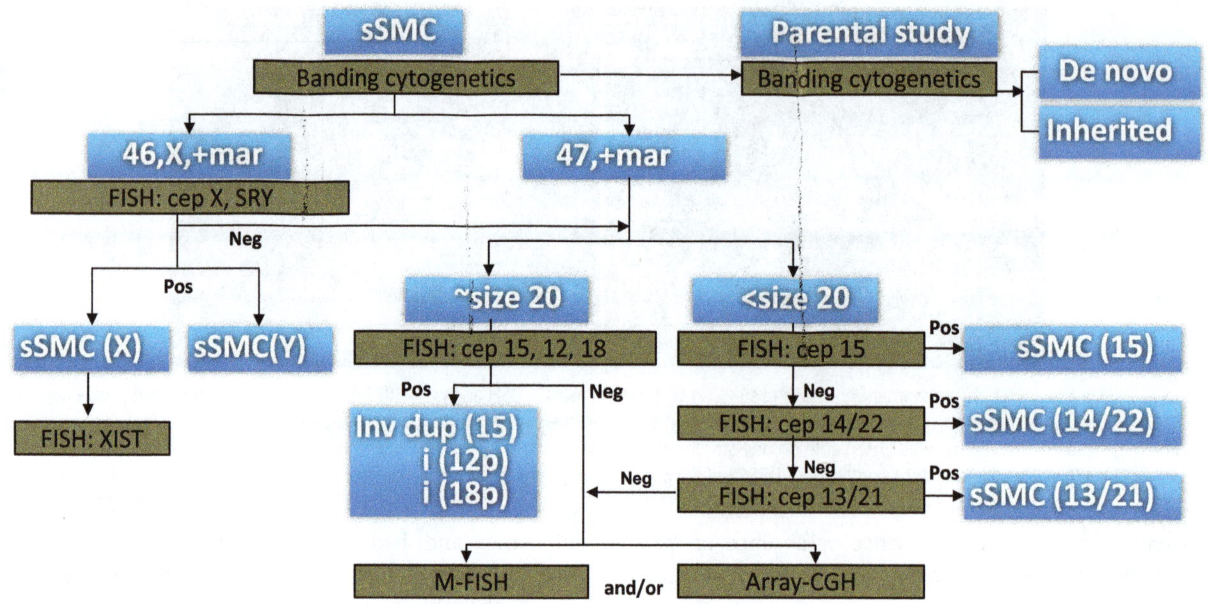

Fig. 8 The algorithm for the determination of chromosomal origin of marker chromosomes

case 12, we have assumed that the sSMC(2) was maternal in origin so the sSMC itself is harmless. However, for case 13, in addition to the sSMC(2), a duplication of 7q11.23 was identified by array CGH, and the genotype-phenotype correlation of sSMC(2) was not evident for this case. Marker chromosomes derived from non-acrocentric autosomes such as chromosome 6, 16, and 19 are also very rare (0.6–1.4 %) and the phenotype associated with each marker is not well established [6].

Marker chromosomes are found in 7-16 % of patients with TS and the marker chromosome is mainly from sex chromosomes, and only rarely from autosomes [18]. Screening of Y chromosome material in sSMC of TS patients is important because of its associated risk of gonadoblastoma [19]. Also, when sSMC is derived from X chromosome in TS patients, depending on the size and content of the sSMC(X)s, lack of the *XIST* locus (Xq13.2) may be associated with a more severe phenotype that includes mental retardation [18]. Although we did not perform FISH for the *XIST* gene, case 1 had no mental retardation, suggesting that her sSMC(X) contained *XIST*.

The extra derivative chromosome produced by the exchange of genomic material between two or more chromosomes is also very rare, except in ES. As shown in our case, parental karyotyping becomes relevant in tracing the origins of sSMCs. To our knowledge, this is the first reported case associating derivative marker chromosome involving chromosome 12 and 18. This patient with trisomy 12p and trisomy 18p showed incomplete cleft palate, developmental coordination disorder and development delay.

There are only a few well-established clinical syndromes associated with sSMCs originating from chromosomes 12, 15, 18 and 22 [20]. And the clinical outcome of the majority of marker chromosomes is highly variable, depending on their origin, size, euchromatin content, co-occurrence of uniparental disomy, and prevalence of aneuploidy in mosaic cases [21]. Generally, while there is no discernibly increased risk for fetal abnormalities if the marker has been inherited from a phenotypically normal parent, the risk for an abnormal phenotype in prenatally ascertained de novo cases is given as ~13 % [22]. Therefore the clinical management and genetic counseling depend on the characteristics of marker chromosomes and parental origin. In this regard, molecular cytogenetics, in combination with banding cytogenetics can provide precise information of the breakpoints of the marker chromosomes and accurate delineation of chromosomal content. The algorithm followed in this study proved as a straightforward and efficient strategy that can be used in most diagnostic molecular cytogenetic laboratories for characterization of sSMCs. Using this algorithm acrocentric sSMCs can be characterized in 2 days, and non-acrocentric sSMCs requiring M-FISH or array CGH can be characterized in 5 days.

Conclusion

This report is the largest study on sSMCs in Korea and expands the spectrum of sSMCs that are molecularly characterized. The stepwise application of molecular cytogenetic methods proved as both practical and efficient strategy that allowed straightforward and accurate characterization of sSMCs. And an accurate identification of the genetic content of sSMCs should provide more information on genotype-phenotype correlation and for genetic counseling.

Abbreviations
array CGH, array comparative genomic hybridization; CES, cat-eye syndrome; ES, Emanuel syndrome; FISH, fluorescence *in situ* hybridization; ISCN 2013, international system for human cytogenetic nomenclature (2013); M-FISH, whole chromosome painting multicolor-FISH; OMIM, online mendelian inheritance in man; sSMCs, small supernumerary marker chromosomes; TS, Turner syndrome

Acknowledgments
The authors are grateful to the patients and their parents, and The Catholic Genetic Laboratory Center for assisting us to carry out this study and compiling this report.

Funding
This study was supported by Research Fund of Seoul St. Mary's Hospital, The Catholic University of Korea.

Authors' contributions
HC, MK, and YK designed and coordinated the study. JK carried out microarray analysis. JS, SCK, and BKK performed the karyotyping and FISH studies. WJ, HC, MK, YK, IYP and IKS participated in drafting and critical review of the manuscript. All authors read and approved the final manuscript.

Competing interests
The authors declare that they have no competing interests.

Author details
[1]Department of Laboratory Medicine, College of Medicine, The Catholic University of Korea, Seoul, Korea. [2]Catholic Genetic Laboratory Center, Seoul St. Mary's Hospital, College of Medicine, The Catholic University of Korea, Seoul, Korea. [3]Department of Obstetrics and Gynecology, College of Medicine, The Catholic University of Korea, Seoul, Korea. [4]Department of Pediatrics, College of Medicine, The Catholic University of Korea, Seoul, Korea. [5]Department of Laboratory Medicine, Seoul St. Mary's Hospital, College of Medicine, The Catholic University of Korea, 222 Banpo-daero, Seocho-gu, Seoul 137-701, Korea.

References
1. Shaffer L, McGowan-Jordan J, Schmid M. ISCN 2013. An International System for Human Cytogenetic Nomenclature (2013). Basel: Karger; 2013.
2. Liehr T, Claussen U, Starke H. Small supernumerary marker chromosomes (sSMC) in humans. Cytogenet Genome Res. 2004;107:55–67.
3. Liehr T, Weise A. Frequency of small supernumerary marker chromosomes in prenatal, newborn, developmentally retarded and infertility diagnostics. Int J Mol Med. 2007;19:719–31.
4. Paoloni-Giacobino A, Morris MA, Dahoun SP. Prenatal supernumerary r(16) chromosome characterized by multiprobe FISH with normal pregnancy outcome. Prenat Diagn. 1998;18:751–2.
5. Woo HY, Cho HJ, Kong SY, Kim HJ, Jeon HB, Kim EC, et al. Marker chromosomes in Korean patients: incidence, identification and diagnostic approach. J Korean Med Sci. 2003;18:773–8.
6. Liehr T, Ewers E, Kosyakova N, Klaschka V, Rietz F, Wagner R, et al. Handling small supernumerary marker chromosomes in prenatal diagnostics. Expert Rev Mol Diagn. 2009;9:317–24.
7. Liehr T, Trifonov V, Polityko A, Brecevic L, Mrasek K, Weise A, et al. Characterization of small supernumerary marker chromosomes by a simple molecular and molecular cytogenetics approach. Balkan J Med Genet. 2007;10:33–7.
8. Liehr T. Small Supernumerary Marker Chromosomes (sSMC): A Guide for Human Geneticists and Clinicians. Springer Berlin Heidelberg: Springer; 2012.
9. Bundey S, Hardy C, Vickers S, Kilpatrick MW, Corbett JA. Duplication of the 15q11-13 region in a patient with autism, epilepsy and ataxia. Dev Med Child Neurol. 1994;36:736–42.
10. Burnside RD, Pasion R, Mikhail FM, Carroll AJ, Robin NH, Youngs EL, et al. Microdeletion/microduplication of proximal 15q11.2 between BP1 and BP2: a susceptibility region for neurological dysfunction including developmental and language delay. Hum Genet. 2011;130:517–28.
11. Liehr T, Starke H, Weise A, Lehrer H, Claussen U. Multicolor FISH probe sets and their applications. Histol Histopathol. 2004;19:229–37.
12. Qi M, Zhao Y, Wang Y, Li T. A new small supernumerary marker chromosome involving 14pter – > q12 in a child with severe neurodevelopmental retardation: case report and literature review. Gene. 2013;531:457–61.
13. Balkan M, Isi H, Gedik A, Erdemoglu M, Budak T. A small supernumerary marker chromosome, derived from chromosome 22, possibly associated with repeated spontaneous abortions. Genet Mol Res. 2010;9:1683–9.
14. McDermid HE, Morrow BE. Genomic disorders on 22q11. Am J Hum Genet. 2002;70:1077–88.
15. Stankiewicz P, Bocian E, Jakubow-Durska K, Obersztyn E, Lato E, Starke H, et al. Identification of supernumerary marker chromosomes derived from chromosomes 5, 6, 19, and 20 using FISH. J Med Genet. 2000;37:114–20.
16. Crolla JA. FISH and molecular studies of autosomal supernumerary marker chromosomes excluding those derived from chromosome 15: II. Review of the literature. Am J Med Genet. 1998;75:367–81.
17. Mrasek K, Starke H, Liehr T. Another small supernumerary marker chromosome (sSMC) derived from chromosome 2: towards a genotype/ phenotype correlation. J Histochem Cytochem. 2005;53:367–70.
18. Wolff DJ, Van Dyke DL, Powell CM, Working Group of the ALQAC. Laboratory guideline for Turner syndrome. Genet Med. 2010;12:52–5.
19. Oliveira RM, Verreschi IT, Lipay MV, Eca LP, Guedes AD, Bianco B. Y chromosome in Turner syndrome: review of the literature. Sao Paulo Med J. 2009;127:373–8.
20. Starke H, Nietzel A, Weise A, Heller A, Mrasek K, Belitz B, et al. Small supernumerary marker chromosomes (SMCs): genotype-phenotype correlation and classification. Hum Genet. 2003;114:51–67.
21. Melo JB, Backx L, Vermeesch JR, Santos HG, Sousa AC, Kosyakova N, et al. Chromosome 5 derived small supernumerary marker: towards a genotype/ phenotype correlation of proximal chromosome 5 imbalances. J Appl Genet. 2011;52:193–200.
22. Warburton D. De novo balanced chromosome rearrangements and extra marker chromosomes identified at prenatal diagnosis: clinical significance and distribution of breakpoints. Am J Hum Genet. 1991;49:995–1013.

9

Isolation and characterization of chromosomal markers in *Poa pratensis*

Yanyan Zhao, Feng Yu, Ruijuan Liu and Quanwen Dou*[iD]

Abstract

Background: *Poa pratensis* L. is a turf grass and forage crop used worldwide. Being a facultative apomictic species, *P. pratensis* has a highly variable chromosome number. Chromosomal markers constitute a powerful tool for chromosome identification and for various aspects of genomic research. However, currently, no chromosomal markers are available for *P. pratensis*.

Results: Four novel chromosome markers were isolated from a screen of Cot-1 DNA libraries, combined with fluorescence in situ hybridization (FISH) in *Poa pratensis*. Three tandemly repetitive sequences (*Pp*TR-1, *Pp*TR-2, and *Pp*TR-3) were characterized as subtelomeric. Monomers of 318 bp, 189 bp and 189 bp were identified in *Pp*TR-1, *Pp*TR-2, and *Pp*TR-3, respectively. One tandemly repetitive sequence (*Pp*CR-1) was shown to be centromeric or pericentromeric, and it had a monomer of 27 bp. The distribution patterns of *Pp*TR-1, *Pp*TR-2, and *Pp*TR-3 were highly conserved across different *P. pratensis* cultivars and in the distantly related *Poa* species, whereas *Pp*CR-1 was conserved across different *P. pratensis* cultivars, but less conserved across *Poa* species.

Conclusion: In this study, we report the identification and characterization of four novel chromosomal markers in *P. pratensis*. These chromosomal markers are powerful tools for accurate assessment of chromosome count, genomic and phylogenetic analyses, as well as studies of apomixis in *P. pratensis*.

Keywords: *Poa pratensis*, Repetitive sequence, Chromosomal markers

Background

Poa pratensis L. (Kentucky bluegrass), which belongs to the *Gramineae* family, is a perennial herbaceous plant with strong regenerative ability, high fecundity, cold resistance, drought tolerance, and rapid colonization [1]. It is used worldwide as a temperate turf grass and forage crop [2, 3]. Through facultative apomixis, this species can propagate diverse and odd ploidy levels, resulting in a wide range of chromosome numbers [4–6].

Traditionally, the ploidy levels in *Poa* were determined by conducting chromosome counts of root tip cells. However, given their relatively small size, high preponderance and morphological similarity, the chromosome number of *P. pratensis* is difficult to accurately quantify [7]. Flow cytometry is the commonly used method for the measurement of DNA content in somatic cells of *P. pratensis* to determine the ploidy level [8]. This approach has been used effectively in *P. pratensis* as an accurate method to evaluate ploidy level in a large number of individual plants [9, 10]. However, quantification of chromosome counts would still be indispensable, particularly, if confirmation of ploidy level is required [11].

The repetitive sequences are commonly used as probes in FISH (fluorescence in situ hybridization) assay for various applications, including identification of individual chromosomes, study of karyotype evolution, and screening for chromosome aberrations [12–14]. Among the 10 tested repetitive sequences, pTa535 was shown to be the most valuable, allowing A-genome chromosome identification and species discrimination across different diploid and polyploid wheat [12]. *Brachypodium pinnatum* chromosomes could be accurately identified using rDNA-based and species-crossing BAC-based FISH probes [13]. However, to date, no information on chromosomal markers is available for *P. pratensis*.

Cot-1 DNA is enriched with highly and moderately repetitive sequences. The labelled Cot-1 DNA could be used (as a probe) to localize heterochromatin in chromosomes

* Correspondence: douqw@nwipb.cas.cn
Key Laboratory of Adaptation and Evolution of Plateau Biota, Northwest Institute of Plateau Biology, the Chinese Academy of Sciences, Xining 810008, China

[14]. A number of previous studies have shown that chromosomal markers could be developed through construction and screening of Cot-1 libraries [15–18]. For example, 11 tandemly repetitive sequences were identified from a Cot-1 library by FISH, followed by sequence analysis of alfalfa (*Medicago sativa*), and this approach was shown to be the most accurate to identify alfalfa chromosomes [18].

In this study, we first constructed a *P. pratensis* Cot-1 library and subsequently conducted FISH screening with labelled clones on mitotic chromosomes. The clones showing strong hybridization signals were further investigated and several distinct chromosomal markers were identified. In this paper, we discuss the application of these chromosomal markers for the determination of ploidy level, assessment of genome composition, phylogenetic analysis, and identification of different types of apomixis.

Methods

Plant materials

Three local *Poa* cultivars and five introduced *P. pratensis* cultivars were used in this study (Table 1). Seeds were germinated at room temperature. The germinated plants were transplanted to the pots and grown at 20 °C in an artificial climate chamber with 12 h light and 12 h darkness.

Cot-1 DNA library construction

The procedure for Cot-1 DNA library construction was adopted from Yu et al. [18], with minor modifications. Genomic DNA of *P. pratensis* 'Qinghai' was autoclaved at 120 °C for 8 min and digested with S1 nuclease for 18 min 50 S. Thereafter, the fragmented DNA was enriched for 100-bp to 400-bp fragments. Subsequently, purified Cot-1 DNA fragments were ligated into the pGEM-T easy vector. Transformed *E. coli* cells (DH5α) were identified by blue/white screening, as per the manufacturer's instructions.

Table 1 Materials used in this study

No.	Cultivar	Source
1	*P. pratensis* 'Qinghai'	Qinghai, China
2	Park	Jacklin, USA
3	Geronimo	DLF-pickseeds, USA
4	Rhythm	DLF-pickseeds, USA
5	Midnight	DLF-pickseeds,USA
6	Kentucky	Jacklin, USA
7	*P. pratensis* var. *anceps* 'Qinghai'	Qinghai, China
8	*P. crymophila* 'Qinghai'	Qinghai, China

Probe preparation

The 5S rDNA was amplified by polymerase chain reaction (PCR) using genomic DNA of *P. pratensis*, as described by Fukui et al. [19]. Inserts of the candidate clones from the constructed Cot-1 library were amplified by PCR, using T7 and SP6 primers. Purified PCR products of 5S rDNA and clone inserts were labelled with tetramethyl-rhodamine-5-dUTP (red) or fluorescein-12-dUTP (green) (Roche Diagnostics) by a random primer labelling method, described by Dou et al. [20]. The pWrrn (clone which contains fragments of wheat 45S rDNA) provided by Professor Tsujimoto (Tottori University, Japan) were labelled by a nick-translation method.

Chromosome preparation

Root tips, with a length of approximately 1–2 cm, were excised and pre-treated in ice-cold water at 0 °C for 24 h, and fixed in ethanol:glacial acetic acid (3:1, v/v) for 24 h at room temperature. Each root tip was squashed in a drop of 45% acetic acid. The slides were kept at -80 °C in the Ultra-low temperature freezer for more than half an hour.

FISH and microphotometry

FISH experiments were carried out as described by Dou et al. [20], with minor modifications. Samples on prepared slides were denatured in 0.2 M NaOH in 70% ethanol at room temperature for 10 min, rinsed in 100% cold ethanol (stored at minus 20 °C) for approximately 30 min, and allowed to air dry. The hybridization was carried out at 37 °C overnight in 10 uL of a mixture containing 10–15 ng of each labeled DNA probe, 5–10 mg of sonicated salmon sperm DNA, 50% formamide, 2 × SSC, and 10% dextran sulfate. After hybridization, the cover glass was removed gently, and the slide was washed with distilled water at room temperature. Chromosomes were stained with 4',6-diamidino-2-phenylindole (DAPI). Slides were observed using a fluorescence microscope (DM R HC, Leica). Images were captured using a cooled CCD camera (Photometrics CoolSNAP) by means of Meta Imaging System (Universal Imaging Corporation). Finally, the images were optimized by contrast adjustment using Adobe Photoshop 6.0.

DNA sequencing and data analysis

Cot-1 DNA cloned products were sequenced by Sangon Biotech Co., Ltd. (Shanghai, China). The DNAman software package (Lynnon Biosoft, Quebec, Canada) was used to analyse the sequence data. Sequence similarities were queried against the NCBI nucleotide database using BLASTN.

Results

Screening and characterization of Cot-1 clones using FISH

Cot-1 DNA is enriched for highly and moderately repetitive DNA sequences. The Cot-1 DNA clones contained highly repeated DNA sequences that often produced a discernible "block" or "dot" signal on chromosomes when visualized by FISH. Firstly, a total of 396 positive Cot-1 clones were screened from 477 clones. The PCR product sizes of the positive clones ranged from 500 to 300 bp. Secondly, 44 Cot-1 positive clones, which were randomly picked, were amplified by PCR and fluorescently labelled. Subsequently, the fluorescent probes made from the insert fragments were hybridized to *P. pratensis* interphase nuclei and mitotic metaphase chromosomes. The results showed that 14 clones, accounting for 31.8% of those tested, produced distinct "dot" or "block" hybridization signals on the chromosomes. To characterize the signals, we categorized the positive clones into two types, according to their chromosomal distribution (Table 2).

Type 1 showed hybridization signals around the centromere and included 1 clone (7.1%). Type 2 showed hybridization signals on the subtelomeric or telomeric regions; most of the clones (92.3%) belonged to this group.

Sequencing and characterization of the screened clones

All 14 clones that we screened were subjected to sequencing. To characterize the sequences of the inserts, we performed homology searches against the existing nucleotide sequences in the NCBI database. The search results revealed no significant sequence similarities. Sequence comparisons revealed that some screened clones had high homology to each other. Finally, data analysis revealed four unique sequences among the 14 positive clones, namely, clone 1, clone 6, clone 23 and clone 94.

Obtaining whole repetitive monomers

The Cot-1 clones contained partial or complete sequences from the same repetitive sequence family. Thus, it was necessary to perform further experiments to determine the length of the repeated monomers. Additional PCRs were conducted using genomic DNA as the template. The oligonucleotide primer sequences were designed from the sequencing information for clone 6, clone 1, clone 23, and clone 94, using the

Primer Premier 5.0 software (*PREMIER* Biosoft international, Canada) (Table 3). Electrophoresis of the PCR products of each pair of primers showed smearing, along with several intense amplification products (Fig. 1). This result implies a distribution pattern of tandem repeats of each tested monomer in the *P. pratensis* genome. A PCR product library was constructed and clones containing large fragments were sequenced.

A 751-bp PCR fragment was obtained with the primers for clone 6. Sequence analysis revealed 27-bp monomers, which were repeated 25 times. (KY618839, NCBI Gene-Bank)(Additional file 1: Figure S1). Clone 6 hybridized near centromeric regions of *P. pratensis* chromosomes in previous tests. We named this 27 bp repetitive monomer *Pp*CR-1. A 412-bp fragment was obtained with the primers for clone 1. Sequence analysis showed that the amplified fragment included one integrated 318 bp monomer unit and part of the second repeated motif (KY618838, NCBI GeneBank)(Additional file 1: Figure S2). A 698-bp fragment and a 689-bp fragment were obtained with the primers for clone 23 and clone 94, respectively (KY618840 and KY618841 , NCBI GeneBank)(Additional file 1: Figure S3 and S4). Three complete 189-bp monomers and two partial monomers were found in both sequences. Given that clones 1 23 and 94 were characterized as subtelomeric or telomeric in *P. pratensis* chromosomes by FISH, we designated the 318, 189, and 189 bp monomers derived from the aforementioned clones, as *Pp*TR-1, *Pp*TR-2, and *Pp*TR-3, respectively.

Characterization of newly identified tandem repeats on mitotic chromosomes across *P. pratensis* cultivars

FISH analyses revealed that *Pp*CR-1 was physically mapped near centromeric regions, whereas *Pp*TR-1, *Pp*TR-2 and *Pp*TR-3 were mapped to subtelomeric regions on mitotic chromosomes in the *P. pratensis* 'Qinghai' cultivar in a previous test (Fig. 2b and e). Due to the apomixis and diversity of *P. pratensis*, six *P. pratensis* cultivars, the Chinese cultivar *P. pratensis* 'Qinghai', and the American cultivars 'Park', 'Geronimo', 'Rhythm', 'Midnight', and 'Kentucky' were

Table 2 Chromosomal distribution of clones from *P. pratensis* Cot-1 DNA library

FISH pattern	Clone number	Percentage of the total
Type1 (centromeric sites)	6	7.1%
Type2 (subtelomeric sites)	1,23,37,88,90,91,94,153, 155,208,232,236,265	92.3%

Table 3 PCR primers used in monomer amplification in *P.pratensis*

Monomers	Sequence (5– > 3')	Annealing temperature (°C)
Clone 6-F (*Pp*CR-1)R	ACCGTGAACTCTGCGTCG	53
Clone 6-R (*Pp*CR-1)F	TGGACTACCGACGCAGAGTTCAC	
Clone 1-F (*Pp*TR-1)R	AAGTTCTCAAGGTTTTACCTTCACC	55
Clone 1-R (*Pp*TR-1)F	GGACTACCGACGCAGAGTTCA	
Clone 23-F (*Pp*TR-2)R	AATCACGTCTTGTGACCGAG	55
Clone 23-R (*Pp*TR-2)F	GGCTCGGTCACAAGACG	
Clone 94-F (*Pp*TR-3)R	AAATTGATGCTTGACTAGTTGGTGA	53
Clone 94-R (*Pp*TR-3)F	CAGCAAATACACTACTCCAGC	

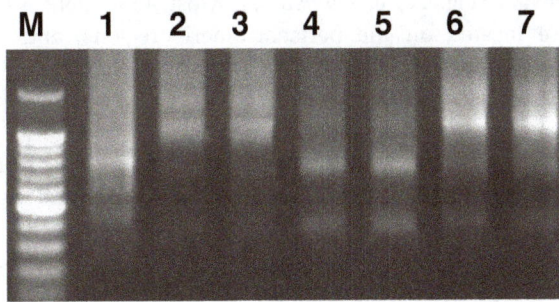

Fig. 1 Patterns of PCR products amplified from designed primers (Table 3). 1, clone 94; 2 and 3, clone 23; 4 and 5, clone 6; 5 and 7, clone 1

examined to assess the extent of evolutionary conservation and variability of the identified repeats between different individuals and across different cultivars. In addition to the four identified repeats, two repetitive DNAs, namely, 5S rDNA and 45S rDNA, which are found universally in plant genomes, were also used in this study as references. Single probes or probe cocktails of different combinations were used for FISH detection on mitotic chromosomes. The distribution information of each repeat was obtained from at least six different individuals of the each tested cultivar.

The repeats, *Pp*TR-1 and *Pp*TR-2, were co-localized in chromosomes of the cultivar 'Qinghai'. Further tests also showed the co-localization of *Pp*TR-1 and *Pp*TR-2 in other *P. pratensis* cultivars (Fig. 2 a). The chromosomal distribution shared between *Pp*TR-1 and *Pp*TR-2 is also shared between different individuals or different cultivars in *P. pratensis*.

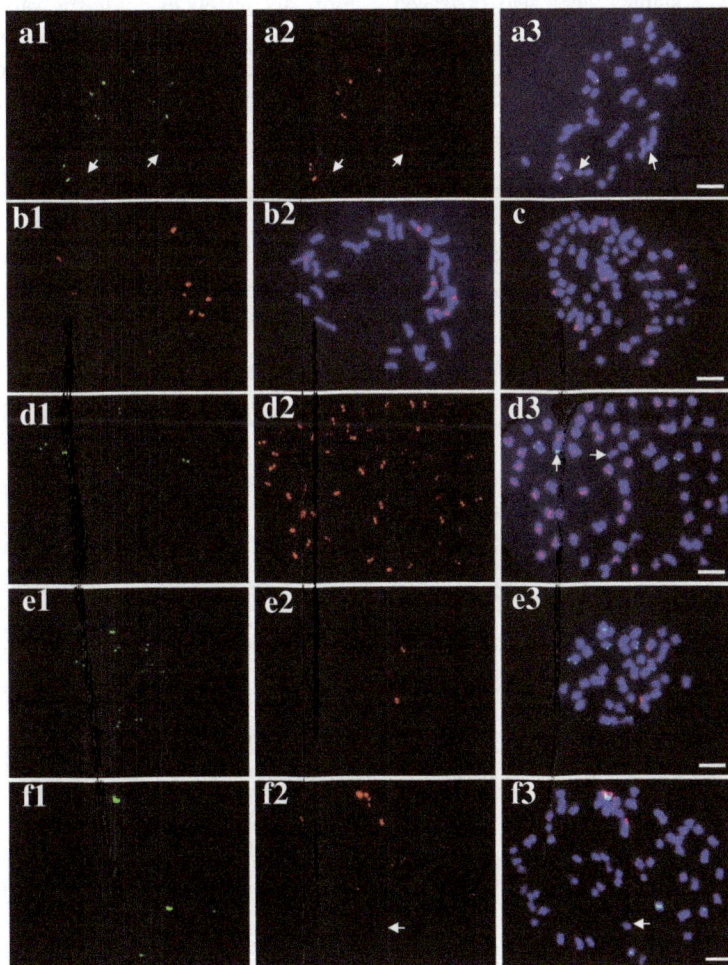

Fig. 2 FISH patterns of mitotic chromosomes of *Poa pratensis* cultivars probed for repetitive sequences: **a1-a3** *Pp*TR-1 (*green*), *Pp*TR-2 (*red*) in 'Park'; **b1-b2** *Pp*CR-1 (*red*) in 'Qinghai'; **c** *Pp*TR-3 (*red*) in 'Midnight'; **d1-d3** *Pp*TR-1 (*green*) and *Pp*CR-1 (*red*) in 'Warrior'; **e1-e3** *Pp*TR-1 (*green*) and *Pp*TR-3 (*red*) in 'Qinghai'; **f1-f3** *Pp*TR-1 (*red*) and 45S rDNA (*green*) in 'Rhythm'. *Arrows* indicate the weak hybridization signals in all, except d3. *Arrows* in d3 indicate chromosomes without *Pp*CR-1 sites. Scale bar =10 μm

The FISH patterns showed that *Pp*CR-1 hybridized on the pericentromeric regions of nearly all chromosomes (chromosomes with hybridization signals corresponding to *Pp*CR-1) across different cultivars, and each targeted chromosome carried only one *Pp*CR-1 hybridization site (Fig. 2 d; Fig. 3b and c). Occasionally, a very small number of chromosomes presenting hybridization signals on the ends of the chromosomes were observed in a few individuals of some cultivars. Because of the highly variable karyotypes of *P. pratensis*, the few chromosomes with a subtelomeric-like distribution of *Pp*CR-1 were mostly telosomic, originating from centromeric fission. Thus, pericentromeric distribution of *Pp*CR-1 in *P. pratensis* was confirmed. The *Pp*TR-1 was physically mapped onto subtelomeric regions of all chromosomes (chromosomes with hybridization signals corresponding to *Pp*TR-1) across different cultivars (Fig. 2d, e, f; Fig. 3a). In most cases, each targeted hybridized chromosome carried a single *Pp*TR-1 site, but one to two chromosomes carrying two *Pp*TR-1 signals were also observed in a few individuals in 'Qinghai' and 'Park'. The single hybridization of *Pp*TR-3 was exclusively detected on the subtelomeric regions of some chromosomes across all

cultivars (Fig. 2c, e; Fig. 3b, d). Most 45S rDNA sites were located on the pericentromeric regions, and 5S rDNA sites were detected in various regions, namely, the pericentromeric, intercalary, or subtelomeric sections across cultivars (Fig. 3c, d).

Highly variable chromosome numbers, ranging from 35 to 112, were observed among individuals and cultivars. The hybridization sites varied from 10 to 89, 7 to 23, and 1 to 23 for *Pp*CR-1, *Pp*TR-1, and *Pp*TR-3, respectively, whereas variable sites from 3 to 11 and 3 to 9 for 45S rDNA and 5S rDNA, respectively, were detected across 6 cultivars (Table 4).

The connection between the number of hybridization sites of each repeat and the variation in total chromosome number was not distinctly revealed due to the complicated facultative apomixis of species of *P. pratensis*. In this study, the percentage of the number of hybridization sites to total chromosome number and the coefficient of variation (CV) were parameters used to more accurately evaluate the variability and conservation of repeat distribution across cultivars. The statistical analyses showed that the cytogenetic characters of 'Qinghai' were significantly different from those of the

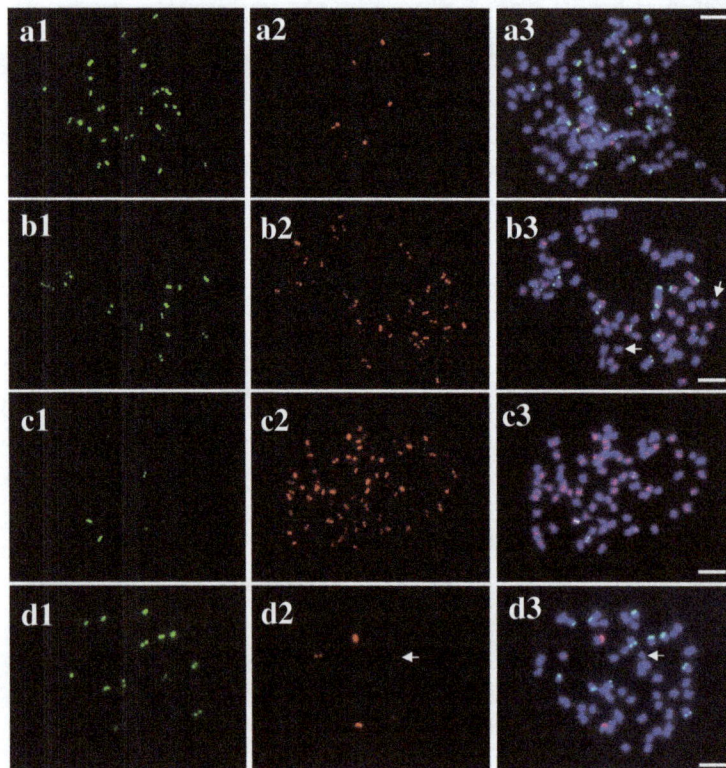

Fig. 3 FISH patterns of mitotic chromosomes of *Poa pratensis* cultivars probed for repetitive sequences: **a1-a3** *Pp*TR-1 (*green*) and 5S rDNA (*red*) in 'Qinghai'; **b1-b3** *Pp*CR-1 (*red*) and *Pp*TR-3 (*green*) in 'Warrior'; **c1-c3** *Pp*CR-1 (*red*) and 45S rDNA (*green*) in 'Park'; **d1-d3** *Pp*TR-3 (*green*) and 5S rDNA (*red*) in 'Kentucky'. *Arrows* in b3 indicates chromosomes without *Pp*CR-1 sites. *Arrows* in d2 and d3 indicate the weak hybridization signals. Scale bar =10 μm

Table 4 Cytogenetic characteristics of *P. pratensis* cultivars and related species

	P. pratensis						Relate species	
	P. pratensis 'Qinghai'	Park	Kentucky	Rhythm	Midnight	Geronimo	P. pratensis var. anceps 'Qinghai'	P. crymophila 'Qinghai'
Chr. No. average	45	60	75	66	70	60	55	28
Chr. No. range	35–112	49–86	52–88	49–98	42–102	32–71	49–63	28
45S sites range (Chr. No. range)	4–8 (35–49)	3–8 (49–86)	5–8 (65–88)	4–9 (56–91)	5–11 (42–102)	3–7 (32–70)	7–9 (49–63)	6–9
5S sites range (Chr. No. range)	5–9 (35–112)	4–8 (49–86)	3–8 (65–84)	4–5 (49–77)	3–8 (42–102)	3–5 (32–70)	6–9 (49–63)	4–5
PpCR-1 sites range (Chr. No. range)	10–19 (32–45)	47–78 (49–79)	69–86 (70–88)	59–89 (63–91)	54–80 (56–84)	45–68 (46–71)	19–24 (49–63)	—
PpTR-1 sites range (Chr. No. range)	12–18 (35–42)	14–23 (49–84)	12–17 (63–85)	11–18 (56–98)	7–16 (56–80)	11–14 (46–71)	5–9 (49–56)	12–18
PpTR-3 range range (Chr. No. range)	1–3 (42–112)	8–20 (49–78)	14–18 (52–81)	12–16 (49–82)	9–17 (50–84)	8–23 (38–70)	2–4 (49–63)	1–2

Chr. Indicates chromosome and No. indicates number

other cultivars (Table 5). The 'Qinghai' cultivar showed the highest percentage of 5S rDNA and *Pp*TR-1 and lowest percentage of *Pp*TR-3, compared with the other cultivars. In addition, the CV of 5S rDNA, *Pp*TR-1, and *Pp*TR-3 in 'Qinghai' were higher than those of the others. These observations are likely due to 'Qinghai' being genetically distant from the other cultivars, and that the samples were collected from wild populations, where nearly no breeding selection was imposed. The percentages of Pp*TR*-1 and Pp*TR*-3 varied from 17.2 to 27.4%, and 18.8 to 26.0%, respectively, while the CV of Pp*TR*-1 and Pp*TR*-3 varied from 7.7 to 18.1% and from 8.6 to 20.0%, respectively, in cultivars from the USA. These results suggest that approximately 20% of all chromosomes in individuals from American cultivars can be estimated to carry hybridization sites for *Pp*TR-1 or *Pp*TR-3. Furthermore, the distribution of *Pp*CR-1 showed the highest percentage, 97.0 to 98.2%, and the lowest CV, 1.3 to 1.7%, across cultivars from the USA. These results imply that nearly 100% of chromosomes carry one *Pp*CR-1 hybridization signal and that the number of *Pp*CR-1 signals can often represent the total chromosome number in individuals of American cultivars.

Characterization of the repeats in *P. pratensis* related species

P. pratensis var. anceps 'Qinghai' presented more similar FISH patterns to *P. pratensis* 'Qinghai' for the tested repeats than to other cultivars (Fig. 4 a, c, e). However, variations between *P. pratensis* 'Qinghai' and *P. pratensis* var. *anceps* 'Qinghai' were still observed. *P. pratensis* 'Qinghai' showed a higher percentage of *Pp*TR-1 and a lower percentage of *Pp*TR-3 than *P. pratensis* var. anceps 'Qinghai' (Table 5).

The cytological characteristics of *P. crymophila* 'Qinghai' were distinctly different from those of *P. pratensis*. The stable chromosome number of 28 identified across the individuals implies that no apomixis occurs in this species (Table 5). Although faint *Pp*CR-1 hybridization signals were occasionally detected in a few chromosomes, clear hybridization sites of *Pp*TR-1 and *Pp*TR-2 were physically mapped exclusively on sub-telomeric regions on a few chromosomes (Fig. 4b, d, f).

Table 5 Statistics results of the percentage of hybridization sites and those of CV across cultivars

	P. pratensis 'Qinghai'	Park	Kentucky	Rhythm	Midnight	Geronimo	P. pratensis var. anceps 'Qinghai'	P. crymophila 'Qinghai'
45S (%)	8.67	9.02	8.42	7.44	12.06	9.28	13.8	26.79
CV(%)	19.07	19.05	11.35	17.71	13.92	9.38	10.71	13.98
5S (%)	13.69	8.29	8.04	7.71	8.12	7.71	11.93	14.88
CV(%)	28.42	17.30	27.54	19.64	16.85	11.29	11.61	9.80
PpCR-1(%)	40.45	98.19	97.08	96.51	97.5	96.96	41.47	—
CV(%)	15.27	1.37	1.57	1.71	1.72	1.73	9.71	
PpTR-1 (%)	37.30	27.41	19.48	18.49	17.17	20.00	13.88	54.17
CV(%)	16.48	7.65	16.15	8.05	18.12	13.25	20.73	13.45
PpTR-3	3.45	18.76	22.43	23.11	20.13	25.93	6.14	4.76
CV(%)	60.52	19.00	15.40	8.55	12.43	19.93	22.6	38.74

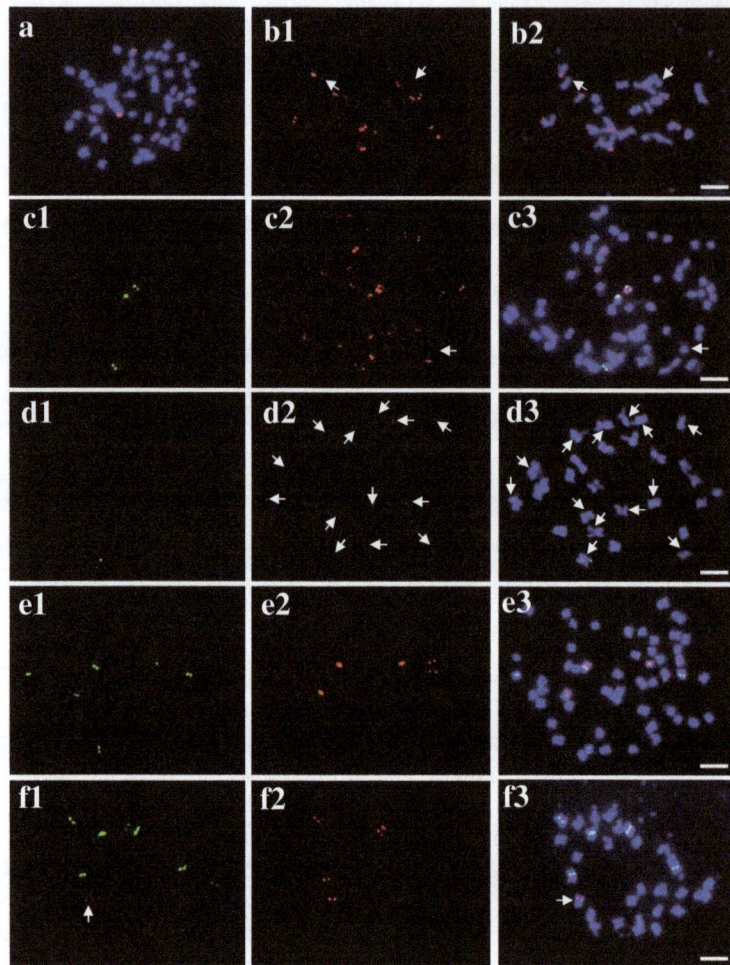

Fig. 4 FISH patterns of mitotic chromosomes of *Poa pratensis* var. anceps 'Qinghai' (a,c and e) and *P. crymophila* 'Qinghai' (b, d, and f) probed with: **a** and **b** *Pp*TR-1 (red); **c** and **d** *Pp*CR-1 (red) + *Pp*TR-3 (green); **e** and **f** 45S rDNA (green) +5S rDNA (red). Arrows indicate the weak hybridization signals. Scale bar =10 μm

Discussion

Variability and conservation of four newly identified chromosomal markers

The repeats *Pp*TR-1, *Pp*TR-2, and *Pp*TR-3 were clearly detected on subtelomeric chromosome regions across different *P. pratensis* cultivars or even other related *Poa* species, although large variations of the number of hybridization signals were identified among cultivars or species. Co-localized distribution was revealed between *Pp*TR-1 and *Pp*TR-2. Co-localization of a few repetitive DNAs was frequently identified in different genomes of the genus *Hordeum* [21, 22]. Although *Pp*TR-3, like *Pp*TR-1 and *Pp*TR-2, was physically mapped in the subtelomeric regions, the discrepancy in the sites between *Pp*TR-3 and *Pp*TR-1 or *Pp*TR-2 implies that their distribution was close rather than intermingled. Furthermore, the exclusive distribution of *Pp*TR-1, *Pp*TR-2 and *Pp*TR-3 not only in the closely related species *P. pratensis* var. *ancep* but also the distantly related species *P. crymophila*

suggests that these sub-telomeric repeats may be highly conserved across different species in the genus *Poa*. A wide distribution of a 120-bp repeat across many different diploid and polyploid species was detected within the Triticeae tribe, and sequence similarity analysis of the repeat suggested that no characteristic genome- or species-specific variants developed during the evolution of the extant genomes [23]. This fact implies that the repeats *Pp*TR-1, *Pp*TR-2 and *Pp*TR-3, being present in the genome of common ancestral species of *Poa*, may have evolved in a similar way as the 120-bp repeat. *Pp*CR-1 is a mini-satellite DNA and was physically mapped at the pericentromeric regions. Plant centromere sequences are characterized by long arrays of highly repetitive satellite sequences that are interspersed frequently with centromeric retrotransposons [24, 25]. In this study, no other repetitive sequences around the centromeres were identified in *P. pratensis*. This result suggests that *Pp*CR-1 may be the main component of the centromeric repetitive sequence. Unlike *Pp*TR-1, *Pp*TR-2 or *Pp*TR-3, *Pp*CR-1 produced only faint and blurry hybridization in the pericentromeric regions of the distantly related species, *P. crymophila*. It can be inferred that *Pp*CR-1 may be more species-specific and may have evolved more rapidly than the subtelomeric repeats.

Chromosome counting assisted by chromosomal markers

The chromosome number of *P. pratensis* is highly variable, with polyploidy and aneuploidy ranging from $2n = 28$ to 154 [3–7]. The overlapped or agglomerated chromosomes in a mitotic chromosome-spread always make chromosome counting difficult, particularly for high-ploidy samples. Ideal chromosomal markers that are highly correlated with chromosome number would facilitate accurate chromosome counting. In this study, chromosomes with *Pp*TR-1, *Pp*TR-2, and *Pp*TR-3 were proportionally detected across different *P. pratensis*. Although total chromosome numbers could be estimated using the number of the chromosomal markers, the variability in relative percentages reduces accuracy. *Pp*CR-1 was detected in nearly all chromosomes (in more than 96% of all chromosomes) in all investigated cultivars except *P. pratensis* 'Qinghai', and *Pp*CR-1 exhibited the lowest percentage of variation. This result suggests that the total chromosome number can be accurately determined by counting *Pp*CR-1 hybridization signals. *Pp*CR-1 is a useful chromosomal marker for chromosome number determination in *P. pratensis*.

Phylogenetic and genome research with chromosomal markers

A basic genome with a chromosome number of seven was determined in *P. pratensis*, despite a highly variable number of chromosomes [6]. Observation of the occurrence of apomixis and the presence of "group segregation" in *P. pratensis* in Missouri, USA suggested an allopolyploid origin of the species [26]. Analysis of chloroplast and nuclear gene sequence data supports the idea that *P. pratensis* is, at least, partly allopolyploid [27]. In this study, *P. pratensis* from Qinghai, China, showed distinctly fewer *Pp*CR-1 and *Pp*TR-3 sites, compared with cultivars from the USA. This result implies a possible large genomic divergence between these cultivars. The genome composition of Qinghai *P. pratensis* presents as more likely to be allopolyploid than those of cultivars from the USA. This observation means that the ability to produce polyploidy with facultative apomictic reproduction may make the genome composition of *P. pratensis* more diverse and complex. Chromosomal markers, using comparative FISH analyses, would be helpful in elucidating plant genome composition in phylogenetic analysis. Comparative karyotyping of *Brachypodium pinnatum* was done using cross- species BAC-FISH [13]. Phylogenetic relationship of A genome between diploid and tetraploid wheat was exclusively uncovered by identification of all A-genome chromosomes, using a set of chromosomal markers [12]. Thus, comparative cytogenetic analysis of the many other *Poa* species using the chromosomal markers identified in this study may provide valuable information about the origin of *P. pratensis*.

Evaluation of reproductive mode and analysis of inheritance of apomixis assisted by chromosomal markers

Poa pratensis has been described as an aposporous and pseudogamous facultative apomictic species [28]. Flow cytometry analysis has revealed that five routes of seed formation and four reproductive pathways define the reproductive mode of *P. pratensis* plants in *P. pratensis* cultivars and core accessions [10, 29]. The inheritance of apomixis in *P. pratensis* has been confirmed in a five-locus model with differences in gene expressivity and penetrance [30]. However, which individual gene is linked to apospory and/or parthenogenesis still remains elusive. Despite their small size and high count, the identification of these chromosomes could be greatly improved using newly identified chromosomal markers, combined with 5S rDNA and 45S rDNA. This fact suggests that the reproductive mode of *P. pratensis* plants can be molecularly and cytogenetically studied by comparing the cytotypes of the parents and progeny, and apomictic inheritance analysis may be aided by finding apomixis-associated chromosomes or chromosome regions.

Conclusions

In this study, we report four novel chromosome markers that were developed by screening Cot-1 DNA libraries, combined with FISH assay in *Poa pratensis*. Three (*Pp*TR-1, *Pp*TR-2, and *Pp*TR-3) were characterized as subtelomeric, and one (*Pp*CR-1) was centromeric or pericentromeric. The chromosomal markers, *Pp*TR-1, *Pp*TR-2, and *Pp*TR-3, were stably detected across different *P. pratensis* cultivars and in the distantly related *Poa* species. However, *Pp*CR-1 was conserved across various *P. pratensis* cultivars but less conserved across *Poa* species. These chromosomal markers will be powerful tools for chromosome counting, genomic and phylogenetic analyses, and studies of apomixis in *P. pratensis*.

Abbreviations
CR: Centromeric repeat; *Pp*: *Poa pratensis*; TR: Telomeric repeat

Acknowledgements
Not applicable.

Funding
This research was sponsored by the Agricultural Science and Technology Achievements Transformation and Promotion Plan of Qinghai (no. 2013-N-515) and the Natural Science Foundation of Qinghai Province (no. 2015-ZJ-903).

Authors' contributions

QD: Designed the study; wrote the manuscript. YZ: Performed most of the experiments; corrected the manuscript; FY,RL: Participated in the experiments; corrected the manuscript. All authors read and approved the final version of the manuscript.

Competing interests

The authors declare that they have no competing interests.

References

1. Soreng RJ, Barrie FR. Proposal to conserve the name *Poa pratensis* (Gramineae) with a conserved type. Taxon. 1999;48:57–159.
2. Balasko JA, Evers GW, Duell RW. Bluegrasses, ryegrasses, and bentgrasses. In: Barnes BF, Miller DA, Nelson CJ, Collins M, Moore KJ, editors. Forages. Vol. 1. An introduction to grassland agriculture forages. Ames: Iowa State Univ. Press; 1995. p. 357–71.
3. Huff DR. Kentucky bluegrass. In: Casler MD, Duncan RR, editors. Turfgrass biology, genetics, and breeding. NJ: Wiley; 2003. p. 27–38.
4. Akerberg E. Apomictic and sexual seed formation in *Poa pratensis* L. Hereditas. 1939;25:359–70.
5. Grazi F, Umaerus M, Akerberg E. Observations on the mode of reproduction and the embryology of *Poa pratensis* L. Hereditas. 1961;47:489–541.
6. Müntzing A. Apomictic and sexual seed production in *Poa*. Hereditas. 1933; 17:131–54.
7. Speckmann GJ, Van Dijk GE. Chromosome number and plant morphology in some ecotypes of *Poa pratensis* L. Euphytica. 1972;21(2):171–80.
8. Arumuganathan K, Earle ED. Estimation of nuclear DNA contents of plants by flow cytometry. Plant Mol Biol Rep. 1991;9:229–41.
9. Eaton TD, Curley J, Williamson RC, Jung G. Determination of the level of variation in polyploidy among Kentucky bluegrass cultivars by means of flow cytometry. Crop Sci. 2004;44(6):2168–74.
10. Wieners RR, Fei S, Johnson RC. Characterization of a USDA Kentucky bluegrass (*Poa pratensis* L.) core collection for reproductive mode and DNA content by flow cytometry. Gen Res Crop Evol. 2006;53:1531–41.
11. Kelley AM, Johnson PG, Waldron BL, et al. A Survey of apomixis and ploidy Levels among Poa L. (Poaceae) using flow cytometry. Crop Sci. 2009;49(4): 1395–402.
12. Badaeva ED, Amosova AV, Goncharov NP, Macas J, Ruban AS, Grechishnikova IV, et al. A set of cytogenetic markers allows the precise identification of all A-genome chromosomes in diploid and polyploid wheat. Cytogenet Genome Res. 2015;146(1):71–9.
13. Wolny E, Fidyk W, Hasterok R. Karyotyping of *Brachypodium pinnatum* (2 n = 18) chromosomes using cross-species BAC–FISH. Genome. 2013;56(4):239–43.
14. Breda E, Wolny E, Hasterok R. Intraspecific polymorphism of ribosomal DNA loci number and morphology in *Brachypodium pinnatum* and *Brachypodium sylvaticum*. Cell Mol Biol Lett. 2012;17(4):526–41.
15. Zwick MS, Hanson RE, Islam-Faridi MN, Stelly DM, Wing RA, Price HJ, McKnight TD. A rapid procedure for the isolation of C0t-1 DNA from plants. Genome. 1997;40:138–42.
16. Begum R, Alam SS, Menzel G, Schmidt T. Comparative molecular cytogenetics of major repetitive sequence families of three *Dendrobium* species (Orchidaceae) from Bangladesh. Ann Bot. 2009;104:863–72.
17. Zhang L, Xu C, Yu W. Cloning and characterization of chromosomal markers from a Cot-1 library of peanut (*Arachis hypogaea* L.). Cytogenet Genome Res. 2012;137:31–41.
18. Yu F, Lei Y, Li Y, Dou Q, Wang H, Chen Z. Cloning and characterization of chromosomal markers in alfalfa (*Medicago sativa* L.). Theor Appl Genet. 2013;126(7):1885–96.
19. Fukui K, Kamisugi Y, Sakai F. Physical mapping of 5S rDNA loci by direct-cloned biotinylated probes in barley chromosomes. Genome. 1994;37:105–11.
20. Dou QW, Chen ZG, Liu YA, Tsujimoto H. High frequency of karyotype variation revealed by sequential FISH and GISH in plateau perennial grass forage *Elymus nutans*. Breed Sci. 2009;59:651–6.
21. Cuadrado A, Jouve N. The nonrandom distribution of long clusters of all possible classes of trinucleotide repeats in barley chromosomes. Chromosom Res. 2007;15(6):711–20.
22. Dou Q, Liu R, Yu F. Chromosomal organization of repetitive DNAs in *Hordeum bogdanii* and *H. brevisubulatum* (Poaceae). Comp Cytogenet. 2016; 10(4):465–81.
23. Contento A, Heslop-Harrison JS, Schwarzacher T. Diversity of a major repetitive DNA sequence in diploid and polyploid Triticeae. Cytogenet Genome Res. 2005;109(1-3):34–42.
24. Cheng Z, Dong F, Langdon T, Ouyang S, Buell CR, Gu M, Blattner FR, Jiang J. Functional rice centromeres are marked by a satellite repeat and a centromere-specific retrotransposon. Plant Cell. 2002;14:1691–704.
25. Jin W, Melo JR, Nagaki K, Talbert PB, Henikoff S, Dawe RK, Jiang J. Maize centromeres: organization and functional adaptation in the genetic background of oat. Plant Cell. 2004;16:571–81.
26. Brown WL. Chromosome complements of five species of *Poa* with an analysis of variation in *Poa pratensis*. Am J Bot. 1939;6:717–23.
27. Patterson JT, Larson SR, Johnson PG. Genome relationships in polyploid Poa pratensis and other Poa species inferred from phylogenetic analysis of nuclear and chloroplast DNA sequences. Genome. 2005;48(1):76–87.
28. Müntzing A. Further study on apomixis and sexuality in *Poa*. Hereditas. 1940;26:115–90.
29. Matzk F, Meister A, Schubert I. An efficient screen for reproductive pathways using mature seeds of monocots and dicots. Plant J. 2000;21(1):97–108.
30. Matzk F, Prodanovic S, Bäumlein H, Schubert I. The inheritance of apomixis in *poa pratensis* confirms a five locus model with differences in gene expressivity and penetrance. Plant Cell. 2005;17(1):13–24.

10

Preferential Y-Y pairing and synapsis and abnormal meiotic recombination in a 47,XYY man with non obstructive azoospermia

Caiyun Wu[1,2†], Liu Wang[3,4†], Furhan Iqbal[3,5], Xiaohua Jiang[3,4], Ihtisham Bukhari[3,4], Tonghang Guo[6], Gengxin Yin[7], Howard J. Cooke[3,4], Zhenyi Cao[2], Hong Jiang[1,2*] and Qinghua Shi[3,4*]

Abstract

Back ground: Men with 47, XYY syndrome are presented with varying physical attributes and degrees of infertility. Little information has been documented regarding the meiotic progression in patients with extra Y chromosome along with the synapses and recombination between the two Y chromosomes.

Methods: Spermatocyte spreading and immunostaining were applied to study the behavior of the extra Y chromosome during meiosis I in an azoospermia patient with 47, XYY syndrome and results were compared with five healthy controls with proven fertility.

Results: The extra Y chromosome was present in all the studied spermatocytes of the patient and preferentially paired and synapsed with the other Y chromosome. Consistently, gamma-H2AX staining completely disappeared from the synapsed regions of Y chromosomes. More interestingly, besides recombination on short arms, recombination on the long arms of Y chromosomes was also observed. No pairing and synapsis defects between homologous autosomes were detected, while significantly reduced recombination frequencies on autosomes were observed in the patient. The meiotic prophase I progression was disturbed with significantly increased proportion of leptotene, zygotene cells and decreased pachytene spermatocytes in the patient when compared with the controls.

Conclusions: These findings highlight the importance of studies on meiotic behaviors in patients with an abnormal chromosomal constitution and provide an important framework for future studies, which may elucidate the impairment caused by extra Y chromosome in mammalian meiosis and fertility.

Keywords: Sex chromosomes, Meiosis, Meiotic sex chromosome inactivation (MSCI), XYY syndrome

Background

The 47,XYY sex chromosome variation is the most common sex chromosome anomaly after Klinefelter syndrome [1–3], occurring in approximately 1 out of 1000 live male births [4]. To account for the increased proportion of paternally derived 47,XXY males as compared to other trisomies it has been suggested that the XY bivalent, with its reduced region of homology, is particularly susceptible to non-disjunction [5]. Paternal non-disjunction at meiosis II resulting in sperm with an extra Y chromosome produces a 47,XYY karyotype in the affected offspring. Majority of the patients with 47,XYY have a delayed diagnosis, with a median age of 17.1 years at diagnosis [6]. Although most XYY boys have no phenotypic abnormalities, they are at greater risk for behavioral problems, mild learning disability, delayed speech/language development and usually with a tall stature [2].

* Correspondence: jiangh105@sina.com; qshi@ustc.edu.cn
†Equal contributors
1The Reproductive Medicine Center, Clinical College of People's Liberation Army Affiliated to Anhui Medical University, Hefei, Anhui, China
3Molecular and Cell Genetics Laboratory, The CAS Key Laboratory of Innate Immunity and Chronic Diseases, Hefei National Laboratory for Physical Sciences at Microscale, School of Life Sciences, University of Science and Technology of China, Hefei, Anhui 230027, China
Full list of author information is available at the end of the article

An association between 47,XYY and fertility problems has been reported in several studies with an increased incidence of chromosomally abnormal spermatozoa in the semen of men with 47,XYY syndrome [7–13]. This greater prevalence of hyper haploid sperm results in an increased risk of passing the extra Y chromosome to offspring [2]. Men with 47,XYY syndrome can have variable sperm counts, ranging from normal to azoospermia [2, 10, 14–16].

Considerable attention has been given to the somatic abnormalities associated with 47,XYY conditions but less is known about their meiotic behaviors; that is, how sex chromosome imbalance influence the meiotic progression, and homologous pairing, synapsis and recombination. In this study, we applied Immnunofluorescence technique to study meiosis in a 47, XYY patient. We used immunostaining of SYCP3 and SYCP1 to study the sex chromosome configurations, MLH1 to detect recombination and γH2AX to determine meiotic sex chromosome inactivation (MSCI) in pachytene cells from the testis of our 47,XYY patient. We observed that the extra Y chromosome was present in all the studied spermatocytes of the patient, preferentially paired and synapsed with another Y chromosome, and associated with X chromosome, which may have affected the meiotic prophase I progression.

Methods

Patient and karyotype analysis

A 27 year old male was presented to Provincial Hospital affiliated with Anhui Medical University, Hefei, Anhui, People's Republic of China. Semen analysis was carried out according to World Health Organization (WHO laboratory manual for the examination of human semen and semen-cervical interaction, 2010) and no sperm were observed in his semen. After obtaining written informed consent, testicular tissues were sampled from the patient. Five fertile men of Han ethnicity having at least one healthy child were recruited as normal controls for this study, and similar experiments were performed on them as mentioned for the patient. All the procedures of this study were approved by the institutional review board and ethical committee of the University of Science and Technology of China.

Histological analysis

Testicular tissues were fixed overnight in 4 % PFA for histological examination. Serial testicular sections were made and positioned on microscope slides, stained with hematoxylin and eosin for histopathology analysis.

Spermatocyte spreading and immunostaining

Testicular tissues were processed as we described previously [17, 18]. Rabbit anti-SYCP3 (Abcam, Cambridge, UK), human anti-CREST (Immunovision, Springdale, AR), mouse anti-MLH1 (BD Pharmingen Biosciences,

San Diego, CA), mouse anti-γ-H2AX (Millipore, Billerica, MA) and Goat anti-SYCP1 (SantaCruz Biotechnology, CA, USA) were used as primary antibodies. These antibodies were detected using the following secondary antibodies: Alexa 555 donkey anti-rabbit (Molecular Probes, Carlsbad, CA), Alexa 488 goat anti-mouse (Molecular Probes, Carlsbad, CA), Alexa 488 donkey anti-goat (Molecular Probes, Carlsbad, CA), Alexa 488 donkey anti-mouse (Molecular Probes, Carlsbad, CA) and 1-amino-4-methyl-coumarin-3-acetic acid (AMCA) donkey anti-human (Jackson Immunoresearch, West Grove, PA), respectively.

Fluorescence in situ hybridization (FISH)

To identify the Y chromosomes in spermatocytes,,FISH was performed as we previously reported on the spermatocyte spreads immunostained for meiotic analyses in previous experiments using a DNA probe specific to the long arm of human Y chromosome(A generous gift from Professor Mingrong Wang, Cancer Institute and Hospital, Chinese Academy of Medical Sciences, Beijing, China). The Y probe was labeled with Spectrum Green dUTP (Vysis, 02N32-050) using a nick translation procedure following the manufacturer's instructions. After the cover slips were moved, the slides were washed in PBS for 5 min, followed by dehydration in ethanol grades (70, 80, 90 and 100 %). After drying, the probes were added to the slides, co-denatured on a hotplate at 80 °C for 10 min and then the slides were incubated overnight in a humid chamber. Cover slips were moved and slides were washed in 0.4XSSC/0.3%NP-40 at 45°Cfor 45 min followed by 2XSSC/0.1 % NP-40 for 20 min at room temperature. After air drying in the dark, antifade and cover slips were added to the slides. Cells were analysed and imaged using an epifluorescence microscope Olympus BX61 (Olympus Inc., Tokyo, Japan) and Image Pro-Plus version 5.1 software (Media Cybernetics Inc., Bethesda, MD).

Statistical analysis

Statistical analyses were performed using SPSS 13.0 software (SPSS Inc., Chicago, IL). A chi-square test was applied to compare the meiotic progression between the patient and controls. The Mann–Whitney test was applied for the comparison of MLH1 foci per cell between the patient and controls.

Results

Analysis of the semen revealed that the patient was suffering from azoospermia. Karyotyping on G-banded metaphases of peripheral blood lymphocytes revealed a karyotype of 47, XYY in all the 100 studied cells of the patient. FISH using a DNA probe specific to human Y chromosome on spermatocyte spreads indicated that all the 71 analyzed pachytene spermatocytes had a XYY constitution (Fig. 1).

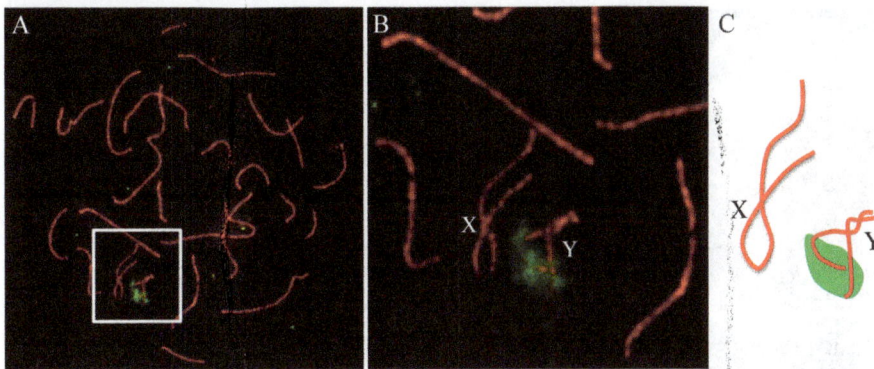

Fig. 1 The extra Y chromosome was present in spermatocytes of the 47, XYY patient. **a** Image of a representative pachytene spermatocyte immunostained for SYCP3 (*Red*) showed two partially paired Y chromosomes identified by FISH using a DNA probe specific to the q arm of human Y chromosome (*Green*). **b** Enlarged area from A. **c** A schematic configuration of the sex chromosomes from the cell shown in **a** and **b**

Prevalence of YY pairing and XY association in spermatocytes of the 47, XYY patient

A total of 71 pachytene spermatocytes were analyzed for the pairing between homologous chromosomes. No abnormalities in pairing between homologous autosomes were observed in all the cells analyzed. For sex chromosomes, 42 out of 71 (or 59.2 %) cells showed pairing in whole Yp and partial Yq, while in the remaining 29 (or 40.8 %) cells the pairing extended to the whole length of Y chromosomes (Fig. 2; Table 1). Notably, in none of the studied pachytene cells, X was found to pair with Y (Fig. 2; Table 1).

In more than 62.1 % spermatocytes analyzed, the Y chromosomes were found to be associated with X chromosome (Table 1). There was no significant difference in the frequency of cells showing XY association between partially and completely paired YY-containing cells (Table 1). In all the 45 spermatocytes displaying XY association, 36 (or 80 %), 3 (or 7 %) and 6 (or 13 %) cells showed an association of Xp with Yp, Xp with Yq and Xq with Yq, respectively.

Abnormal sex chromosome synapsis the 47, XYY patient

To detect synapsis between homologous chromosomes, SYCP1, a central element of synaptonemal complexes, were detected by immunostaining in pachytene spermatocyte spreads of the 47,XYY patient (Fig. 3). In all the 71 spermatocytes analyzed, no synapsis defects were observed for autosomes. For the two Y chromosomes, partialand complete synapsis was observed in 52 and 19 studied spermatocytes, respectively (Table 3). Higher frequency of Y-Y synapsis was observed in those spermatocytes where Y chromosomes were found associated with X chromosomes in all the 45 studied spermatocytes (Table 3). X chromosome was found associated with the Y chromosomes in 45 of the studied spermatocytes but synapses of X with Y chromosome was not observed in any of the studied pachytene spermatocytes (Fig. 3).

Reduced recombination on sex chromosomes and autosomes of the 47, XYY patient

In order to determine effects of presence of two Y chromosomes on recombination during meiosis, the MLH1 foci, the meiotic recombination markers, were counted in pachytene spermatocytes of the patient. All the 65 spermatocytes with partial or complete YY synapsis were analyzed. Recombination between two the Y chromosomes was observed in 27 out of 65 or 41.5 % cells. In spermatocytes with partial YY synapsis, recombination was observed to occur between the two Yp in 21 out of 47 (or 44.7 %) cells (Fig. 2; Table 2), while in those with complete YY synapsis, recombination between the two Yp was seen as expected but at a lower frequency (4 out of 18, or 22.2 %, Table 2). More interestingly, recombination between the two Yq was also observed in 2 out of 18 (or 11.1 %) spermatocytes with complete YY synapsis (Fig. 4; Table 2). It was noted that the frequency of recombination between Yp arms was higher when two Y chromosomes were partially synapsed. More strikingly, MLH1 foci were not detected on remaining 38 cells although the two Y chromosomes were synapsed (Fig. 2; Table 2).

Recombination frequency of autosomes in the 47, XYY patient was determined in71 pachytene spermatocytes and compared to those in 437 spermatocytes from five controls. The mean number of MLH1 foci per cell in the patient was significantly lower than those in the controls (44.9 ± 4.6, vs.48.1 ± 5.8; $P < 0.001$, Mann–Whitney test).

Meiotic sex chromosome inactivation (MSCI) in the 47, XYY, male

It has been documented that the chromosome or chromosome's regions that had not experienced synapsis undergo inactivation and are decorated by γ-H2AX signals in spermatocytes [19, 20]. We immunostained mid-late pachytene spermatocytes of the patient and controls for the meiotic sex chromosome inactivation (MSCI) marker,

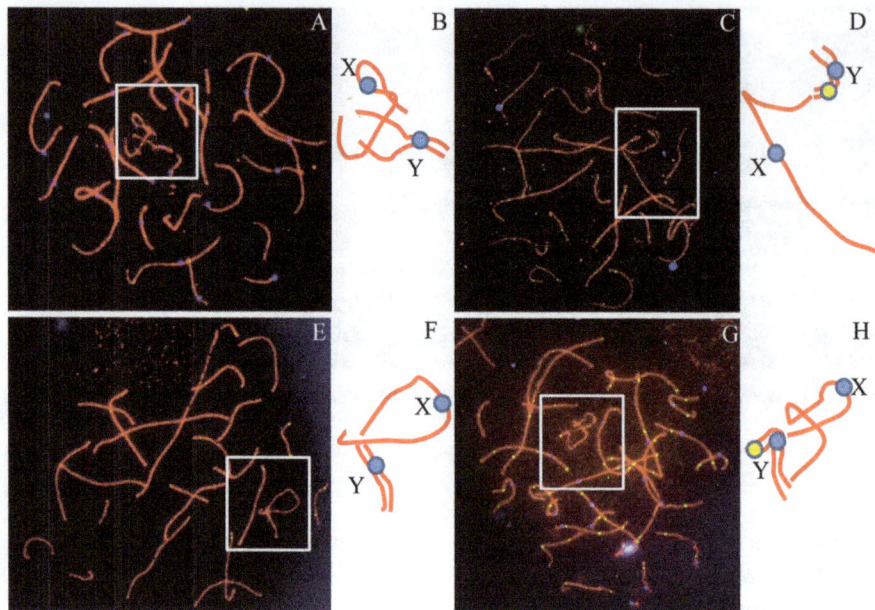

Fig. 2 Sex chromosome pairing and recombination in the 47, XYY patient. Representative pachytene spermatocytes immunostained for CREST (*Blue*), SYCP3 (*Red*) and MLH1 (*Green*). **a** Two Y chromosomes partially paired and associated with X chromosome. There is no recombination on the sex chromosomes. **c** Two Y chromosomes partially paired and associated with chromosome X. Notably there is a recombination focus on the short arm of Y bivalent. **e** Two Y chromosomes completely paired and associated with X chromosome at the end of short arms. Notably there is no recombination on the sex chromosomes. **g** Two Y chromosomes completely paired and associated with chromosome X. Notably there is a recombination focus on the short arm of Y bivalent. **b**, **d**, **f** and **h** are the schematic configurations of the sex chromosomes from the cell shown in **a**, **c**, **e** and **g**, respectively

phosphorylated H2AX (γH2AX), and the axial element protein SYCP3. In spermatocytes where two Y chromosomes were partially synapsed, γ-H2AX signals were detected around unsynapsed regions of two Y chromosomes and X chromosomes as expected (Fig. 4a-d). Interestingly, the γ-H2AX signals were only visible only on X chromosome in the spermatocytes where two Y chromosomes were completely paired and synapsed (Fig. 4e-g). These results indicate that synapsis can indeed occur between the two Y chromosomes.

Meiotic progression was disturbed in 47, XYY male

To determine whether the meiotic progression was distorted in our 47,XYY patient, a total of 210 spermatocytes in different sub-stages of meiotic prophase I were studied in the patient and the results were compared with the controls (1117 spermatocytes from 5 normal men). An increase in leptotene (P <0.001, chi-square test) and zygotene (P <0.001, chi-square test) but decrease in the pachytene spermatocytes (P <0.001, chi-square test) were observed in our patient (Fig. 5).

Decreased germ cells in the testicular sections of the 47, XYY male

Histological examination of the H&E stained testicular sections revealed normal spermatogenesis with a lot of typical sperm in testicular tubules of a control male (Fig. 6a). However, reduced number of germ cells and no mature sperm were observed in testicular sections of the 47,XYY patient (Fig. 6b).

Discussion

A lot of variation has been reported regarding the presence of the extra Y chromosome in germ cells, spermatogenesis

Table 1 Sex chromosome pairing in pachytene spermatocytes in the 47, XYY patient

Cell type	No. of cells analyzed	No. (%[a]) of cells showing Y associated with X	No. (%[a]) of cells not showing Y associated with X
YY partially paired	42	27(64.3 %)[a]	15(35.7 %)[a]
YY completely paired	29	18(62.1 %)[a]	11(37.9 %)[a]
XY + Y	0	0	0
Total (%)	71	45(63.4 %)[a]	26(36.6 %)[a]

Sex chromosomes pairing was determined by over lapping SYCP3 signals
[a]The percentages were calculated by dividing the number of cells showing Y associated or not associated with X (respectively) with the corresponding number of cells analyzed

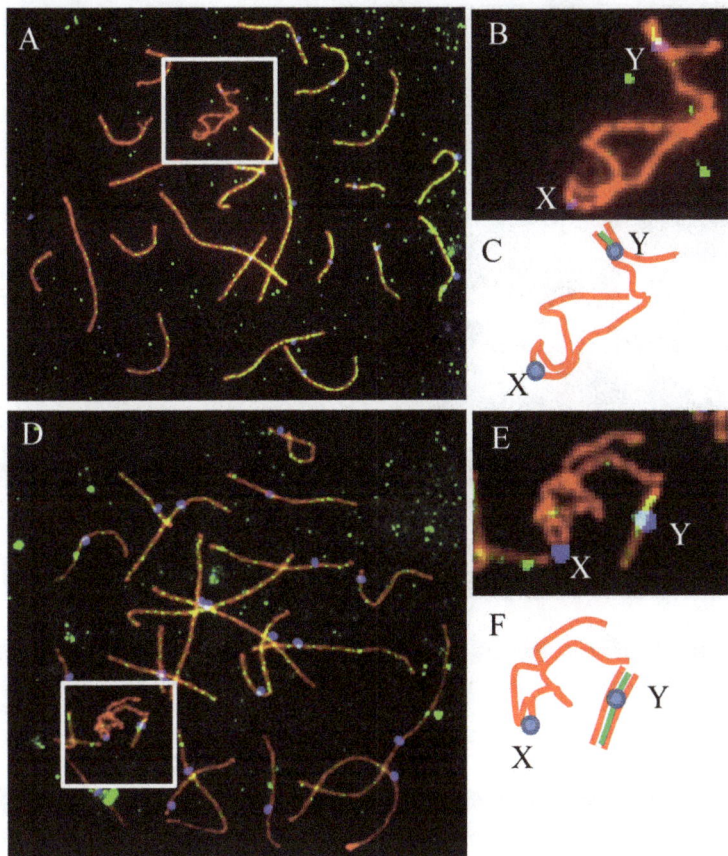

Fig. 3 Synapsis between the two Y chromosomes in spermatocytes of the 47, XYY patient. Images of representative pachytene spermatocytes immunostained for CREST (*Blue*), SYCP3 (*Red*) and SYCP1 (*Green*). **a** Two Y chromosomes partially synapsed with one Y chromosome being associated with the X chromosome at the end of q arm. **b** Enlarged area from (**a**). **c** A schematic configuration of the sex chromosomes from the cell shown in **a** and **b**. **d**) Two Y chromosomes completely synapsed. **e** Enlarged area from (**d**). **f** A schematic configuration of the sex chromosomes from the cell shown in **d** and **e**

and sperm counts in 47,XYY patients. Many men with 47,XYY karyotype has normal meiotic progression and are fertile. It has been suggested in some studies that the extra Y chromosome is lost before meiosis thus conserving fertility in these patients [2, 12, 15, 21]. In the present study, the extra Y chromosome was not lost in primary spermatocytes and XYY constitution was seen in all the 71 studied spermatocytes of our patient (Fig. 1; Table 1). This 47, XYY man showed disturbed meiotic progression and suffered from azoospermia with few germ cells in testicular tubules

(Fig. 6b). Blanco et al. [22] reported that most (95.9 %) premeiotic cells and 57.9 % pachytenespermatocytes showed XYY chromosomal constitution, and 42.1 % of post-reductional germ cells were XY in their 47,XYY patient who was oligoasthenoteratozoospermia. Solari and Valzacchi [23] observed XYY constitution in all studied spermatocytes of a 47,XXY patient with severe oligozoospermia. Both of these studies concluded that the arrest point for the genetically abnormal germ cells may reside at the primary and secondary spermatocyte or spermatid

Table 2 Sex chromosome synapsis in pachytene spermatocytes in the 47, XYY patient

Cell type	No. of cells analyzed	No. (%[a]) of cells showing Y associated with X	No. (%[a]) of cells not showing Y associated with X
YY partially synapsed	52	35(67.3 %)[a]	17(32.7 %)[a]
YY completely synapsed	19	10(52.6 %)[a]	9(47.4 %)[a]
XY + Y	0	0	0
Total (%)	71	45(63.4 %)[a]	26(36.6 %)[a]

Sex chromosomes synapsis was determined by over lapping SYCP1 signals
[a]The percentages were calculated by dividing the number of cells showing Y associated or not associated with X (respectively) with the corresponding number of cells analyzed

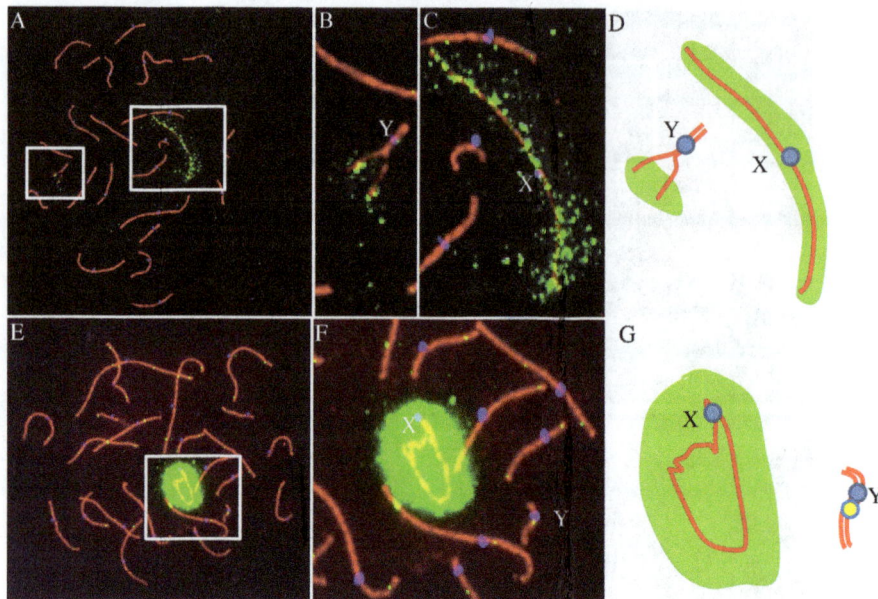

Fig. 4 Unsynapsed regions of the sex chromosomes are stained positive for γH2AX while synapsed regions remained unstained in spermatocytes of 47,XYY male. Pachytene spermatocytes immunostained for γ-H2AX (*Green*), MLH1 (*Green*), CREST (*Blue*) and SYCP3 (*Red*). **a** γ-H2AX signals are not detected in the region of synapsed YY, but detected in unsynapsed regions of Y chromosomes and X chromosome. **b, c** Enlarged area from (**a**). **d** A schematic configuration of the sex chromosomes from the cell shown in **b** and **c**. **e** γ-H2AX signals are not visible on the completely synapsed YY but visible around X chromosome. **f** Enlarged area from (**e**). **g** A schematic configuration of the sex chromosomes from the cell shown in **e** and **f**

stages leading to a continuous elimination of these cells during spermatogenesis. Solari and Valzacchi [23] observed a high level of germ cell death at or immediately after the meiotic divisions. Milazzo et al. [24] reported that two 47,XYY patients with severe oligozoospermia showed extra Y chromosome in 60.0 and 39.6 % of analyzed pachytene spermatocytes, respectively. They observed large number of apoptotic round spermatids and impaired meiotic division and cytokinesis failure leading to diploid (mainly 47,XYY cells) and tetraploid (94,XXYYYY) meiocytes, when present. Thus, the presence of the extra Y chromosomes in spermatocytes may disturb spermatogenesis and result in infertility of 47,XYY males.

We have observed abnormal pair and synapsis of sex chromosomes in our 47,XYY patient. A predominant pair and synapsis pattern observed was a partially or completely paired and synapsed YY bivalent associated with X chromosome, which forming a trivalent in 45 of 71, or 63.4 % of studied spermatocytes (Figs. 2 and 3; Tables 1 and 3). The minor pair and synapsis pattern was an YY bivalent and a univalent X in 26 of 71, or 36.6 % of the studied cells, while in none of the studied cells, X and Y were found associated with each other (Figs. 2 and 3; Tables 1 and 3). Several other studies on pachytene cells have also reported that the two Y-chromosomes preferentially pair and synapsis [2, 22, 23]. Solari and Valzacchi [23] had found a complete absence of normal XY pachytene spermatocytes and 86 % spermatocytes showed Y-Y bivalent plus a univalent X in

their XYY patient. We thus conclude that pair and synapsis occur preferentially between two Y chromosomes to form X+YY configuration in XYY spermatocytes.

The preferential pairing and synapsis of the Y-chromosomes is may be due to their greater homology compared with the X chromosome. X+YY cells are likely to be lethal due to the escape of Y genes and prevention of X genes from meiotic sex chromosome inactivation (MSCI), which normally silences the unsynapsed sex chromosomes [25] and result in a low sperm count [2, 23, 24, 26]. In consistence, we observed that synapsis took place along at least entire short arms and partial long arms of the two Y chromosomes, but never between X and Y chromosomes, in all the studied pachytene spermatocytes (Fig. 3), and the γ-H2AX signals were only visible on X and distal part of Yq (Fig. 4). γ-H2AX signals were not detected in the region where YY were synapsed YY while γ-H2AX signals were detectable in unsynapsed regions of Y and X chromosomes (Additional file 1: Figure S1) indicating that synapsis of the Y chromosomes can afford protection of the Y chromosome from γ-H2AX phosphorylation preventing MSCI.

It has been established that each pair of homologous chromosomes must have at least one recombination between them, and the recombination only occurs on the pseudo autosomal region (PAR) of X and Y chromosomes in normal spermatocytes [27, 28]. In our 47,XYY patient, we observed recombination between two Y chromosomes in 27 of 65, or 41.5 % cells analyzed, in which 25

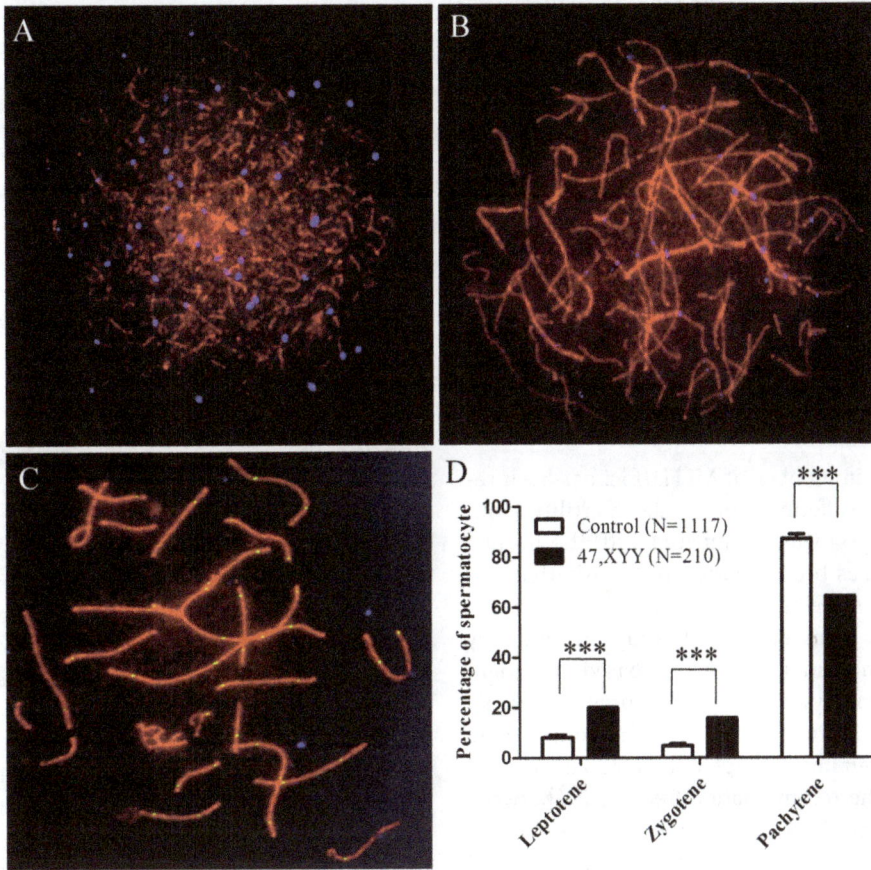

Fig. 5 Meiotic progression was disturbed in the 47, XYY patient. Representative images show (**a**) Leptotene, (**b**) Zygotene and (**c**) Pachytene spermatocytes immunostained for SYCP3 (*Red*), MLH1 (*Green*) and CREST (*Blue*). **d** An increase in leptotene and zygotene, and decrease in pachytene spermatocytes were observed in the 47, XYY patient. N, The number of cells analysed; *** *P* <0.001, chi-square test

spermatocytes showed recombination between two Yp arms while 2 showed recombination between two Yq arms. This indicates at least that long arm of Y chromosome also has the property to pair, synapse and recombine between each other during meiosis. MLH1 foci were not detected on remaining 38 cells although the two Y chromosomes were paired (Fig. 2; Table 2), the reason for this remains unknown. To our surprise, the number of MLHI foci on autosomes were also significantly reduced in our 47,XYY patient when compared to the controls (Table 2),

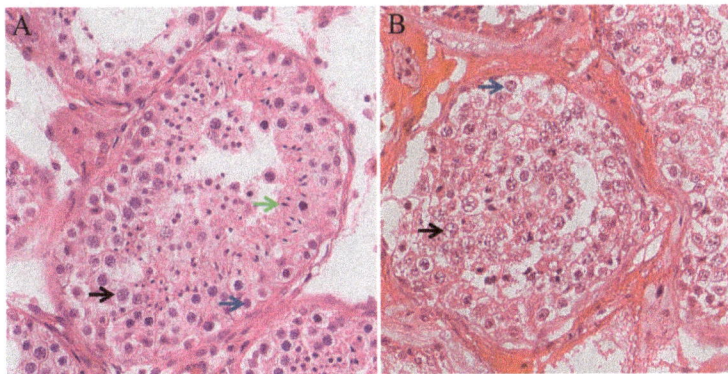

Fig. 6 Decreased number of early germ cells and absence of sperm in the testicular sections of the 47, XYY male. H&E staining of testicular sections showed (**a**) normal histology and spermatogenesis in control and (**b**) reduced number of early germ cells and absence of sperm in the 47, XYY patient. *Blue arrow*, spermatogonia; *black arrow*, spermatocytes; *green arrow*, sperm

Table 3 Recombination on YY bivalents in the 47, XYY patient

Cell type	No. of cells analyzed	No. (%[a]) of cells with recombination in Yp	No. (%[a]) of cells with recombination in Yq	Total recombination in YY bivalent (%)
YY partially synapsed	47	21 (44.7 %)[a]	0	44.7%[a]
YY completely synapsed	18	4(22.2 %)[a]	2 (11.1 %)[a]	33.3%[a]
Total (%)	65	25 (38.5 %)[a]	2 (3.0 %)[a]	41.5%[a]

Sex chromosomes recombination was determined by MLH1 signals
[a]The percentages were calculated by dividing the number of cells showing recombination on Y chromosomes with the number of cells analyzed

which indicates presence of an inter-chromosomal effect (ICE). This ICE was probably due to activation of pachytene checkpoint that delays pachytene progression when either the process required for crossover is defective or when there are defects in the structure of meiotic chromosome axis [29].

A huge variation in number of MLH1 foci has been reported in subjects suffering from male infertility (with variety of phenotypes) when compared with the normal fertile controls. It has been reported previously that status and age of the subjects did not affect the recombination frequencies. Lynn et al. [30] did not find any difference in recombination frequencies based on patient status (e.g., cancers, cystic fibrosis, or previous vasectomy) and age. This study shows that the control data we have used in our manuscript is reliable and can be used to compare the recombination frequencies between the patient and controls. Regarding the counts of MLH1 foci in control and patient spermatocytes and the % of cells with MLH1 on XY chromosomes, individual variations has been reported for both patients and controls. Sun et al. [31] has reported mean frequency of 49.8 ± 4.3 of autosomal recombination foci in a 47 year old control having 73 % recombination focus in XY bivalent. While Codina-Pascual et al. [32] has studied the meiotic progression in 4 patients with azoospermia and 6 patients suffering from oligoasthenozoospermia. They have reported that the mean MLH1 foci per cell were similar in patients (47.3) and controls (48.8). Upon comparison of MLH1 foci in sex chromosomes they observed decreased mean MLH1 foci (% cells) in patients (59.2 %) as compared to controls (69.9 %). It was observed that number of MLH1 foci on X-Y chromosome was different in patients suffering from azoospermia (61.7 %) and oligoasthenozoospermia (59.2 %) indicating that MLH1 foci number varies with the underlying type of infertility. Sun et al. [33] has also reported decreased mean MLH1 foci (% cells) in 7 patients with non obstructive azoospermia (77.7 %) as compared to controls (86.2 %). The mean number of MLH1 foci (% cells) in this study is higher for both patients and controls than the data we have presented in the submitted manuscript and Sun et al. [33] has reported that despite having 77.7 % MLH1 foci on sex chromosomes, the patients suffered from reduced meiotic recombination on the XY bivalent

confirming that there is no specific range for MLH1 foci per cell for both autosomes as well as sex chromosomes and the number of MLH1 foci varies from person to person.

Conclusion

In conclusion, we have reported that the extra Y chromosome was present in all the studied pachytene spermatocytes of a 47, XYY patient. Presence of this extra Y chromosome has resulted in abnormal sex chromosome pairing, synapsis and recombination and prevented the meiotic sex chromosome inactivation, leading to disturbed spermatogenesis, germ cell loss and consequently azoospermiain our patient. Hence, this work provides an important framework for future studies, which may elucidate the impairment caused by extra Y chromosome in mammalian meiosis and fertility.

Competing interest
All the authors declare that they have no conflict of interest of any sort with anyone.

Authors' contributions
LW and QS conceived the idea and coordinated the project. THG and LW collected the samples. LW, IB, HJ and CW conducted the experiments related to meiotic progression. GXY and ZYC performed the karyotyping. LW analyzed the data. QS and FI wrote the manuscript. All authors read and approved the final manuscript before submission.

Acknowledgements
We gratefully acknowledge the subjects for sample donation to this study.

Funding
This work was supported by the National Basic Research Program (2013CB947902 and 2014CB943101) of China (973), by grants from National Natural Science Foundation of China (31371519, 31301227 and 313111245) and the Knowledge Innovation Program of the Chinese Academy of Sciences (KSCX2-EW-R-07).

Author details
[1]The Reproductive Medicine Center, Clinical College of People's Liberation Army Affiliated to Anhui Medical University, Hefei, Anhui, China. [2]The Reproductive Medicine Center, 105 Hospital of People's Liberation Army, Hefei, Anhui, China. [3]Molecular and Cell Genetics Laboratory, The CAS Key Laboratory of Innate Immunity and Chronic Diseases, Hefei National Laboratory for Physical Sciences at Microscale, School of Life Sciences, University of Science and Technology of China, Hefei, Anhui 230027, China. [4]Collaborative Innovation Center of Genetics and Development, Fudan University, Shanghai 200438, China. [5]Institute of Pure and Applied Biology, Bahauddin Zakariya University, Multan 60800, Pakistan. [6]Center for Reproductive Medicine, Anhui Medical University, Affiliated Provincial Hospital, Hefei, China. [7]Anhui Provincial Family Planning Institute of Science and Technology, Hefei, China.

References

1. Gekas J, Thepot F, Turleau C, Siffroi JP, Dadoune JP, Briault S, et al. Chromosomal factors of infertility in candidate couples for ICSI: an equal risk of constitutional aberrations in women and men. Hum Reprod. 2001;16:82–90.
2. Rives N, Milazzo JP, Miraux L, North MO, Sibert L, Mace B. From spermatocytes to spermatozoa in an infertile XYY male. Int J Androl. 2005; 28:304–10.
3. Shi Q, Martin RH. Aneuploidy in human spermatozoa: FISH analysis in men with constitutional chromosomal abnormalities, and in infertile men. Reproduction. 2001;121:655–66.
4. Morel F, Roux C, Bresson JL. Sex chromosome aneuploidies in sperm of 47,XYY men. Arch Androl. 1999;43:27–36.
5. Shi Q, Spriggs E, Field LL, Ko E, Barclay L, Martin RH. Single sperm typing demonstrates that reduced recombination is associated with the production of aneuploid 24,XY human sperm. Am J Med Genet. 2001;99:34–8.
6. Stochholm K, Juul S, Gravholt CH. Diagnosis and mortality in 47,XYY persons: a registry study. Orphanet J Rare Dis. 2010;5:15.
7. Speed RM, Faed MJW, Batstone PJ, Baxby K, Barnetson W. Persistence of 2 Y-Chromosomes through Meiotic Prophase and Metaphase-I in an Xyy Man. Hum Genet. 1991;87:416–20.
8. Blanco J, Rubio C, Simon C, Egozcue J, Vidal F. Increased incidence of disomic sperm nuclei in a 47,XYY male assessed by fluorescent in situ hybridization (FISH). Hum Genet. 1997;99:413–6.
9. Chevret E, Rousseaux S, Monteil M, Usson Y, Cozzi J, Pelletier R, et al. Meiotic behaviour of sex chromosomes investigated by three-colour FISH on 35,142 sperm nuclei from two 47,XYY males. Hum Genet. 1997;99:407–12.
10. Lim AS, Fong Y, Yu SL. Analysis of the sex chromosome constitution of sperm in men with a 47, XYY mosaic karyotype by fluorescence in situ hybridization. Fertil Steril. 1999;72:121–3.
11. Gonzalez-Merino E, Hans C, Abramowicz M, Englert Y, Emiliani S. Aneuploidy study in sperm and preimplantation embryos from nonmosaic 47,XYY men. Fertil Steril. 2007;88:600–6.
12. Wong EC, Ferguson KA, Chow V, Ma S. Sperm aneuploidy and meiotic sex chromosome configurations in an infertile XYY male. Hum Reprod. 2008;23:374–8.
13. Shi Q, Martin RH. Multicolor fluorescence in situ hybridization analysis of meiotic chromosome segregation in a 47,XYY male and a review of the literature. Am J Med Genet. 2000;93:40–6.
14. Egozcue S, Blanco J, Vendrell JM, Garcia F, Veiga A, Aran B, et al. Human male infertility: chromosome anomalies, meiotic disorders, abnormal spermatozoa and recurrent abortion. Hum Reprod Update. 2000;6:93–105.
15. Moretti E, Anichini C, Sartini B, Collodel G. Sperm ultrastructure and meiotic segregation in an infertile 47, XYY man. Andrologia. 2007;39:229–34.
16. Abdel-Razic MM, Abdel-Hamid IA, ElSobky ES. Nonmosaic 47, XYY syndrome presenting with male infertility: case series. Andrologia. 2012;44:200–4.
17. Jiang H, Wang L, Cui Y, Xu Z, Guo T, Cheng D, et al. Meiotic chromosome behavior in a human male t(8;15) carrier. J Genet Genomics. 2014;41:177–85.
18. Pan ZZ, Yang QL, Ye N, Wang L, Li JH, Yu D, et al. Complex relationship between meiotic recombination frequency and autosomal synaptonemal complex length per cell in normal human males. Am J Med Genet A. 2012; 158A:581–7.

19. Turner JM, Mahadevaiah SK, Fernandez-Capetillo O, Nussenzweig A, Xu X, Burgoyne PS. Silencing of unsynapsed meiotic chromosomes in the mouse. Nat Genet. 2005;37:41–7.
20. Mahadevaiah SK, Turner JM, Baudat F, Rogakou EP, de Boer P, Blanco-Rodríguez J, et al. Recombinational DNA double-strand breaks in mice precede synapsis. Nat Genet. 2001;27:271–6.
21. El-Dahtory F, Elsheikha HM. Male infertility related to an aberrant karyotype, 47,XYY: four case reports. Cases J. 2009;2:28.
22. Blanco J, Egozcue J, Vidal F. Meiotic behaviour of the sex chromosomes in three patients with sex chromosome anomalies (47,XXY, mosaic 46,XY/47,XXY and 47,XYY) assessed by fluorescence in-situ hybridization. Hum Reprod. 2001;16:887–92.
23. Solari AJ, Rey VG. The prevalence of a YY synaptonemal complex over XY synapsis in an XYY man with exclusive XYY spermatocytes. Chromosom Res. 1997;5:467–74.
24. Milazzo JP, Rives N, Mousset-Simeon N, Mace B. Chromosome constitution and apoptosis of immature germ cells present in sperm of two 47,XYY infertile males. Hum Reprod. 2006;21:1749–58.
25. Turner JM. Meiotic sex chromosome inactivation. Development. 2007;134: 1823–31.
26. Roeder GS, Bailis JM. The pachytene checkpoint. Trends Genet. 2000;16: 395–403.
27. Hinch AG, Altemose N, Noor N, Donnelly P, Myers SR. Recombination in the human pseudoautosomal region PAR1. Plos Genetics. 2014;10(7):e1004503.
28. Flaquer A, Rappold GA, Wienker TF, Fischer C. The human pseudoautosomal regions: a review for genetic epidemiologists. Eur J Hum Genet. 2008;16:771–9.
29. Subramanian VV, Hochwagen A. The meiotic checkpoint network: step-by-step through meiotic prophase. Cold Spring Harb Perspect Biol. 2014;6(10):a016675.
30. Lynn A, Koehler KE, Judis L, Chan ER, Cherry JP, Schwartz S, et al. Covariation of synaptonemal complex length and mammalian meiotic exchange rates. Science. 2002;296:2222–5.
31. Sun F, Oliver-Bonet M, Liehr T, Starke H, Ko E, Rademaker A, et al. Human male recombination maps for individual chromosomes. Am J Hum Genet. 2004;74:521–31.
32. Codina-Pascual M, Oliver-Bonet M, Navarro J, Campillo M, Garcia F, Egozcue S, et al. Synapsis and meiotic recombination analyses: MLH1 focus in the XY pair as an indicator. Hum Reprod. 2005;20:2133–9.
33. Sun F, Mikhaail-Philips M, Oliver-Bonet M, Ko E, Rademaker A, Turek P, et al. Reduced meiotic recombination on the XY bivalent is correlated with an increased incidence of sex chromosome aneuploidy in men with non-obstructive azoospermia. Mol Hum Reprod. 2008;14:399–404.

11

Karyotype alteration generates the neoplastic phenotypes of SV40-infected human and rodent cells

Mathew Bloomfield and Peter Duesberg[*]

Abstract

Background: Despite over 50 years of research, it remains unclear how the DNA tumor viruses SV40 and Polyoma cause cancers. Prevailing theories hold that virus-coded Tumor (T)-antigens cause cancer by inactivating cellular tumor suppressor genes. But these theories don't explain four characteristics of viral carcinogenesis: (1) less than one in 10,000 infected cells become cancer cells, (2) cancers have complex individual phenotypes and transcriptomes, (3) recurrent tumors without viral DNA and proteins, (4) preneoplastic aneuploidies and immortal neoplastic clones with individual karyotypes.

Results: As an alternative theory we propose that viral carcinogenesis is a form of speciation, initiated by virus-induced aneuploidy. Since aneuploidy destabilizes the karyotype by unbalancing thousands of genes it catalyzes chain reactions of karyotypic and transcriptomic evolutions. Eventually rare karyotypes evolve that encode cancer-specific autonomy of growth. The low probability of forming new autonomous cancer-species by random karyotypic and transcriptomic variations predicts individual and clonal cancers. Although cancer karyotypes are congenitally aneuploid and thus variable, they are stabilized or immortalized by selections for variants with cancer-specific autonomy. Owing to these inherent variations cancer karyotypes are heterogeneous within clonal margins. To test this theory we analyzed karyotypes and phenotypes of SV40-infected human, rat and mouse cells developing into neoplastic clones. In all three systems we found (1) preneoplastic aneuploidies, (2) neoplastic clones with individual clonal but flexible karyotypes and phenotypes, which arose from less than one in 10,000 infected cells, survived over 200 generations, but were either T-antigen positive or negative, (3) spontaneous and drug-induced variations of neoplastic phenotypes correlating 1-to-1 with karyotypic variations.

Conclusions: Since all 14 virus-induced neoplastic clones tested contained individual clonal karyotypes and phenotypes, we conclude that these karyotypes have generated and since maintained these neoplastic clones. Thus SV40 causes cancer indirectly, like carcinogens, by inducing aneuploidy from which new cancer-specific karyotypes evolve automatically at low rates. This theory explains the (1) low probability of carcinogenesis per virus-infected cell, (2) the individuality and clonal flexibility of cancer karyotypes, (3) recurrence of neoplasias without viral T-antigens, and (4) the individual clonal karyotypes, transcriptomes and immortality of virus-induced neoplasias - all unexplained by current viral theories.

Keywords: Cancer-specific reproductive autonomy, Immortality, Preneoplastic aneuploidy, Individuality of cancer phenotypes and transcriptomes, Clonal karyotypes of cancers, Speciation theory of carcinogenesis

* Correspondence: duesberg@berkeley.edu
Department of Molecular and Cell Biology, Donner Laboratory, University of California at Berkeley, Berkeley, CA, USA

Background

The DNA tumor viruses SV40 and Polyoma are very efficient carcinogens in immune-tolerant animals and in cultured animal and human cells [1–3]. But, despite over 50 years of research the mechanism of viral carcinogenesis is still unclear. The currently prevailing theories hold that non-structural viral proteins, termed Tumor (T)-antigens, cause cancer by inactivating cellular tumor suppressor genes [4–7]. However, these viral theories do not explain the following four characteristics of viral carcinogenesis.

1) *Less than 1 in 10,000 virus-infected cells form an immortal neoplastic clone.* Even under optimal experimental conditions SV40 transforms only one in over 10,000 infected human (if any [8]) or animal cells into an immortal neoplastic clone [2, 3, 8–25] (see also Results). According to their clonal origins new neoplastic clones only manifest in infected cultures after delays of several weeks to months following infection [9, 10, 12, 13, 15, 16, 26–28] (see also Results). Likewise tumors develop in animals only 3 to 24 months after injection of viruses [1, 29–31], or after transfection with cloned viral DNAs [32], or after the birth of animals with transgenic viral genes [33–35]. The low probability and late appearance of immortal neoplastic clones indicate that viral genes are not sufficient for neoplastic transformation and immortalization. But the rare clonogenic event that generates and immortalizes clonal cancers from mortal somatic cells is still unknown.

2) *Virus-induced tumors and neoplastic clones have individual rather than virus-coded phenotypes and transcriptomes.* Paradoxically, in view of the virus-cancer theory, viral tumors [1, 30, 36–38] and neoplastic clones formed in vitro [3, 9, 10, 12, 13, 15, 16, 27, 28, 39–44] have complex individual clonal phenotypes and transcriptomes, rather than common virus-specific phenotypes. The individuality of Polyoma- and SV40 virus-induced tumors even from the same tissue of origin is in fact the reason why the two viruses were surnamed 'Polyoma viruses' - many (= poly) different types of carcinomas [1, 3, 45, 46]. Accordingly, we show below that the same SV40 virus induces in primary rat and mouse cells from the same tissue of origin, very different neoplastic clones with individually different morphologies and growth rates.

3) *Virus-induced tumors and neoplastic clones without viral proteins and genes.* In searching for a viral role in carcinogenesis over 20 studies have found no viral T-antigen and no viral DNA in neoplastic clones induced by Polyoma virus [10, 47–50] and SV40 [2, 11, 12, 27, 51–59]. These results were initially

described as "perplexing exceptions" in an influential review of the virus-cancer theory [2]. Subsequently, it was found that tumors induced in mice with transcriptionally controllable transgenic SV40 T-antigens do not revert to normal, when their T-antigens are switched off [33]. Moreover, there are recurrent reports that tumors from mice with transgenic viral T-antigens are free of T-antigen or viral genes or both [34, 35, 60–62]. One such study from our lab found that four of nine tumors of mice with transgenic SV40-T-antigen genes lacked viral T-antigens and mRNAs of T-antigen altogether [35]. Another study even found "increased oncogenicity" after the loss of T-antigen [62]. In addition tumors of transgenic mice were found to be heterogeneous, containing both T-antigen-negative and positive cells by others and us [35, 63, 64] (see also Results). It follows that viral genes and proteins are not necessary to maintain neoplastic phenotypes such as cancer-specific reproductive autonomy and immortality. This explains, why SV40 and polyoma viruses with conditional transforming genes, which would allow neoplastic clones to revert to normal cells under non-permissive conditions, were never found - despite enormous efforts [2, 3, 33, 46, 65–68].

4) *Viruses induce preneoplastic aneuploidy and neoplasias with abnormal karyotypes and transcriptomes.* Unexpectedly, it was discovered in 1962 that SV40 induces proliferation of human cells with heterogeneous aneuploidies and abnormal cell morphologies within days after infection [39, 40, 51, 69–73]. This discovery was immediately seen as a breakthrough in cancer research. Accordingly Shein and Enders wrote in 1962: "Accelerated growth, abnormal growth pattern, and chromosomal aberrations exhibited by E cells (SV40-transformed human epithelial cells) are characteristics commonly associated with rapidly growing tumors and with "continuous" lines of cells in culture." [39]. Subsequently, abnormal karyotypes and / or transcriptomes and phenotypes were found in human cell lines "immortalized" by virus or by transfection with genes of viral T-antigens [12–18, 25, 42–44, 74–86]. Abnormal karyotypes and / or transcriptomes were also found in neoplastic clones arising from cultures of SV40 and Polyoma virus-infected primary hamster [9, 10, 27, 87], rat [3, 12, 41, 88] and mouse cells [37, 38, 89]. And were also found in tumors induced by Polyoma virus in mice [30] and by transgenic SV40 T-antigens in rats [90] and in mice [35, 37, 38]. Since a majority of clonal tumors from transgenic mice were T-antigen-free, we concluded in 2010 that these clonal karyotypes

have neoplastic function [35]. Surprisingly, none of the currently prevailing virus-cancer theories cited above [4–7] mentions the abnormal karyotypes and / or transcriptomes of SV40 and Polyoma virus-infected or transfected preneoplastic cells and of the immortal neoplastic clones and tumors that arise from such cells.

Alternative theory of virus-induced neoplastic transformation based on karyotype alteration

Given these four unexplained characteristics of viral carcinogenesis, particularly the preneoplastic aneuploidy of virus-infected cells and the individual abnormal karyotypes and the immortality of virus-induced neoplastic clones or tumors, we speculated that viral carcinogenesis might be a form of speciation [91–95] - much like non-viral carcinogenesis [96–99].

Accordingly, we propose that SV40 induces cancer indirectly by inducing preneoplastic aneuploidy at high rates (m1, in Fig. 1). Since aneuploidy destabilizes the karyotype by unbalancing thousands of genes, it catalyzes chain reactions of karyotypic and transcriptomic evolutions, also at high rates (m2, in Fig. 1). Eventually rare karyotypes evolve that encode cancer-specific

autonomy of growth, at very low rates (m3, Fig. 1). The low probability of forming new autonomous cancer-species by random karyotypic and transcriptomic variations predicts individual and clonal cancers. Although cancer karyotypes are congenitally aneuploid and thus variable, they are stabilized or immortalized by selections for variants with cancer-specific autonomy. Owing to these inherent variations cancer karyotypes are heterogeneous within clonal margins (shaded in Fig. 1) [100–102]. The resulting spread of quasi-clonal karyotypes is illustrated below in 'karyotype arrays' in which multiple individual karyotypes of the same cancer are compared (see Results).

In sum this karyotypic theory proposes that SV40 and Polyoma viruses generate clonal immortal cancers indirectly by inducing aneuploidy, which catalyzes the rare evolution of new cancer-causing karyotypes.

To test the karyotypic theory of viral carcinogenesis, we analyzed here the karyotypes and phenotypes of virus-infected (1) human mesothelial, (2) rat lung, and (3) mouse embryo cells from the time of infection to the origins of immortal neoplastic clones. As we show below, we found in each of these three systems, (1) preneoplastic heterogeneous aneuploidies, (2) neoplastic clones with

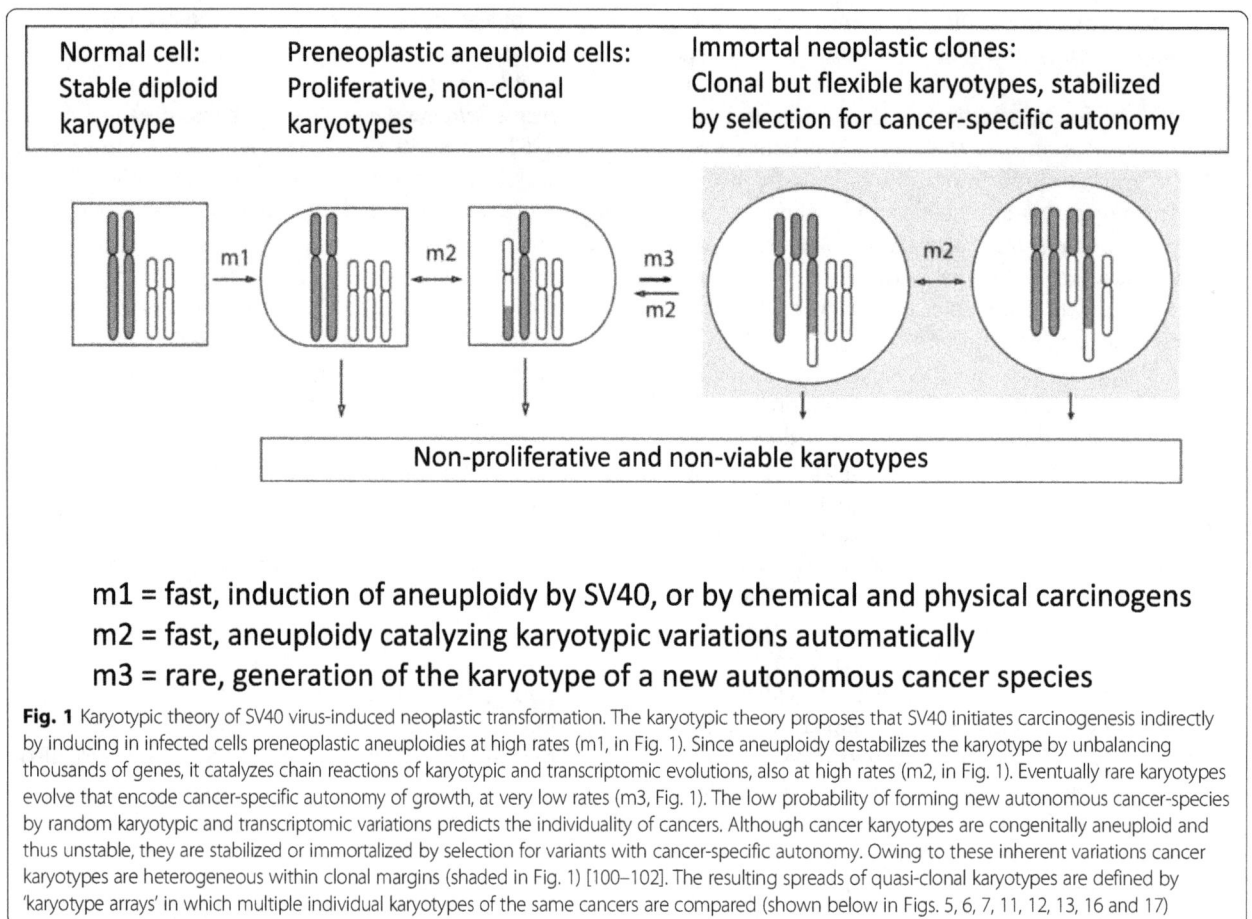

m1 = fast, induction of aneuploidy by SV40, or by chemical and physical carcinogens
m2 = fast, aneuploidy catalyzing karyotypic variations automatically
m3 = rare, generation of the karyotype of a new autonomous cancer species

Fig. 1 Karyotypic theory of SV40 virus-induced neoplastic transformation. The karyotypic theory proposes that SV40 initiates carcinogenesis indirectly by inducing in infected cells preneoplastic aneuploidies at high rates (m1, in Fig. 1). Since aneuploidy destabilizes the karyotype by unbalancing thousands of genes, it catalyzes chain reactions of karyotypic and transcriptomic evolutions, also at high rates (m2, in Fig. 1). Eventually rare karyotypes evolve that encode cancer-specific autonomy of growth, at very low rates (m3, Fig. 1). The low probability of forming new autonomous cancer-species by random karyotypic and transcriptomic variations predicts the individuality of cancers. Although cancer karyotypes are congenitally aneuploid and thus unstable, they are stabilized or immortalized by selection for variants with cancer-specific autonomy. Owing to these inherent variations cancer karyotypes are heterogeneous within clonal margins (shaded in Fig. 1) [100–102]. The resulting spreads of quasi-clonal karyotypes are defined by 'karyotype arrays' in which multiple individual karyotypes of the same cancers are compared (shown below in Figs. 5, 6, 7, 11, 12, 13, 16 and 17)

individual clonal karyotypes and phenotypes, which arose from one in 10,000 infected cells and survived over 200 generations, (3) spontaneous and drug-induced phenotypic variations of neoplastic clones that correlated 1-to-1 with karyotypic variations, but no consistent correlations with SV40 genes.

Since all 14 virus-induced neoplastic clones tested contained individual quasi-clonal karyotypes, we concluded that these karyotypes generate the complex individual phenotypes and transcriptomes of neoplastic clones, rather than common viral genes, which are not present in dozens of neoplastic clones (Results and Background). It would follow that the carcinogenic action of SV40 virus is indirect, as an initiator of the evolution of cancer causing karyotypes.

Results and discussion

In the following we have tested the karyotypic theory of viral transformation in SV40-infected primary human (I), rat (II) and mouse cells (III).

I. Transformation of human cells by SV40

To test the theory that SV40 transforms normal human cells to neoplastic cells indirectly by inducing preneoplastic aneuploidy (see Fig. 1), we have used an established system of viral transformation described by Bocchetta et al. in 2000 [21]. In this system SV40 induces enhanced growth and preneoplastic transformation in primary human mesothelial cells within two weeks after infection and rare neoplastic clones from less than one of 10,000 infected cells two to three months after infection [21].

Phenotypes and karyotypes of SV40-infected preneoplastic human mesothelial cells
Phenotypes of SV40-infected preneoplastic cells
To determine the phenotypes of preneoplastic SV40-infected mesothelial cells, we infected a sub-confluent culture of primary mesothelial cells with SV40 at a multiplicity of infection of 10 and kept an un-infected control under the same conditions. Comparison of infected and uninfected cells by light microscopy two weeks after infection indicated that the infected cells had formed dense multilayers of polymorphic cells with rounded and oval shapes, as described by Bocchetta et al. [21] and shown in Fig. 2a. In parallel with enhanced growth, the infected mesothelial culture also shed a relatively large minority of infected cells, which would not reattach to a new culture dish. This SV40-induced enhanced proliferation and degeneration of cells also confirms previous observations of Bochetta et al. and many others [8, 13, 21, 31, 39, 51]. By contrast, the uninfected culture consisted of partly spindle-shaped and partly rounded cells and barely reached confluence under the same conditions (Fig. 2b).

Karyotypes of SV40-infected preneoplastic cells
To test for the predicted aneuploidies of preneoplastic cells (Fig. 1), we analyzed the karyotypes of the SV40-infected human mesothelial cells shown in Fig. 2 one and two months after infection. As shown in Table 1, we found that 65 % (13 of 20) of the infected human cells carried heterogeneous, near-diploid aneuploidies at one month after infection. At two months after infection 95 % (19 per 20) of these cells carried heterogeneous

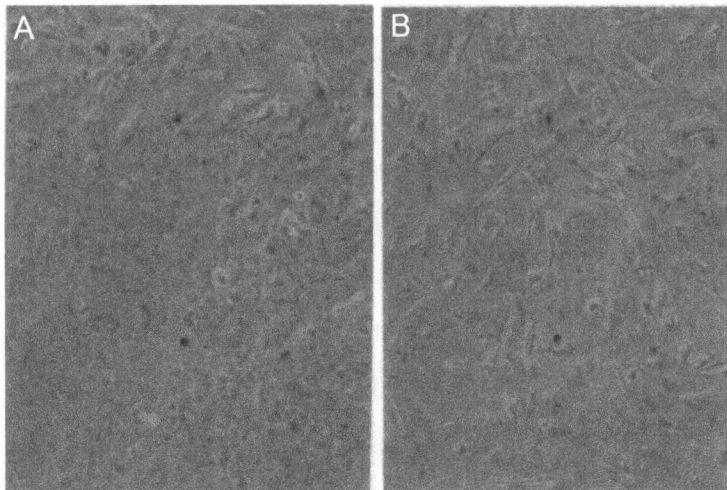

Fig. 2 Phenotypes of human mesothelial cells three weeks after infection by SV40 compared to an uninfected control. A subconfluent culture of human mesothelial cells was infected with SV40 at a multiplicity of 10. In parallel an uninfected culture was maintained under the same conditions (see text). **a** A 120X magnification of the infected culture three weeks after infection shows highly increased cell density and "pre-transformed" cell morphologies [13], compared to the uninfected control shown in (**b**). It follows that SV40 transforms the morphology and raises the density of cultures of mesothelial cells shortly after infection

Table 1 Karyotypes of mesothelial cells 1 month after infection with SV40: 13 aneuploid per 20

Karyotypes	1	2	3	4	5	6	7	8	9	10	11	12	13
Total no of chromosomes	47	45	45	47	49	45	45	47	47	44	48	46	42
Chromosomes													
1	2	2	2	2	2	1	2	2	2	2	2	2	2
2	2	2	2	2	2	2	2	2	2	3	2	2	2
3	2	2	2	2	2	2	2	2	2	2	2	2	1
4	2	2	2	2	2	2	2	2	2	2	2	2	2
5	2	2	2	2	2	2	2	3	3	2	2	3	2
6	2	2	2	2	2	2	2	2	2	2	2	2	1
7	2	2	2	2	2	2	1	2	2	2	2	2	2
8	2	2	2	2	2	2	2	2	2	2	2	2	1
9	2	2	2	2	2	2	2	2	2	2	3	2	2
10	2	2	2	2	2	2	2	2	2	2	2	2	2
11	2	2	2	2	2	2	2	2	2	2	2	1	2
12	2	2	2	2	2	2	2	2	2	2	2	2	2
13	2	2	2	2	2	2	2	2	2	2	2	3	2
14	2	2	2	2	2	2	2	2	2	2	2	2	2
15	2	2	2	3	2	2	2	2	2	2	2	2	2
16	2	2	2	2	2	2	2	2	2	1	2	2	2
17	2	2	2	2	3	2	2	2	2	1	2	2	2
18	2	2	2	2	2	2	2	2	2	2	2	1	2
19	2	2	2	2	3	2	2	2	2	2	2	2	2
20	2	2	2	2	2	2	2	2	2	1	3	2	2
21	2	1	2	2	3	2	1	2	2	1	2	2	2
22	2	2	2	2	2	2	2	2	2	2	2	2	2
X	2	2	1	2	2	2	2	2	2	2	2	2	1
Y	0	0	0	0	0	0	0	0	0	0	0	0	0
der(7;21)?	0	0	0	0	0	0	1	0	0	0	0	0	0
der(7)	1	0	0	0	0	0	0	0	0	0	0	0	0
i(21q)	0	0	0	0	0	0	0	0	0	1	0	0	0

aneuploidies, of which three had near tetraploid karyotypes, as is shown in Table 2. By contrast, the uninfected mesothelial controls could not even be karyotyped for lack of mitoses.

We conclude from the high percentages of aneuploidization of cells early after infection, that the virus induces aneuploidy directly, probably by the viral T-antigen. Accordingly, T-antigen induces aneuploidy either by binding randomly to chromosomes, or to specific mitosis proteins as suggested by others [85, 86].

With these results we confirmed that SV40 alters the phenotypes, the growth rate, the karyotype and also kills a fraction of the infected human cells within weeks after infection. These results are thus compatible with the theory that SV40-induced aneuploidies with proliferative phenotypes enhance growth and alter cellular phenotypes. Simultaneously virus-induced aneuploidies with

lethal phenotypes would kill cells (Fig. 1) in addition to lytic infections [3].

Phenotypes and karyotypes of two neoplastic lines from SV40-infected mesothelial cells

To test the theory that individual clonal karyotypes, rather than viral genes, generate and immortalize new neoplastic clones with individual phenotypes (see Fig. 1), we have analyzed the phenotypes and karyotypes of two immortal lines derived from SV40-infected mesothelial cells. These lines or clones have been isolated from infected mesothelial cells and termed F1 and F4 by Bocchetta et al. [21]. Bocchetta et al. also proved that these lines are immortal by demonstrating that the lines survived over 200 generations in culture. Neoplastic lines are designated "immortal", "permanent" or "continuous" in the literature, if they have survived over 100 generations

Table 2 Karyotypes of mesothelial cells two months after infection with SV40: 19 aneuploid per 20

Karyotypes	1	2	3	4	5	6	7	8	9	10	11	12	13	14	15	16	17	18	19
Total no of chromosomes	45	46	46	43	46	46	47	47	46	47	47	47	47	48	49	60	75	75	83
Chromosomes																			
1	2	2	2	2	2	2	2	2	1	1	2	2	2	2	2	2	3	4	4
2	1	2	2	2	2	2	2	2	2	2	2	2	2	2	2	3	1	4	3
3	2	2	2	2	2	2	2	2	2	2	3	2	2	2	2	2	3	4	3
4	2	2	2	2	2	2	2	2	2	2	2	2	2	3	2	4	2	3	4
5	2	2	2	2	3	2	3	2	2	1	2	2	3	2	3	1	5	3	4
6	1	2	2	2	2	2	2	3	2	2	2	2	2	3	2	2	3	4	2
7	2	2	2	2	2	2	2	2	2	2	2	2	2	2	2	2	4	2	3
8	2	2	2	2	2	2	2	2	2	2	2	2	2	2	2	3	3	2	3
9	2	2	2	2	2	2	2	2	1	2	2	2	2	2	2	3	3	2	3
10	2	1	2	2	2	2	2	2	2	3	2	2	2	2	2	2	4	4	4
11	2	2	2	2	2	2	2	2	2	2	2	2	2	2	2	2	3	3	3
12	2	2	2	2	2	2	2	2	2	2	2	2	2	2	2	3	4	3	4
13	2	2	2	2	2	2	2	2	2	2	2	2	2	2	2	2	4	3	3
14	2	2	1	1	1	2	2	2	2	2	2	2	2	2	2	2	4	4	4
15	2	2	2	1	2	1	2	2	2	1	2	2	2	2	2	4	4	3	4
16	2	2	2	1	2	2	2	2	2	2	2	2	2	2	2	4	2	3	2
17	2	2	2	2	1	2	2	2	2	2	2	2	2	2	2	1	4	4	3
18	2	2	2	2	2	2	2	2	2	2	2	2	1	3	2	2	3	2	2
19	2	2	2	2	2	2	2	2	1	1	2	2	2	1	3	2	3	3	4
20	2	1	2	2	2	2	2	2	2	2	2	2	2	2	3	4	4	4	4
21	2	2	2	2	2	2	2	2	2	2	2	2	2	2	2	1	2	3	3
22	2	2	2	2	2	2	2	2	2	2	2	2	2	2	2	4	2	3	2
X	2	2	2	2	2	2	2	2	2	2	2	2	2	2	2	1	3	3	4
Y	0	0	0	0	0	0	0	0	0	0	0	0	0	0	0	0	0	0	0
der(1q)	0	0	0	0	0	0	0	0	1	1	0	0	0	0	0	0	0	0	0
der(18) long	0	0	0	0	0	0	0	0	0	0	0	0	1	0	0	0	0	1	0
der(9;6;9;6)	0	0	0	0	0	0	0	0	0	0	0	0	0	0	0	0	0	0	1
der(17;18)	0	0	0	0	0	0	0	0	0	0	0	0	0	0	0	0	0	0	1
der(22;7)	0	0	0	0	0	0	0	0	0	0	0	0	0	0	0	0	0	0	1
der(16;8;3)	0	0	0	0	0	0	0	0	0	0	0	0	0	0	0	0	0	0	1
der(8;3)	0	0	0	0	0	0	0	0	0	0	0	0	0	0	0	0	0	0	1
der(22;16)	0	0	0	0	0	0	0	0	0	0	0	0	0	0	0	0	0	0	1
min(3?)	0	0	0	0	0	0	0	0	0	0	0	0	0	0	0	0	0	0	1
der(8)	0	0	0	0	0	0	0	0	0	0	0	0	0	0	0	0	0	0	1
der(1;17)	0	0	0	0	0	0	0	0	0	0	0	0	0	0	0	1	0	0	0
der(17;12)	0	0	0	0	0	0	0	0	0	0	0	0	0	0	0	1	0	0	0
der(22) small	0	0	0	0	0	0	0	0	0	0	0	0	0	0	0	1	0	0	0
min(19)	0	0	0	0	0	0	0	0	0	0	0	0	0	0	0	1	0	0	0
der(19q)	0	0	0	0	0	0	0	0	1	0	0	0	0	0	0	0	0	0	0
der(9;13?;9)	0	0	0	0	0	0	0	0	1	0	0	0	0	0	0	0	0	0	0
der(16q)	0	0	0	0	0	0	0	0	0	0	0	0	0	0	0	0	2	0	0
der(19;14)	0	0	0	0	0	0	0	0	0	1	0	0	0	0	0	0	0	0	0

Table 2 Karyotypes of mesothelial cells two months after infection with SV40: 19 aneuploid per 20 *(Continued)*

der(1)	0	0	0	0	0	0	0	0	0	1	0	0	0	0	0	0	0	0	0
dic(5;15)	0	0	0	0	0	0	0	0	0	1	0	0	0	0	0	0	0	0	0
i(14q)	0	0	1	0	0	0	0	0	0	0	0	0	0	0	0	0	0	0	0
dic(2;6)	1	0	0	0	0	0	0	0	0	0	0	0	0	0	0	0	0	0	0
der(13) small	0	0	0	0	0	0	0	0	0	0	0	1	0	0	0	0	0	0	0
der(15;3)	0	0	0	0	0	1	0	0	0	0	0	0	0	0	0	0	0	0	0
der(12;9)	0	0	0	0	0	0	0	0	0	0	0	0	0	0	0	0	0	1	0
der(10q)	0	1	0	0	0	0	0	0	0	0	0	0	0	0	0	0	0	0	0
der(20) long	0	1	0	0	0	0	0	0	0	0	0	0	0	0	0	0	0	0	0
der(17)	0	0	0	0	1	0	0	0	0	0	0	0	0	0	0	0	0	0	0

in culture or as transplants in animals [5, 7, 13, 14, 17, 89, 103]. By contrast, normal cells fail to survive over 50 generations in these conditions [104].

Phenotype of the neoplastic F1 line

As can be seen in Fig. 3a, the F1 line formed a dense, mostly single-layered culture of cells with rather uniform, F1-specific round to oval morphologies, which differed from the heterogeneous cell morphologies of the preneoplastic mass culture, shown in Fig. 2a. This result supports the theory that the F1 cells are encoded by a clonal F1-specific genotype, which would be a karyotype in the light of our theory.

'Karyotype array' of the neoplastic F1 line

Next we asked, whether the F1 line has the predicted F1-specific clonal karyotype (see Fig. 1). For this purpose we have stained metaphase chromosomes of F1 with chromosome-specific color-coded DNA probes and arranged the chromosomes based on these colors into a conventional human karyotype with a computer-assisted microscope, following published procedures (Methods) [101, 102]. The resulting karyotype shows in Fig. 4a that F1 has indeed a specific, abnormal human karyotype with a total number of 54 chromosomes, which include 20 cancer-specific hybrid or marker chromosomes, instead of the normal 46 human chromosomes.

But to determine, whether the F1-karyotype shown in Fig. 4a is indeed clonal, multiple karyotypes of the same putative clone must be compared. To meet this end, we have used the recently developed 'karyotype arrays,' which are designed to compare multiple karyotypes of the same clone [101, 102]. Karyotype-arrays are three-dimensional tables of typically 20 karyotypes, which list

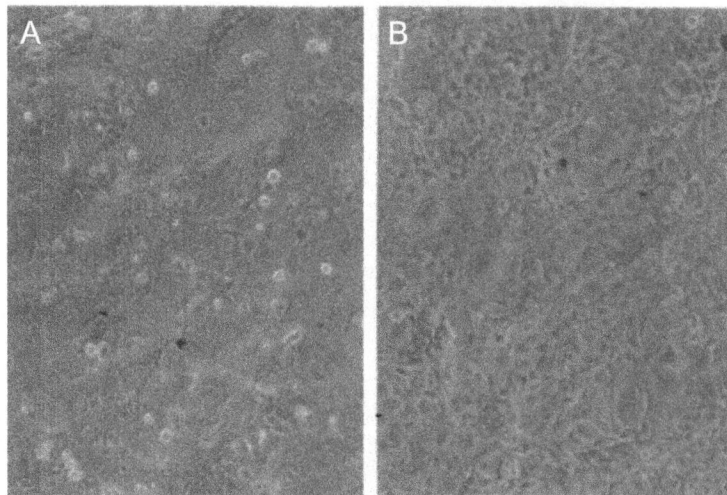

Fig. 3 Cell morphologies of the immortal cell lines F1 and F4 derived from SV40-infected human mesothelial cells. The karyotypic cancer theory predicts that neoplastic karyotypes encode the individual phenotypes of SV40-transformed neoplastic clones. To test this prediction we have compared at 120X magnifications cultures of the immortal neoplastic cell lines F1 and F4, which arose from SV40-infected human mesothelial cells. It can be seen in the micrographs shown in (**a**) that the F1 line formed a dense monolayer of cells and in (**b**) that the F4 line formed a multilayer of cells. The micrographs also show that both lines consisted of round to oval polymorphic cells, and that the F4-cells were on average larger than the F1 cells. This result revealed phenotypic cellular similarity but sociological dissimilarity of the two cell lines

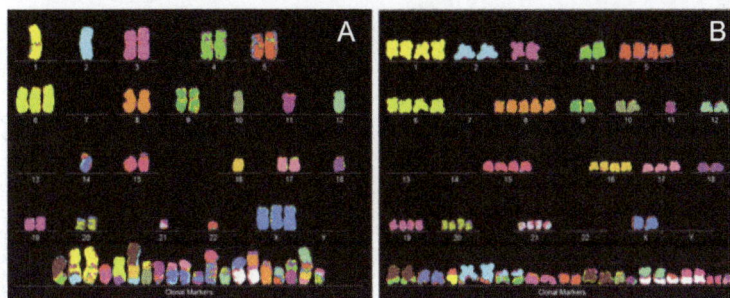

Fig. 4 Karyotypes of the immortal cell lines F1 and F4 derived from a common culture of SV40-infected human mesothelial cells. To test, whether the karyotypes of F1and F4 would explain the individual but related phenotypes of F1 and F4, we compared their karyotypes. The karyotypes were prepared from metaphase chromosomes stained with chromosome-specific fluorescent colors following published procedures (Methods). As shown in (**a**), F1 has a hyper-diploid, aneuploid karyotype with 56 including 36 normal and 20 marker chromosomes. The karyotype shown in (**b**) indicates that F4 has a hypo-tetraploid karyotype with 81 including 56 normal and 25 marker chromosomes. However, a close comparison of the copy numbers of the ten F1-chromosomes, 2, 5, 10, 11, 12, 15, 18, 19, 20 and of one shared marker chromosome (the first on the list of marker chromosomes), with their F4-counterparts reveals that the F1-copy numbers are exactly duplicated in F4. This suggests that F4 probably originated from F1 by some form of karyotype duplication (see text)

the chromosome numbers of each karyotype on the x-axis, the copy numbers of each chromosome on the y-axis, and the number of karyotypes arrayed on the z-axis. Such arrays are specifically useful to define the degree of clonality and individuality of the inherently flexible karyotypes of cancers (see Fig. 1) for two reasons: Firstly, they reveal at a glance the degree of clonality, or lack of it, by parallel lines that are formed by the chromosomes of karyotypes with the same copy numbers. Secondly, arrays also reveal at a glance the individuality of clones in comparison with others, by forming individual patterns of clonal chromosome copy numbers, which are readily distinguishable from those of other clones.

As shown in Fig. 5a and the attached table, the karyotype array of F1 consists of an average number of 56 chromosomes (confirming Fig. 4a), which are 70 to 100 % clonal. Accordingly, the 56 F1-chromosomes formed the quasi-clonal, F1-specific karyotype array that is shown in Fig. 5a. In addition the F1-array also showed the 0-30 % of F1-chromosomes with non-clonal copy numbers, which reflect the inherent flexibility of cancer karyotypes (see above, Fig. 1).

In sum, we have demonstrated that the immortal F1 line has an individual (compared to normal) clonal karyotype and phenotype. The clonality and individuality of the F1-karyotype array confirm the prediction of the karyotypic theory that this karyotype has generated and since maintained the phenotype of the F1 line for over 200 generations.

The individuality and high complexity of the transcriptomes of SV40-transformed human neoplastic clones, which consist of hundreds of abnormally expressed mRNAs [43, 44], directly confirm the view that complex individual karyotypes, rather than common viral genes, encode the complex individual phenotypes of SV40-induced neoplastic clones.

We conclude that the F1 karyotype is either sufficient for neoplastic transformation or is necessary and possibly also dependent SV40 genes. If SV40-transformation were indeed dependent on SV40-genes, those genes would have to be present in all viral tumors and neoplastic clones, which we tested below (See, *Non-correlations between SV40 T-antigen and the cells of the immortal clones F1 and F4*, and Background).

Karyotypic variations of the neoplastic F1 line generate phenotypically distinct sub-clones

Variation of the F1 line to the phenotypically distinct F4 line
In an effort to confirm the predicted individuality of new neoplastic clones like F1, we compared the F1 line with a second immortal neoplastic line from SV40-infected human mesothelial cells, which was also isolated by Bocchetta et al. and named the F4 line [21].

The F4 phenotype To determine, whether F4 has an individual clonal phenotype, as predicted for an independent neoplastic clone by the karyotypic theory, we set up parallel cultures of F4 and F1, in which F1 served as a standard of comparison. As can be seen in Fig. 3b, the F4 line formed a multi-layered culture, which was distinct from the mostly mono-layered culture of F1 shown in Fig. 3a. But, the comparison also showed that both clones consist of cells with round to oval morphologies. These results thus indicated that the two lines are distinct sociologically, but have very similar cellular morphologies. According to our theory that cancer karyotypes encode cancer phenotypes, this result predicts that the karyotypes of F1 and F4 are related, yet distinct. This predicted karyotypic relationship of F1 and F4 was tested next.

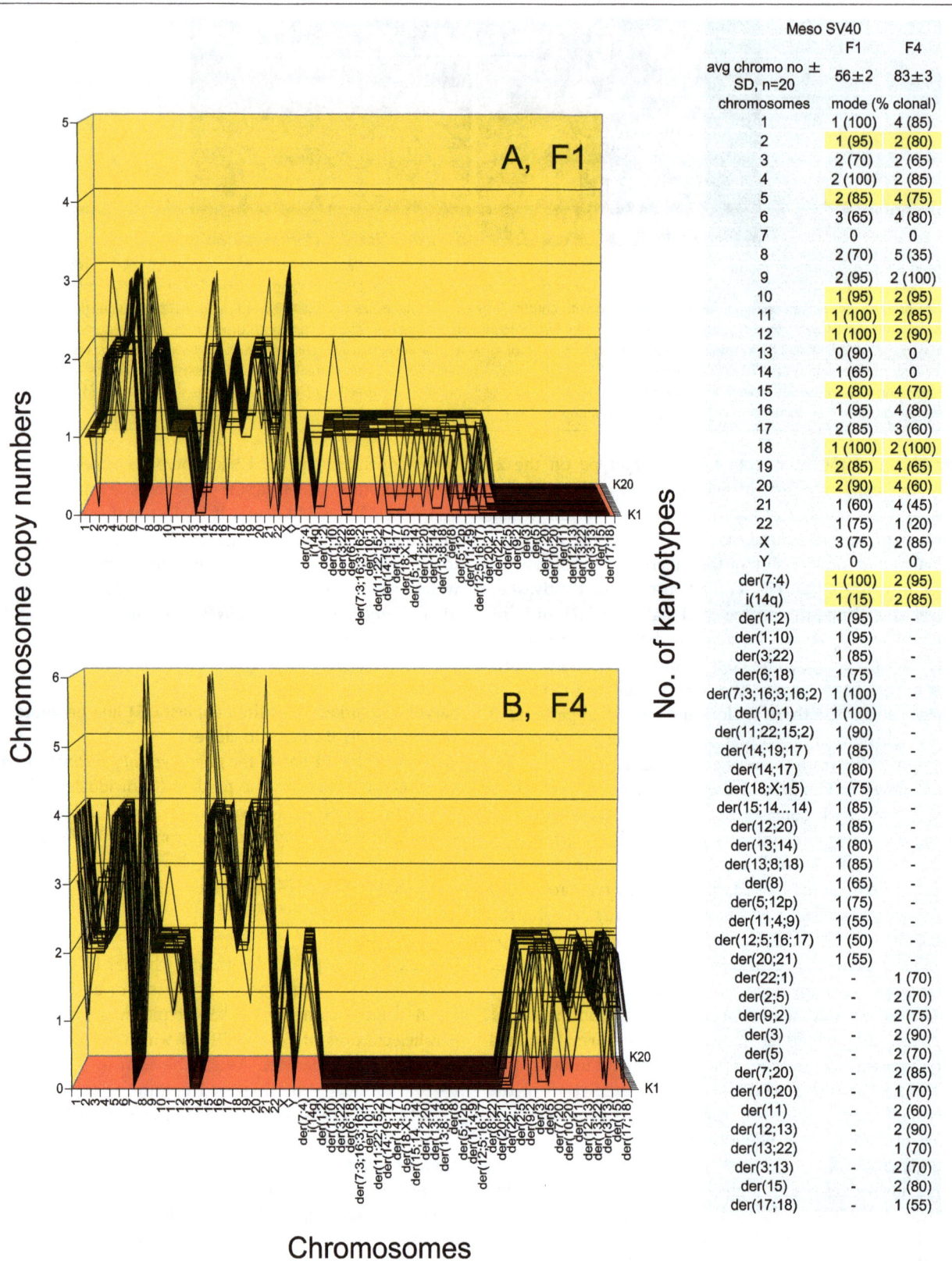

	Meso SV40	
	F1	F4
avg chromo no ± SD, n=20	56±2	83±3
chromosomes	mode (% clonal)	
1	1 (100)	4 (85)
2	1 (95)	2 (80)
3	2 (70)	2 (65)
4	2 (100)	2 (85)
5	2 (85)	4 (75)
6	3 (65)	4 (80)
7	0	0
8	2 (70)	5 (35)
9	2 (95)	2 (100)
10	1 (95)	2 (95)
11	1 (100)	2 (85)
12	1 (100)	2 (90)
13	0 (90)	0
14	1 (65)	0
15	2 (80)	4 (70)
16	1 (95)	4 (80)
17	2 (85)	3 (60)
18	1 (100)	2 (100)
19	2 (85)	4 (65)
20	2 (90)	4 (60)
21	1 (60)	4 (45)
22	1 (75)	1 (20)
X	3 (75)	2 (85)
Y	0	0
der(7;4)	1 (100)	2 (95)
i(14q)	1 (15)	2 (85)
der(1;2)	1 (95)	-
der(1;10)	1 (95)	-
der(3;22)	1 (85)	-
der(6;18)	1 (75)	-
der(7;3;16;3;16;2)	1 (100)	-
der(10;1)	1 (100)	-
der(11;22;15;2)	1 (90)	-
der(14;19;17)	1 (85)	-
der(14;17)	1 (80)	-
der(18;X;15)	1 (75)	-
der(15;14...14)	1 (85)	-
der(12;20)	1 (85)	-
der(13;14)	1 (80)	-
der(13;8;18)	1 (85)	-
der(8)	1 (65)	-
der(5;12p)	1 (75)	-
der(11;4;9)	1 (55)	-
der(12;5;16;17)	1 (50)	-
der(20;21)	1 (55)	-
der(22;1)	-	1 (70)
der(2;5)	-	2 (70)
der(9;2)	-	2 (75)
der(3)	-	2 (90)
der(5)	-	2 (70)
der(7;20)	-	2 (85)
der(10;20)	-	1 (70)
der(11)	-	2 (60)
der(12;13)	-	2 (90)
der(13;22)	-	1 (70)
der(3;13)	-	2 (70)
der(15)	-	2 (80)
der(17;18)	-	1 (55)

No. of karyotypes

Chromosomes

Fig. 5 (See legend on next page.)

The F4 karyotype Comparisons of the karyotypes and the karyotype arrays of F1 and F4 are shown in Figs. 4 and 5. As can be seen in Figs. 4b and 5b and the attached tables, the F4 line has a hypo-tetraploid karyotype with an average number of 83 chromosomes. The copy numbers of these chromosomes were 60-100 % clonal. Accordingly the F4-chromosomes formed a quasi-clonal F4-specific karyotype array, which is different from, but is also similar to that of the F1 line with only 56 chromosomes (compare Fig. 5a and b).

Accordingly, a close examination of the arrays of F1 and F4 revealed that 11 F4-chromosomes including one shared marker chromosome are exact duplications of the copy numbers of the corresponding F1-chromosomes (marked yellow in the table of Fig. 5). In addition the comparison shows that F1 and F4 also share two clonal nullisomies of chromosomes 7 and 13. Furthermore, several F4-chromosomes with non-duplicated copy numbers, compared to F1, were also increased in F4, but not exactly two-fold.

As a result the karyotype of F4 can be said to be an approximately two-fold amplification or tetraploidization of that of F1. Obviously this tetraploidization occurred together with the gain of 13 F4-specific markers and the loss of 19 F1-specific marker chromosomes, as can be seen in Figs. 4 and 5. We deduce from these karyological data that the F4 clone branched off from the original F1 clone by an approximate tetraploidization, including losses of F1-specific and gains of new F4-specific marker chromosomes. It is also consistent with our results that F4 and F1 derived from a common unknown, but near-diploid F1-like precursor of F1 and F4, and that each clone subsequently diverged individually.

Thus the F4 line is a variant of the F1 line, rather than an independent clone as initially expected [21]. This karyotypic relationship between F1 and F4 explains directly their phenotypic relationship that is shown in Fig. 3.

To test the view that SV40-induced neoplastic clones undergo spontaneous variations, we searched for additional, experimentally controllable variations of cancer phenotypes by karyotypic variations. For this purpose we studied next karyotype variations correlating with experimentally induced drug-resistance of F1 and F4.

Variation of F1 to a puromycin-resistant F1-variant

A puromycin-resistant variant of the F1 line was generated by selection of survivors at increasing concentrations of puromycin up to 2 μg per ml medium following published procedures [97, 102, 105]. The karyotype of the puromycin-resistant F1 was then compared with that of the parental F1 based on the karyotype arrays shown in Figs. 5a and 6.

As can be seen in Fig. 6, the puromycin-resistant F1 line has a hyper-tetraploid karyotype with an average number of 105 chromosomes, which are 45–100 % clonal. Accordingly, these 105 chromosomes formed an individual quasi-clonal karyotype array that is different from, but also similar to that of the hyper-diploid parental F1 line, shown above in Fig. 5a.

Moreover, a close comparison of the chromosome copy numbers of the puromycin-resistant F1-variant with the parental F1 line revealed that the copy numbers of 14 F1-chromosomes are exactly duplicated and six are increased to lesser or higher degrees in the puromycin-resistant F1 variant, compared to the parental clone. These duplications and concomitant near two-fold increases of chromosome copy numbers are marked yellow in the table of Fig. 6.

Thus the puromycin-resistant F1 is indeed a karyotypic variant of F1, rather than an independent clone. The underlying karyotypic variation was once more based on an approximate tetraploidization of the F1 karyotype (as in the variation from F1 to F4 described above). This tetraploidization coincided with the generation of 29 new resistance-specific marker chromosomes, the loss of three parental marker chromosomes and changed copy numbers of some shared non-duplicated chromosomes, marked yellow in the table of Fig. 6. The karyotypic variation that sets apart F1 from

Chromosome copy numbers

F1 rPuro

No. of karyotypes

Chromosomes

K20

K1

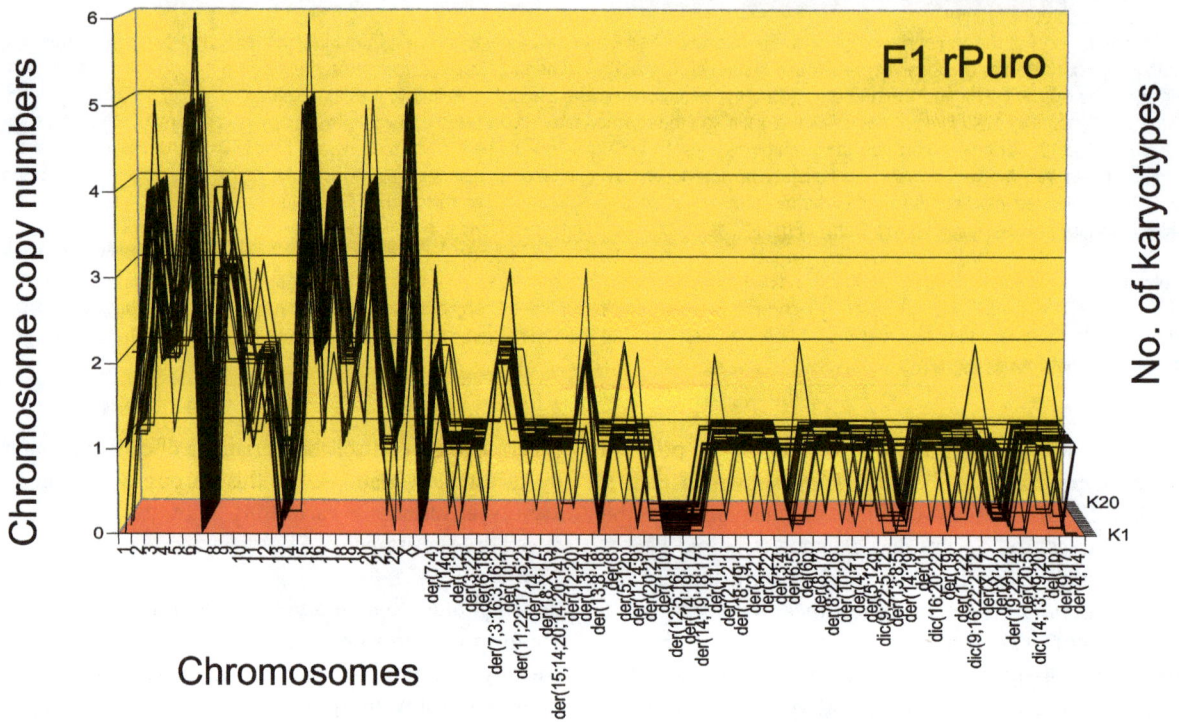

Comparison of the karyotypes of the puromycin-resistant F1 line with the parental neoplastic line.

avg ± SD, n=20 chromosomes	F1 56±2 mode (% clonal)	F1 rPuro 105±5 mode (% clonal)	clonal markers	F1 mode (% clonal)	F1 rPuro mode (% clonal)	clonal markers	F1 mode (%clonal)	F1 rPuro mode (%clonal)
1	1 (100)	1 (80)	der(7;4)	1 (100)	2 (80)	der(2;22)	-	1 (95)
2	1 (95)	2 (85)	i(14q)	1 (15)	1 (75)	der(3;4)	-	1 (95)
3	2 (70)	4 (80)	der(1;2)	1 (95)	1 (90)	der(6;5)	-	1 (35)
4	2 (100)	2 (90)	der(3;22)	1 (85)	1 (100)	del(6p)	-	1 (75)
5	2 (85)	3 (60)	der(6;18)	1 (75)	1 (90)	der(8;17)	-	1 (95)
6	3 (65)	5 (60)	der(7;3;16;3;16;2)	1 (100)	2 (90)	der(8;22;18)	-	1 (90)
7	0	0	der(10;1)	1 (100)	2 (80)	der(10;21)	-	1 (95)
8	2 (70)	3 (60)	der(11;22;17;15;2)	1 (90)	1 (90)	der(4;11)	1 (5)	1 (90)
9	2 (95)	3 (75)	der(14;17)	1 (80)	1 (95)	der(5;12q)	1 (5)	1 (85)
10	1 (95)	2 (60)	der(18;X;15)	1 (75)	1 (100)	dic(9;22;5;12)	-	1 (80)
11	1 (100)	2 (65)	der(15;14...14)	1 (85)	1 (90)	der(13;8;5)	-	1 (70)
12	1 (100)	2 (90)	der(12;20)	1 (85)	1 (90)	der(14;19)	1 (5)	1 (30)
13	0 (90)	0 (75)	der(13;14)	1 (80)	2 (75)	der(1)	-	1 (95)
14	1 (65)	1 (80)	der(13;8;18)	1 (85)	1 (50)	dic(16;20;22)	-	1 (95)
15	2 (80)	5 (70)	der(8)	1 (65)	1 (100)	der(19)	-	1 (95)
16	1 (95)	2 (85)	der(5;12p)	1 (75)	1 (85)	der(17;22)	-	1 (90)
17	2 (85)	4 (85)	der(11;4;9)	1 (55)	1 (85)	dic(9;16;22;2;12)	-	1 (90)
18	1 (100)	2 (80)	der(20;21)	1 (55)	1 (80)	der(X;17)	-	1 (90)
19	2 (85)	2 (80)	der(1;10)	1 (95)	-	der(X;12)	-	1 (65)
20	2 (90)	4 (80)	der(12;5;16;17)	1 (50)	-	der(19;22;14)	-	1 (25)
21	1 (60)	2 (65)	der(14;19;17)	1 (85)	-	der(20;5)	-	1 (80)
22	1 (75)	1 (85)	der(14;19;18;17)	-	1 (30)	dic(14;13;19;20)	1 (5)	1 (95)
X	3 (75)	5 (50)	der(11;1)	-	1 (90)	del(1p)	-	1 (80)
Y	0	0	der(21;2;1)	-	1 (90)	der(9;17)	-	1 (65)
			der(18;19;1)	-	1 (100)	der(4;14)	-	1(85)
			der(2;21)	1 (5)	1 (95)			

Fig. 6 (See legend on next page.)

the puromycin-resistant variant provides thus a consistent explanation for the corresponding phenotypic variation, namely the acquisition of the new puromycin-resistant phenotype.

Variation of F4 to a puromycin-resistant F4-variant

In the following the karyotype of F4, itself a variant of F1 (see Fig. 5 above), was compared to the karyotype of a variant of F4 that was resistant to puromycin at 2 µg per ml medium. The puromycin-resistant F4 line was prepared as described for the puromycin-resistant variant of F1 above.

As shown in Fig. 7 and the attached table, the puromycin-resistant F4 has a hypo-tetraploid karyotype with an average number of 80 chromosomes, which were 70–100 % clonal. Accordingly the chromosomes of drug-resistant F4 formed a clonal puromycin-resistant F4-specific karyotype array. This drug-resistant-F4 array is visibly related to, but also different from that of the parental F4 array, shown in Fig. 5b. Close comparisons of the two arrays indicate that the resistant F4 clone shared with the parental F4 clone 23 chromosomes with the same copy numbers including three rare nullisomies. The comparison further shows that the resistant clone differed from the parental clone randomly in the copy numbers of 13 intact chromosomes, the gain of two resistance-specific marker chromosomes and the loss of four parental marker chromosomes. Hence, the karyotypic variation that sets apart the puromycin-resistant F4-variant from the parental F4 is again consistent with the acquisition of puromycin-resistance by karyotypic variation, rather than being an independent clone.

In sum, all three examples of phenotypic variations of the original neoplastic F1 line support the theory that karyotype variations of neoplastic clones cause phenotype variations.

Karyotypic variation and origination: two distinct mechanisms generating new neoplastic clones

As a result of our comparative karyotypic analyses of immortal neoplastic clones derived from SV40-infected human mesothelial cells, we have now before us two distinct mechanisms that generate new neoplastic clones with distinct individual phenotypes:

1) The independent generation of new neoplastic clones with new individual clonal karyotypes and phenotypes from preneoplastic SV40-infected, aneuploid cells at very low rates (i.e., m3 in Fig. 1). Examples are the F1 clone from human mesothelial cells and 10 other neoplastic clones from SV40-infected rat and mouse cells described below (Sections II and III).

2) The generation of new neoplastic clones by variations of the karyotypes of existing neoplastic clones at rather high rates (i.e., m2 in Fig. 1). Examples are the three variants or sub-clones of the mesothelial F1 stem line described in Figs. 5, 6 and 7. We have described previously additional examples of karyotypic variants with new phenotypes derived from other established primary cancers, such as drug-resistant variants [105, 106] and metastatic variants [97, 107].

It may be argued, however, that the complex new individual karyotypes and transcriptomes of neoplastic clones are not sufficient to generate, maintain and vary their neoplastic phenotypes and that SV40-genes are also necessary. To test this possibility, we have asked whether viral proteins are consistently present in the virus-induced neoplastic line F1 and its derivative variants.

Non-correlations between SV40 T-antigen and the cells of the immortal lines F1 and F4

Our evidence that specific karyotypes generate and maintain the phenotypes of SV40 virus-induced neoplastic clones and of their variants raises the question, whether the initiating SV40 has any direct etiological role in maintaining and varying neoplastic clones. If so, all virus-induced neoplastic clones should contain SV40 genes, particularly the genes of the viral T-antigens [4–7].

To answer this question, we have reacted cultures of the immortal F1 and F4 clones with primary mouse antibodies against the T-antigen of SV40 and green-fluorescent secondary goat antibodies following the manufacturer's protocol (Abcam Inc., Cambridge, MA). In addition we have also counter-stained the same cultures with the blue-fluorescent DNA-specific dye Diamidino-2-Phenylindole (DAPI) to detect all cells of the F1 and F4 cultures, independent of the presence of T-antigen. As can be seen in

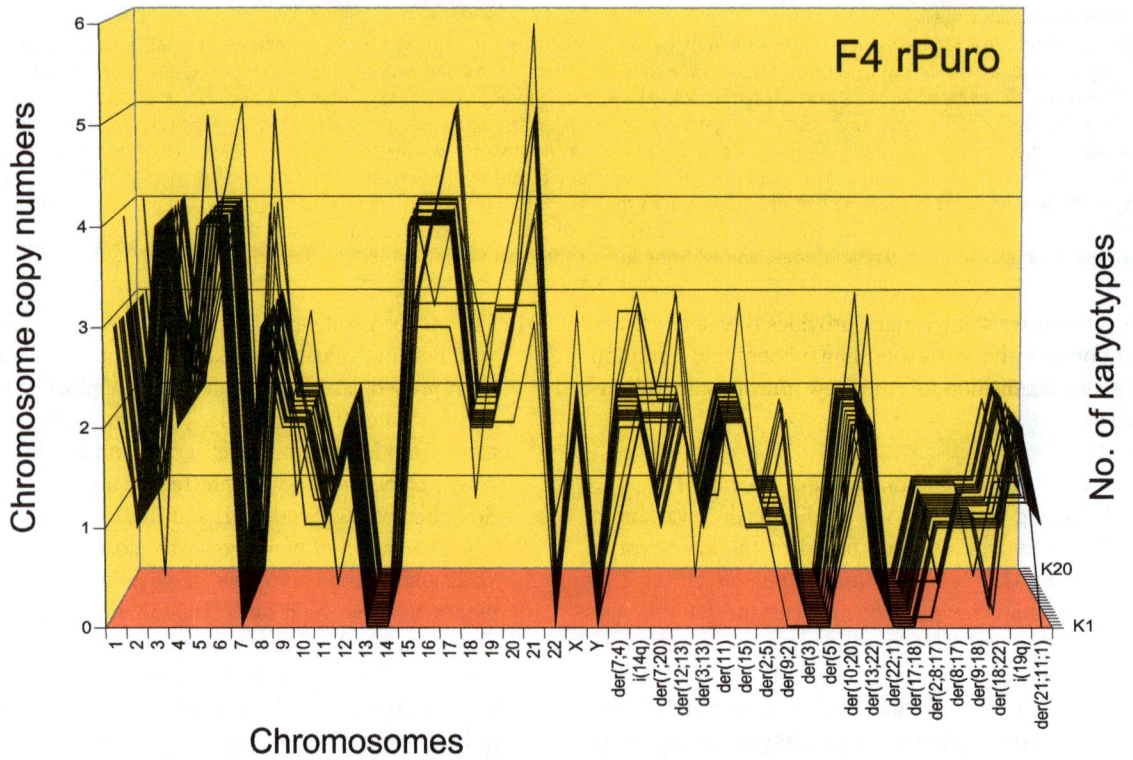

Comparison of the karyotypes of the puromycin-resistant F4 line with the parental F4 cell line.

avg ± SD, n=20	F4 83±3	F4 rPuro 80±2	clonal markers	F4	F4 rPuro
chromosomes	mode (% clonal)		der(7;4)	2 (95)	2 (80)
1	4 (85)	3 (80)	i(14q)	2 (85)	2 (85)
2	2 (80)	1 (95)	der(7;20)	2 (85)	1 (55)
3	2 (65)	4 (85)	der(12;13)	2 (90)	2 (85)
4	2 (85)	2 (100)	der(3;13)	2 (70)	1 (95)
5	4 (75)	4 (75)	der(11)	2 (60)	2 (95)
6	4 (80)	4 (90)	der(15)	2 (80)	2 (80)
7	0	0	der(2;5)	2 (70)	1 (100)
8	5 (35)/4 (30)	3 (80)	der(9;2)	2 (75)	1 (75)
9	2 (100)	2 (85)	der(3)	2 (90)	-
10	2 (95)	2 (80)	der(5)	2 (70)	-
11	2 (85)	1 (95)	der(10;20)	1 (70)	2 (70)
12	2 (90)	2 (95)	der(13;22)	1 (70)	2 (85)
13	0	0	der(22;1)	1 (70)	-
14	0	0	der(17;18)	1 (55)	-
15	4 (70)	4 (65)	der(2;8;17)	1 (15)	1 (90)
16	4 (80)	4 (85)	der(8;17)	1 (5)	1 (85)
17	3 (60)	4 (75)	der(9;18)	1 (15)	1 (100)
18	2 (100)	2 (85)	der(18;22)	1 (20)	1 (75)
19	4 (65)	2 (80)	i(19q)	-	2 (80)
20	4 (60)	3 (90)	der(21;11;1)	-	1 (95)
21	4 (45)	5 (70)			
22	0 (80)	0 (95)			
X	2 (85)	2 (95)			
Y	0	0			

Fig. 7 (See legend on next page.)

(See figure on previous page.)
Fig. 7 Comparison of the karyotype array of the F4 line with that of a puromycin-resistant derivative. To determine whether resistance to puromycin of the F4 line was acquired by karyotypic variation, as was found in Fig. 6, the karyotype array of a puromycin-resistant F4 variant was compared to that of the parental F4 line. The array of the drug-resistant F4 shows a hypo-tetraploid karyotype consisting of 80 chromosomes that were 55–100 % clonal. Accordingly, these chromosomes formed a quasi-clonal array, which is distinct from, but visibly related to from the parental F4 line, shown in Fig. 5b. Specifically, the puromycin-resistant F4 variant differs from the parental line in the copy numbers of 15 of their 34-shared chromosomes (marked yellow in Fig. 7), the gain of two resistance-specific marker chromosomes and the loss of four parental marker chromosomes. We conclude that the F4 line acquired resistance to puromycin by karyotypic variation, as was the case with the puromycin-resistant variant of the F1 clone described in Fig. 6

Fig. 8a, about 30 % of the F1-cells were negative for T-antigen. In the remaining cells the concentrations of T-antigen ranged from relatively low to high. Similarly, Fig. 8b shows that about 50 % of the F4-cells were negative for T-antigen. In the T-antigen-positive F4 cells the concentrations of the antigen also ranged from relatively low to high. Prior studies of negative and heterogeneous expressions of T-antigen in immortal clones from SV40-infected human cells are consistent with our observation [13, 35, 51, 63, 86] (see also Background).

We conclude from the non-correlations of T-antigen with the immortal neoplastic clones studied by us here and previously by others (Background), that T-antigen is not necessary to maintain neoplastic transformation and immortality. If the T-antigen were necessary for neoplastic transformation and immortality, then it should be present in all cells of a clone, just like the individual clonogenic karyotypes described above. Moreover, its level should have been equalized for optimal neoplastic concentration in all cells of the immortal F1 and F4 lines after selections for autonomy over the 200 generations since their isolation (see above).

The over 20 previous studies listed in the Background, which reported SV40-induced neoplastic human, hamster, mouse and rat clones without viral genes and T-antigens lend further definitive support to this conclusion.

In the following we have tested the generality of the theory that SV40 transforms cells indirectly by inducing aneuploidy, which catalyzes spontaneous karyotypic evolutions of rare immortal neoplastic clones in rat and mouse cells.

II. Transformation of rat cells by SV40

Next we tested, whether the karyotypic mechanism of transformation described for human mesothelial cells also applies to the formation of neoplastic clones from SV40-infected rat cells. For this purpose we studied primary rat lung cells infected with SV40 virus at a multiplicity of two, as described above for human cells and previously by others for primary rat cells [3, 41, 88].

Karyotypes of SV40-infected preneoplastic rat lung cells

To test SV40-infected lung cells for the preneoplastic aneuploidy predicted by the karyotypic theory, the karyotypes of infected cells were determined three weeks after infection. This time point was chosen, because confluent cultures of rat lung cells infected at a multiplicity two and passaged twice at 3-fold dilutions formed foci three weeks after infection (see next paragraph). At that time we analyzed the karyotypes of the non-transformed, inter-focal regions of the infected culture for virus-induced

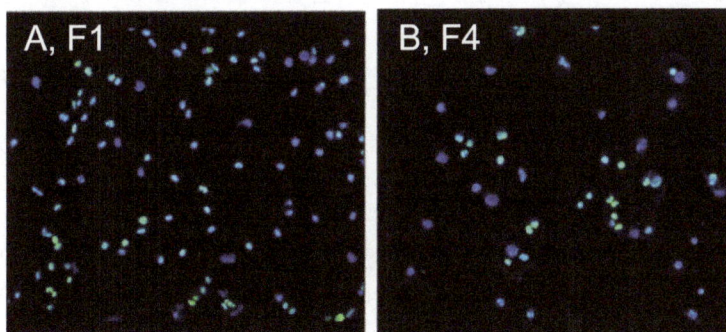

Fig. 8 Non-correlations between SV40 T-antigen and the cells of the immortal clones F1 and F4. To answer the question whether clonal cancer karyotypes are sufficient to generate and maintain neoplastic clones or are also dependent on T-antigen, we analyzed the immortal neoplastic clones F1 and F4 for the presence of viral T- antigen. For this purpose F1 and F4 cell cultures were reacted with mouse anti-T-antigen antibodies-linked to a green fluorescent dye and counter-stained with the blue fluorescent DNA dye, 'DAPI,' to detect nuclear DNA irrespective of T-antigen (Methods). **a** shows that about 30 % of the cells of the F1 line were T-antigen negative, while the remaining 70 % were heterogeneous for T-antigen expression ranging from very low to relatively high levels. **b** shows that about 50 % of the cells of F4 were T-antigen negative, whereas the rest of the cells were heterogeneous ranging from very low to relatively high T-antigen levels, similar to the F1 culture. We conclude that T-antigen is not necessary to maintain neoplastic transformation of F1 and F4 lines

preneoplastic aneuploidy. As can be seen in Table 3, 65 % of the infected, non-transformed rat cells contained randomly aneuploid karyotypes at that time, by contrast un-infected controls were 95 % diploid (not shown). This result extended the findings of high percentages of preneo-plastic aneuploidies in SV40-infected human mesothelial cells, described above in Tables 1 and 2 and in the Background. We conclude that SV40 induces preneoplastic aneuploidy in rat cells, just as it did in the human cells described above.

Phenotypes and karyotypes of focal colonies of transformed rat cells

Three weeks after infection of 10^6 rat lung cells and their subsequent expansion to confluent cultures, as described above, a total of 108 foci of morphologically transformed cells arose from three confluent 10-cm dishes of infected rat cells. This time course from infection to focus formation in rat cells confirms and extends prior studies [39, 83]. A typical focus arising from the confluent background of the virus-infected rat cells is

Table 3 Karyotypes of rat lung cells 3 weeks after infection with SV40: 13 aneuploid per 20

Karyotypes	1	2	3	4	5	6	7	8	9	10	11	12	13
Total no of chromosomes	45	42	43	43	43	44	42	43	43	44	42	70	86
Chromosomes													
1	2	2	2	2	2	2	2	2	2	2	2	3	4
2	2	2	2	2	2	2	1	2	2	2	2	4	4
3	2	3	2	2	3	2	3	3	2	2	2	3	6
4	2	2	2	2	2	2	2	2	2	2	2	2	4
5	2	2	2	2	2	2	2	2	2	2	1	4	4
6	2	2	2	2	2	2	2	2	2	2	2	4	4
7	2	2	2	2	2	2	2	2	2	2	2	4	4
8	2	2	2	2	2	2	2	2	2	2	2	4	4
9	2	2	2	2	2	2	2	2	2	2	2	4	4
10	1	2	2	2	2	2	2	2	2	2	2	4	4
11	3	2	2	2	2	2	2	2	2	2	2	2	4
12	1	2	2	2	2	2	2	2	2	2	2	3	4
13	2	2	2	2	2	2	2	2	2	2	2	3	4
14	2	2	2	2	2	2	2	2	2	2	2	2	4
15	2	2	2	2	2	2	2	2	2	2	2	3	4
16	2	1	2	2	2	2	2	2	2	2	2	3	4
17	2	2	2	2	2	2	2	2	2	2	2	2	4
18	2	2	2	2	2	2	2	2	2	2	2	4	4
19	2	2	2	2	2	2	2	2	2	2	2	4	4
20	2	2	2	2	2	2	1	2	2	2	2	4	4
X	2	2	2	2	2	2	1	2	2	2	2	4	4
Y	0	0	0	0	0	0	0	0	0	0	0	0	0
der(3;12)	0	0	0	0	0	1	0	0	1	0	0	0	0
del(2)(q?)	0	0	0	0	0	0	1	0	0	0	0	0	0
dic(X;20)	0	0	0	0	0	0	1	0	0	0	0	0	0
der(5)	0	0	0	0	0	0	0	0	0	0	1	0	0
der(12;10)	1	0	0	0	0	0	0	0	0	0	0	0	0
der(10)	1	0	0	0	0	0	0	0	0	0	0	0	0
dic(11;17)	1	0	0	0	0	0	0	0	0	0	0	0	0
del(17q)	1	0	0	0	0	0	0	0	0	0	0	0	0
mar(?)	0	0	1	1	0	1	0	0	0	0	0	0	0
der(3;2)	0	0	0	0	0	0	0	0	0	1	0	0	0
del(14q)	0	0	0	0	0	0	0	0	0	1	0	0	0

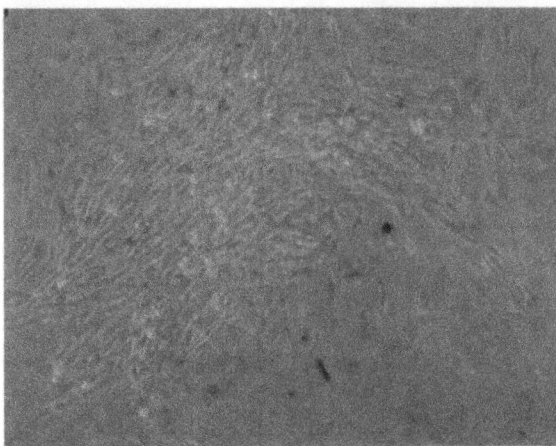

Fig. 9 Focus of transformed cells from a culture of rat lung cells three weeks after infection with SV40. This focus was one of 108 that arose in confluent secondary cultures of rat lung cells three weeks after infection of a primary culture with SV40 virus. The micrograph was taken at 120X magnification. Details of preparing the culture are described in the text

shown in Fig. 9. The yield of 108 focal colonies of transformed cells corresponds to clonogenic transformation of only one in 10,000 of the 10^6 originally infected cells. This low probability of neoplastic transformation of SV40-infected rat cells is also consistent with that observed in prior studies of neoplastic transformation of rat [41, 88] and of human mesothelial cells described by others including Bochetta et al., who prepared the F1 an F4 lines studied above [21], (see also Background).

Morphologically distinct phenotypes of neoplastic rat clones
To determine, whether the focal colonies of SV40-infected rat cells contain the predicted individual clonal phenotypes, cultures of six colonies termed, F8, F33, F3, F100, F10 and FC1 were investigated. Micrographs at 120X magnification of these six cultures show in Fig. 10 that each colony had its own, rather uniform and thus quasi-clonal cell morphology. This result also confirmed previous descriptions of clonal individualities [41, 88]. Moreover, the estimated growth rates of individual colonies were clone-specific like those described previously by others [3, 17, 41, 88]. The growth rate of the F100 clone was stable over 50 passages corresponding to over 100 cell generations, consistent with neoplastic immortality. In sum, these results confirmed the prediction of the karyotypic theory that individual neoplastic clones have individual clonal phenotypes (Fig. 1).

Individual karyotypes of neoplastic rat clones
To test for the predicted clonal karyotypic origins of the six rat colonies F8, F33, F3, F100, F10 and FC1 shown in Fig. 10, we used the karyotype array technique that was introduced for this purpose above in Fig. 5 and Section I. The karyotype arrays of these six neoplastic rat colonies are shown below in three figures, each depicting the arrays of two of the six rat colonies with the following results:

Figure 11a and the attached table shows that F8 contains a near-diploid karyotype with 41 chromosomes, which were 85–100 % clonal. (The normal Norwegian rat contains 42 chromosomes.) Accordingly the F8-chromosomes formed a quasi-clonal F8-specific karyotype array. In addition F8 contained several partially clonal and several non-clonal

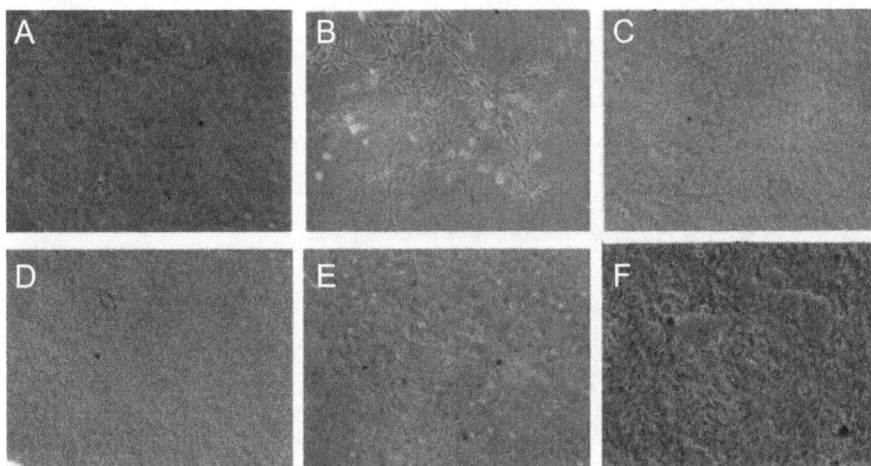

Fig. 10 Individual cell morphologies of six focal colonies from cultured primary rat lung cells, three weeks after infection with SV40. To test the theory that the karyotypes of individual neoplastic clones encode individual phenotypes, we analyzed the cellular morphologies of six focal colonies from SV40-infected rat lung cells (see example in Fig. 9). As can be seen by the 120X magnification of cultures of the six focal colonies, F8 (**a**), F33 (**b**), F3 (**c**), F100 (**d**), F10 (**e**) and FC1 (**f**), all clones had individual cell morphologies. This result indicates that individual karyotypes, rather than common viral genes, encode the individual phenotypes of the distinct neoplastic clones

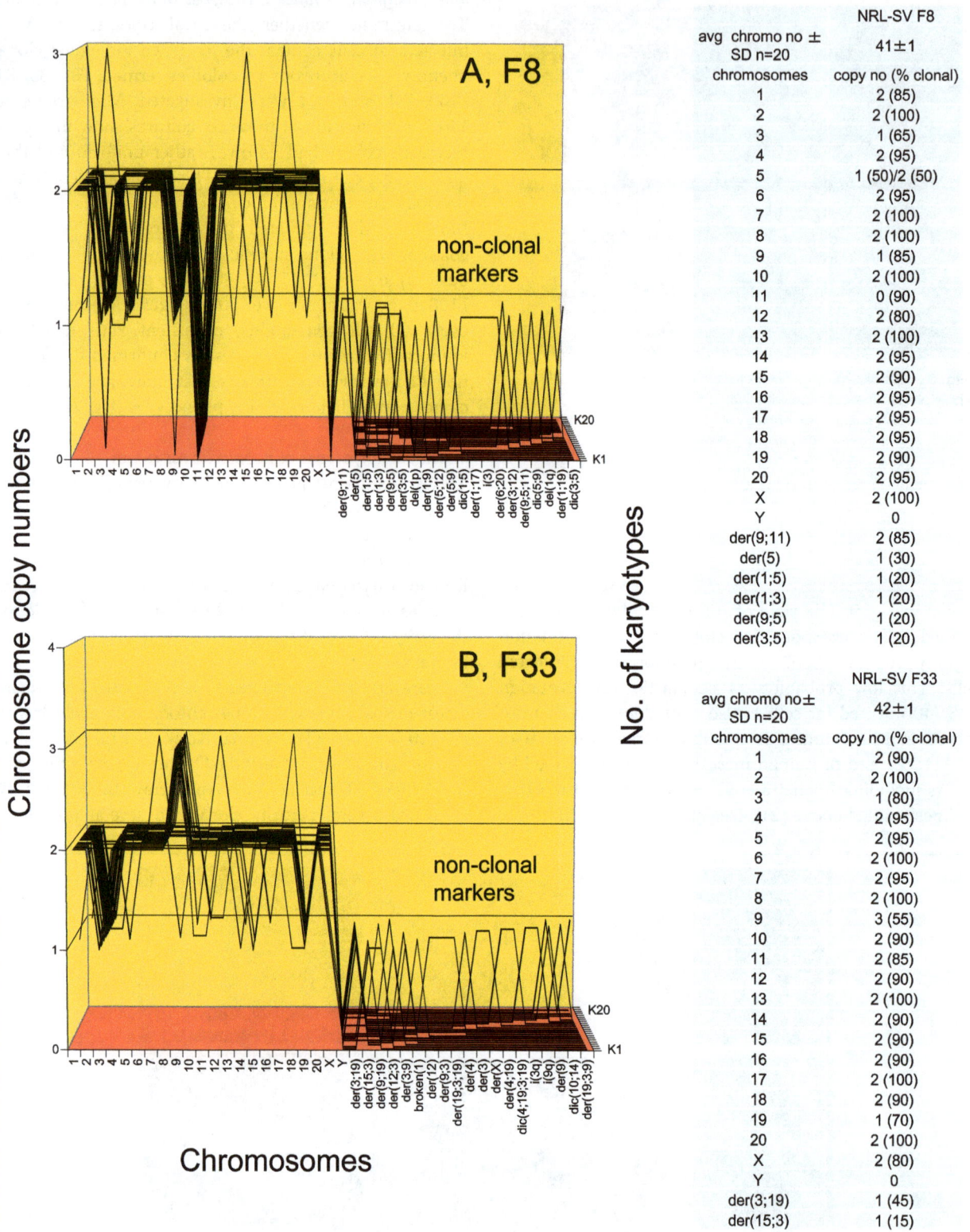

	NRL-SV F8
avg chromo no ± SD n=20	41±1
chromosomes	copy no (% clonal)
1	2 (85)
2	2 (100)
3	1 (65)
4	2 (95)
5	1 (50)/2 (50)
6	2 (95)
7	2 (100)
8	2 (100)
9	1 (85)
10	2 (100)
11	0 (90)
12	2 (80)
13	2 (100)
14	2 (95)
15	2 (90)
16	2 (95)
17	2 (95)
18	2 (95)
19	2 (90)
20	2 (95)
X	2 (100)
Y	0
der(9;11)	2 (85)
der(5)	1 (30)
der(1;5)	1 (20)
der(1;3)	1 (20)
der(9;5)	1 (20)
der(3;5)	1 (20)

	NRL-SV F33
avg chromo no± SD n=20	42±1
chromosomes	copy no (% clonal)
1	2 (90)
2	2 (100)
3	1 (80)
4	2 (95)
5	2 (95)
6	2 (100)
7	2 (95)
8	2 (100)
9	3 (55)
10	2 (90)
11	2 (85)
12	2 (90)
13	2 (100)
14	2 (90)
15	2 (90)
16	2 (90)
17	2 (100)
18	2 (90)
19	1 (70)
20	2 (100)
X	2 (80)
Y	0
der(3;19)	1 (45)
der(15;3)	1 (15)

Fig. 11 (See legend on next page.)

marker chromosomes, indicative of ongoing karyotypic variation (explained in Fig. 1). Fig. 11b shows that F33 contains a pseudo-diploid karyotype with 42 chromosomes that were 70–100 % clonal. Accordingly the F33 chromosomes also formed an individual quasi-clonal karyotype array, which was different from that of F8. The distinct individualities of these two karyotype arrays thus support the theory that neoplastic clones have individual karyotypes that encode individual phenotypes.

Figure 12a shows that F3 contains a near-diploid karyotype of 41 chromosomes that were 70-100 % clonal. Accordingly, the F3-chromosomes formed an individual quasi-clonal F3-specific karyotype array, which was different from those of F8 and F33 shown in Fig. 11. A third of the F3 cells had near-tetraploid karyotypes that appeared to be duplications of the predominant near-diploid F3 karyotypes. Figure 12b shows that F100 also contains a near-diploid karyotype with 43 chromosomes that were 95-100 % clonal. The very high clonality of the F100 colony may be a result of stabilizing selections during its long passage history. F100 dates from an early pilot experiment conducted before the other rat clones were prepared. Accordingly the F100-chromosomes also formed an individual clonal F100-specific karyotype array, which was different from those of F3, F8 and F33. Thus, the karyotypes of four distinct neoplastic rat clones support the theory that individual karyotypes encode the individual phenotypes of neoplastic clones.

Figure 13a shows that F10 contains a near-diploid karyotype with an average number of 41 chromosomes that were between 70 and 100 % clonal. Accordingly they formed a quasi-clonal array, which was different from those of colonies F8, F33, F3 and F100. The F10 clone also included a minor (15 %) tetraploid variant, similar to that found in clone F3 described above (Fig. 12a). Fig. 13b shows that clone FC1 contains a near triploid karyotype with 64 chromosomes that were between 55 and 100 % clonal. Accordingly the FC1 chromosomes formed an individual quasi-clonal array, which differed from those of all five sister colonies described above and in Figs. 11 and 12.

In sum, the individual karyotype arrays of all six morphologically distinct rat clones support the theory that individual clonal karyotypes generate and encode the individual phenotypes of neoplastic clones.

Non-correlations between SV40 T-antigen and the cells of the neoplastic rat clones F3 and F100

It may be argued as above (Fig. 8) that the individual clonal karyotypes of virus-induced neoplastic rat clones may depend on SV40 genes for neoplastic transformation. In view of this we tested the neoplastic clones F3 and F100 for the presence of T-antigen, as described above for Fig. 8. As shown in Fig. 14a, we found that SV40 T-antigen is heterogeneously distributed among the cells of the F3 clone: some cells were T-antigen-free and others contained various low to high levels of T-antigen. By contrast, we found no T-antigen in F100 cells under our conditions, as shown in Fig. 14b. The absence of the karyotype-destabilizing effect of the T-antigen may also explain the high clonality of F100 (see Fig. 12b).

Because of these non-correlations between T-antigen and neoplastic rat cells prepared here and those observed above with neoplastic human cells (Fig. 8), we conclude that T-antigen is not necessary for the neoplastic proliferation of SV40-induced immortal human and rat clones (Section I, Fig. 8). This conclusion is supported by dozens of other studies describing SV40-induced neoplastic clones of human or rodent cells that either contain fractions of T-antigen-negative cells or are entirely T-antigen-free (Background).

In sum karyotypic analysis of neoplastic transformation of rat cells by SV40 virus confirms karyotypic theory of viral transformation

The karyotypic clonality and individuality of six focal rat colonies thus confirms once more the prediction of the karyotypic theory that individual karyotypes are the genetic origins of these neoplastic clones and maintain the individualities of these clones via complex transcriptomes [37, 38, 43, 44]`– independent of SV40 genes. Since viral genes are not cancer-specific, not likely to generate individuality, not present in all neoplastic cells and are too few to explain the endless individualities of virus-induced neoplastic clones and tumors described

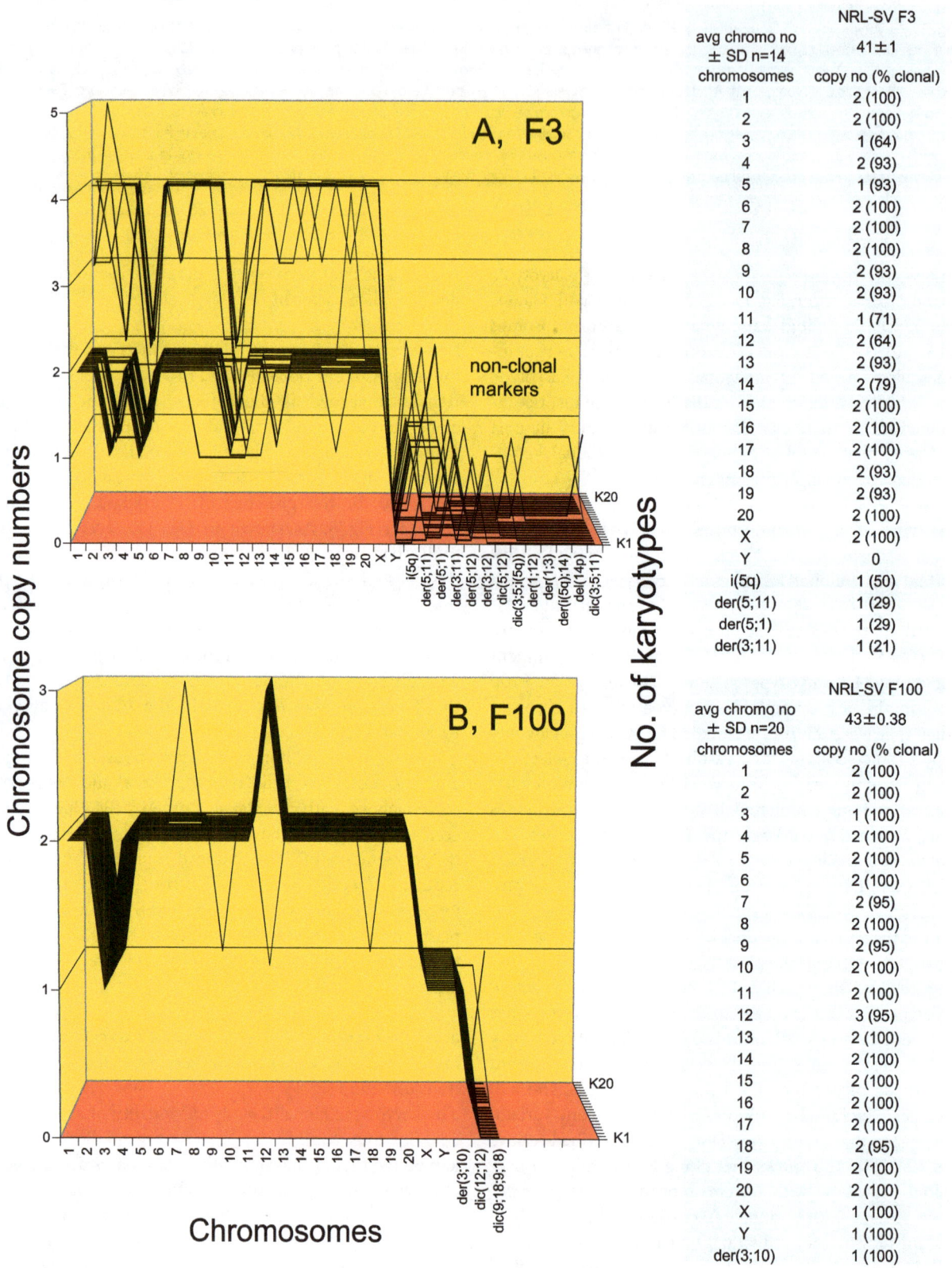

Fig. 12 (See legend on next page.)

(See figure on previous page.)
Fig. 12 Karyotype arrays of six morphologically distinct focal colonies from SV40-infected rat lung cells: second pair of three. To test the theory that individual clonal karyotypes encode the individual phenotypes, two more of the six morphologically distinct rat clones described in Fig. 10 were compared. **a** shows that F3 has a near-diploid karyotype of 41 chromosomes that were 70–100 % clonal. Accordingly, the F3 chromosomes formed an individual, quasi-clonal karyotype array, which was different from those of F8 and F33 shown in Fig. 11. A third of the F3 cells had near-tetraploid karyotypes that appeared to be duplications of the predominant near-diploid F3 karyotypes. **b** shows that F100 has a near-diploid karyotype with 43 chromosomes that were 95–100 % clonal. Accordingly the F100 chromosomes also formed a quasi-clonal F100 karyotype array, which was different from those of F3, F8 and F33. Thus the karyotypes of four distinct neoplastic rat clones support the theory that individual karyotypes encode the individual phenotypes of neoplastic clones

here and previously (Background), we conclude that the individual clonal karyotypes of SV40-induced neoplastic clones are sufficient for neoplastic transformation.

In the following we have tested the karyotypic theory of viral transformation in SV40-infected mouse embryo cells.

III. Transformation of mouse embryo cells by SV40

Last we test whether the karyotypic mechanism of transformation described for human mesothelial and rat lung cells also applies to the formation of neoplastic clones from SV40-infected mouse embryo cells. For this purpose we studied mouse embryo cells infected with SV40 virus, as described above for rat cells and previously for mouse lung and tail cells [89].

Karyotypes of SV40-infected preneoplastic mouse embryo cells

To determine, whether SV40 induces preneoplastic aneuploidy in mouse cells as predicted by the karyotypic theory, we examined cultures derived from 10^6 mouse embryo cells infected with SV40 at a multiplicity of two as described above for the infection of rat cells. About three weeks after infection, when rare foci of transformed cells first appeared (see next paragraph), we karyotyped the non-transformed, inter-focal regions of the SV40-infected mouse embryo cultures to test for the predicted preneoplastic aneuploidy.

As shown in Table 4, 65 % or 13 of 20 cells of the infected, non-transformed mouse cells contained randomly aneuploid karyotypes at that time, compared to less than 5 % in uninfected controls (not shown). This high level of aneuploidization of mouse cells by SV40 is very similar to those described above for SV40-infected human and rat cells at this stage of infection (Tables 1, 2 and 3; See also Background). At variance with human and rat cells, 77 % or 10 of the 13 karyotypes of aneuploid mouse cells were near tetraploid.

Phenotypes and karyotypes of focal colonies of transformed mouse cells

Between three and four weeks after infection of the primary culture of 10^6 mouse embryo cells about 50 distinct foci of morphologically transformed cells appeared in confluent subcultures, which were expanded and maintained as described above for the rat cultures. This yield of 50 foci corresponded to clonogenic neoplastic transformation of about one per 20,000 of the one million originally infected cells. This low yield of clonogenic transformation is in close agreement with the yields of about one or less per 10,000 SV40-infected rat and human mesothelial cells described above and in Background.

Phenotypes of neoplastic mouse clones

We selected four of these foci, F1, F9, F10 and F11 to determine whether they contain the individual clonal phenotypes and karyotypes predicted by the karyotypic theory. As can be seen in Fig. 15, all four focal colonies from SV40-infected mouse cells had individual and clonal cell morphologies, as was the case for the rat colonies described above in Fig. 10. These focal mouse colonies also grew at individual rates. For example, the growth rate of F9 was relatively low compared to those of F10 and F11. Moreover, preliminary tests of the predicted immortality of F10 (Fig. 1) showed that this clone survived over 40 cell generations in culture without any loss of viability. In fact the growth rate of F10 seemed to increase during these passages in culture confirming reports that transformation to autonomous growth and immortality is easier to achieve with SV40-infected mouse cells than with human cells [13, 17, 108].

Karyotypes of neoplastic mouse clones

To test for the predicted clonal karyotypic origins of the four transformed colonies F1, F9, F10 and F11 of SV40-infected mouse embryo cells shown in Fig. 15, we prepared their karyotype arrays as described above for Figs. 5, 6, 7, 11, 12 and 13. The results are shown in the following two Figures, each depicting the arrays of two of the four focal colonies.

Figure 16a and the attached table shows that the F1 mouse colony has a near diploid karyotype with an average number of 39 chromosomes, which were 82 to 100 % clonal. (The normal mouse contains 40 chromosomes.) Accordingly, the 39 F1-chromosomes formed a quasi-clonal F1-specific karyotype array, which is shown

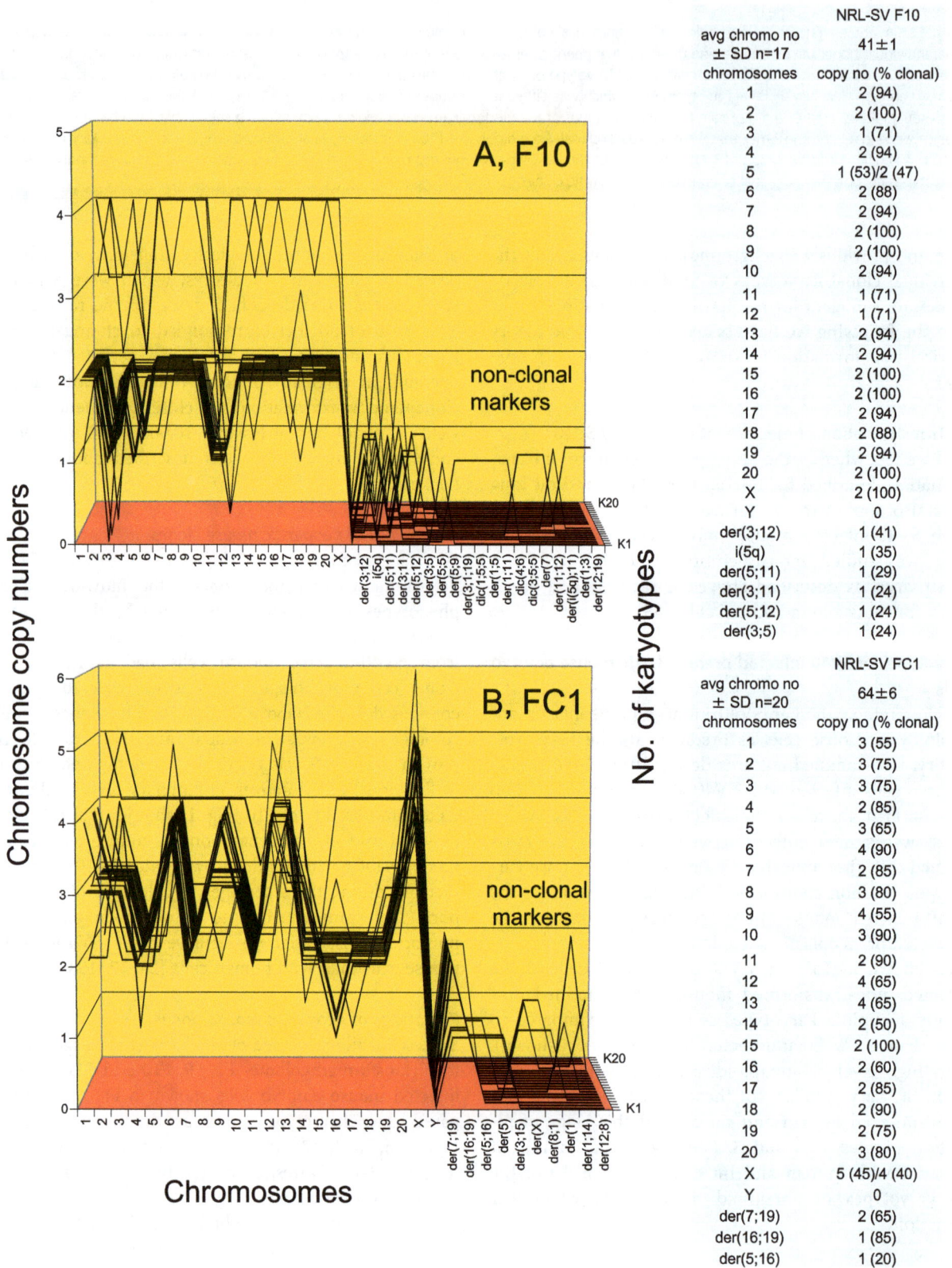

Fig. 13 (See legend on next page.)

(See figure on previous page.)

Fig. 13 Karyotype arrays of six morphologically distinct focal colonies derived from SV40-infected rat lung cells: third pair of three. To test the theory that individual clonal karyotypes encode individual phenotypes, we analyzed and compared the arrays of a third pair of six individually distinct rat focal colonies. **a** shows that F10 has a near-diploid karyotype with an average number of 41 chromosomes that were between 70 and 100 % clonal. Accordingly they formed a quasi-clonal F10-specific array, which is different from those of the F8, F33, F3 and F100 colonies. The F10 clone also includes a minor (15 %) tetraploid variant, similar to that found in clone F3 described above (Fig. 12a). **b** shows that clone FC1 has a near triploid karyotype with 64 chromosomes that were between 55 and 100 % clonal. Accordingly they formed a quasi-clonal FC1-specific array, which differs from those of all five sister colonies described above and in Figs. 11 and 12. Thus the individual karyotypes of the six phenotypically distinct rat clones support the theory that individual karyotypes encode the individual phenotypes of neoplastic clones

in Fig. 16a. The F1 colony also included a minor (15 %) tetraploid variant, much like the two rat clones described above in Figs. 11a and 12a. Figure 16b shows that the F9 colony has a hypo-tetraploid karyotype with an average number of 76 chromosomes, which were 65 to 95 % clonal. Accordingly the F9-chromosomes also formed an individual quasi-clonal F9-specific array, which was different from that of F1.

Figure 17a and the attached table shows that the F10 mouse colony has a hyper-tetraploid karyotype with an average number of 96 chromosomes, which were 70 to 100 % clonal. Accordingly the F10-chromosomes formed an individual quasi-clonal F10-specific array, which differed from those of F1 and F9. Figure 16b shows that F11 has a near-tetraploid karyotype with an average of 78 chromosomes, which were 85 to 100 % clonal with the exception of chromosome 4 that was only 55 % clonal. Accordingly, the F11-chromosomes also formed an individual, quasi-clonal F11-specific array, which differed from those of all three sister clones.

In sum karyotypic analysis of neoplastic transformation of mouse cells by SV40 virus confirms the karyotypic theory of viral transformation

Thus all four morphologically distinct focal colonies of SV40-infected mouse cells analyzed formed highly clonal, individual karyotype arrays – similar to the individual neoplastic clones of SV40-infected human and rat cells described above. Moreover, there is also evidence in the literature that virus-induced neoplastic mouse clones each have highly complex, individual transcriptomes [37, 38], which directly confirms the view that individual karyotypes encode the individual phenotypes of neoplastic clones via individual transcriptomes. The clonality and individuality of the karyotypes of four focal mouse colonies thus confirms once more the prediction of the karyotypic theory that individual karyotypes are the genetic origins of these neoplastic clones, and maintain the individualities of these clones – rather than common viral T-antigens, which are present in all pre-neoplastic cells and which are unlikely to encode the complex individual transcriptomes and phenotypes of neoplastic clones.

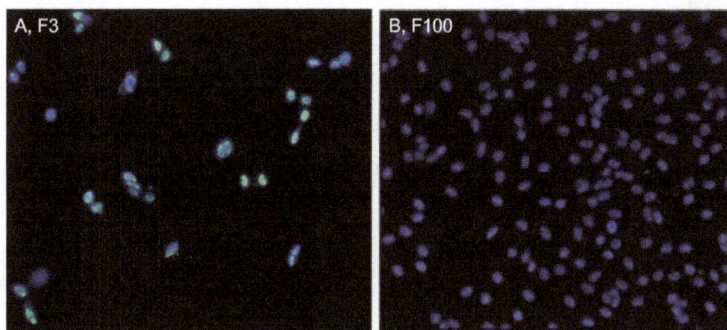

Fig. 14 Non-correlations between the cells of two SV40-induced neoplastic clones of rat lung cells and SV40 T-antigen. To test the prediction of the karyotypic theory that the clonal karyotypes of SV40-induced neoplastic clones are sufficient to generate and maintain neoplastic clones, independent of the viral T-antigen, we analyzed the cells of the SV40-induced neoplastic rat clones F3 and F100 (described in Figs. 10 and 12) for the presence of viral T-antigen with green-labeled antibodies, as described above for Fig. 8. **a** shows that about 30 % of the F3 cells were T-antigen negative, while the remaining 70 % were heterogeneous, expressing T-antigen between very low to relatively high levels. **b** shows that all cells of the neoplastic rat clone F100 were T-antigen negative under the conditions of our test (Methods). We concluded from the absence of detectable T-antigen in F100 and the absence or heterogeneous presence of T-antigen in F3 cells that T-antigen is not necessary to maintain neoplastic transformation of SV40-induced neoplastic rat clones, as predicted by the karyotypic theory

Table 4 Karyotypes of mouse embryonic cells 3 weeks after infection with SV40: 13 aneuploid per 20

Karyotypes	1	2	3	4	5	6	7	8	9	10	11	12	13
Total no of chromosomes	36	40	39	74	74	81	79	78	79	79	78	79	80
Chromosomes													
1	2	1	1	4	3	4	4	4	4	4	4	4	4
2	2	2	2	4	4	4	4	4	4	4	4	4	4
3	2	2	2	3	3	4	4	4	4	4	3	4	4
4	2	2	2	3	3	4	4	4	4	3	4	4	4
5	2	2	1	3	4	4	4	4	4	4	4	4	4
6	1	2	2	4	3	4	4	2	4	4	4	4	4
7	2	2	2	4	4	4	4	4	4	4	4	4	4
8	2	2	2	4	4	4	4	4	4	4	4	4	4
9	1	1	1	3	3	4	4	4	4	4	4	4	4
10	2	1	1	4	3	4	4	4	4	4	4	4	4
11	2	2	1	3	4	4	4	4	4	4	4	4	4
12	1	2	2	4	4	4	4	4	4	4	4	3	4
13	2	2	2	4	4	4	4	4	4	4	4	5	4
14	1	2	2	4	4	4	4	4	4	4	3	4	4
15	2	2	2	4	4	4	4	4	4	4	4	4	4
16	2	2	2	3	4	4	4	4	4	4	4	4	4
17	1	2	2	4	4	5	4	4	4	4	4	3	4
18	2	2	2	4	4	4	3	4	4	4	4	4	4
19	2	2	2	4	3	4	4	4	4	4	4	4	4
X	1	1	1	2	2	2	2	2	2	2	2	2	2
Y	1	1	1	2	2	2	2	2	1	2	2	2	2
dup(Xq)	0	0	0	0	1	0	0	0	0	0	0	0	0
del(9)(q)	1	0	0	0	0	0	0	0	0	0	0	0	0
der(1;9)	0	1	1	0	0	0	0	0	0	0	0	0	0
der(10;11)	0	1	0	0	0	0	0	0	0	0	0	0	0
der(10)	0	1	1	0	0	0	0	0	0	0	0	0	0
der(5)	0	0	1	0	0	0	0	0	0	0	0	0	0
der(11)	0	0	1	0	0	0	0	0	0	0	0	0	0

Moreover, the facts that (1) three of the four neoplastic mouse clones were near tetraploid and a fourth was partially tetraploid, and that (2) the majority of preneoplastic karyotypes of SV40-infected mouse cells was also tetraploid (Table 4) support the prediction of our theory that cells with preneoplastic aneuploidies are the precursors of neoplastic clones (Fig. 1).

Conclusions

This study was undertaken to test the theory that SV40 induces cancer indirectly by inducing preneoplastic aneuploidy, much like conventional carcinogens [97, 101, 109, 110]. Since aneuploidy unbalances thousands of genes,

it destabilizes the karyotype and thus catalyzes automatic evolutions of new karyotypes and transcriptomes including rare cancer-specific karyotypes and transcriptomes at very low rates [97]. This theory is outlined in the Background and graphically summarized in Fig. 1. The theory predicts that despite their destabilizing congenital aneuploidies cancer karyotypes are stabilized or immortalized within narrow karyotype-specific margins of variations by selections for cancer-specific autonomy of growth [97, 101, 102], (Fig. 1). Moreover, the theory predicts that the abnormal karyotypes of cancers generate highly complex, individual transcriptomes with hundreds of abnormally expressed mRNAs and thus highly complex new phenotypes. This

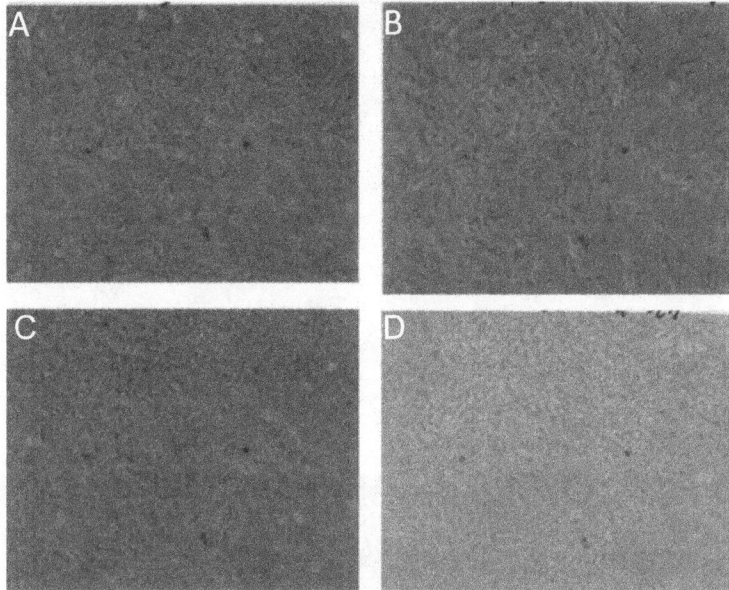

Fig. 15 Distinct cell morphologies of four Individual focal colonies from SV40-infected mouse embryo cells. To test the theory that individual karyotypes encode neoplastic clones with individual phenotypes, we analyzed the cellular morphologies of four focal colonies that arose from SV40-infected mouse embryo cells. As seen by 125-fold magnification of cultures of four such colonies, F1 (**a**), F9 (**b**), F10 (**c**) and F11 (**d**), each clone had an individual and apparently clonal cell morphology. This result indicates that individual genotypes, rather than common SV40 genes encode the morphologies of these virus-induced colonies

prediction has already been confirmed in several studies of SV40-induced neoplastic clones of human and mouse cells [37, 38, 43, 44].

To test this karyotypic virus-cancer theory, we have analyzed the karyotypes and phenotypes of SV40-infected human, rat, and mouse cells from infection to the evolution of rare immortal neoplastic clones. In all three systems we found the predicted (1) preneoplastic aneuploidies, (2) neoplastic transformation at low rates, namely less than one of 10,000 infected cells, which is incompatible with direct viral transformation, (3) neoplastic clones with individual clonal karyotypes, which define the genetic origin [101, 102] and maintain the complex individual phenotypes of neoplastic clones via complex individual transcriptomes [37, 38, 43, 44], (4) variations of cancer phenotypes, such as cell morphology and drug-resistance, that correlated 1-to-1 with variations of karyotypes, and (5) immortality of virus-induced neoplastic clones surviving over 200 generations, which is cancer-specific [89] and is analogous to the immortality of non-viral cancers [89, 97] – and indeed to the immortality of all normal species [92–95]. But, we found no consistent correlations between neoplastic cells and SV40 T-antigen.

We also tested our theory for its ability to explain as yet unclear roles of viruses in two other cancer systems:

First, our theory confirmed the "assumption" of Rous and Beard studying Shope rabbit fibroma virus in 1935, "The virus is the immediate cause for carcinosis; yet compatible with the assumption that it merely provides an essential, preliminary cell disturbance." [111]. Not surprisingly, in view of the karyotypic theory, Palmer [112] and subsequently McMichael, Wagner, Nowell and Hungerford [113] found in 1959 and 1963 that the carcinomas induced by the Shope-fibroma virus have individual karyotypes. But without a theory for the karyotypic individuality of cancers McMichael et al. thought "their significance with respect to the subsequent development of malignancy remains obscure" [113].

Second, the karyotypic theory predicts a testable target for the poorly defined "hit-and-run" hypothesis of human Adenovirus-induced but Adenovirus-free experimental tumors and neoplastic clones [114, 115] – namely clonal cancer-specific karyotypes like those identified here in SV40-induced but SV40-free and T-antigen-free neoplastic clones and tumors. In addition our theory provides a plausible explanation for the induction of preneoplastic aneuploidy also induced by Adenoviruses in human cells [116, 117].

In view of our experimental and theoretical tests of the karyotypic theory, we conclude that SV40 and likely Shope-fibroma and Adeno-viruses induce cancers indirectly, by inducing preneoplastic aneuploidy, which catalyzes spontaneous evolution of virus-independent cancer karyotypes at low rates – much like conventional carcinogens induce carcinogen-independent cancers by inducing preneoplastic aneuploidy [101].

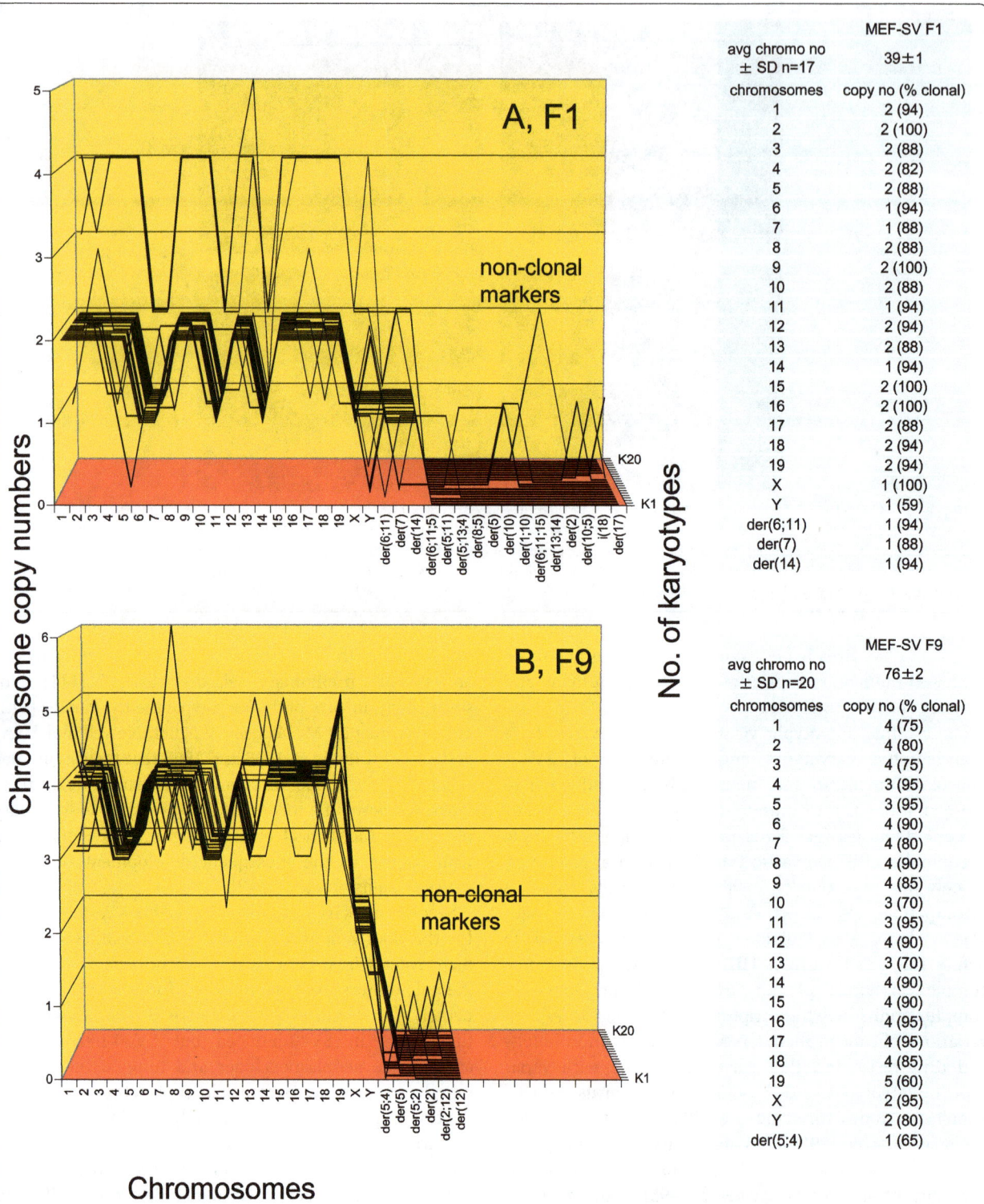

MEF-SV F1	
avg chromo no ± SD n=17	39±1
chromosomes	copy no (% clonal)
1	2 (94)
2	2 (100)
3	2 (88)
4	2 (82)
5	2 (88)
6	1 (94)
7	1 (88)
8	2 (88)
9	2 (100)
10	2 (88)
11	1 (94)
12	2 (94)
13	2 (88)
14	1 (94)
15	2 (100)
16	2 (100)
17	2 (88)
18	2 (94)
19	2 (94)
X	1 (100)
Y	1 (59)
der(6;11)	1 (94)
der(7)	1 (88)
der(14)	1 (94)

MEF-SV F9	
avg chromo no ± SD n=20	76±2
chromosomes	copy no (% clonal)
1	4 (75)
2	4 (80)
3	4 (75)
4	3 (95)
5	3 (95)
6	4 (90)
7	4 (80)
8	4 (90)
9	4 (85)
10	3 (70)
11	3 (95)
12	4 (90)
13	3 (70)
14	4 (90)
15	4 (90)
16	4 (95)
17	4 (95)
18	4 (85)
19	5 (60)
X	2 (95)
Y	2 (80)
der(5;4)	1 (65)

Fig. 16 Karyotype arrays of four morphologically distinct neoplastic colonies derived from SV40-infected mouse embryo cells: first two of four. To test the theory that individual clonal karyotypes encode the phenotypes of individual neoplastic clones from SV40-infected mouse cells, the karyotype arrays of the four focal mouse colonies F1, F9, F10 and F11, shown in Fig. 15 were compared to each other in two separate figures, namely 16 and 17. **a** shows that F1 has a near diploid karyotype with 39 chromosomes including three marker chromosomes, which were 88–100 % clonal. Accordingly the F1 chromosomes formed a quasi-clonal F1-specific karyotype array. **b** shows that F9 has a hypo-tetraploid karyotype with 76 chromosomes, which 60–95 % clonal. Accordingly the F9 chromosomes formed a quasi-clonal F9-specific karyotype array, which is different from that of F1. The 1-to-1 karyotype-phenotype correlation of F1 and F9 thus supports the theory that individual karyotypes, rather than common viral genes, encode the individual phenotypes of the SV40-induced neoplastic mouse clones

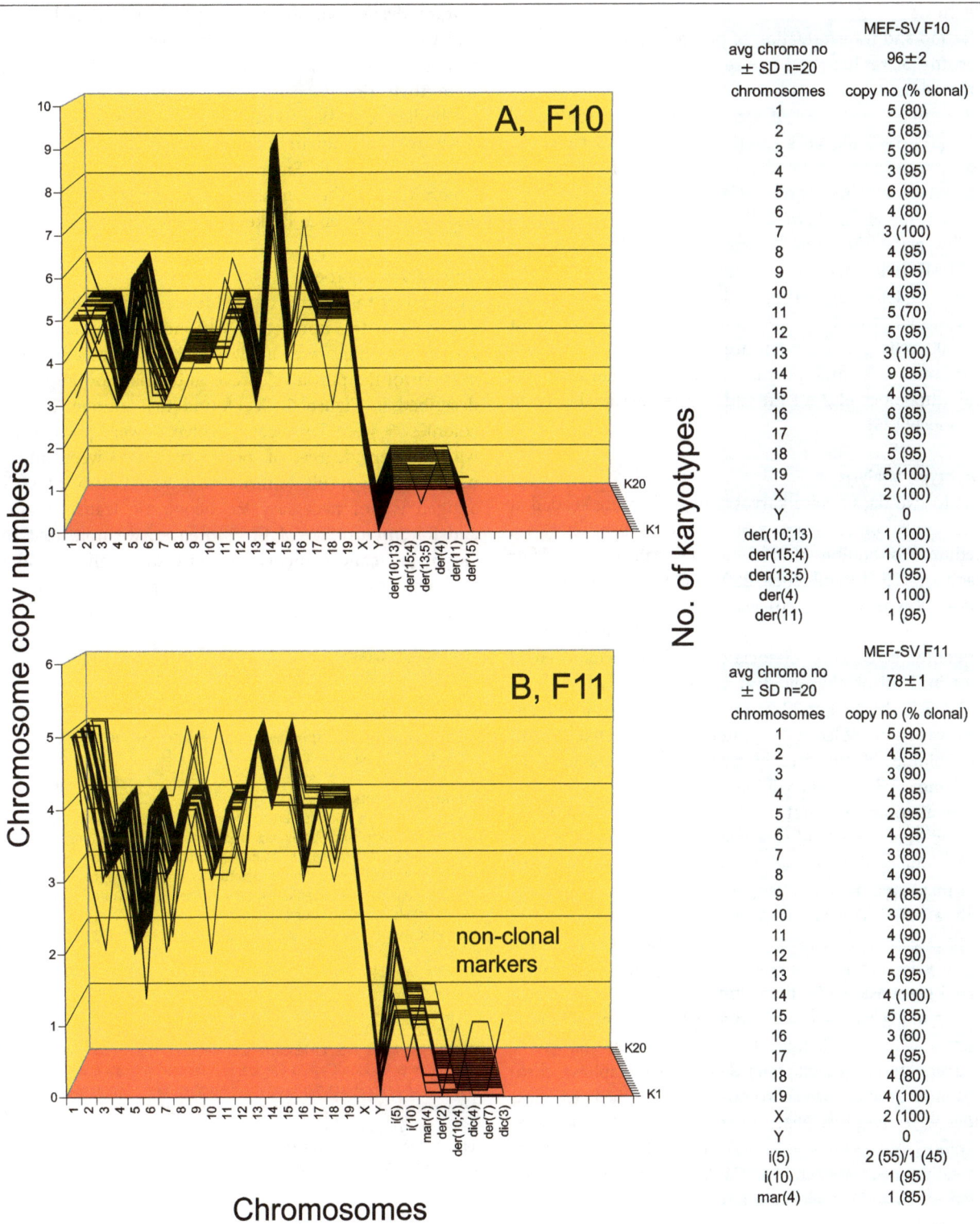

MEF-SV F10	
avg chromo no ± SD n=20	96±2
chromosomes	copy no (% clonal)
1	5 (80)
2	5 (85)
3	5 (90)
4	3 (95)
5	6 (90)
6	4 (80)
7	3 (100)
8	4 (95)
9	4 (95)
10	4 (95)
11	5 (70)
12	5 (95)
13	3 (100)
14	9 (85)
15	4 (95)
16	6 (85)
17	5 (95)
18	5 (95)
19	5 (100)
X	2 (100)
Y	0
der(10;13)	1 (100)
der(15;4)	1 (100)
der(13;5)	1 (95)
der(4)	1 (100)
der(11)	1 (95)

MEF-SV F11	
avg chromo no ± SD n=20	78±1
chromosomes	copy no (% clonal)
1	5 (90)
2	4 (55)
3	3 (90)
4	4 (85)
5	2 (95)
6	4 (95)
7	3 (80)
8	4 (90)
9	4 (85)
10	3 (90)
11	4 (90)
12	4 (90)
13	5 (95)
14	4 (100)
15	5 (85)
16	3 (60)
17	4 (95)
18	4 (80)
19	4 (100)
X	2 (100)
Y	0
i(5)	2 (55)/1 (45)
i(10)	1 (95)
mar(4)	1 (85)

Fig. 17 Karyotype arrays of four morphologically distinct neoplastic colonies derived from SV40-infected mouse embryo cells: second pair of two. To test the theory that individual clonal karyotypes encode individual phenotypes, the karyotypes of two of four mouse colonies, namely F10 and F11 were compared here. **a** shows that F10 has a hyper-tetraploid karyotype with 96 chromosomes that were 70–100 % clonal. Accordingly, the F10 chromosomes formed an F10-specific quasi-clonal array, which is different from those of F1 and F9. **b** shows that F11 has a near tetraploid karyotype with an average number of 78 chromosomes, which were 55–100 % clonal. Accordingly the F11 chromosomes also formed an individual quasi-clonal array, which is different from those of all three sister colonies, F1, F9, and F10 tested above. The individual karyotypes of the four phenotypically distinct mouse clones thus support the theory that individual karyotypes encode the individual phenotypes of neoplastic clones

Methods

Infection and transformation of primary human mesothelial, rat lung and mouse embryo cells with SV40 tumor virus

Subconfluent cultures of primary human mesothelial cells [21], rat lung cells (prepared from a 0.5 to 1-year old Sprague Dawley rat from the Office of Laboratory Animal Care (University of California at Berkeley) and primary mouse embryo cells from the Tissue Culture Facility at UC Berkeley (Barker Hall, UCB) were grown in RPMI 1640 medium (Sigma Co.) supplemented with 3 to 5 % fetal calf serum and antibiotics as described previously [101, 102]. Subconfluent cultures of about 500,000 cells per 5 cm-culture dishes in 3 ml medium were infected at multiplicities of 10 for human cells and at multiplicities of 2 for rat and mouse cells as described previously [25].

Karyotype analysis

One to two days before karyotyping, cells were seeded at about 50 % confluence in a 5-cm culture dish with 3 ml medium containing 3 to 5 % fetal calf serum. After reaching ~75 % confluence, 250 ng colcemid in 25 µl solution (KaryoMax, Gibco) was added to 3 ml medium. The culture was then incubated at 37 °C for 4–8 h. Subsequently cells were dissociated with trypsin, washed once in 3 ml of physiological saline and then incubated in 0.075 molar KCl at 37 °C for 15 min. The cell suspension was then cooled in ice-water, mixed ('prefixed') with 0.1 volume of the freshly mixed glacial acetic acid-methanol (1:3, vol. per vol.) and centrifuged at 800 g for 6 min at room temperature. The cell pellet was then suspended in about 100 µl supernatant and mixed drop-wise with 5 ml of the ice-cold acetic acid-methanol solution and incubated at room temperature for 15 min or overnight at -20C. This cell suspension was then pelleted once more as above and re-suspended in a small volume of the acetic acid-methanol solution. An aliquot of a visually turbid suspension was then transferred with a micropipette tip to a glass microscope slide, allowed to evaporate at room and inspected under the microscope at x200 for a an adequate non-overlapping density of metaphase chromosomes. Metaphase chromosomes attached to glass slides were then hybridized to color-coded, chromosome-specific DNA probes as described by the manufacturer (MetaSystems, Newton, MA 02458). Karyotypes were analyzed under a fluorescence microscope as described by us previously [17, 49].

T-antigen staining

Anti-SV40 T antigen antibody and Alexa Fluor 488 goat anti-mouse IgG were purchased from Abcam (Boston, MA). The SV40-transformed human and rat cell lines that we tested were grown on microscope slides or cell culture dishes, washed with phosphate-buffered saline, and wet cultures were fixed with freshly prepared, cold methanol-acetic acid (3:1) for 15 minutes. The cultures were then rinsed again with saline and reacted with antibodies according to the manufacturer's protocol.

All work on human and animal cell cultures has been approved by the Environmental Health and Safety Committee of the University of California at Berkeley and by the Lawrence Berkeley Laboratory at Berkeley.

Note added in proof

In an effort to confirm our evidence for T-antigen-negative cells of the immortal SV40-induced human mesothelial F1 line, we analyzed 25 single-cell-derived colonies of the puromycin-resistant variant of the F1-line described in Figure 6. We found that among 25 such colonies, 5 were T-antigen positive, 7 were positive but with different degrees of positivity and 13 were entirely negative. This result confirms that, based on our test, T-antigen is not necessary for neoplastic transformation and for immortality of F1. Moreover, we note that the karyotypic cancer theory explains the high individual multiplicities of over- and under-expressed cellular proteins of SV40-transformed neoplastic cells [118].

Competing interests
The authors declare that they have no competing interests.

Authors' contributions
MB and PD carried out experimental work and prepared the manuscript and approved the final manuscript.

Acknowledgments
We are indebted to Michele Carbone (Cancer Research Center of Hawaii at Honolulu) for providing SV40-infected and uninfected human mesothelial cells, and the immortal clones F1 and F4, which were derived from SV40-infected mesothelial cells. We are grateful to Fang Qi (from the Carbone lab) for initial help with the infection of mesothelial cells by SV40. Further we thank Michele Carbone, Robert Hoffman (AntiCancer Inc. and UC San Diego) and Peter Walian (Lawrence Berkeley National Laboratory, Donner Lab, Berkeley CA) for critical reviews of this manuscript and for stimulating discussions and ideas. We further thank Alfred Boecking (Heinrich Heine University, Duesseldorf, Germany), Peter Bullock (Tufts University, Boston), Christian Fiala (GynMed Ambulatorium, Vienna, Austria), Andreas Klein and Annette Hildmann (Charite – Universitaetsmedizin Berlin), David Rasnick (Oakland CA, former visiting scholar at UC Berkeley), Mark Vincent (Department of Medical Oncology, London Regional Cancer Center, London, Ontario, Canada) for valuable information, inspiring questions and critical comments on the manuscript. Bong-Gyoon Han (Lawrence Berkeley National Laboratory, Donner Lab) is specifically thanked for drafting and designing Fig. 1. Our study would not have been possible without the generous support of the philanthropists Robert Leppo (San Francisco), Christian Fiala, Rajeev and Christine Joshi (London, UK), Peter Rozsa of the Taubert Memorial Foundation (Los Angeles) and several anonymous private sources.

References
1. Gross L. Oncogenic Viruses. 2nd ed. Oxford, UK: Pergamon; 1970.
2. Butel JS, Tevethia SS, Melnick JL. Oncogenicity and cell transformation by papovavirus SV40: the role of the viral genome. Adv Cancer Res. 1972;15:1–55.
3. Tooze J. The Molecular Biology of Tumour Viruses. Cold Spring Harbor: Cold Spring Harbor Laboratorty; 1973.

4. Cheng J, DeCaprio JA, Fluck MM, Schaffhausen BS. Cellular transformation by Simian Virus 40 and Murine Polyoma Virus T antigens. Semin Cancer Biol. 2009;19(4):218–28.

5. Levine AJ. The common mechanisms of transformation by the small DNA tumor viruses: The inactivation of tumor suppressor gene products: p53. Virology. 2009;384(2):285–93.

6. Alberts B, Johnson A, Lewis J, Raff M, Roberts K, Walter P. Molecular Biology of the Cell. New York: Garland; 2014.

7. Weinberg RA. The biology of cancer. 2nd ed. London: Garland Science; 2014.

8. Gotoh S, Gelb L, Schlessinger D. SV40-transformed human diploid cells that remain transformed throughout their limited lifespan. J Gen Virol. 1979;42(2):409–14.

9. Vogt M, Dulbecco R. Steps in the neoplastic transformation of hamster embryo cells by polyoma virus. Proc Natl Acad Sci U S A. 1963;49:171–9.

10. Defendi V, Lehman JM. Transformation of hamster embryo cells in vitro by polyoma virus: morphological, karyological, immunological and transplantation characteristics. J Cell Physiol. 1965;66(3):351–409.

11. Gaffney EV, Fogh J, Ramos L, Loveless JD, Fogh H, Dowling AM. Established lines of SV40-transformed human amnion cells. Cancer Res. 1970;30(6):1668–76.

12. Sack Jr GH. Human cell transformation by simian virus 40–a review. In Vitro. 1981;17(1):1–19.

13. Huschtscha LI, Holliday R. Limited and unlimited growth of SV40-transformed cells from human diploid MRC-5 fibroblasts. J Cell Sci. 1983;63:77–99.

14. Canaani D, Naiman T, Teitz T, Berg P. Immortalization of xeroderma pigmentosum cells by simian virus 40 DNA having a defective origin of DNA replication. Somat Cell Mol Genet. 1986;12(1):13–20.

15. Shay JW, Wright WE. Quantitation of the frequency of immortalization of normal human diploid fibroblasts by SV40 large T-antigen. Exp Cell Res. 1989;184(1):109–18.

16. Shay JW, Van Der Haegen BA, Ying Y, Wright WE. The frequency of immortalization of human fibroblasts and mammary epithelial cells transfected with SV40 large T-antigen. Exp Cell Res. 1993;209(1):45–52.

17. Jha KK, Banga S, Palejwala V, Ozer HL. SV40-Mediated immortalization. Exp Cell Res. 1998;245(1):1–7.

18. Akoum A, Lavoie J, Drouin R, Jolicoeur C, Lemay A, Maheux R, et al. Physiological and cytogenetic characterization of immortalized human endometriotic cells containing episomal simian virus 40 DNA. Am J Pathol. 1999;154(4):1245–57.

19. Butel JS, Lednicky JA. Cell and molecular biology of simian virus 40: implications for human infections and disease. J Natl Cancer Inst. 1999;91(2):119–34.

20. Butel JS. Viral carcinogenesis: revelation of molecular mechanisms and etiology of human disease. Carcinogenesis. 2000;21(3):405–26.

21. Bocchetta M, Di Resta I, Powers A, Fresco R, Tosolini A, Testa JR, et al. Human mesothelial cells are unusually susceptible to simian virus 40-mediated transformation and asbestos cocarcinogenicity. Proc Natl Acad Sci U S A. 2000;97(18):10214–9.

22. Kendall SD, Linardic CM, Adam SJ, Counter CM. A network of genetic events sufficient to convert normal human cells to a tumorigenic state. Cancer Res. 2005;65(21):9824–8.

23. Mahale AM, Khan ZA, Igarashi M, Nanjangud GJ, Qiao RF, Yao S, et al. Clonal selection in malignant transformation of human fibroblasts transduced with defined cellular oncogenes. Cancer Res. 2008;68(5):1417–26.

24. Carbone M, Pannuti A, Zhang L, Testa JR, Bocchetta M. A novel mechanism of late gene silencing drives SV40 transformation of human mesothelial cells. Cancer Res. 2008;68(22):9488–96.

25. Li L, McCormack AA, Nicholson JM, Fabarius A, Hehlmann R, Sachs RK, et al. Cancer-causing karyotypes: chromosomal equilibria between destabilizing aneuploidy and stabilizing selection for oncogenic function. Cancer Genet Cytogenet. 2009;188(1):1–25.

26. Medina D, Sachs L. Cell-virus interactions with the polyoma virus: the induction of cell transformation and malignancy in vitro. Br J Cancer. 1961;15(4):885–904.

27. Diamandopoulos GT, Enders JF. Studies on transformation of Syrian hamster cells by simian virus 40 (SV40): acquisition of oncogenicity by virus-exposed cells apparently unassociated with the viral genome. Proc Natl Acad Sci U S A. 1965;54(4):1092–9.

28. Diamandopoulos GT, Dalton-Tucker MF, van der Noordaa J. Early in-vitro SV40-mediated morphologic transformation of primary hamster cells. Its correlation with the development of the oncogenic state. Am J Pathol. 1969;57(2):199–213.

29. Eddy BE, Stewart SE, Young R, Mider GB. Neoplasms in hamsters induced by mouse tumor agent passed in tissue culture. J Natl Cancer Inst. 1958;20(4):747–61.

30. Hellstroem KE, Hellstroem I, Sjoegren HO. Further studies on karyotypes of a variety of primary and transplanted mouse polyoma tumors. J Natl Cancer Inst. 1963;31:1239–53.

31. Girardi AJ, Jensen FC, Koprowski H. Sv40-induced transformation of human diploid cells: crisis and recovery. J Cell Physiol. 1965;65:69–83.

32. Fabarius A, Li R, Yerganian G, Hehlmann R, Duesberg P. Specific clones of spontaneously evolving karyotypes generate individuality of cancers. Cancer Genet Cytogenet. 2008;180(2):89–99.

33. Ewald D, Li M, Efrat S, Auer G, Wall RJ, Furth PA, et al. Time-sensitive reversal of hyperplasia in transgenic mice expressing SV40 T antigen. Science. 1996;273(5280):1384–6.

34. Foster BA, Gingrich JR, Kwon ED, Madias C, Greenberg NM. Characterization of prostatic epithelial cell lines derived from transgenic adenocarcinoma of the mouse prostate (TRAMP) model. Cancer Res. 1997;57(16):3325–30.

35. Klein A, Li N, Nicholson JM, McCormack AA, Graessmann A, Duesberg P. Transgenic oncogenes induce oncogene-independent cancers with individual karyotypes and phenotypes. Cancer Genet Cytogenet. 2010;200(2):79–99.

36. Eddy BE, Borman GS, Berkeley WH, Young RD. Tumors induced in hamsters by injection of rhesus monkey kidney cell extracts. Proc Soc Exp Biol Med. 1961;107:191–7.

37. Klein A, Guhl E, Zollinger R, Tzeng YJ, Wessel R, Hummel M, et al. Gene expression profiling: cell cycle deregulation and aneuploidy do not cause breast cancer formation in WAP-SVT/t transgenic animals. J Mol Med. 2005;83(5):362–76.

38. Cantalupo PG, Saenz-Robles MT, Rathi AV, Beerman RW, Patterson WH, Whitehead RH, et al. Cell-type specific regulation of gene expression by simian virus 40 T antigens. Virology. 2009;386(1):183–91.

39. Shein HM, Enders JF. Transformation induced by siminian virus 40 in human renal cell cultures, I. Morpholgy and growth characteristics. Proc Natl Acad Sci U S A. 1962;48:1164–72.

40. Koprowski H, Ponten JA, Jensen F, Ravdin RD, Moorehead PS, Saksela E. Transformation of cultures of human tissue infected with simian virus SV40. J Cell Comp Physiol. 1962;59:281–92.

41. Botchan M, Topp W, Sambrook J. The arrangement of simian virus 40 sequences in the DNA of transformed cells. Cell. 1976;9(2):269–87.

42. Hoffschir F, Ricoul M, Dutrillaux B. SV40-transformed human fibroblasts exhibit a characteristic chromosomal pattern. Cytogenet Cell Genet. 1988;49(4):264–8.

43. Greco D, Vellonen KS, Turner HC, Hakli M, Tervo T, Auvinen P, et al. Gene expression analysis in SV-40 immortalized human corneal epithelial cells cultured with an air-liquid interface. Mol Vis. 2010;16:2109–20.

44. Danielsson F, Skogs M, Huss M, Rexhepaj E, O'Hurley G, Klevebring D, et al. Majority of differentially expressed genes are down-regulated during malignant transformation in a four-stage model. Proc Natl Acad Sci U S A. 2013;110(17):6853–8.

45. Dulbecco R. Viral carcinogenesis. Cancer Res. 1961;21:975–80.

46. Dulbecco R. Cell transformation by viruses and the role of viruses in cancer. The eleventh Marjory Stephenson Memorial Lecture. J Gen Microbiol. 1973;79(1):7–17.

47. Israel MA, Chowdhury K, Ramseur J, Chandrasekaran K, Vanderryn DF, Martin MA. Tumorigenicity of polyoma virus in hamsters. Cold Spring Harb Symp Quant Biol. 1980;44(Pt 1):591–6.

48. Moore JL, Chowdhury K, Martin MA, Israel MA. Polyoma large tumor antigen is not required for tumorigenesis mediated by viral DNA. Proc Natl Acad Sci U S A. 1980;77(3):1336–40.

49. Lania L, Gandini-Attardi D, Griffiths M, Cooke B, De Cicco D, Fried M. The polyoma virus 100 K large T-antigen is not required for the maintenance of transformation. Virology. 1980;101(1):217–32.

50. Lania L, Hayday A, Fried M. Loss of functional large T-antigen and free viral genomes from cells transformed in vitro by polyoma virus after passage in vivo as tumor cells. J Virol. 1981;39(2):422–31.

51. Shein HM, Enders JF, Levinthal JD. Transformation induced by simian virus 40 in human renal cell cultures. II. Cell-virus relationships. Proc Natl Acad Sci U S A. 1962;48:1350–7.

52. van der Noordaa J, Enders JF. Early effects by SV40 on growth in vitro of hamster and human tissue cells. Proc Soc Exp Biol Med. 1966;122(4):1144–9.

53. Levine AS, Oxman MN, Henry PH, Levin MJ, Diamandopoulos GT, Enders JF. Virus-specific deoxyribonucleic acid in simian virus 40-exposed hamster cells: correlation with S and T antigens. J Virol. 1970;6(2):199–207.

54. Santoli D, Wroblewska Z, Gilden D, Koprowski H. Establishment of continuous multiple sclerosis brain cultures after transformation with PML-SV40 virus. J Neurol Sci. 1975;24(3):385–90.

55. Seif R, Martin RG. Simian virus 40 small t antigen is not required for the maintenance of transformation but may act as a promoter (cocarcinogen) during establishment of transformation in resting rat cells. J Virol. 1979;32(3):979–88.

56. Seif R, Seif I, Wantyghem J. Rat cells transformed by simian virus 40 give rise to tumor cells which contain no viral proteins and often no viral DNA. Mol Cell Biol. 1983;3(6):1138–45.

57. de Lapeyriere O, Hayot B, Imbert J, Courcoul M, Arnaud D, Birg F. Cell lines derived from tumors induced in syngeneic rats by FR 3 T3 SV40 transformants no longer synthesize the early viral proteins. Virology. 1984;135:74–86.

58. Discroll K, Carter J, Iype P, Kumari H, Crosbty L, Aardema M, et al. Establishment of immortalized alveolar type ii epithelial cell lines from adult rats. In Vitro Cell Dev Biol-Animal. 1995;31:516–27.

59. Herrmann J, Gressner AM, Weiskirchen R. Immortal hepatic stellate cell lines: useful tools to study hepatic stellate cell biology and function? J Cell Mol Med. 2007;11(4):704–22.

60. Bell Jr RH, Memoli VA, Longnecker DS. Hyperplasia and tumors of the islets of Langerhans in mice bearing an elastase I-SV40 T-antigen fusion gene. Carcinogenesis. 1990;11(8):1393–8.

61. Tzeng YJ, Zimmermann C, Guhl E, Berg B, Avantaggiati ML, Graessmann A. SV40 T/t-antigen induces premature mammary gland involution by apoptosis and selects for p53 missense mutation in mammary tumors. Oncogene. 1998;16(16):2103–14.

62. Salewski H, Bayer TA, Eidhoff U, Preuss U, Weggen S, Scheidtmann KH. Increased oncogenicity of subclones of SV40 large T-induced neuroectodermal tumor cell lines after loss of large T expression and concomitant mutation in p53. Cancer Res. 1999;59(8):1980–6.

63. Sepulveda AR, Finegold MJ, Smith B, Slagle BL, DeMayo JL, Shen RF, et al. Development of a transgenic mouse system for the analysis of stages in liver carcinogenesis using tissue-specific expression of SV40 large T-antigen controlled by regulatory elements of the human alpha-1-antitrypsin gene. Cancer Res. 1989;49(21):6108–17.

64. O'Connell K, Landman G, Farmer E, Edidin M. Endothelial cells transformed by SV40 T antigen cause Kaposi's sarcomalike tumors in nude mice. Am J Pathol. 1991;139(4):743–9.

65. Fried M. Cell-transforming ability of a temperature-sensitive mutant of polyoma virus. Proc Natl Acad Sci U S A. 1965;53:486–91.

66. Eckhart W. Properties of temperature-sensitive mutants of polyoma virus. Cold Spring Harb Symp Quant Biol. 1975;39(Pt 1):37–40.

67. Tegtmeyer P. Function of simian virus 40 gene A in transforming infection. J Virol. 1975;15(3):613–8.

68. Rassoulzadegan M, Perbal B, Cuzin F. Growth control in simian virus 40-transformed rat cells: temperature-independent expression of the transformed phenotype in tsA transformants derived by agar selection. J Virol. 1978;28(1):1–5.

69. Yerganian G, Shein HM, Enders JF. Chromosomal disturbances observed in human fetal renal cells transformed in vitro by simian virus 40 and carried in culture. Cytogenetics. 1962;1:314–24.

70. Moorhead PS, Saksela E. Non-random chromosomal aberrations in Sv 40-transformed human cells. J Cell Physiol. 1963;62:57–83.

71. Todaro GJ, Wolman SR, Green H. Rapid transformation of human fibroblasts with low growth potential into established cell lines by SV40. J Cell Comp Physiol. 1963;62:257–65.

72. Wolman S, Hirschhorn K, Todaro G. Early chromosomal changes in SV40-infected human fibroblast cultures. Cytogenetic and Genome Research. 1964;3(1):45–61.

73. Moorhead PS, Saksela E. The Sequence of chromosome aberrations during SV40 transformation of a human diploid cell strain. Hereditas. 1965;52:271–84.

74. Hoffman RM, Jacobsen SJ, Erbe RW. Reversion to methionine independence in simian virus 40-transformed human and malignant rat fibroblasts is associated with altered ploidy and altered properties of transformation. Proc Natl Acad Sci U S A. 1979;76(3):1313–7.

75. Begovich A, Francke U. Karyotype evolution of the simian virus 40-transformed human cell line LNSV. Cytogenet Cell Genet. 1979;23(1–2):3–11.

76. Wolman SR, Steinberg ML, Defendi V. Simian virus 40-induced chromosome changes in human epidermal cultures. Cancer Genet Cytogenet. 1980;2:39–46.

77. Walen KH, Arnstein P. Induction of tumorigenesis and chromosomal abnormalities in human amniocytes infected with simian virus 40 and Kirsten sarcoma virus. In Vitro Cell Dev Biol. 1986;22(2):57–65.

78. Liu J, Li H, Nomura K, Dofuku R, Kitagawa T. Cytogenetic analysis of hepatic cell lines derived from SV40-T antigen gene-harboring transgenic mice. Cancer Genet Cytogenet. 1991;55(2):207–16.

79. Stewart N, Bacchetti S. Expression of SV40 large T antigen, but not small t antigen, is required for the induction of chromosomal aberrations in transformed human cells. Virology. 1991;180(1):49–57.

80. Ray FA, Meyne J, Kraemer PM. SV40 T antigen induced chromosomal changes reflect a process that is both clastogenic and aneuploidogenic and is ongoing throughout neoplastic progression of human fibroblasts. Mutat Res. 1992;284(2):265–73.

81. Reddel RR, Ke Y, Gerwin BI, McMenamin MG, Lechner JF, Su RT, et al. Transformation of human bronchial epithelial cells by infection with SV40 or adenovirus-12 SV40 hybrid virus, or transfection via strontium phosphate coprecipitation with a plasmid containing SV40 early region genes. Cancer Res. 1988;48(7):1904–9.

82. Li R, Sonik A, Stindl R, Rasnick D, Duesberg P. Aneuploidy vs. gene mutation hypothesis of cancer: recent study claims mutation but is found to support aneuploidy. Proc Natl Acad Sci U S A. 2000;97(7):3236–41.

83. Li R, Rasnick D, Duesberg P. Correspondence re: D. Zimonjic et al., Derivation of human tumor cells in vitro without widespread genomic instability. Cancer Res., 61: 8838–8844, 2001. Cancer Res. 2002;62(21):6345–8. discussion 6348–6349.

84. Nicholson JM, Duesberg P. On the karyotypic origin and evolution of cancer cells. Cancer Genet Cytogenet. 2009;194(2):96–110.

85. Hein J, Boichuk S, Wu J, Cheng Y, Freire R, Jat PS, et al. Simian virus 40 large T antigen disrupts genome integrity and activates a DNA damage response via Bub1 binding. J Virol. 2009;83(1):117–27.

86. Hu L, Filippakis H, Huang H, Yen TJ, Gjoerup OV. Replication stress and mitotic dysfunction in cells expressing simian virus 40 large T antigen. J Virol. 2013;87(24):13179–92.

87. Cooper HL, Black PH. Cytogenetic studies of hamster kidney cell cultures transformed by the simian vacuolating virus (SV40). J Natl Cancer Inst. 1963;30:1015–43.

88. Pollack R, Risser R, Conlon S, Rifkin D. Plasminogen activator production accompanies loss of anchorage regulation in transformation of primary rat embryo cells by simian virus 40. Proc Natl Acad Sci U S A. 1974;71(12):4792–6.

89. Duesberg P, McCormack A. Immortality of cancers: a consequence of inherent karyotypic variations and selections for autonomy. Cell Cycle. 2013;12(5):783–802.

90. Kappler R, Pietsch T, Weggen S, Wiestler OD, Scherthan H. Chromosomal imbalances and DNA amplifications in SV40 large T antigen-induced primitive neuroectodermal tumor cell lines of the rat. Carcinogenesis. 1999;20(8):1433–8.

91. Goldschmidt RB. The material basis of evolution. New Haven, CT: Yale University Press; 1940.

92. White MJD. Modes of speciation. San Francisco: W H Freeman and Co.; 1978.

93. King M. Species evolution: the role of chromosome change. Cambridge: Cambridge University Press; 1993.

94. Cairns-Smith AG. Chp 2, The immortal germline. In: Marsh J, Goode J, editors. Ciba Foundation Symposium 182 - Germline Development. Norvatis: Cambridge University Press; 2007.

95. Lepperdinger G. Open-ended question: is immortality exclusively inherent to the germline?–A mini-review. Gerontology. 2009;55(1):114–7.

96. Van Valen L, Maiorana V. HeLa, a new microbial species. Evolutionary Theory. 1991;10:71–4.

97. Duesberg P, Mandrioli D, McCormack A, Nicholson JM. Is carcinogenesis a form of speciation? Cell Cycle. 2011;10(13):2100–14.

98. Vincent MD. Cancer: beyond speciation. Adv Cancer Res. 2011;112:283–350.

99. Heng HH, Stevens JB, Bremer SW, Liu G, Abdallah BY, Ye CJ. Evolutionary mechanisms and diversity in cancer. Adv Cancer Res. 2011;112:217–53.

100. Duesberg PH. Does aneuploidy destabilize karyotypes automatically? Proc Natl Acad Sci U S A. 2014;111:E974.

101. Bloomfield M, McCormack A, Mandrioli D, Fiala C, Aldaz CM, Duesberg P. Karyotypic evolutions of cancer species in rats during the long latent periods after injection of nitrosourea. Mol Cytogenet. 2014;7(1):71.

102. McCormack A, Fan JL, Duesberg M, Bloomfield M, Fiala C, Duesberg P. Individual karyotypes at the origins of cervical carcinomas. Mol Cytogenet. 2013;6(1):44.
103. Smith HS, Wolman SR, Dairkee SH, Hancock MC, Lippman M, Leff A, et al. Immortalization in culture: occurrence at a late stage in the progression of breast cancer. J Natl Cancer Inst. 1987;78(4):611–5.
104. Hayflick L. The limited in vitro lifetime of human diploid cell strains. Exp Cell Res. 1965;37:614–36.
105. Duesberg P, Li R, Sachs R, Fabarius A, Upender MB, Hehlmann R. Cancer drug resistance: the central role of the karyotype. Drug Resist Updat. 2007;10(1–2):51–8.
106. Li R, Hehlman R, Sachs R, Duesberg P. Chromosomal alterations cause the high rates and wide ranges of drug resistance in cancer cells. Cancer Genet Cytogenet. 2005;163(1):44–56.
107. Duesberg P, Iacobuzio-Donahue C, Brosnan JA, McCormack A, Mandrioli D, Chen L. Origin of metastases: subspecies of cancers generated by intrinsic karyotypic variations. Cell Cycle. 2012;11(6):1151–66.
108. Holliday R. Neoplastic transformation: the contrasting stability of human and mouse cells. Cancer Surv. 1996;28:103–15.
109. Oshimura M, Barrett JC. Chemically induced aneuploidy in mammalian cells: mechanisms and biological significance in cancer. Environ Mutagen. 1986;8(1):129–59.
110. Duesberg P, Li R, Rasnick D, Rausch C, Willer A, Kraemer A, et al. Aneuploidy precedes and segregates with chemical carcinogenesis. Cancer Genet Cytogenet. 2000;119(2):83–93.
111. Rous P, Beard JW. The progression to carcinoma of virus-induced rabbit papillomas (Shope). J Exp Med. 1935;62(4):523–48.
112. Palmer CG. The cytology of rabbit papillomas and derived carcinomas. J Natl Cancer Inst. 1959;23:241–9.
113. McMichael H, Wagner JE, Nowell PC, Hungerford DA. Chromosome studies of virus-induced rabbit papillomas and derived primary carcinomas. J Natl Cancer Inst. 1963;31:1197–215.
114. Nevels M, Tauber B, Spruss T, Wolf H, Dobner T. "Hit-and-run" transformation by adenovirus oncogenes. J Virol. 2001;75(7):3089–94.
115. Pfeffer A, Schubbert R, Orend G, Hilger-Eversheim K, Doerfler W. Integrated viral genomes can be lost from adenovirus type 12-induced hamster tumor cells in a clone-specific, multistep process with retention of the oncogenic phenotype. Virus Res. 1999;59(1):113–27.
116. Caporossi D, Bacchetti S. Definition of adenovirus type 5 functions involved in the induction of chromosomal aberrations in human cells. J Gen Virol. 1990;71(Pt 4):801–8.
117. Zur Hausen H. Induction of specific chromosomal aberrations by adenovirus type 12 in human embryonic kidney cells. J Virol. 1967;1(6):1174–85.
118. Fransen L, Van Roy F, Fiers W. Changes in gene expression and protein phosphorylation in murine cells, transformed or abortively infected with wild type and mutant simian virus 40. J Biol Chem. 1983;258(8):5276–5290.

12

Clinicohematological and cytogenetic profile of myelodysplastic syndromes

Nida Anwar*, Aisha Arshad, Muhammad Nadeem, Sana Khurram, Naveena Fatima, Sumaira Sharif, Saira Shan and Tahir Shamsi

Abstract

Background: Myelodysplastic syndromes (MDS) are clonal stem cell disorders exhibiting cytopenias, ineffective hematopoiesis and morphological dysplasia. Bone marrow cytogenetics, inspite of being incorporated as mandatory tool in diagnosis are done less frequently due to limited availability of this technique in Pakistan. The aim of the study was to study baseline clinicohematological and cytogenetic characteristics of patients presenting with de novo MDS.

Results: A retrospective cross sectional study was done at National Institute of Blood Diseases and Bone Marrow Transplantation, Karachi, Pakistan from 2010 to 2016. Total of 177 patients were included in the study having median age 51 years and male to female ratio of 3:1. Pancytopenia was observed in 80 (45%) patients and bicytopenia in 74 (42%). Mean Hb% was 7.8 ± 2.18 g/dl, total leukocyte count (TLC) $8.8 \pm 13.6 \times 10^9$/l, platelet count was $82 \pm 95.7 \times 10^9$/l. Of total 170 (96%) were transfusion dependent. Refractory cytopenias with multilineage dysplasia (RCMD) was the most common world health organization (WHO) category. Karyotype was done in 98 (55%) patients out of which 44 (45%) had abnormal karyotype, complex karyotype (CK) was most commonly observed in 12 (12.2%) followed by monosomy 7 in 7 (7.1%).

Conclusions: We found younger median age at diagnosis, higher mean TLC and no significant history of recurrent infections. CK and monosomy 7 carry bad prognostic implications and early disease transformation to acute myeloid leukemia (AML). Monosomy 7 being associated with bad overall survival, such patients must be identified early with close clinical follow up and offered stem cell transplant. This is the largest cohort of patients of MDS evaluated for baseline clinical and cytogenetic characteristics in our country.

Keywords: Myelodysplastic syndromes, Clinicohematological characteristics, Cytogenetics, Karyotype

Background

Myelodysplastic syndromes (MDS) are group of clonal hematopoietic stem cell disorders exhibiting ineffective hematopoiesis, morphological dysplasia and progressive tendency to evolve into acute myeloid leukemia (AML) [1–5]. The exact pathogenesis is not completely understood [3]. However, proposed pathogenic causes include increased apoptosis, immunological abnormalities along with clonal basis [5]. The disease can be classified into primary (de novo) and secondary MDS, whether it is de novo or arise as result of previous radiochemical

exposure [1]. Consensus International Prognostic Scoring System (IPSS) is used for predicting outcome and planning therapy in MDS which includes number of cytopenias, percentage of bone marrow blast and cytogenetics [5]. Thus the role of cytogenetics with respect to diagnosis and prognosis has been well established in this clonal disorder [5]. However in developing countries like Pakistan, with poor socioeconomic status of patients, clinicians have very limited availability of sophisticated techniques like cytogenetics inspite of this being incorporated as mandatory tool for the diagnosis [5]. Thus most of the cases of refractory cytopenias are not diagnosed for MDS. Impact of racial difference on disease biology and clinical behavior was evaluated in previous Asian study but has

* Correspondence: drnidairfan@yahoo.com
National Institute of Blood Disease and Bone Marrow Transplantation (NIBD), St 2/A block 17 Gulshan-e-Iqbal KDA scheme 24, Karachi, Pakistan

not been well established [6]. Keeping this in mind, this study was done to assess the baseline clinicohematological characteristics of patients presenting with MDS, evaluate their cytogenetic profile and compare our analysis to what has been reported previously. This is the largest cohort of patients diagnosed with MDS and evaluated for their baseline hematological, clinical and cytogenetic profile in our country.

Methods

This retrospective cross sectional study was conducted at National Institute of Blood Diseases and Bone Marrow Transplantation, Karachi Pakistan from June 2010 to June 2016. Baseline investigations done included complete blood counts, serum vitamin B 12, serum and RBC folate levels. Clinical parameters were recorded. Bone marrow biopsy samples were taken from posterior superior iliac spine through jamshidi needle and were stained by leishman's stain. Perl's (Iron) stain was carried out on each bone marrow sample by commercially provided kits from merck diagnostic according to manufacturer's instructions. Cytogenetic analysis was performed on overnight, 24-h un-stimulated and 72-h stimulated bone marrow cultures using standard procedures. The GTG (G-bands via trypsin using Giemsa) banding technique was applied, karyotypes were described according to the International System for Human Cytogenetic Nomenclature (ISCN) 2013, karyogram were made using Meta system. Patients were classified according to world health organization (WHO) 2008 classification and IPSS was also calculated. Approval from the Institutional ethics committee was obtained prior to the study.

Inclusion criteria

During the study period, patients diagnosed as de novo MDS based on morphological and/or cytogenetic basis were included in the study. Thorough morphological assessment of peripheral smears and bone marrow biopsy was done along with bone marrow cytogenetic analysis.

Exclusion criteria

Patients presenting with cytopenias and normocytic/macrocytic anemia due to other non malignant causes, patients having history of prior chemotherapy or irradiation and patients having organomegaly or lymphadenopathy were excluded from the study.

Statistical analysis

Statistical analysis was done by statistical package for the social sciences version 22.0 (SPSS Inc, Chicago, IL, USA). Descriptive variables were calculated as mean, standard deviation (SD), frequencies and percentages.

Results

A total of 177 consecutive patients diagnosed with MDS were included in the study. The median age of patient was 51 (range 3 to 90 years). The male to female ratio was 3:1. Frequency of all patients according to WHO classification 2008 is shown in (Fig. 1). IPSS scoring of patients is given in (Fig. 2). Mean hemoglobin (Hb), total leukocyte count (TLC), platelets, MCV at baseline and subtypes of MDS as per WHO classification in comparison with other national and international studies is shown in Table 1 [1–3, 6–15].

Comparison of cytogenetic profile of our patients with other national and international data is shown in Table 2 [1–3, 6–15].

Moreover, we observed the cytogenetics of our patients in each WHO category which is summarized in Table 3.

In our patients the most common presenting complaint was loss of appetite in 173 (98%) followed by weakness 141 (80%) and fever 83 (47%). Absolute neutophil count (ANC) of <1.8 was found in 78 (44%) and >1.8 was found in 99 (56%) of patients. Pancytopenia was observed in 80 (45%) and bicytopenia in 74 (42%) (anemia and thrombocytopenia). However, 23 (13%) had cytopenia of one cell lineage. One hundred and seventy (96%) patients were transfusion dependent. History of recurrent infection was found in 21 (12%). Bacterial infections were observed to be the most common cause followed by viral and fungal infections. Co morbidities were observed in 116 (66%) of patients including hypertension in 61 (35%), diabetes mellitus in 55 (31%) while 61 (34%) had no known co morbid. Iron grading was done on all the bone marrow aspirate samples by Perl's

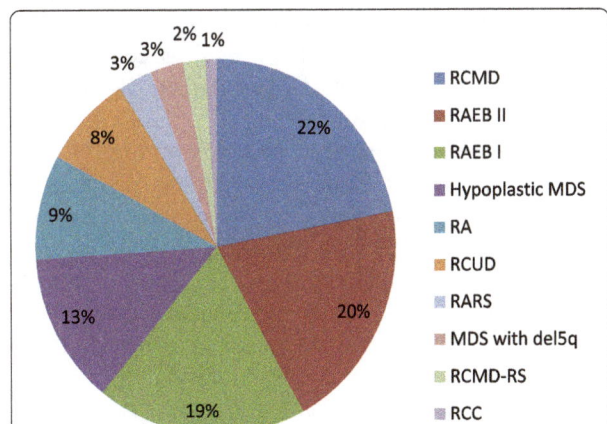

Fig. 1 Frequency of MDS patients according to WHO subtype. RCMD = Refractory Cytopenia(s) with Multilineage Dysplasia. RAEB II = Refractory Anemia with Excess Blasts II. RAEB I = Refractory Anemia with Excess Blast I. RA = Refractory Anemia, RCUD = Refractory Cytopenias with Unilineage Dysplasia, RARS = Refractory Anemia with Ringed Sideroblasts, RCMD-RS = Refractory Cytopenias with Multilineage Dysplasia and Ringed Sideroblasts, RCC = Refractory Cytopenias of Childhood

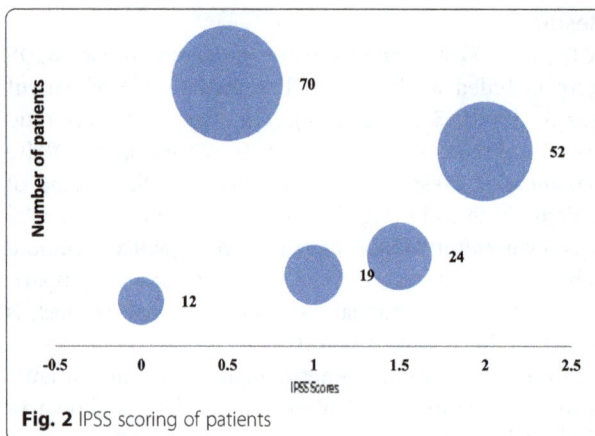

Fig. 2 IPSS scoring of patients

staining method. Grade III iron was found to be frequent, seen in 57 (32%) followed by grade IV in 38 (21.5%) and grade I in 36 (20.3%). Bone marrow myelofibrosis (MF) was done according to WHO 2008 myelofibrosis grading system and found to be MF -0 in 77 (44%), MF -I in 70 (39.5%) and MF-II in 30 (16.9%). Out of all patients, 97 (55%) were alive, 80 (45%) had died by the end of study period. The cause of death for 30 (38%) patients could not be ascertained whereas in rest of the patients the causes of death were septicemia in 19 (23.7%), severe anemia in 10 (12.5%), cardiac arrest in 15 (18.7%) and intracranial bleeding in 6 (7.5%) patients.

Discussion

Myelodysplastic syndromes are characterized by ineffective hematopoiesis with blood cytopenias and morphological dysplasia [1–5]. MDS is generally considered a preleukemic disorder and is prevalent in elder individuals in western world [5]. However, median age at diagnosis in our study was younger which concurs with other studies done in Asia [1–4, 6–8] as compared to the studies from west with higher median age in MDS (Greece, Germany, Poland) [10, 14, 15]. In our study we observed male predominance which is universally seen in this disorder [1–8]. However, male to female ratio was 3:1 which is slightly higher as compared to previous studies [1–4, 6, 7] and somewhat comparable to what has been observed in Greece [10]. The possible explanation of gender in our region could be low literacy rate in our country and male predominant society where females seek medical attention less frequently. The most common presenting complaint in our patients was loss of appetite followed by weakness. In our study mean Hb was 7.7 g/dl which is in concordance with a previous national study [1] and higher as compared to other studies done in Pakistan, China and India [2, 6, 8] and lower as compared to Turkey, Greece and Poland [9, 10, 15]. In our study, mean platelet count was 82 $\times10^9$/l, which is in concordance with a national study and also seen in

India [1, 8]. Interestingly data from Turkey and Greece reveals normal platelet count in MDS [9, 10]. Mean TLC count of 8.8 $\times10^9$/l in our study was higher as compared to other regional and international studies (Table 1) [1, 2, 6, 8, 9, 11, 12].

Anemia was most common presentation in previously reported studies and same was observed in our patients [1, 2]. History of recurrent infections is seen in MDS [5]. However, only 11% of our patients had history of recurrent infections, bacterial infections being most common. In our study 80 (45%) of patients presented with pancytopenia and 74 (42%) with bicytopenia having anemia and thrombocytopenia. Similar trend was observed by previous study done on regional level [1].

In our study refractory cytopenia with multilineage dysplasia (RCMD) was the most common encountered WHO sub category of MDS followed by refractory anemia with excess blast (RAEB) as observed in previous study from Pakistan [3] and the least common WHO sub category was refractory cytopenia with unilineage dysplasia (RCUD) which however contrasts with other national studies [1, 2]. On the other hand refractory anemia (RA) was most commonly observed in China and Greece [6, 10]. In our study, hypoplastic MDS was seen in 23 (13%) which is an interesting finding not observed in previous studies [1–3, 6–15]. Refractory cytopenia of childhood (RCC) was observed in only one of our patients. However we compared the classification with some previous studies in which they have followed French American British (FAB) classification [6, 7, 11–13] which is one of our study limitations.

In this study we found abnormal karyotype in 44 (45%), complex karyotype (CK) being most common in 12 (12.2%) followed by monosomy 7 in 7 (7.1%). Monosomy 7 is not commonly observed in previous studies [3, 6, 9–13, 15] except for one study from India showing higher frequency [8]. CK in our study was observed to be lower as compared to China [6]. Trisomy 8 was seen in 3 (3%), lower as compared to other studies [3, 6, 8, 10, 11]. Patients with RAEB II revealed higher frequency of chromosomal abnormalities, comparable to previously reported data [3]. In one of our patients isolated del(9q) was seen and in other del(9q) was seen along with t(1;9) (q11;q34). Del(9q) is associated with AML but very rarely reported in MDS [16] and to the best of our knowledge and searched literature t(1;9) has not been reported in MDS before. Isolated del(5q) was seen in one of our female patient with RAEB II who presented with pancytopenia which is in contrast to the clinical presentation of MDS with del(5q) syndrome [17].

Cytogenetic studies are done at limited centers in Pakistan, our study could be helpful to outline cytogenetic characteristics of MDS in our region. Karyotypic

Table 1 Hematological characteristics in comparison with national and international studies

Variables	Present study	Pakistan [1]	Pakistan [2]	Pakistan [3]	China [6]	Korea [7]	India [8]	Turkey [9]	Greece [10]	Taiwan [11]	Singapore [12]	Spain [13]	Germany [14]	Poland [15]
Total No. of Patients	177	45	46	71	508	176	40	54	855	189	43	640	216	863
Median age(years)	51.7	64	Mean 43.09	60	49	57	42	67	73.1	56	Mean 64	66	73	70
Mean Hb (g/dl)	7.8	7.7	6.52	–	6.3	–	6.84	9.0	9.5	8.0	7.7	–	–	9.1
Mean MCV (fl)	90	89.4	89.4	–	–	–	–	–	–	–	–	–	–	97
Mean TLC ($\times 10^9$/l)	8.8	5.7	3.4	–	3.0	–	4.45	3.8	7.52	3.3	5.6	–	–	–
Mean Platelet ($\times 10^9$/l)	82	83	60	–	42	–	85	163	158	61	101	–	–	129
MDS Category														
RCMD %	22	53.3	52.2	52	–	37	10	–	14.3	–	–	–	31	28.3
RAEB-II %	19.7	4.4	6.5	23.9	21.1	21	15	30	14.4	18.5	7	12	11	19.6
RAEB-I %	19.2	4.4	6.5	11.3	27	29	18	7	18.9	40.7	16.3	32	8	13.9
Hypoplastic MDS %	13	–	–	–	–	–	–	–	–	–	–	–	–	–
RA %	9	–	–	8.5	43.9	12	37	57	20.6	32.5	38.1	29	9	19.7
RARS %	7.9	–	–	2.8	2.8	–	7.5	–	6.2	8	14	12	4	6.7
RCUD %	3.3	22.2	RCUD–RA 26	–	–	–	–	–	–	–	–	–	–	–
RCMD-RS %	2.8	–	2.2	1.4	–	–	2.5	–	2.8	–	–	–	13	2.1
MDS with 5q %	2.20	–	–	–	–	–	10	6	1.9	–	–	–	2	4.6
RCC %	0.5	–	–	–	–	–	–	–	–	–	–	–	–	–
MDS-U %	–	15.5	6.5	–	–	1	–	–	–	–	–	–	–	5.1

Table 2 Cytogenetic profile in comparison with national and international studies

Variables	Present study	Pakistan[1]	Pakistan[2]	Pakistan[3]	China[6]	Korea[7]	India[8]	Turkey[9]	Greece[10]	Taiwan[11]	Singapore[12]	Spain[13]	Germany[14]	Poland[15]
Cytogenetics available/ Total No. of patients	98/177	–	–	71/71	367/508	–	40/40	54/54	591/855	175/189	40/43	640/640	–	276/863
Normal Karyotype %	55	–	–	57.7	62.9	–	53	85	61.6	53.1	52.5	49	–	44.6
Abnormal Karyotype %	44	–	–	42.3	37.1	–	47	15	38.4	46.8	47.5	51	–	55.4
Complex Karyotype %	12	–	–	15.5	38.9	–	–	–	7.6	17.2	20	14	–	6.4
Monosomy 7%	7.1	–	–	–	–	–	32	–	–	–	–	–	–	–
Del(5q) %	6.1	–	–	2.8	12.5	–	–	6	2.7	9.1	15	5	–	19
Del(7q) %	2	–	–	4.2	4.4	–	–	–	3	14.9	7.5	4	–	1.8
Trisomy 8%	3	–	–	9.9	25.7	–	16	9	8.3	12	10	5	–	2.2
Del(20q) %	4	–	–	1.4	14.7	–	–	–	2.2	6.3	–	1	–	0.3
Trisomy 21%	1	–	–	–	–	–	–	–	–	–	–	–	–	–
t(1;9) (q11;q34) along with Del(9q)[a] %	1	–	–	–	–	–	–	–	–	–	–	–	–	–
Trisomy 8 with Del(7q)[b] %	1	–	–	–	–	–	–	–	–	–	–	–	–	–
t(6;9) (p23;q23)[b] %	1	–	–	–	–	–	–	–	–	–	–	–	–	–
Monosomy 7,8[b] %	1	–	–	–	–	–	–	–	–	–	–	–	–	–
Del(9q)[b] %	2	–	–	–	–	–	–	–	–	–	–	–	–	–

[a] unique cytogenetic findings in our study
[b] rare cytogenetics

Table 3 Cytogenetics of patients in each WHO category

WHO subtype:	Total No. of cytogenetic performed N = 98 (%)	Normal karyotype N = 54 (%)	Abnormal karyotype N = 44 (%)	Chromosomal Abnormalities (N)
RCMD	22.4	10.2	12.2	t(6;9) (p23;q23) (1) Del(20q) (2) +8 (1) −7 (4) 46,XY,+3,del(5q),del(10q) (1) 48,XY,del(5q),+8 + 11,del (20q) (1) 47,XY,del(5q),+8,del(20q) (1) 49,XY,del(5q),del(7q),+8 + 11 + 17,del(20q) (1)
RAEB II	27.5	13.2	14.20	Del(9q) (1),del(5q) (1), del(7q) (2), del(20q) (2) +8 (1) −7 (1),−8 (1),−11 (1) 45,XY,t(6;9) (P23;q34),−3,+17 (1) 46,XY,t(1;9),del(9q),+11 (1) 47,XY,del(5q), +8 del(20q) (1) 49,XY,del(5q),del(7q),+8,del(11q),+17,del(20q) (1)
RAEB-I	16.32	7.14	9.1	Del(9q) (1), Del(20q) (1) +8 (1) −7 (2),−7,8 (1) 45,XY,del(5q),del(7q),-Y (1) 47,XX,t(3;12) (q26.2;q22),del(7q),+15 (1) 47,XY,+11 + 17,−22 (1)
Hypoplastic MDS	11.2	9.1	2.04	+8 with del(7q) (1) +12 (1)
RA	7.14	6.12	1.02	47,XY,+11,+17,del(20q) (1)
RCUD	5.1	4.08	1.02	t(1;9) (q11;q34) along with del(9q) (1)
RARS	2.04	2.04		–
RCMD-RS	2.04	2.04		–
MDS with 5q	5.10		5.10	Del5q (5)
RCC	1.02	1.02		–

abnormalities exhibit a significant role in diagnosis and prognosis of MDS. We observed CK and monosomy 7 frequent in our study which carries poor overall survival and early transformation to AML. Such patients must be identified early in the disease course. Since our study was retrospective, future prospective studies are needed to ascertain the findings.

Conclusion

In our study we observed younger median age of disease presentation, higher mean TLC count and no significant history of recurrent infections. RCMD was the most common WHO category and CK was most common abnormal karyotype followed by monosomy 7. Since both carry adverse prognostic implications, early identification of such patients with close clinical follow up and upfront allogenic stem cell transplant must be considered keeping in view the younger age in our cohort at time of presentation. This study was done retrospectively yet represents a large cohort of MDS in our country. In future, prospective studies are needed to be done to further elaborate disease biology and clinical outcome of the baseline adverse

disease characteristics observed in our study. Also molecular testing in MDS must be incorporated since nowadays diagnostic spectrum of MDS is moving rapidly towards molecular analysis and its relation to disease outcome.

Abbreviations

AML: Acute myeloid leukemia; ANC: Absolute neutophil count; GTG: G-bands via trypsin using Giemsa; Hb: Hemoglobin; IPSS: International Prognostic Scoring System; ISCN: International system for human cytogenetic nomenclature; MDS: Myelodysplasticsyndromes; RA: Refractory anemia; RAEB I: Refractory anemia with excess blast I; RAEB II: Refractory anemia with excess blasts II; RARS: Refractory anemia with ringed sideroblasts; RCC: Refractory cytopenia of childhood; RCMD: Refractory cytopenia(s) with multilineage dysplasia; RCMD-RS: Refractory cytopenias with multilineage dysplasia and ringed sideroblasts; RCUD: Refractory cytopenias with unilineage dysplasia; TLC: Total leukocyte count; WHO: World Health Organization

Acknowledgements

All the authors gratefully acknowledge all our MDS patients for their cooperation throughout the study period and the ethics committee for their approval to conduct this study.

Funding

No funding.

Authors' contributions

NA had the main idea of the study and contributed in literature search and manuscript writing, AA contributed in literature search and collection of patient's data. MN critically reviewed and revised the manuscript. SK contributed in manuscript writing. NF contributed in statistical analysis. SS contributed in collection of patient's data. SaS performed the cytogenetics of patients. TS contributed in editing and critically reviewed the manuscript. All authors read and approved the final manuscript.

Competing interests

The authors declare that they have no competing interests.

References

1. Sultan S, Irfan SM. Adult primary myelodysplastic syndrome: experience from a tertiary care center in Pakistan. APJCP. 2016;17(3):1535–7.
2. Ehsan A, Aziz M. Clinico-haematological characteristics in pakistani patients of primary myelodysplastic syndrome according to World Health Organization classification. JCPSP. 2010;20(4):232–6.
3. Rashid A, Khurshid M, Shaikh U, Adil S. Chromosomal abnormalities in primary myelodysplastic syndrome. JCPSP. 2014;9:632–5.
4. Sultan S, Irfan SM, Jawed SN. Spectrum of the WHO CLassification *De Novo* myelodysplastic syndrome: experience from Southern Pakistan. APJCP. 2016; 17(3):1049–52.
5. Malcovati L, Hellström-Lindberg E, Bowen D, Adès L, Cermak J, Del Cañizo C, et al. Diagnosis and treatment of primary myelodysplastic syndromes in adults: recommendations from the European LeukemiaNet. Blood. 2013; 122(17):2943–64.
6. Chen B, Zhao WL, Jin J, Xue YQ, Cheng X, Chen XT, et al. Clinical and cytogenetic features of 508 Chinese patients with myelodysplastic syndrome and comparison with those in Western countries. Leukemia. 2005;19(5):767–75.
7. Lee JH, Shin YR, Lee JS, Kim WK, Chi HS, Park CJ, et al. Application of different prognostic scoring systems and comparison of the FAB and WHO classifications in Korean patients with myelodysplastic syndrome. Leukemia. 2003;17(2):305–13.
8. Chaubey R, Sazawal S, Dada R, Mahapatra M, Saxena R. Cytogenetic profile of Indian patients with de novo myelodysplastic syndromes. Ind J Med Res. 2011;134(4):452–7.
9. Demirkan F, Alacacioglu I, Piskin O, Ozsan HG, Akinci B, Ozcan AM, et al. The clinical, haematological and morphological profile of patients with myelodysplastic syndromes: a single institution experience from Turkey. Leuk Lymph. 2007;48(7): 1372–8.
10. Avgerinou C. The incidence of myelodysplastic syndromes in Western Greece is increasing. Ann Hematol. 2013;92:877–87.
11. Huang T-C. Comparison of hypoplasticmyelodysplastic syndrome (MDS) with normo-/hypercellular MDS by international prognostic scoring system, cytogenetic and genetic studies. Leukemia. 2008;22:544–50.
12. Lau LG. Clinico-pathological analysis of Myelodysplastic syndromes according to French-American-British Classification and International Prognostic Scoring System. Ann Acad Med Singapore. 2004;33:589–95.
13. Sole F, Espinet B, Sanz GF, Cervera J, Calasanz MJ, Luno, et al. Incidence, characterization and prognostic significance of chromosomal abnormalities in 640 patients with primary myelodysplastic syndromes. Br J Haematol. 2000;108:346–56.
14. Neukirchen J, Schoonen WM, Strupp C, Gattermann N, Aul C, Haas R, et al. Incidence and prevalence of myelodysplastic syndromes: data from the düsseldorf MDS-registry. Leuk Res. 2011;35:1591–6.
15. Mądry K, Machowicz R, Waszczuk-Gajda A, Drozd-Sokołowska J, Hołowiecka BS, Wiater E, et al. Demographic, hematologic, and clinical feature of myelodysplastic syndrome patients: results from the first polish myelodysplastic syndrome registry. Acta Haematol. 2015;134:125–34.
16. Vigue F. del(9q) solely. Atlas Genet Cytogenet Oncol Haematol. 1998;2(2):55–6.
17. Boultwood J, Fidler C, Strickson AJ, Watkins F, Gama S, Kearney L, et al. Narrowing and genomic annotation of the commonly deleted region of the 5q- syndrome. Blood. 2002;99:4638–41.

13

CANPMR syndrome and chromosome 1p32-p31 deletion syndrome coexist in two related individuals affected by simultaneous haplo-insufficiency of *CAMTA1* and *NIFA* genes

Emanuele G. Coci[1*], Udo Koehler[2], Thomas Liehr[3], Armin Stelzner[1], Christian Fink[4], Hendrik Langen[1] and Joachim Riedel[1]

Abstract

Background: Non-progressive cerebellar ataxia with mental retardation (CANPMR, OMIM 614756) and chromosome 1p32-p31 deletion syndrome (OMIM 613735) are two very rare inherited disorders, which are caused by mono-allelic deficiency (haplo-insufficiency) of calmodulin-binding transcription activator 1 (*CAMTA1*) and, respectively, nuclear factor 1 A (*NFIA*) genes. The yet reported patients affected by mono-allelic *CAMTA1* dysfunction presented with neonatal hypotonia, delayed and ataxic gait, cerebellar atrophy, psychological delay and speech impairment, while individuals carrying a disrupted *NFIA* allele suffered from agenesis/hypoplasia of the corpus callosum, ventriculomegaly, developmental delay and urinary tract abnormalities. Both disorders were not seen in one patient together before.

Results: In this study two related individuals affected by a complex clinical syndrome, characterized by cognitive, neurological and nephrological features were studied for the underlying genetic disorder(s) by molecular cytogenetics. The two individuals present dysmorphic facies, macrocephaly, generalized ataxia, mild tremor, strabismus, mild mental retardation and kidney hypoplasia. Moreover, neuro-radiological studies showed hypoplasia of corpus callosum. Genetic investigations revealed a paracentric inversion in the short arm of one chromosome 1 with breakpoints within *CAMTA1* and *NFIA* coding sequences.

Conclusions: To the best of our knowledge, this is the first report of two patients harboring the simultaneous mono-allelic disruptions and consequent haplo-insufficiencies of two genes due to an inversion event. Disruption of *CAMTA1* and *NFIA* genes led to neuro-psychological and nephrological dysfunctions, which comprised clinical features of CANPMR syndrome as well as chromosome 1p32-p31 deletion syndrome.

Keywords: NFIA, Chromosome 1p32-p31 deletion syndrome, CAMTA1, CANPMR syndrome, Paracentric inversion on short arm of chromosome 1

* Correspondence: Emanuele.Coci@akh-celle.de
[1]Center of Social Pediatrics and Pediatric Neurology, General Hospital of Celle, 29221 Celle, Germany
Full list of author information is available at the end of the article

Background

Non-progressive cerebellar ataxia with mental retardation (CANPMR, OMIM 614756) is a very rare neuro-developmental disorder, belonging to the heterogeneous family of genetically determined cerebellar ataxias [1, 2] with recessive [3] and dominant [4] pattern of inheritance. The affected patients present with ataxic gait, dysmetries, variable mental retardation, cerebellar abnormalities and dysmorphic facies with heterogeneous penetrance. To date few genes/loci have been associated to autosomal recessive forms of cerebellar ataxias: *ATCAY* [5], chromosome 20q11-q13 locus [6], *VLDLR* [7], *ZNF592* [8], *SPTBN2* [9], *CWF19L1* [10], *PMPCA* [11]. Calmodulin-binding transcription activator 1 (*CAMTA1*) maps on chromosome 1p36, carries 23 exons and encodes 2 protein isoforms in mammalians. The brain-specific transcription factor CAMTA1 functions as homodimeric complex binding to gene promoters' CGCG box thorough CG-1 domain, supporting the assembly of other transcription factors (e.g. Nkx2-5) and enhancing transcription of effector genes (e.g. Fbxl4) [12–14]. *CAMTA1* dysfunction has been associated to human pathology by Thevenon et al. [15], who reported five patients affected by *CAMTA1* haploinsufficiency due to deletions or duplications in the gene region coding for CG-1 domain, which plays a pivotal role in the whole CAMTA1 function. As mentioned above, the reported patients suffered from ataxia, broad-based gait, tremor, intellectual impairment and speech delay, cerebellar abnormalities (atrophy of lobes and/or vermis) and facial dysmorphisms (strabismus, large forehead, wide and broad nose, small ears).

The clinical features of chromosome 1p32-p31 deletion syndrome (OMIM 613735) were firstly described by Campbell et al. [16]. Some years later, Lu et al. proposed the causal association between this malformation syndrome and Nuclear Factor 1 A (*NFIA*) haplo-insufficiency [17]. *NFIA* maps on 1p31.2, carries 11 exons and produces at least 9 different protein isoforms [18–20]. The protein is functionally divided in two sections: a 200 amino acid long N-terminal DNA binding and dimerization domain, mainly encoded by exon 2, and C-terminal transactivation and repression domains, mainly encoded by exons 3 to 11. The first one binds to the nucleotide consensus sequence $TTGGC(N)_5GCCAA$ within the promoter region of several genes. The latter ones operate by directly activating basal transcription factors at transcription start sites, by displacing repressive histones from target genes, by interacting with other co-activator proteins [20]. All five individuals reported by Lu et al. (three of which previously described by Campbell et al.) presented with hypoplastic or absent corpus callosum, ventriculomegaly with or without relevant hydrocephalus and development delay; some of them carried urinary tract abnormalities (3 patients),

epileptic seizures (3 patients), tethered spinal cord (4 patients) and Chiari malformation (3 patients). Although the chromosomal abnormalities [a translocation t(1;20), a translocation t(1;2), a 2.2 Mb deletion in 1p31-p32, a 12 Mb deletion in 1p31-p32] differed and the deleted regions comprised different genes among the five patients, only *NFIA* gene was either disrupted or fully deleted in all five patients, thus underpinning the association between *NFIA* haplo-insufficiency and the common CNS abnormalities (hypoplasia of corpus callosum, ventriculomegaly and hydrocephalus). A strong confirmation on their pathophysiological hypothesis was given by the clinical and histopathological findings of $Nfia^{-/-}$ mouse model [17, 21]. A detailed study of the genome expression profile in murine $Nfia^{-/-}$ brain at embryonic and post-natal stages showed a very strong imbalance in time-related expression of several genes playing a pivotal role in oligodendrocyte differentiation (e.g. *Mag, Mal, Mobp, Mog, Sox2, Sox4, Sox11, Dio2, Myef2*) as well as in axonal growth/guidance (e.g. *Clusterin, aFGF, Ndrg2, EphrinB2, Crmp1*) [22]. The essential role of transcription factor Nfib and Nfic in brain, tooth and lung development was already described in the corresponding mouse models [23, 24]. Few further reports described heterogeneous clinical findings associated with deletions mapping on chromosome 1p31 and 1p32 and encompassing several other genes [25, 26].

We describe the first family (Fig. 1) with two related individuals (II.1 and III.1) carrying simultaneous disruptions

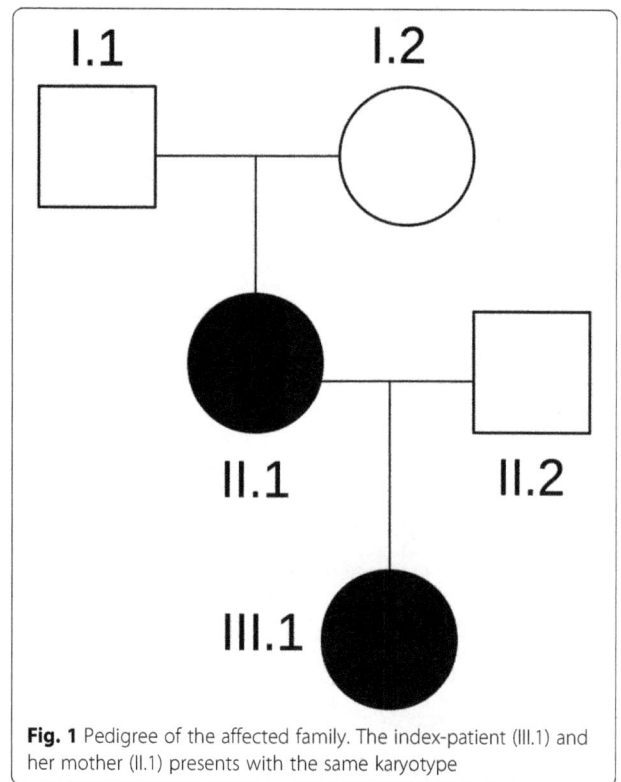

Fig. 1 Pedigree of the affected family. The index-patient (III.1) and her mother (II.1) presents with the same karyotype

and consequent haplo-insufficiencies of *NFIA* and *CAMTA* genes due to a paracentric inversion in the short arm of chromosome 1 and presenting with clinical signs of CANPMR syndrome as well as chromosome 1p32-p31 deletion syndrome.

Results and discussion
Patient 1
Since the first months of life the index-patient (III.1) presented with generalized hypotonia, reduced muscular strength, particularly evident at trunk und pelvis, normal tendon reflexes, large head (> P90), prominent forehead, strabismus divergens and light bilateral ptosis. The patient could sit at 11 months and walk at 23 months of age. Gowers' sign was through-out positive. Light dyskinesias and ataxia appeared at 3 years and, respectively, 6 years of age. She could speak the first words at about 30 months of age.

She slowly improved her motor, cognitive and language skills. Now, at the age of 7 years she can walk unassisted, climb stairs and speak short sentences. Her daily skills are compromised and she attends a special care kindergarten. Her intelligence quotient (IQ) score of 51 (Snijders-Oomen Non-Verbal test, SON-R) indicates a severe intellectual impairment (Table 1).

The electroencephalogram (EEG) did not show epileptic discharges. The brain MR investigations at 2 and 6 ½ years of age revealed hypoplasia of corpus callosum, while the cerebellum was structurally normal (Fig. 2). Organ ultrasound did not show any structural abnormalities of kidneys and urinary tract, although the patient suffered from recurrent urine infections starting from 18 months of age.

Patient 2 and other individuals of pedigree
The mother (II.1) of the index patient (28 years) presents with a similar clinical constellation of III.1, whereby she suffered from neonatal hypotonia, but sat unassisted at 8 months, walked at 14 months and spoke the first words at 12 months of age. She presents with a moderate ataxia, gait instability and dysmetria, which does not strongly impair the daily skills. Her IQ score of 65 (SON-R test) revealed a mental retardation. She has not completed any job training course and is currently unemployed. The brain MR scan, performed at 28 years of age, revealed hypoplasia of corpus callosum (Fig. 2).

Since the early childhood, she suffered from recurrent urinary tract infections due to vesicoureteral reflux (VUR) and from hypoplasia of the right kidney. The father (II.2) of the index patient carries a normal male karyotype and is a healthy individual. The maternal grandparents (I.1 and I.2) are healthy individuals; nevertheless their karyotype could not be analyzed due to missing compliance.

Table 1 Clinical, psychological, radiological features of the affected patients II.1 and III.1

	II.1 (28 years)	III.1 (6 ½ years)
Development parameters		
Sitting age (months)	8	11
Walking age (months)	14	23
Speaking age (months)	12	30
Clinical findings		
Macrocephaly	Yes (P 97)	No (P 90)
Muscle tonus	Normal	Normal
Seizures	No	No
Facies		
Forehead	Large	Large
Strabismus	Yes (divergens)	Yes (divergens)
Nasal bridge	Broad	Broad
Ears form and position	Normal	Normal
Mouth form and occlusion	Normal	Normal
Eye distance	2.5 cm (intercantal) and 6 cm (interpupillar)	2.5 cm (intercantal) and 5.5 cm (interpupillar)
Cerebellar symptoms		
Ataxic gait	Yes	Yes
Instability	Yes	Yes
Dysmetry	Yes	Yes
Dysartria	Yes	Yes
SARA score	6/40	11/40
Kidney and urinary tract defects	Recurrent infections, hypoplasia of the right kidney	Recurrent infections
Intelligence quotient (SON-R scale)	65	51
Brain MRI findings		
Corpus callosum hypoplasia	Hypoplastic	Hypoplastic
Ventriculomegaly or hydrocephalus	No	No
Cerebellar abnormalities	No	No

SARA Scale for the Assessment and Rating of Ataxia

Cytogenetic investigations
The index-patient III.1 harbors a paracentric inversion in the short arm of chromosome 1 with breakpoints within *CAMTA1* (1p36.31) and *NFIA* (1p31.3) genes (Fig. 3).

In correspondence of both breakpoints, two deletions occurred affecting *CAMTA1* exon 5 (deletion length 211 Kb; position 6,936,272 - 7,146,519 Mb, GRCh37/hg19)

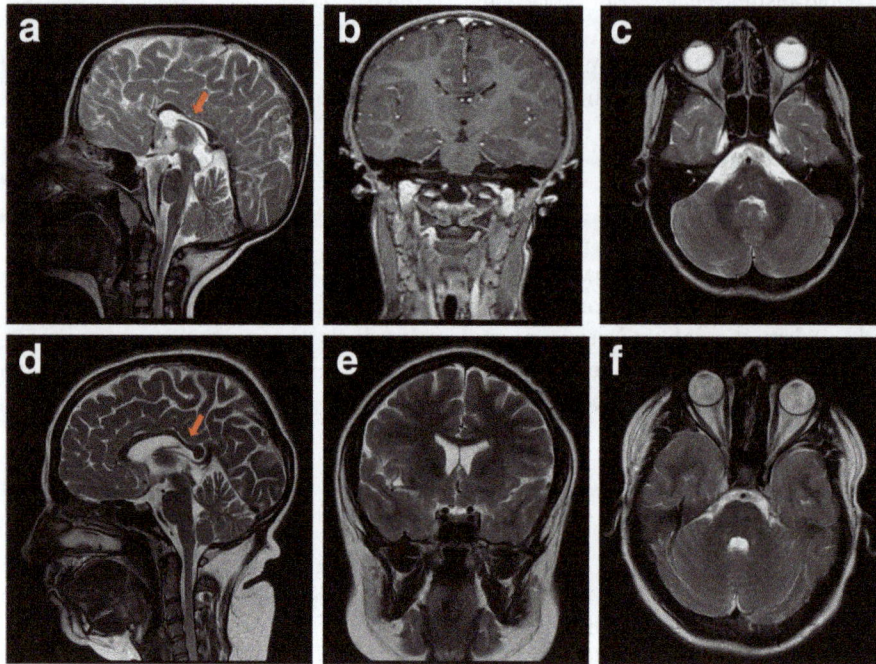

Fig. 2 Brain MR investigation of index-patient (III.1, pictures **a**, **b**, **c**) and her mother (II.1, pictures **d**, **e**, **f**). Hypoplasia of the corpus callosum is revealed in both patients (red arrows). Otherwise no other structural anomalies were observed

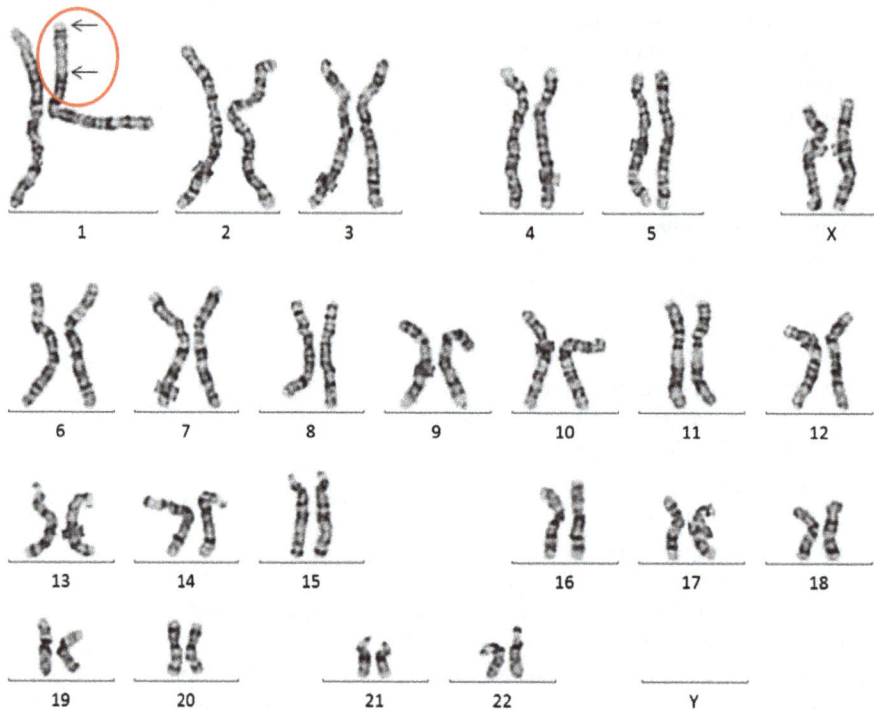

Fig. 3 Karyotype of index-patient (III.1). Karyotyping (GTG-banding) of lymphocytes of peripheral blood revealed an inversion in the short arm of chromosome 1. Breakpoints in 1p31.3 and 1p36.31 (arrows) correspond to two deletions, which have been revealed by SNP array and depicted in Fig. 4

and *NFIA* exons 3-4 (deletion length 217 Kb; position 61,591,640 - 61,807,789 Mb, GRCh37/hg19) in patients II.1 and III1, which could only be resolved by SNP array (Fig. 4).

The resulting genotype is described as [46,XX,inv(1) (p36.31p31.3).arr   1p36.31(6,936,272-7,146,519)x1mat, 1p31.3(61,591,640-61,807,789)x1mat]. Due to the chromosomal inversion, the remaining coding regions of the affected alleles are restricted to exons 1 to 4 for *CAMTA1* and, respectively, exons 1 to 2 for *NFIA*. For *CAMTA1*, C-terminal 2/3 of CG-1 domain is deleted (about 80 out of 120 amino acids) and the other 3 C-terminal domains (TIG, IQ motif and Ankirin) are fully deleted. For *NFIA*, the N-terminal DNA binding domain (encoded by exon 2) is not affected by the deletion, but the C-terminal transactivation and repression domains (including also the proline-rich domain) are absent from the remaining coding sequence. The second affected individual II.1, mother of the index-patient, carries the same chromosomal aberration as her daughter, III.1. The individual II.2, father of III.1, does present a normal male karyotype. We were not able to test the karyotype of I.1 and I.2, grandparents of the index patient, due to their missing compliance; nevertheless, they are healthy individuals without any clinical findings resembling the syndromic features of II.1 and III.1.

Given the similar clinical and genetic findings of both patients the chromosomal aberration occurred de novo

in patient II.1 at embryonic stage and was transmitted to patient III.1.

Conclusions

To our knowledge, our related patients are the unique two described individuals with combined features from two independent syndromes. CANPMR syndrome (OMIM 614756) is a rare genetic disorder of the nervous system presenting with cerebellar ataxia and mild to severe mental retardation, whose genetic cause was recently described to be *CAMTA1* haploinsufficiency [15]. Chromosome 1p32-p31 deletion syndrome (OMIM 613735) presents with hypoplasia/aplasia of the corpus callosum, one of the most common congenital abnormalities of the CNS [27], accompanied by ventriculomegaly with or without hydrocephalus and developmental delay. The haploinsufficiency of *NFIA* was implied by Lu et al [17] to be the molecular cause of this syndrome.

According to the last insights on the genetic pathophysiology of these two syndromes [15, 17], the complex disorder affecting our two related patients is very likely caused by the simultaneous haplo-insufficiencies of *NFIA* and *CAMTA1*, which are the breakpoints of a paracentric inversion in the short arm of chromosome 1. The inversion-associated disruption of *NFIA*'s and *CAMTA1*'s reading frames causes very likely the decay of the remaining mRNA strains (corresponding to *NFIA* exons

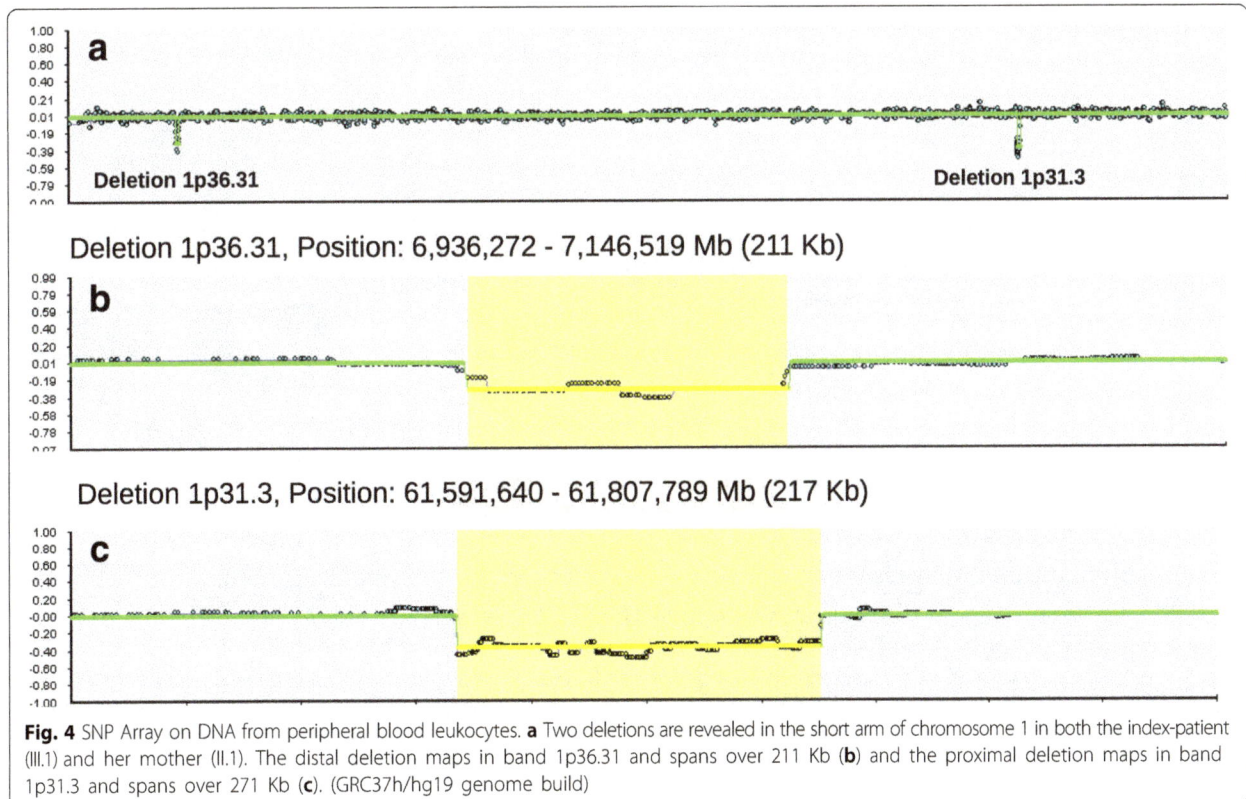

Fig. 4 SNP Array on DNA from peripheral blood leukocytes. **a** Two deletions are revealed in the short arm of chromosome 1 in both the index-patient (III.1) and her mother (II.1). The distal deletion maps in band 1p36.31 and spans over 211 Kb (**b**) and the proximal deletion maps in band 1p31.3 and spans over 271 Kb (**c**). (GRC37h/hg19 genome build)

1–2 and, respectively *CAMTA1* exons 1–4), which are transcribed from the affected alleles of both genes.

If a truncated NFIA protein is synthesized, the C-terminal transactivation and repression domains would completely lack and therefore the truncated NFIA protein would be unable to exert his effector function. The absence of seizures in our two patients may exclude that *NFIA* haplo-insufficiency causes epileptic seizures, which were described in 3 out of 5 patients reported by Lu et al. On the contrary, the urinary tract abnormalities and VUR in 3 out of 5 patients from Lu et al and in our 2 patients (carrying mono-allelic *NFIA* disruption) seem to reinforce the view that NFIA plays a major role in the human urinary tract development. Remarkably, our patients carry mono-allelic disruptions of only two genes in comparison with the patients reported by Lu et al. [17] and Koehler et al. [25], which harbored larger deletions encompassing several other genes apart from *NFIA* (Fig. 5). This fortuitous genetic condition strengthens the casual association between *NFIA* haplo-insufficiency and some clinical findings described in our study.

The pathogenic insights on *CAMTA1* haploinsufficiency are enforced by the clinical findings of our two patients. Ataxic and delayed gait, dysmetric movements, instability, macrocephaly and ventriculomegaly, cerebellar and cortical abnormalities at MR scans strengthen the clinical stigmata of CANPMR syndrome. While all former patients reported by Thevenon et al carried intragenic deletions and duplications disrupting the N-terminal CG-1 domain (short deletion of exon 4 in familiy 1, duplication of exons 3 to 5 in family 2, short deletion of exon 3 in familiy 3), the chromosomal inversion harbored by our 2 patients represents the first report on mono-allelic deletion of C-terminal domains TIG, IQ motif and Ankirin from *CAMTA1* reading frame and shows the patho-physiological consequence of this genetic event. Among 11 patients from 3 families reported by Thevenon et al, 9 out of 11 patients are reported to have a pathologic intelligence quotient (IQ) between 40 and 67 and a mild to severe intellectual disability (ID), like our 2 patients.

Although an inversion-dependent imbalance on the expression of neighboring genes, located nearby to inversion breakpoints, cannot be theoretically excluded as co-factor responsible for the clinical phenotype, such positional effect seems to be very unlikely in our cases.

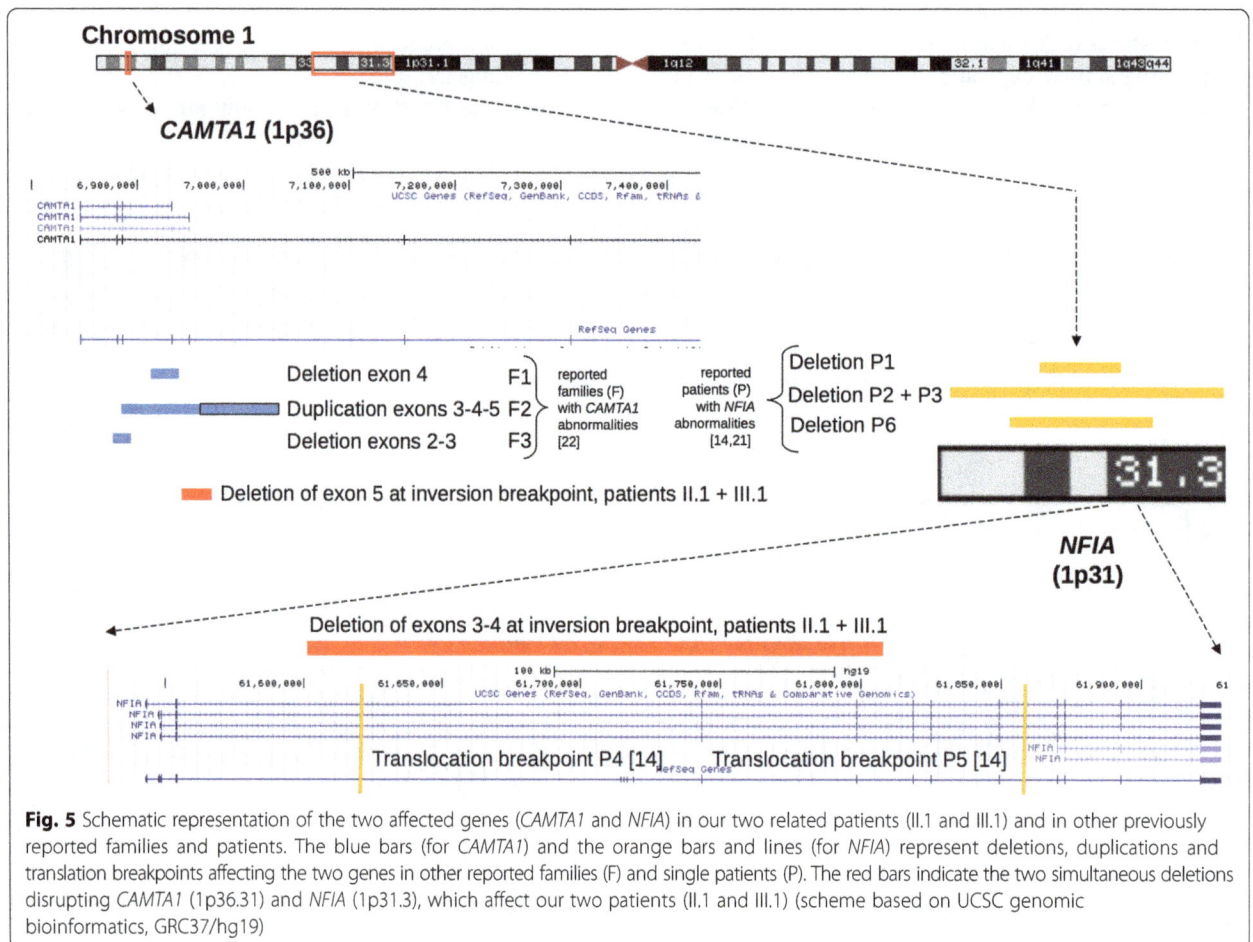

Fig. 5 Schematic representation of the two affected genes (*CAMTA1* and *NFIA*) in our two related patients (II.1 and III.1) and in other previously reported families and patients. The blue bars (for *CAMTA1*) and the orange bars and lines (for *NFIA*) represent deletions, duplications and translation breakpoints affecting the two genes in other reported families (F) and single patients (P). The red bars indicate the two simultaneous deletions disrupting *CAMTA1* (1p36.31) and *NFIA* (1p31.3), which affect our two patients (II.1 and III.1) (scheme based on UCSC genomic bioinformatics, GRC37/hg19)

In fact, no gene mapping in the proximity of deletion 1p36.31 (e.g. *DNAJC11, THAP3, PHF13, VAMP3, PER3, UTS2*) or in the proximity of the deletion 1p31.3 (e.g. *CYP2J2, HOOK1, FGGY, TM2D1, INADL, KANK*) was associated with brain and urinary tract abnormalities to date.

Taken together, in our two patients the study of the mono-allelic and simultaneous disruption of genes *CAMTA1* and *NFIA*, whose haploinsufficiencies were already associated to two independent pathological phenotypes [15, 17], sheds further light on the clinical and genetic features of the rare developmental disorders CANPMR syndrome and chromosome 1p32-p31 deletion syndrome.

Methods
Upon extraction of DNA from total peripheral blood leucocytes, conventional karyotyping was performed using G-banding techniques on stimulated blood lymphocytes with standard cytogenetic methods and analyzed at 500–550 band resolution. Karyotypes were described according to the International System for Human Cytogenetic Nomenclature (ISCN 2013).

SNP array was performed using an Infinium CytoSNP-850 K microarray (Illumina, San Diego, CA, USA) with an average resolution of 18Kb and a practical resolution in genes *CAMTA1* and *NFIA* of 1 Kb according to the manufacturer's protocol. The data analysis was done using BlueFuse V4.2 software. The gene alignment was done using the University of California Santa Cruz (UCSC) genomic bioinformatics browser. The two deleted regions were mapped using the Genome Research Consortium Build 37 human/human genome 19 (GRCh37/hg19). The GenBank, Ensembl and OMIM browser accession numbers for *CAMTA1* are NM_015215, ENST00000303635, ENSG00000171735, MIM 611501 and for *NFIA* are NM_001134673, ENST00000403491, ENSG 00000162599, MIM 600727.

Cerebral MRI was performed on clinical 1.5 T MRI systems (Magnetom Avanto and Aera, Siemens Medical, Germany) using standardized MRI protocols including multiplanar T1 and T2-weighted MR-sequences.

Patient consent
The authors obtained the patient consent for the publication of the data.

Abbreviations
CANPMR: cerebellar ataxia non progressive with mental retardation; SARA: scale for the assessment and rating of ataxia; SON-R: Snijders-Oomen non-verbal test.

Competing interests
The authors declare that they have no competing interests.

Authors' contributions
EC, TL, AS, HL, JR participated in the design of the study and analyzed the patients' phenotype. EC and UK perfomed the genetic studies. CF performed the neuro-radiological investigations. All authors drafted and approved the final manuscript.

Acknowledgements
The authors express our deep gratitude to the family for the full collaboration throughout the project.

Author details
[1]Center of Social Pediatrics and Pediatric Neurology, General Hospital of Celle, 29221 Celle, Germany. [2]Medizinisch Genetisches Zentrum, 80335 Munich, Germany. [3]Institute of Human Genetics, Friedrich Schiller University, Jena University Hospital, 07743 Jena, Germany. [4]Department of Radiology, General Hospital of Celle, 29223 Celle, Germany.

References
1. Steinlin M, Zangger B, Boltshauser E. Non-progressive congenital ataxia with or without cerebellar hypoplasia: a review of 34 subjects. Dev Med Child Neurol. 1998;40:148–54.
2. Yapici Z, Eraksoy M. Non-progressive congenital ataxia with cerebellar hypoplasia in three families. Acta Paediatr. 2005;94:248–53.
3. Guzzetta F, Mercuri E, Bonanno S, Longo M, Spano M. Autosomal recessive congenital cerebellar atrophy. A clinical and neuropsychological study. Brain Dev. 1993;15:439–45.
4. Imamura S, Tachi N, Oya K. Dominantly inherited early-onset non-progressive cerebellar ataxia syndrome. Brain Dev. 1993;15:372–6.
5. Bomar JM, Benke PJ, Slattery EL, Puttagunta R, Taylor LP, Seong E, et al. Mutations in a novel gene encoding a CRAL-TRIO domain cause human Cayman ataxia and ataxia/dystonia in the jittery mouse. Nat Genet. 2003;35:264–9.
6. Tranebjaerg L, Teslovich TM, Jones M, Barmada MM, Fagerheim T, Dahl A, et al. Genome-wide homozygosity mapping localizes a gene for autosomal recessive non-progressive infantile ataxia to 20q11-q13. Hum Genet. 2003; 113:293–5.
7. Boycott KM, Flavelle S, Bureau A, Glass HC, Fujiwara TM, Wirrell E, et al. Homozygous deletion of the very low density lipoprotein receptor gene causes autosomal recessive cerebellar hypoplasia with cerebral gyral simplification. Am J Hum Genet. 2005;77:477–83.
8. Nicolas E, Poitelon Y, Chouery E, Salem N, Levy N, Mégarbané A, et al. CAMOS, a nonprogressive, autosomal recessive, congenital cerebellar ataxia, is caused by a mutant zinc-finger protein, ZNF592. Eur J Hum Genet. 2010; 18:1107–13.
9. Lise S, Clarkson Y, Perkins E, Kwasniewska A, Sadighi Akha E, Schnekenberg RP, et al. Recessive mutations in SPTBN2 implicate β-III spectrin in both cognitive and motor development. PLoS Genet. 2012;8(12):e1003074. doi:10.1371/journal.pgen.1003074.
10. Burns R, Majczenko K, Xu J, Peng W, Yapici Z, Dowling JJ, et al. Homozygous splice mutation in CWF19L1 in a Turkish family with recessive ataxia syndrome. Neurology. 2014;83:2175–82.
11. Jobling RK, Assoum M, Gakh O, Blaser S, JRaiman JA, Mignot C, et al. PMPCA mutations cause abnormal mitochondrial protein processing in patients with non-progressive cerebellar ataxia. Brain. 2015;138:1505–17.
12. Finkler A, Ashery-Padan R, Fromm H. CAMTA1s: calmodulin-binding transcription activators from plants to human. FEBS Lett. 2007;581:3893–8.
13. Han J, Gong P, Redding K, Mitra M, Guo P, Li HS. The fly CAMTA transcription factor potentiates deactivation of rhodopsin, a G protein-couples light receptor. Cell. 2006;127:847–58.
14. Gong P, Han L, Redding K, Li HS. A potential dimerization region of dCAMTA is critical termination of fly visual response. J Biol Chem. 2007;282:21253–8.
15. Thevenon J, Lopez E, Keren B, Heron D, Mignot C, Altuzarra C, et al. Intragenic CAMTA1 rearrangements cause non-progressive congenital ataxia with or without intellectual disability. J Med Genet. 2012;49:400–8.
16. Campbell CG, Wang H, Hunter GW. Interstitial microdeletion of chromosome 1p in two siblings. Am J Med Genet. 2002;111:289–94.
17. Lu W, Quintero-Rivera F, Fan Y, Alkuraya FS, Donovan DJ, Xi Q, et al. NFIA haploinsufficiency is associated with a CNS malformation syndrome and urinary tract defects. PLoS Genet. 2007;3:830–43.
18. Qian F, Kruse U, Lichter P, Sippel AE. Chromosomal localization of the four genes (NFIA, B, C, and X) for the human transcription factor nuclear factor I by FISH. Genomics. 1995;28:66–73.

19. Grunder A, Qian F, Ebel TT, Mincheva A, Lichter P, Kruse U, et al. Genomic organization, splice products and mouse chromosomal localization of genes for transcription factor Nuclear Factor One. Gene. 2003;304:171–81.

20. Gronostajski RM. Roles of the NFI/CTF gene family in transcription and development. Gene. 2000;249:31–45.

21. Das Neves L, Duchala CS, Godinho F, Haxhiu MA, Colmenares C, Macklin WB, et al. Disruption of the murine nuclear factor I-A gene (Nfia) results in perinatal lethality, hydrocephalus, and agenesis of the corpus callosum. PNAS. 1999;96:11946–51.

22. Wong YW, Schulze C, Streichert T, Gronostajski RM, Schachner M, Tilling T. Gene expression analysis of nuclear factor I-A deficient mice indicates delayed brain maturation. Genome Biol. 2007;8:R72.

23. Steele-Perkins G, Butz KG, Lyons GE, Zeichner-David M, Kim HJ, Cho MI, et al. Essential role of NFI-C/CTF transcription-replication factor in tooth root development. Mol Cell Biol. 2003;23:1075–84.

24. Steele-Perkins G, Plachez C, Butz KG, Yang G, Bachurski CJ, Kinsman SL, et al. The transcription factor gene Nfib is essential for both lung maturation and brain development. Mol Cell Biol. 2005;25:685–98.

25. Koehler U, Holinski-Feder E, Ertl-Wagner B, Kunz J, von Moers A, von Voss H, et al. A novel 1p31.3p32.2 deletion involving the NFIA gene detected by array CGH in a patient with macrocephaly and hypoplasia of the corpus callosum. Eur J Pediatr. 2010;169:463–8.

26. Nyboe D, Kreiborg S, Kirchhoff M, Hove HB. Familial craniosynostosis associated with a microdeletion involving the NFIA gene. Clin Dysmorphol. 2015;24:109–12.

27. Paul LK, Brown WS, Adolphs R, Tyszka JM, Richards LJ, Mukherjee P, et al. Agenesis of the corpus callosum: genetics, development and functional aspects of the connectivity. Nat Rev Neurosci. 2007;8:287–99.

14

Copy number changes and methylation patterns in an isodicentric and a ring chromosome of 15q11-q13

Qin Wang[1], Weiqing Wu[1,2], Zhiyong Xu[1], Fuwei Luo[1], Qinghua Zhou[2,3], Peining Li[2] and Jiansheng Xie[1*]

Abstract

Background: The low copy repeats (LCRs) in chromosome 15q11-q13 have been recognized as breakpoints (BP) for not only intrachromosomal deletions and duplications but also small supernumerary marker chromosomes 15, sSMC(15)s, in the forms of isodicentric chromosome or small ring chromosome. Further characterization of copy number changes and methylation patterns in these sSMC(15)s could lead to better understanding of their phenotypic consequences.

Methods: Routine G-band karyotyping, fluorescence in situ hybridization (FISH), array comparative genomic hybridization (aCGH) analysis and methylation-specific multiplex ligation-dependent probe amplification (MS-MLPA) assay were performed on two Chinese patients with a sSMC(15).

Results: Patient 1 showed an isodicentric 15, idic(15)(q13), containing symmetrically two copies of a 7.7 Mb segment of the 15q11-q13 region by a BP3::BP3 fusion. Patient 2 showed a ring chromosome 15, r(15)(q13), with alternative one-copy and two-copy segments spanning a 12.3 Mb region. The defined methylation pattern indicated that the idic(15)(q13) and the r(15)(q13) were maternally derived.

Conclusions: Results from these two cases and other reported cases from literature indicated that combined karyotyping, aCGH and MS-MLPA analyses are effective to define the copy number changes and methylation patterns for sSMC(15)s in a clinical setting. The characterized genomic structure and epigenetic pattern of sSMC(15)s could lead to further gene expression profiling for better phenotype correlation.

Keywords: Isodicentric chromosome, Ring chromosome, 15q11-q13, Array comparative genomic hybridization (aCGH), Methylation-specific multiplex ligation-dependent probe amplification (MS-MLPA)

Background

The low copy repeats (LCRs) clustered in the chromosome 15q11-q13 region are known breakpoints 1 to 5 (BP1-5) for meiotic non-allelic homologous recombination which results in interstitial deletions and duplications [1]. Deletions of this region account for approximately 70 % of patients with Prader-Willi syndrome (PWS, OMIM#176270) and Angelman syndrome (AS, OMIM#105830). Reciprocal duplications of 15q11-q13 can cause autism, developmental delays, intellectual disability, ataxia, seizures, and behavioral problems (OMIM#608636). The PWS/AS critical region (PWACR) of 15q11-q13 contains many imprinting genes and shows the parental-origin effects [2]. In addition to intrachromosomal rearrangements, small supernumerary marker chromosomes 15, sSMC(15)s, in the forms of an inverted duplication (inv dup) or an isodicentric chromosome (idic) and a small ring chromosome, were also derived from rearrangements of the LCRs of 15q11-q13 [3]. The phenotypic consequences of these sSMC(15) are associated with their genomic structure, parental-origin imprinting effects and level of mosaicism [4].

---

* Correspondence: jsxieszmch@aliyun.com
[1]Shenzhen Maternity and Child Healthcare Hospital, 3012 Fuqiang Road, Shenzhen, Guangdong, China
Full list of author information is available at the end of the article

Most sSMC(15)s take the form of a dicentric inv dup and can be classified into two groups: small sSMC(15)s and large sSMC(15)s. The small sSMC(15)s have breakpoints at the BP1 or BP2 proximal to the critical region and usually clinically irrelevant, while the large sSMC(15)s frequently extend beyond the BP3 to include the critical region and are frequently associated with abnormal phenotypes [5–17]. However, unexpected level of structural complexity including asymmetrical breakpoints, unequal size of inverted arms, and multiple types of atypical rearrangements among sSMC(15)s were noted [9, 12, 14, 15]. Previous studies showed that *de novo* sSMC(15)s characterized molecularly were of maternal origin [5, 7, 9, 10, 17]. It has been recognized that maternal duplication of this region will produce abnormal phenotype but paternal duplication carriers are commonly unaffected. However, recent studies showed that patients with paternal duplication of 15q11-q13 may also have mild abnormal phenotype [8, 17]. In addition to the genomic structure and parental origin, the level of mosaicism might also alter the risk associated with an abnormal phenotype. A mitigate effect correlating the mild phenotype of motor and speech development delay with the percentage and the type of cell lineages containing the sSMC(15) was suggested [10, 13, 15]. However, results from a large case series showed that about 60 % percent mosaic sSMC cases with clinical abnormalities had no direct correlation to the level of mosaicism in the peripheral blood and there is no simple relationship between clinical abnormalities and sSMC mosaicism [4].

The application of array comparative genomic hybridization (aCGH) analysis has proven very effective in defining the breakpoints, copy number changes, and gene content for sSMC(15)s [11, 12, 14–17]. Recently, methylation-specific multiplex ligation-dependent probe amplification (MS-MLPA), a rapid and cost-effective technique with high specificity and sensitivity, has been introduced for genetic analysis of copy number changes and methylation patterns [18–21]. In this study, we present copy number changes and methylation pattern from an isodicentric chromosome 15 and a small ring chromosome 15. Review of literature found five reports with combined copy number and methylation analyses on 34 cases of sSMC(15)s and two cases of small ring chromosome 15 [17, 22–25]. These results demonstrate that combined karyotype, FISH, aCGH and MS-MPLA analyses could be used in a clinical setting effectively to define genomic structure, parental origin and level of mosaicism for sSMC(15)s.

Results

Patient 1 is a 3-year-old girl. She was born at 41 weeks of gestation from an uneventful pregnancy and delivered by Caesarean section. Her birth weight was 3,550 g (75th percentile) and birth length was 51 cm (85th percentile). She showed head control at 6 months, standing with aid at 18 months, and walking not steadily at 26 months. Her verbal language was nearly absent and no visual contact. The daily life was completely taken care by the family. She showed no dysmorphic features and no record of seizures but was hypotonia and impulsive. She failed to follow instructions and lacked response to commands. Electroencephalography (EEG) study and nuclear magnetic resonance imaging (MRI) were normal. The parents were healthy and non-consanguineous. The father was 40-year-old and the mother was 42-year-old at the time of her birth. Parental chromosome studies were normal.

For patient 1, karyotyping analysis showed a supernumerary isodicentric chromosome 15, 47,XX,+idic(15)(pter → q13.1::q13.1 → pter), in all cells examined (Fig. 1a). FISH test was performed using dual color probes for the SNRPN gene at 15q11.2 and a control locus at 15qter. Of the 20 metaphase cells analyzed, the normal chromosomes 15 showed positive hybridization signals on the targeted loci from both probes and the idic(15) had two strong signals from the SNRPN probe but no signal from the control probe. Of the 50 interphases examined, four signals for the SNRPN probe and two signals for the control probe were noted (Fig. 1b). The result confirmed that the idic(15) contained two copies of the *SNRPN* gene region. The aCGH result indicated a 7.7 Mb duplication of chromosome 15q11-q13 (chr15:18,362,355-26,110,139) including genes from *A26B1* to *HERC2*. The $\log_2$ ratio (L2R) was 0.885, indicating that the idic(15)(q13.1) was composed of two copies of the 15q11-q13 region with a breakage-fusion event occurred at BP3 (Fig. 1c). The MLPA result showed four copies for this chromosomal fragment by an increased mean peak height ratio of 2.0 (Fig. 1d). For the MS-MLPA in a normal control, the four probes for the *SNRPN* gene (a maternally methylated sequence containing a *HhaI* restriction site) decreased half of the peak height ratio, indicating the presence of one *Hha I* digested paternal unmethylated copy and another *Hha I* undigested maternal methylated copy. In patient 1, the MS-MLPA result showed a one-fourth decrease of the peak height ratio after *Hha I* digestion, indicating the presence of one copy unmethylated paternal *SNRPN* and three copies of methylated maternal *SNRPN* (Fig. 1e). These results indicated that the idic(15) was symmetric and of maternal origin.

Patient 2 was a six-year-old girl. She was born at 39 weeks of gestation from an uneventful pregnancy and delivered by Caesarean section. She could sit without aid at age one year but walk clumsy and stumbled at 25 months. Her language ability was limited. She attended special educational training but made no much

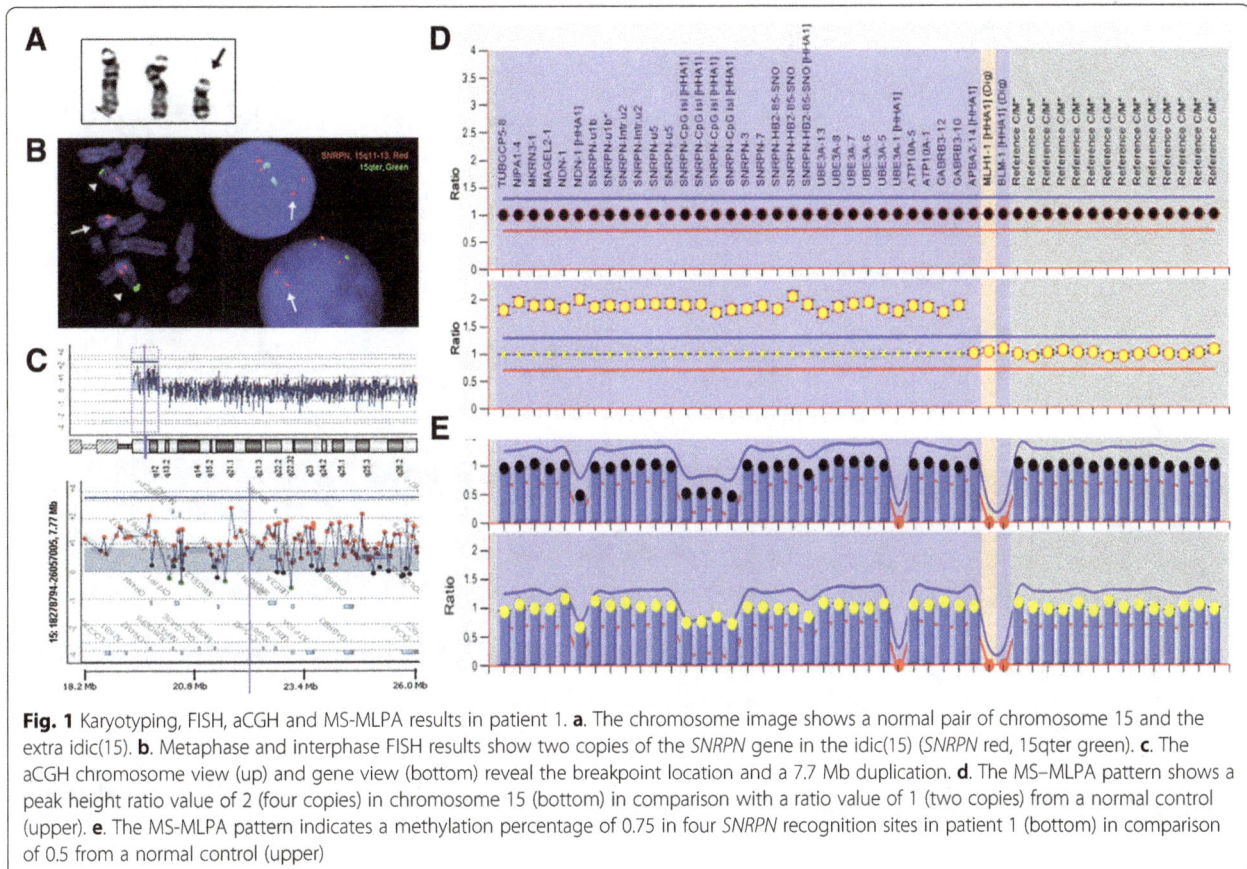

Fig. 1 Karyotyping, FISH, aCGH and MS-MLPA results in patient 1. **a**. The chromosome image shows a normal pair of chromosome 15 and the extra idic(15). **b**. Metaphase and interphase FISH results show two copies of the *SNRPN* gene in the idic(15) (*SNRPN* red, 15qter green). **c**. The aCGH chromosome view (up) and gene view (bottom) reveal the breakpoint location and a 7.7 Mb duplication. **d**. The MS–MLPA pattern shows a peak height ratio value of 2 (four copies) in chromosome 15 (bottom) in comparison with a ratio value of 1 (two copies) from a normal control (upper). **e**. The MS-MLPA pattern indicates a methylation percentage of 0.75 in four *SNRPN* recognition sites in patient 1 (bottom) in comparison of 0.5 from a normal control (upper)

progress. She had intellectual disability, autistic like behaviors, hyperphagia and hyperactivity but no dysmorphic features. Sleep problem and epileptic seizure were not known in patient history. According to her parents, the girl could follow simple instructions and fetch small things. She could eat almost by herself but never achieved sphincter control. Her parents were healthy and they were 23-year-old at the time of her birth.

For patient 2, chromosome analysis performed on 100 metaphase cells from cultured peripheral blood lymphocytes showed a mosaic pattern for a supernumerary small ring chromosome 15, 47,XX,+r(15)(q13)[32]/46,XX[68] (Fig. 2a). The aCGH analysis revealed unique copy number changes in the 12.3 Mb region of 15q11-q13 (chr15:18,362,355-30,701,573) encompassing genes from *A26B1* to *CHRNA7*. Starting from the proximal to the distal end at BP5, a 1.571 Mb tetrasomic segment of 15q11.1-q11.2 (chr15:18,362,355-19,934,192, L2R:1.000, proximal to BP1 with polymorphic copy number variants), a 2.404 Mb trisomic segment at 15q11.2 (chr15:20,418,129-22,821,963, L2R:0.360, from BP1 to between BP2/BP3), a 4.974 Mb tetrasomic segment of 15q11.2-q13.1 (chr15:23,020,445-27,994,906, L2R:0.727, from BP2/BP3 to BP3/BP4), followed by a 1.791 Mb trisomic segment (chr15: 28,910,278-30,701,573, L2R:0.350, from

BP4 to BP5) were delineated (Fig. 2b). The MLPA result revealed an increased mean peak height ratio of 1.5 in segment from gene *TUBGCP5* to *SNRPN* and a ratio of 2.0 in segment from *UBE3A* to *APBA2*. The results indicated that the r(15) had alternative two-copy and one-copy segments (Fig. 2c). The MS-MLPA result showed a one-fourth decrease of the peak height ratio after digestion, indicating that the duplication segment within the r(15) was methylated and of maternal origin (Fig. 2d).

Discussion and conclusion

Currently, more than 1300 similar sSMC(15) cases (published or not) are collected in the online sSMC database (http://ssmc-tl.com/sSMC.html). Carefully checking the website and review of literatures found five reports with combined karyotype, aCGH/SNP and methylation analyses on 34 cases of idic(15) and two cases of small r(15) [17, 22–25]. The genomic structures and methylation patterns from these cases and our two cases are summarized in Table 1. For the formation of *de novo* idic(15), different types of breakage-fusion events including symmetrical BP3::BP3 and BP4::BP4 and asymmetric BP3::BP4, BP3::BP5 and BP4::BP5 were noted (Table 1). These observations indicated that the *de novo* idic(15)s

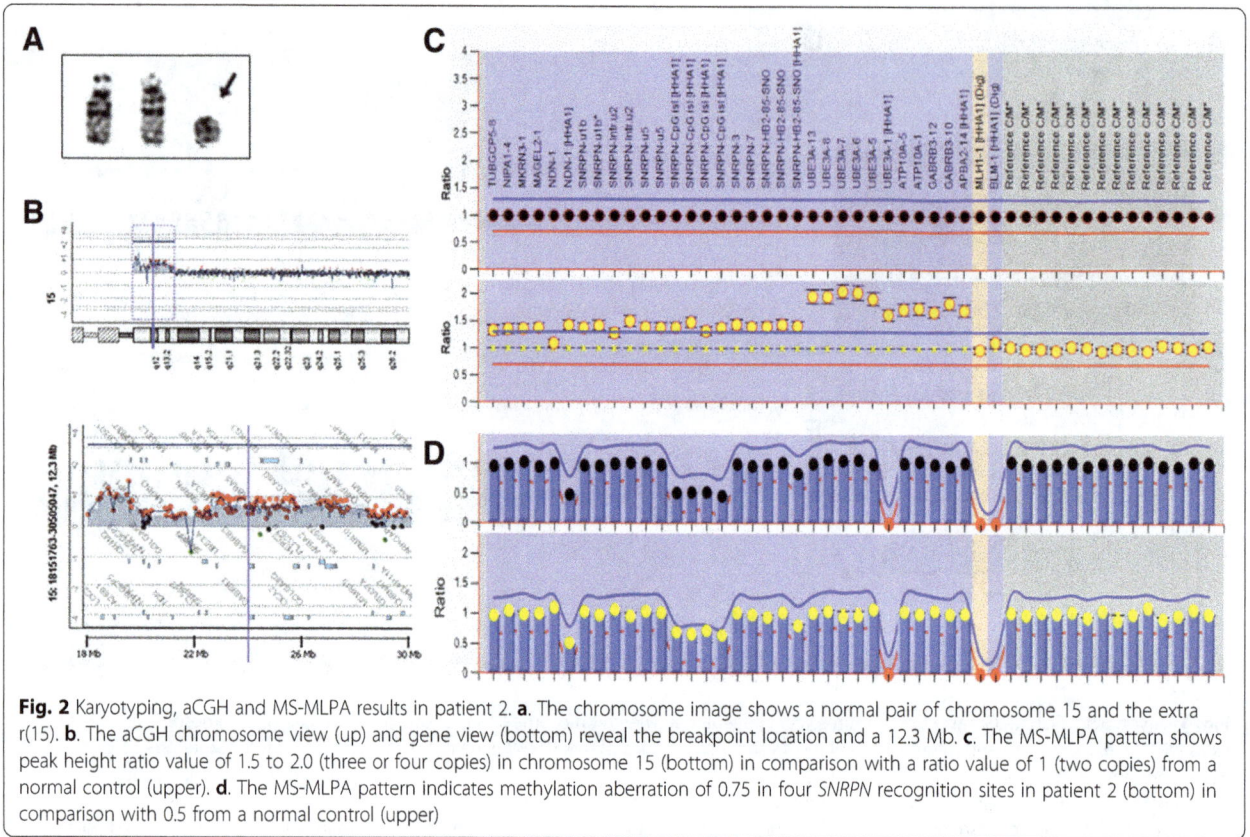

Fig. 2 Karyotyping, aCGH and MS-MLPA results in patient 2. **a.** The chromosome image shows a normal pair of chromosome 15 and the extra r(15). **b.** The aCGH chromosome view (up) and gene view (bottom) reveal the breakpoint location and a 12.3 Mb. **c.** The MS-MLPA pattern shows peak height ratio value of 1.5 to 2.0 (three or four copies) in chromosome 15 (bottom) in comparison with a ratio value of 1 (two copies) from a normal control (upper). **d.** The MS-MLPA pattern indicates methylation aberration of 0.75 in four SNRPN recognition sites in patient 2 (bottom) in comparison with 0.5 from a normal control (upper)

Table 1 A summary of sSMC(15) defined by karyotype, aCGH or SNP, and methylation analyses

SMC15	Test Methods				Patient Number	Age	Gender	Inheritance	BP Fusion	Methylation	References
	G-banding	aCGH/SNP	FISH	Methylation							
trc(15), idic(15)	+	Nimblegen	+	MS-SB	2	11y, 26y	M, F	de novo	BP3::BP3, BP4::BP5	Maternal	[22] Hogart A, et al., 2009
rea(15), inv dup(15)	+	Affymetrix	+	MS-PCR	2	5y, 9y	M, M	de novo	BP4::BP5, BP4::BP5	Maternal	[23] Yang J, et al. 2013
inv dup(15) or idic(15)	+	Agilent & Illumina	+	MS-MLPA	8	1.7y-14.5y	M(3), F(5)	de novo	BP3::BP3,BP2-BP3::	Maternal	[17] Ageeli EA, et al. 2014
der(15)t(15q;6p)					1	7y	M	paternal carrier	BP2-BP3::	Paternal	
del(15)[14]/psu dic(15)[4]	+	Agilent	+	MS-PCR	1	2y	F	de novo	BP3::BP3	Maternal	[24] Tan E-S, et al. 2014
idic(15)	+	Agilent	+	MS-MLPA	20	3 m-23y	M(13), F(7)	1 de novo, 19 unk	BP3::BP3 or BP4, BP4::BP4 or BP5	Maternal	[25] Aypar U, et al. 2014
idic(15)	+	Agilent	+	MS-MLPA	1	3y	F	de novo	BP3::BP3	Maternal	This report
r(15)	+	Agilent	+	MS-MLPA	2	1d, 7y	M, M	unk	BP2/BP3::,BP3::BP3	Maternal	[25] Aypar U, et al. 2014
r(15)	+	Agilent	-	MS-MLPA	1	6y	F	de novo	BP5::BP5> > BP2/BP3::BP3/BP4	Maternal	This report

Abbreviations: *MS* methylation sensitive, *SB* Southern blot; + = yes; – = not; m = month; y = year; unk, unknown

originated from maternal meiotic crossing-over event between paired or mis-paired LCRS of homologous chromosomes in pachytene and followed by non-disjunction in the subsequent divisions [3]. Several modes of formation for inv dup or idic chromosome have been proposed. The most plausible mode of formation is the U-type exchange resulting from crossover mistakes of chromatids of two homologous chromosomes during meiosis [3] (Fig. 3a). Supernumerary small ring chromosome for the 15q11-q13 is an uncommon chromosomal abnormality and also likely derived from breakage and fusion event at the LCRs of 15q11-q13. However, the small r(15) from the two cases in the literature and our patient 2 showed break-fusions occurred between BPs (BP2/BP3 or BP3/BP4). The complex copy number changes and the variable breakage-fusion points within the r(15) may be explained by a two-step process including initial ring formation by a break-fusion event at the LCRs, an intermediate double ring from ring DNA replication, and a secondary asymmetric break-fusion event to introduce segmental duplications and deletions between BPs (Fig. 3b) [26, 27]. Therefore, for small supernumerary r(15), ring structure instability and secondary rearrangements should be considered.

Our two cases and almost all reported *de novo* cases of idic(15)s showed a genomic structure including PWACR and a methylation pattern of maternal origin [5–17, 22–25]. As reported from previous analyses, clinical phenotypes for sSMC(15)s are related with the duplication region containing the PWACR and the maternally derived homologue of chromosome 15q [13, 17]. A comparison of clinical features between our patients and among those previously reported cases with similar size of duplication noted that patient 2 showed a relatively mild phenotype despite a larger size containing genes from BP1 to BP5. The presence of normal cells from the mosaic ring sSMC(15) might alleviate the severity of the clinical manifestation. Since routine karyotyping analysis was only done for cells from peripheral blood culture, the percentage of the mosaic r(15) in other tissues was not known. Micro-invasive methods to access other types of tissues, especially muscular and neurologic

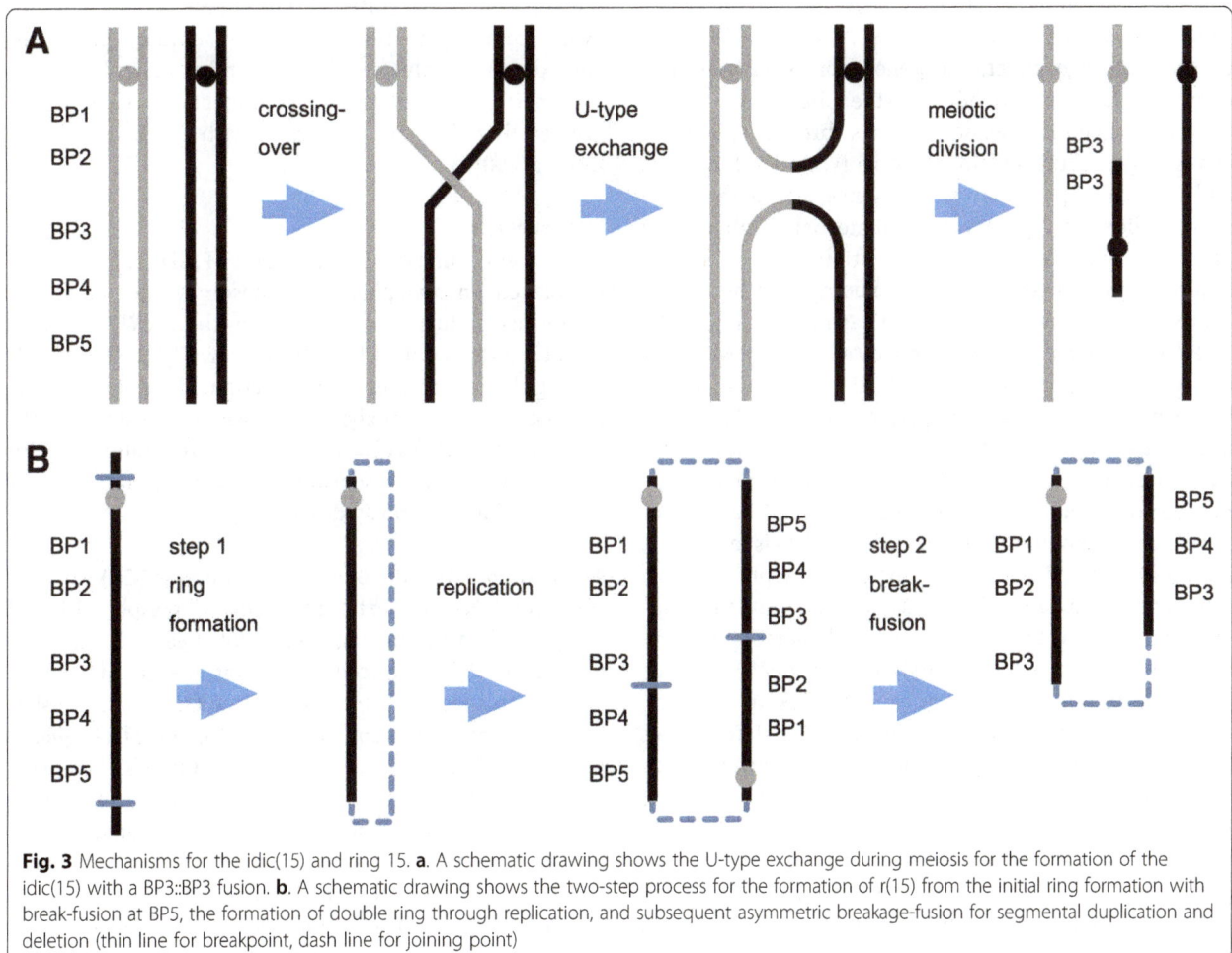

Fig. 3 Mechanisms for the idic(15) and ring 15. **a.** A schematic drawing shows the U-type exchange during meiosis for the formation of the idic(15) with a BP3::BP3 fusion. **b.** A schematic drawing shows the two-step process for the formation of r(15) from the initial ring formation with break-fusion at BP5, the formation of double ring through replication, and subsequent asymmetric breakage-fusion for segmental duplication and deletion (thin line for breakpoint, dash line for joining point)

tissues, are needed to evaluate the mosaic pattern for sSMC(15)s. The gene content within sSMC(15)s and the parental-origin imprinting effects could be the determine factors affecting the phenotype [22, 28]. Patient 1 had a 7.7 Mb BP1-BP3 duplication which contains genes involving in developmental or neurological diseases. The BP1-BP2 region contains *NIPA1, NIPA2* and *CYFIP1* genes which are associated with the central nervous system development or function [29–31]. The BP2-BP3 region contains paternally expressed genes *MKRN3, MAGEL2, NDN* and *SNRPN*; these four genes are implicated in the autism disorder [17, 32]. The maternally expressed *UBE3A* gene is exclusively-expressed in brain tissue and the neurodevelopmental complexities are associated with increased *UBE3A* in dup15q syndrome [33, 34]. The *NDN* gene is an imprinted gene expressed exclusively from the paternal allele, which is associated with neurological and muscular disorder and implicated as a negative growth regulator in human cancer [35, 36]. Patient 2 had a 12.3 Mb duplication involving BP1-BP5 region that extending to gene *CHRNA7*. The clinical phenotype like speech delay, hyperphagia, hyperactivity, mental retardation, no facial dysmorphism and no epilepsy may be influenced by gain of dosage of *CHRNA7* [17, 37, 38]. In addition to the gene dosage effect, the gene expression may also contribute to the variability of the phenotypes which were influenced in unexpected ways through epigenetic changes [22]. Further elucidation of cellular functions and molecular pathways of the genes within the BP1-BP5 duplication region will facilitate better phenotype prediction and therapeutic intervention.

Several molecular methods including Southern blot analysis on methylation sensitive restriction sites, MS-PCR, sequencing of bisulfate-treated DNA, MS-PCR and MS-MLPA, have been introduced to define methylation pattern for sSMC(15)s [21, 22, 39]. Southern blot and sequencing methods are more time consuming and expensive. MS-PCR may show more variation in copy number quantitation. The present study and several reports have demonstrated that MS-MLPA is a robust, high-throughput, rapid and inexpensive approach with high specificity and sensitivity [22–25]. It provides an efficient way to simultaneously detect copy number changes and DNA methylation within 15q11-q13 in a semi-quantitative manner [39]. Taken together, combined cell-based karyotyping and FISH to detect the chromosome structure and mosaic pattern with DNA-based aCGH and MS-MLPA for copy number changes and methylation patterns should be recommended for clinical analysis of sSMC(15). Practice guidelines for PWS/AS and analytic algorithms for sSMC(15)s using this combined methods have been proposed [25, 39].

In conclusion, we have defined the copy number changes and methylation pattern in an idic(15) and a r(15) from two Chinese patients by karyotyping, aCGH, and MS-MLPA analysis. The results revealed that the idic(15) with a BP3::BP3 fusion and a r(15) likely resulting from secondary breakage-fusion between BP2/BP3 and BP3/BP4 were maternally derived. Variable spectrum of neurodevelopmental phenotype might be explained by the gene dosage and epigenetic imprinting effects from these sSMC(15)s.

Methods

Patients

Two patients were referred for genetic evaluation of developmental delay, speech retardation and intellectual disabilities at the genetic counseling clinic in Shenzhen Maternal and Child Healthcare Hospital. This study was approved by the hospital's Institutional Review Board and written informed consents were obtained from their parents.

Karyotype analysis

Chromosome analysis was performed on G-banded metaphases from cultured peripheral blood lymphocytes according to the laboratory's standard protocols. An extended analysis of 100 G-banded metaphase cells was performed to allow the detection of equal or greater than 3 % of mosaicism with 95 % confidence interval [40].

FISH analysis

Fluorescence in situ hybridization (FISH) analysis was performed on metaphase chromosomes and interphase nuclei using dual color probes for the *SNRPN* gene at 15q11.2 and a control locus at 15qter (Cytocell Inc.) following the manufacturer's instruction. Hybridization signal patterns were analyzed on twenty metaphase cells and 50 interphase cells. FISH probe preparation, in situ hybridization, signal scoring, and image capture were performed as previously described [41].

Array comparative genomic hybridization (aCGH)

Genomic DNA was extracted from the peripheral blood using the Gentra Puregene Blood kit (Qiangen, Valencia, CA, USA). DNA concentration was measured using a NanoDrop spectrophotometer (ND-1000, Thermo Fisher Scientific Inc., Waltham, Mass., USA), and DNA quality was verified by agarose gel electrophoresis. For each case, 2 ug of patient genomic DNA was used following the protocol from the SurePrint G3 Human CGH 8x60K Microarray Kit (Agilent Technologies, Santa Clara, CA, USA). DNA labeling, sex-matched test/control hybridization, post hybridization washes, image scanning, and data analysis were processed as previously described [39]. The base pair positions for detected genomic imbalances were designated according to the March 2006 Assembly (NCBI36/hg18) in the UCSC Human Genome browser (http://genome.ucsc.edu/).

MS-MLPA

MLPA reagents were obtained from MRC-Holland (Amsterdam, The Netherlands; SALSA MLPA kit ME028). The ME028 Kit can be used to detect copy number changes and to analyze the CpG island methylation of the 15q11 region in a semi-quantitative manner. The Kit contains 32 probes specific for sequences in the PWACR and 14 reference probes outside the region. Four of the PWACR specific probes in the *SNRPN* gene contain a recognition site for the methylation sensitive *HhaI* enzyme and can be used for the presence of aberrant methylation patterns in the 15q11 locus. The *NDN* gene also contains methylation probes while it has a known tendency to over-digest resulted in variable results. The experiment procedures were performed following the manufacturer's protocol [18, 42]. The MS-MLPA data was imported into the software Coffalyser.Net (designed by MRC-Holland) to analyze both the copy number variation and the methylation profile.

Competing interests
The authors declare that they have no competing interests.

Authors' contributions
WQ, performed chromosome analysis, data analysis, literature review and drafted the manuscript; WW, performed MS-MLPA and literature review; FL, performed chromosome analysis; ZQ/XZ, performed aCGH analysis; PL, reviewed aCGH result and revised the manuscript; XJ, organized this study, reviewed clinical and laboratory data, and finalized this manuscript. All authors read and approved the final manuscript.

Acknowledgements
This work was supported by the National Natural Science Foundation of China (31471204). The authors appreciate the families to take part in this study. We also thank Audrey Meusel for checking and editing this manuscript.

Author details
[1]Shenzhen Maternity and Child Healthcare Hospital, 3012 Fuqiang Road, Shenzhen, Guangdong, China. [2]Department of Genetics, Yale School of Medicine, New Haven, CT, USA. [3]First Affiliated Hospital, Biomedical Translational Research Institute, Jinan University, Guangzhou, Guangdong, China.

References
1. Zody MC, Garber M, Sharpe T, Young SK, Rowen L, O'Neill K, et al. Analysis of the DNA sequence and duplication history of human chromosome 15. Nature. 2006;440:671–5.
2. Horsthemke B, Buiting K. Imprinting defects on human chromosome 15. Cytogenet Genome Res. 2006;113:292–9.
3. Liehr T, Claussen U, Starke H. Small supernumerary marker chromosomes (sSMC) in humans. Cytogenet Genome Res. 2004;107:55–67.
4. Liehr T, Mrasek K, Weise A, Dufke A, Rodríguez L, Martínez Guardia N, et al. Small supernumerary marker chromosomes–progress towards a genotype-phenotype correlation. Cytogenet Genome Res. 2006;112:23–34.
5. Crolla JA, Harvey JF, Sitch FL, Dennis NR. Supernumerary marker 15 chromosomes: a clinical, molecular and FISH approach to diagnosis and prognosis. Hum Genet. 1995;95:161–70.
6. Huang B, Crolla JA, Christian SL, Wolf-Ledbetter ME, Macha ME, Papenhausen PN, et al. Refined molecular characterization of the breakpoints in small inv dup(15) chromosomes. Hum Genet. 1997;99:11–7.
7. Webb T, Hardy CA, King M, Watkiss E, Mitchell C, Cole T. A clinical, cytogenetic and molecular study of ten probands with supernumerary inv dup (15) marker chromosomes. Clin Genet. 1998;53:34–43.
8. Eggermann K, Mau UA, Bujdoso G, Koltai E, Engels H, Schubert R, et al. Supernumerary marker chromosomes derived from chromosome 15: analysis of 32 new cases. Clin Genet. 2002;62:89–93.
9. Roberts SE, Maggouta F, Thomas NS, Jacobs PA, Crolla JA. Molecular and fluorescence in situ hybridization characterization of the breakpoints in 46 large supernumerary marker 15 chromosomes reveals an unexpected level of complexity. Am J Hum Genet. 2003;73:1061–72.
10. Maggouta F, Roberts SE, Dennis NR, Veltman MW, Crolla JA. A supernumerary marker chromosome 15 tetrasomic for the Prader-Willi/Angelman syndrome critical region in a patient with a severe phenotype. J Med Genet. 2003;40:e84.
11. Locke DP, Segraves R, Nicholls RD, Schwartz S, Pinkel D, Albertson DG, et al. BAC microarray analysis of 15q11–q13 rearrangements and the impact of segmental duplications. J Med Genet. 2004;41:175–82.
12. Wang NJ, Liu D, Parokonny AS, Schanen NC. High-resolution molecular characterization of 15q11-q13 rearrangements by array comparative genomic hybridization (Array CGH) with detection of gene dosage. Am J Hum Genet. 2004;75:267–81.
13. Dennis NR, Veltman MWM, Thompson R, Crain E, Bolton PF, Thomas NS. Clinical findings in 33 subjects with large supernumerary marker(15) chromosomes and 3 subjects with triplication of 15q11-q13. Am J Med Genet. 2006;140:434–41.
14. Tsuchiya KD, Opheim KE, Hannibal MC, Hing AV, Glass IA, Raff ML, et al. Unexpected structural complexity of supernumerary marker chromosomes characterized by microarray comparative genomic hybridization. Mol Cytogenet. 2008;1:7.
15. Wang NJ, Parokonny AS, Thatcher KN, Driscoll J, Malone BM, Dorrani N, et al. Multiple forms of atypical rearrangements generating supernumerary derivative chromosome 15. BMC Genet. 2008;9:2.
16. Kleefstra T, de Leeuw N, Wolf R, Nillesen WM, Schobers G, Mieloo H, et al. Phenotypic spectrum of 20 novel patients with molecularly defined supernumerary marker chromosomes 15 and a review of the literature. Am J Med Genet. 2010;152A:2221–9.
17. Al Ageeli E, Drunat S, Delanoë C, Perrin L, Baumann C, Capri Y, et al. Duplication of the 15q11-q13 region: clinical and genetic study of 30 new cases. Eur J Med Genet. 2014;57:5–14.
18. Nygren AO, Ameziane N, Duarte HM, Vijzelaar RN, Waisfisz Q, Hess CJ, et al. Methylation-specific MLPA (MS-MLPA): simultaneous detection of CpG methylation and copy number changes of up to 40 sequences. Nucleic Acids Res. 2005;33:e128.
19. Procter M, Chou LS, Tang W, Jama M, Mao R. Molecular diagnosis of Prader-Willi and Angelman syndromes by methylation-specific melting analysis and methylation-specific multiplex ligation-dependent probe amplification. Clin Chem. 2006;52:1276–83.
20. Bittel DC, Kibiryeva N, Butler MG. Methylation-specific multiplex ligation-dependent probe amplification analysis of subjects with chromosome 15 abnormalities. Genet Test. 2007;11:467–75.
21. Depienne C, Moreno-De-Luca D, Heron D, Bouteiller D, Gennetier A, Delorme R, et al. Screening for genomic rearrangements and methylation abnormalities of the 15q11-q13 region in autism spectrum disorders. Biol Psychiatry. 2009;66:349–59.
22. Hogart A, Leung KN, Wang NJ, Wu DJ, Driscoll J, Vallero RO, et al. Chromosome 15q11-13 duplication syndrome brain reveals epigenetic alterations in gene expression not predicted from copy number. J Med Genet. 2009;46:86–93.
23. Yang J, Yang Y, Huang Y, Hu Y, Chen X, Sun H, et al. A study of two Chinese patients with tetrasomy and pentasomy 15q11q13 including Prader-Willi/Angelman syndrome critical region present with developmental delays and mental impairment. BMC Med Genet. 2013;14:9.
24. Tan ES, Yong MH, Lim EC, Li ZH, Brett MS, Tan EC. Chromosome 15q11-q13 copy number gain detected by array-CGH in two cases with a maternal methylation pattern. Mol Cytogenet. 2014;7:32.
25. Aypar U, Brodersen PR, Lundquist PA, Dawson DB, Thorland EC, Hoppman N. Does parent of origin matter? Methylation studies should be performed

on patients with multiple copies of the Prader-Willi/Angelman syndrome critical region. Am J Med Genet. 2014;164A:2514–20.

26. Sodre CP, Guilherme RS, Meloni VF, Brunoni D, Juliano Y, Andrade JA, et al. Ring chromosome instability evaluation in six patients with autosomal rings. Genet Mol Res. 2010;9:134–43.

27. Zhang HZ, Xu F, Seashore M, Li P. Unique genomic structure and distinct mitotic behavior of ring chromosome 21 in two unrelated cases. Cytogenet Genome Res. 2012;136:180–7.

28. Burnside RD, Pasion R, Mikhail FM, Carroll AJ, Robin NH, Youngs EL, et al. Microdeletion/microduplication of proximal 15q11.2 between BP1 and BP2: a susceptibility region for neurological dysfunction including developmental and language delay. Hum Genet. 2011;130:517–28.

29. Goytain A, Hines RM, El-Husseini A, Quamme GA. NIPA1(SPG6), the basis for autosomal dominant form of hereditary spastic paraplegia, encodes a functional Mg2+ transporter. J Biol Chem. 2007;282:8060–8.

30. Goytain A, Hines RM, Quamme GA. Functional characterization of NIPA2, a selective Mg2+ transporter. Am J Physiol Cell Physiol. 2008;295:944–53.

31. Napoli I, Mercaldo V, Boyl PP, Eleuteri B, Zalfa F, De Rubeis S, et al. The fragile X syndrome protein represses activity-dependent translation through CYFIP1, a new 4E-BP. Cell. 2008;134:1042–54.

32. Chamberlain SJ, Lalande M. Neurodevelopmental disorders involving genomic imprinting at human chromosome 15q11-q13. Neurobiol Dis. 2010;39:13–20.

33. Scoles HA, Urraca N, Chadwick SW, Reiter LT, Lasalle JM. Increased copy number for methylated maternal 15q duplications leads to changes in gene and protein expression in human cortical samples. Mol Autism. 2011;2:19.

34. Smith SE, Zhou YD, Zhang G, Jin Z, Stoppel DC, Anderson MP. Increased gene dosage of Ube3a results in autism traits and decreased glutamate synaptic transmission in mice. Sci Transl Med. 2011;3:103ra97.

35. Jay P, Rougeulle C, Massacrier A, Moncla A, Mattei MG, Malzac P, et al. The human necdin gene, NDN, is maternally imprinted and located in the Prader-Willi syndrome chromosomal region. Nat Genet. 1997;17:357–61.

36. Haviland R, Eschrich S, Bloom G, Ma Y, Minton S, Jove R, et al. Necdin, a negative growth regulator, is a novel STAT3 target gene down-regulated in human cancer. PLoS One. 2011;6:e24923.

37. Gault J, Robinson M, Berger R, Drebing C, Logel J, Hopkins J, et al. Genomic organization and partial duplication of the human alpha7 neuronal nicotinic acetylcholine receptor gene (CHRNA7). Genomics. 1998;52(2):173–85.

38. Xu J, Pato MT, Torre CD, Medeiros H, Carvalho C, Basile VS, et al. Evidence for linkage disequilibrium between the alpha 7-nicotinic receptor gene (CHRNA7) locus and schizophrenia in Azorean families. Am J Med Genet. 2001;105:669–74.

39. Ramsden SC, Clayton-Smith J, Birch R, Buiting K. Practice guidelines for the molecular analysis of Prader Willi and Angelman syndromes. BMC Med Genet. 2010;11:70.

40. Hook EB. Exclusion of chromosomal mosaicism: tables of 90%, 95% and 99% confidence limits and comments on use. Am J Hum Genet. 1977;29:94–7.

41. Zhang HZ, Li P, Wang D, Huff S, Nimmakayalu M, Qumsiyeh M, et al. FOXC1 gene deletion is associated with eye anomalies in ring chromosome 6. Am J Med Genet A. 2004;124a(3):280–7.

42. Xu ZY, Geng Q, Luo FW, Xu F, Li P, Xie JS. Multiplex ligation-dependent probe amplification and array comparative genomic hybridization analyses for prenatal diagnosis of cytogenomic abnormalities. Mol Cytogenet. 2014;7:84.

15

Coexistence of iAMP21 and *ETV6-RUNX1* fusion in an adolescent with B cell acute lymphoblastic leukemia

Jun Gu[1], Alexandra Reynolds[2], Lianghua Fang[3,4], Corrie DeGraffenreid[1], Kenneth Sterns[1], Keyur P. Patel[3], L. Jeffrey Medeiros[5], Pei Lin[5] and Xinyan Lu[2,6*]

Abstract

Background: Intrachromosomal amplification of chromosome 21 (iAMP21) results from breakage-fusion-bridge cycles and chromothripsis is a distinct marker of a subgroup of B cell acute lymphoblastic leukemia (B-ALL) cases associated with a poor prognosis. iAMP21 accounts for 2% of pediatric B-ALL and occurs predominantly in older children or adolescents. *ETV6-RUNX1* fusion, resulting from t(12;21)(p13;q22), is associated with an excellent outcome in younger children with B-ALL. Coexistence of iAMP21 with *ETV6-RUNX1* fusion is extremely rare with limited clinical information available.

Results: We report the case of an 18-year old Caucasian man diagnosed with *ETV6-RUNX1* fusion positive B-ALL. He was treated with intensive chemotherapy and achieved remission for 6 months before relapse, 15 months after the initial diagnosis. G-band karyotyping and Fluorescence in situ hybridization (FISH) analyses performed on bone marrow revealed complex abnormalities: 41,X,-Y,der(3)t(3;20)(p11.2;q11.2),-4,t(5;22)(q32;q11.2),del(9)(p13),dic(9;17)(p13;p11.2),t(12;21)(p13;q22),der(14)t(14;17)(p11.2;q11.2),der(17;22)(q11.2;q11.2),-20,add(21)(q22),-22[4]/46,XY[15] with an iAMP21 and an *ETV6-RUNX1*. Additional molecular studies confirmed *ETV6-RUNX1* fusion and with a *TP53* mutation. High-resolution single nucleotide polymorphism microarray (SNP array) revealed the iAMP21 to be chromothripsis of 21q and subsequent metaphase FISH further delineated complex genomic aberrations. Although the patient received intensive chemotherapy with allogenic stem cell transplant, he died 26 months after initial diagnosis. We searched the literature and identified six cases showing coexisting iAMP21 and *ETV6-RUNX1*. The median age for these six patients was 10 years (range, 2–18) and males predominated. The median overall survival (OS) was 28 months.

Conclusions: Patients with B-ALL associated with both iAMP21 and *ETV6-RUNX1* tend to be older children or adolescents and have a poor prognosis.

Keywords: B-ALL, iAMP21, *RUNX1* amplification, *ETV6-RUNX1* fusion, SNP microarray

* Correspondence: xinyan.lu@northwestern.edu
[2]Department of Hematopathology, The University of Texas MD Anderson Cancer Center, 1515 Holcombe Blvd. Unit 0350, Houston, TX 77030, USA
[6]Department of Pathology, Northwestern University Feinberg School of Medicine, 303 East Chicago Avenue, Tarry 7-723, Chicago, IL 60611, USA
Full list of author information is available at the end of the article

Background

The latest revision to the World Health Organization (WHO) classification of B-cell lymphoblastic leukemia/lymphoma (B-ALL) has added B-ALL with intrachromosomal amplification of chromosome 21 (iAMP21) as an entity in the group of B-ALL with recurrent genetic abnormalities [1]. iAMP21 is a distinct marker that can be readily detected by metaphase FISH [2] and is caused by breakage-fusion-bridge cycles and chromothripsis, which is a phenomenon reported in cancer genomes, resulted from tens to hundreds of genomic rearrangements occur in a cellular crisis. Chromthripsis can involve one or more chromosomes, often with massive copy number aberrations [3]. Recent study suggested that hyperploidy and telomere attrition could be triggering events for chromothripsis and are frequently associated with *TP53* mutation [4].

B-ALL associated with iAMP21 is a poor prognostic subgroup that represents 2% of pediatric B-ALL cases. The median age of patients is 9 years old and there is a prevalence of males. Patients with iAMP21 often show low platelet and low white blood cell counts (WBC) [5–8]. These patients have a relapse rate that is three times higher than other B-ALL patients are and therefore patients often require intensified therapy, particularly in older children or adolescents with B-ALL [9].

The t(12;21)(p13;q22) which results in the formation of the *ETV6-RUNX1* fusion gene accounts for about 25% of pediatric B-ALL. Patients with B-ALL associated with *ETV6-RUNX1* tend to be younger children and patients have a favorable outcome [10]. iAMP21 has been reported rarely in B-ALL associated with *ETV6-RUNX1* [11].

In this study, we describe a patient with B-ALL associated with both iAMP21 with *ETV6-RUNX1* that we have characterized extensively by using molecular and cytogenetic methods. We also reviewed the literature and identified six similar cases [7, 12]. This combination of molecular alterations in B-ALL tends to occur in older male patients who have a poor prognosis.

Results

The patient was an 18-year old Caucasian man who presented initially with pancytopenia. A complete blood count showed: WBC 2.0×10^9/L, platelets 88×10^9/L and hemoglobin 8.3 g/dL. Bone marrow examination showed 61% blasts and the patient was diagnosed with a B-ALL at another institution (Table 1). FISH studies performed on the bone marrow aspirate smears showed *ETV6-RUNX1* fusion in 28% of interphases with no evidence of *BCR-ABL1* or *MLL* gene rearrangements. No concurrent chromosome data were available from the initial bone marrow studies. The patient did not have central nervous system (CNS) involvement and he was treated with the intrathecal cytarabine, daunorubicin, vincristine, intrathecal methotrexate, PEG asparaginase and prednisone (CALGB 10403 regimen) elsewhere. The patient did not respond well initially although he eventually achieved remission for 6 months after a second round of chemotherapy. The patient then began to show minimal residual disease by flow cytometry immunophenotypic analysis 8 months after the initial diagnosis, and eventually relapsed 15 months after the diagnosis. The patient was transferred to our institution at this time (Table 1).

Table 1 Clinical and laboratory data of the patient

Date	10/9/2013	6/24/2014	12/9/2014	12/31/2014	6/8/2015	8/19/2015
Significant event	Initial diagnosis	MRD Positive	1st Relapse	Persistent disease	Post-ASCT[a]	2nd Relapse
BM Blast (%) (0–5)	61	NA	5	54	1	25
WBC (x10⁹/L)	2.0	5.5	4.6	2.8	5.6	2.2
PLT (x10³/μL)	88	383	202	79	133	79
HB (g/dL)	8.3	10.8	13.3	12.9	9.1	11.4
Flow-cytometry analysis	Positive[b]	Positive	Positive[c]	Positive[d]	NA	Positive
G-Band karyotyping	NA[e]	NA	46,XY	Complex	46,XY	46,XY
ETV6-RUNX1/iAMP21 FISH	Positive	Negative	Borderline Negative	Positive	NA	NA
ETV6-RUNX1 by PCR	NA	NA	NA	Positive	NA	NA
Treatment	CALGB[f]	Post- CALGB	Blinatumomab	Hyper-CVAD[g] + Inotuzumab	50 days Post-ASCT	EPOCH[h] + Rituxan

[a]*Post ASCT* post allogeneic stem cell transplantation
[b]CD19lo, CD22+, cytoplasmic CD79a+, HLA-DR+, aberrant CD13 and CD33 expression, CD3-, CD10-, CD20-, surface Ig-, CD34-, CD38-,MPO-
[c]CD10+, CD13+, CD19lo, CD33+/lo, CD9-, CD20-, CD34-, surface Ig-
[d]CD10+, CD13+, CD19+, CD22+,CD33+ (subset), CD45 dim, CD38 dim, CD58, cytoplasmic CD79a, CD81, TdT+, cytoplasmic CD3-, CD15-, CD20-, CD25-, CD34-, CD66c-, CD117-, CRLF2-, cytoplasmic IgM-, MPO-
[e]*NA* not available
[f]CALGB: IT Cytarabine, Daunorubicin, Vincristine, IT Methotrexate, PEG Asparaginase and Prednisone
[g]Hyper-CVAD: Cyclophosphamide, Vincristine, Doxorubicin Hydrochloride, Dexamethasone
[h]EPOCH: Etoposide, Vincristine, Cyclophosphamide, Doxorubicin Hydrochloride

At time of relapse, the complete blood count showed: WBC 2.8×10^9/L, platelets 79×10^9/L and hemoglobin 12.9 g/dL. Bone marrow examination showed 54% blasts. Conventional cytogenetic analysis on the relapsed bone marrow showed a complex karyotype of 41,X,-Y,-3,-4, del(5)(p14),der(5)t(5;22) (q22;q11.2),del(10)(q24q25),-12,-14,-17,add(17)(p11.2),-20,+add(21)(p11.2),der(21)add(21)(p11.2) hsr(?21),der(21)t(12;21)(p13;q22),-22,add(22)(p11.2),+der(?)t (?;5)(?;?)t(?;22)(?;?),+mar[4]/46,XY[15] as initially reported. A nuclear fusion of *ETV6-RUNX1* signal with *RUNX1* amplification were observed in 27.5% of the interphases (Fig. 1). High-resolution SNP microarray revealed losses of chromosomes Yq, 3p, 4, 9p, 17p and 20p, as well as chromothripsis-like pattern of chromosome 21q (Fig. 2). Subsequent metaphase FISH analysis on the G-banded chromosomes targeting *ETV6-RUNX1*, DS523/D5S721/*EGR1*, *CSF1R*, *CDKN2A/CEP9*, *TP53/CEP17* and DS20S108 along with whole chromosome painting (WCP) for chromosomes 17 and 22 (Figs. 3 and 4) showed: 1) a der(3)t(3;20) (p11.2;q11.2)

(D20S108+); 2) a der(5)t(5;22)(q32;q11.2)(WCP22+); 3) a del(9)(p13) (CDKN2A-,D9Z1+), a dic(9;17)(p13;p11.2)(CDKN2A-,D9Z1+;D17Z1+,TP53-,WCP17+); 4) a t(12;21)((p13; (q22)RUNX1+; ETV6+,RUNX1+) and add(21)(RUNX1++ +++); 5) a der(14)t(14;17)(p11.2;q11.2)(WCP17+); 6) a der(17)t(17;22) (TP53+,D17Z1+,WCP17+,WCP22+); 7) der((22)t(5;22)(CSF1R+,WCP22+) (Table 2). By integrating all the SNP array and chromosome and/or metaphase FISH, the above karyotype was further refined to 41,X,-Y,der(3)t(3;20)(p11.2;q11.2),-4,t(5;22)(q32;q11.2), del(9)(p13),dic(9;17)>(p13;p11.2),t(12;21)(p13;q22),der(14)t(14;17)(p11.2;q11.2), der(17;22)(q11.2;q11.2),-20,add(21)(q22),-22[4]/46,XY[15] (Figs. 3 and 4). In addition, sequencing analysis revealed a 10 base pair deletion-insertion mutation in exon 4 of *TP53* (NM_000546(*TP53*): c.310_321delinsGT p.Q104fs), resulting in a loss of *TP53* function. While this specific mutation is not previously reported in the catalogue of somatic mutations in cancer (COSMIC), this region in exon 4 is known to be involved by similar deleterious (frameshift and

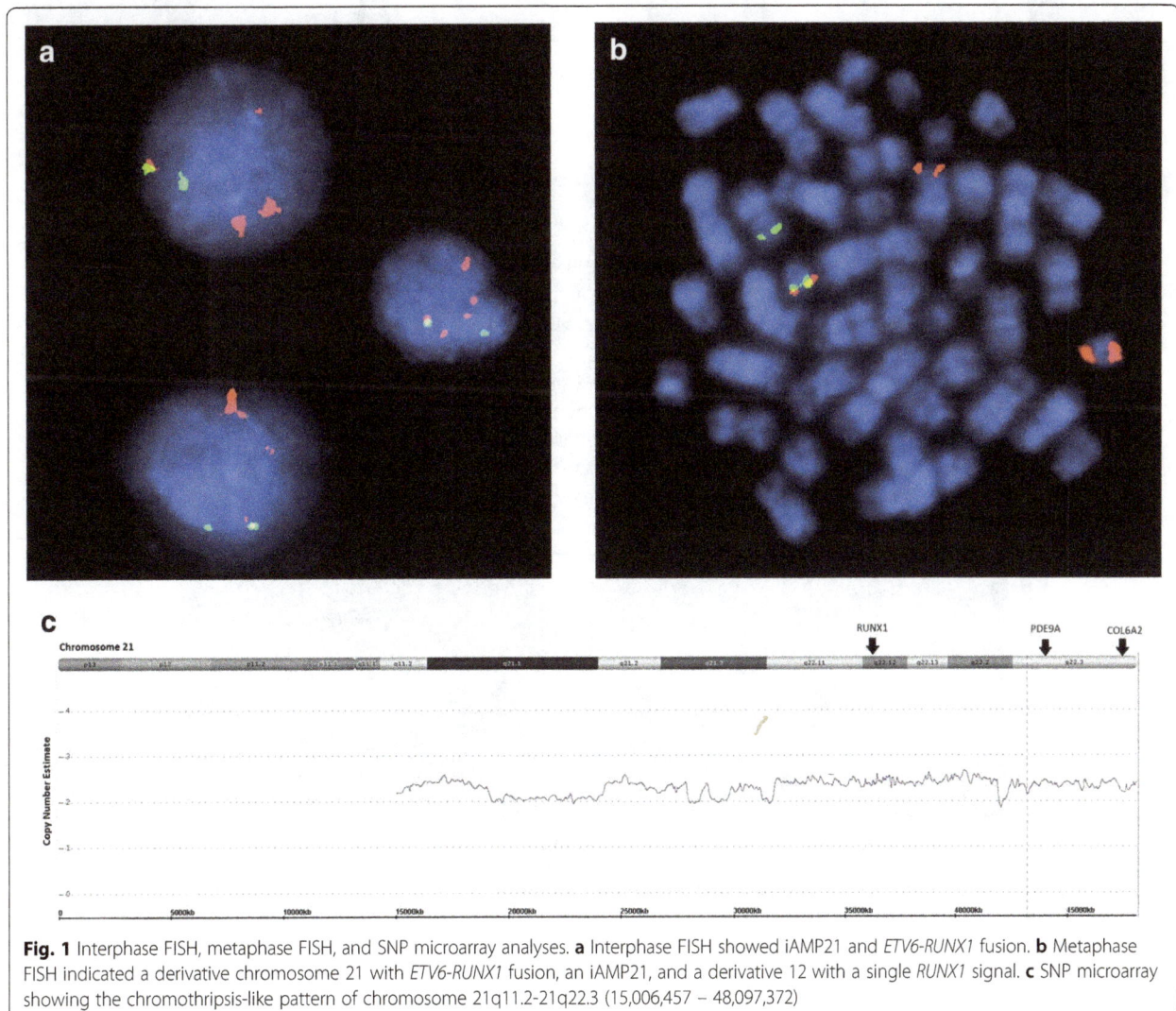

Fig. 1 Interphase FISH, metaphase FISH, and SNP microarray analyses. **a** Interphase FISH showed iAMP21 and *ETV6-RUNX1* fusion. **b** Metaphase FISH indicated a derivative chromosome 21 with *ETV6-RUNX1* fusion, an iAMP21, and a derivative 12 with a single *RUNX1* signal. **c** SNP microarray showing the chromothripsis-like pattern of chromosome 21q11.2-21q22.3 (15,006,457 – 48,097,372)

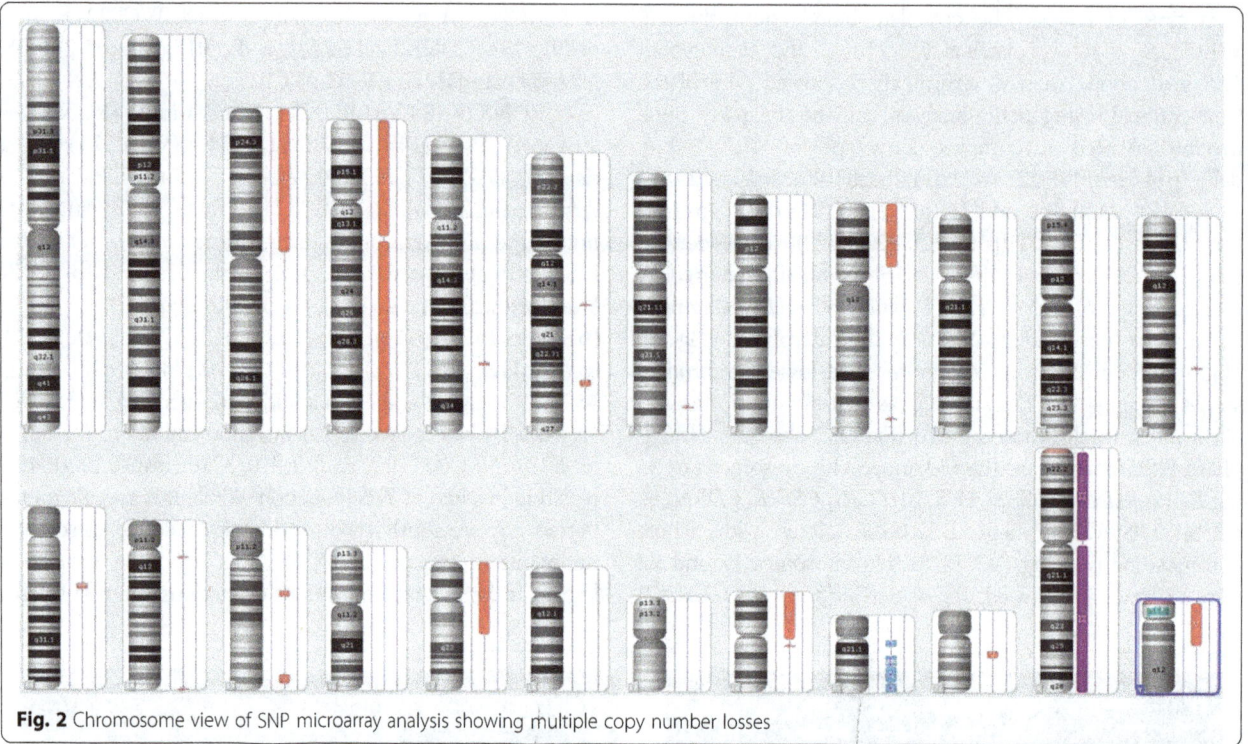

Fig. 2 Chromosome view of SNP microarray analysis showing multiple copy number losses

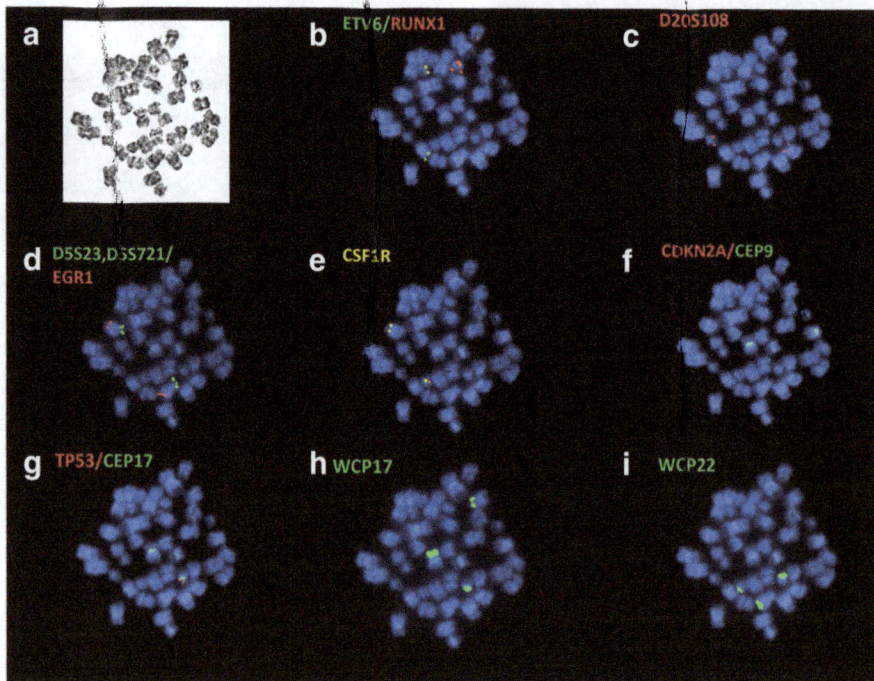

Fig. 3 Sequential G-banding and metaphase FISH was performed to refine initial karyotyping result. **a** G-banded metaphase. **b** Metaphase FISH indicated *ETV6* (green) and *RUNX1* (red) fusion as well as *RUNX1* amplification. **c** No deletions for D20S108/20q12 probe in red, one signal on a normal chromosome 20 and the other signal on the derivative chromosome 3. **d** No deletions for D5S23/D5S721(5p15.2) in green and *EGR1* (5q31) in red). **e** No rearrangement for *CSF1R*/ 5q33–34, however, one copy was translocated to chromosome 22. **f** Homozygous deletion of *CDKN2A* (9p21) in red; centromere 9 in green. **g** Hemizygous deletion of *TP53* (17p13.1) in red; centromeric 17 in green. **h** Whole chromosome painting (WCP) for 17 (green) stained three different chromosomes, indicated translocations. **i** WCP for 22 (green) stained three different chromosomes, indicated translocations

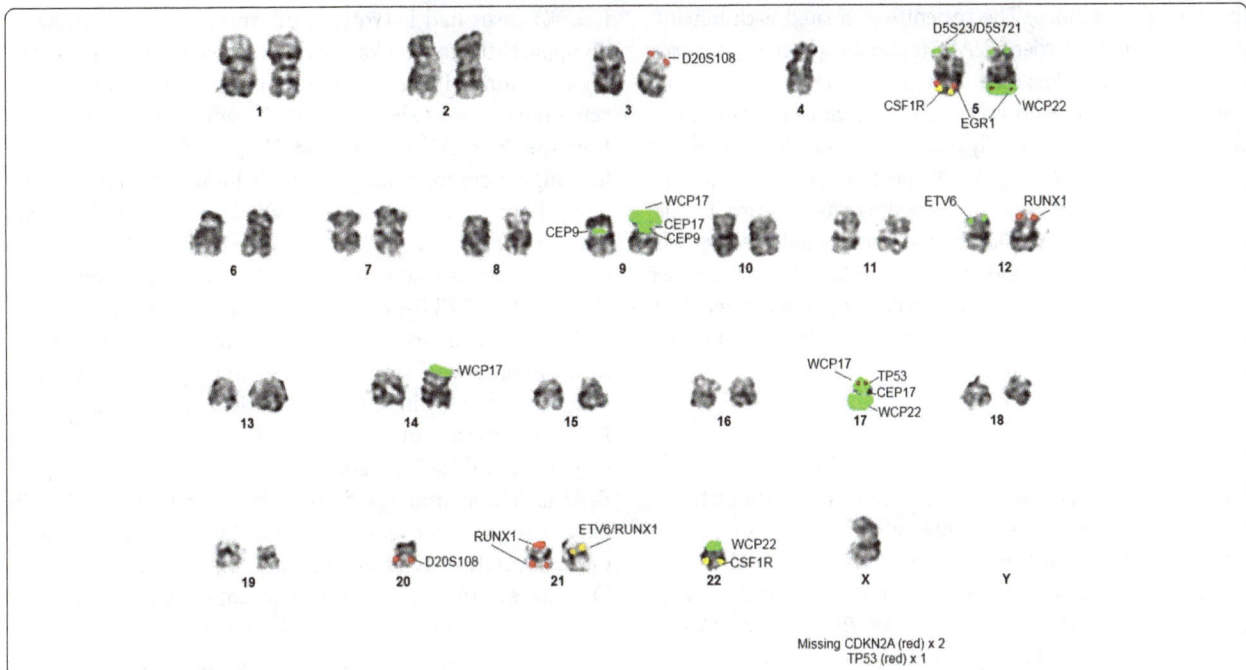

Fig. 4 Refined karyotype of abnormal metaphase displayed in Fig. 3a with co-localized FISH signals indicated a hypodiploid clone with 1) a der(3)t(3;20)(p11.2;q11.2)(D20S108+); 2) a der(5)t(5;22)(q32;q11.2)(WCP22+); 3) a del(9)(p13)(CDKN2A-), a dic(9;17)(p13;p11.2)(D9Z1+,CDKN2A-;D17Z1 +,TP53-,WCP17+); 4) a t(12;21)(p13;q22)(RUNX1+; ETV6+,RUNX1+) and add(21)(RUNX1+++++); 5) a der(14)t(14;17)(p11.2;q11.2)(WCP17+); 6) a der(17)t(17;22) (TP53+,D17Z1+,WCP17+,WCP22+); 7) der(22)t(5;22)(CSF1R+,WCP22+)

Table 2 G-band, FISH, and SNP-array results comparison

Chromosome	G-band	FISH	SNP-array
Y	-Y	ND[a]	Yp11.31q11.23(2,650,140-28,799,937)x0-1
3	der(3)t(3;20)(p11.2;q11.2)	D20S108+	3p26.3p11.2(61,891-87,302,938)x1-2
4	−4	ND	4q13.3q35.2(73,857,745-190,957,473)x1 ~ 2
5	t(5;22)(q22;q11.2)	wcp22+;wcp22+,CSF1R+	
9	del(9)(p13); dic(9;17)(p13;p11.2)	CDKN2A-,D9Z1+ D9Z1+,CDKN2A-;D17Z1+,TP53-,WCP17+	9p24.3p21.3(203,861-21,608,158)x1 ~ 2, 9p21.3(21,617,251-23,426,271)x1 ~ 2, 9p21.3p13.1(23,436,107-38,787,480)x1 ~ 2,
12	t(12;21)	RUNX1+;ETV6+,RUNX1+	
13	NL[b]	ND	13q14.2(47,925,533-48,966,146)x1 ~ 2, 13q14.2(48,984,342-49,177,989)x1 ~ 2, 13q14.2q14.3(49,182,831-51,194,835)x1 ~ 2
14	der(14;17)(p11.2;q11.2)	wcp17+	
17	der(17)t(17;22)	TP53+,D17Z1+,WCP17+,WCP22+	17p13.3q21.32(525-45,059,684)x1 ~ 2
20	−20	disomy for 20q12(D20S108)	20p13q11.21(61,568-29,497,009)x1 ~ 2
21	add(21)(q22)	RUNX1+++++	21q11.2q21.1(15,006,457-19,142,414)x2 ~ 3, 21q21.2q21.3 (24,806,259-27,905,650)x2 ~ 3, 21q21.3(28,498,600-28,835,696)x2 ~ 3, 21q21.3(29,805,880-31,211,807)x2 ~ 3, 21q22.11q22.2(31,795,184-41,909,261)x2 ~ 3, 21q22.2q22.3(42,364,149-48,097,372)x2 ~ 3
22	-22, t(5;22)	t(5;22)(CSF1R+,WCP22+)	

[a]ND not done
[b]NL normal

truncating) mutations. The patient was treated with blinatu-momab and the hyper-CVAD (cyclophosphamide, vincristine, doxorubicin, dexamethasone)/inotuzumab regimen, but only a partial remission was achieved. Due to persistent disease, the patient eventually received a matched unrelated donor allogeneic stem cell transplant (ASCT) 19 months after the initial diagnosis and 6 months after relapse. Unfortunately, the post-transplant course was complicated by liver veno-occlusive disease and relapse of B-ALL. Despite further therapy with R-EPOCH (rituximab, etoposide, vincristine, cyclophosphamide, and doxorubicin) and the patient died 26 months after initial diagnosis.

Discussion

We report the case of an 18-year-old with B-ALL associated with iAMP21 and *ETV6-RUNX1*. The patient had a very poor outcome despite intensified chemotherapy and allogeneic stem cell transplant. We also searched the literature and identified six additional cases of B-ALL with co-existing iAMP21 and the *ETV6-RUNX1* [7, 11–14] (Table 3). The median age of these seven patients was 10 years old (range, 2–18) and the median WBC count was 9.1 ×10^9/L (range, 0.7–34.2 ×10^9/L). Six of seven

(85.7%) cases had karyotypic information with 3 showing an apparently normal karyotype at the diagnosis, likely the result of limited blasts dividing in short-term culture. The remaining 3 cases showed iAMP21 which presented as either the "der(21)" or an "add(21)"; 2 of these cases also had highly complex karyotypes including the current patient. Four of 7 cases had detailed *ETV6/RUNX1* FISH data (Table 3). Case 1 showed the *ETV6-RUNX1* fusion amplification as a sole finding. Patients 2 and 3 apparently showed the *ETV6-RUNX1* fusion as the primary clone and iAMP21 as apparent evidence of a clonal evolution. Interestingly, very similar to the findings as observed in our case (case 7 in Table 3), patient 4 had the *ETV6-RUNX1* fusion only with a normal karyotype at the diagnosis, and had the additional iAMP21 in the relapsed B-ALL. These findings further indicate that iAMP21 is likely a secondary event that results in disease progression. OS information is available for 3 of 7 (42.9%) patients; OS was 34, 28 and 24 months in patients 1, 4 and 7, respectively (Table 3). Patient 1 had a better OS, likely attributable to younger age at the diagnosis. The overall poor prognosis observed in these patients suggests that the adverse clinical impact of iAMP21 overrides the

Table 3 Clinicopathologic features of iAMP21 and *ETV6-RUNX1* fusion positive B-ALL cases

Cases	Age(Yr)/ Gender	WBC Count (10^9/L)	BM Blast %	Additional Abnormalities	Outcome	Treatment	References
1	2/M	9.1	NA[a]	Karyotype: 46,XY. FISH: *ETV6-RUNX1* (4–5 copies) fusion in 80% cells	EFS[b]: 22 months. OS[c]: 34 months	ALL-IC-BFM	Case #4 Haltrich, 2013 [12]
2	10/M	NA	NA	*RUNX1* amplification with *ETV6-RUNX1* fusion in 5.5% cells and without *ETV6-RUNX1* fusion in 88.5% cells	NA	NA	Case #4 Ma, 2001 [14]
3	2/F	78	98	*ETV6-RUNX1* fusion with *RUNX1* amplification in 56% cells and without *RUNX1* amplification in 23% cells. Karyotype: 46,XX	NA	NA	Case #23 Mikhail, 2002 [13]
4	7/M	34.2	NA	At diagnosis: *ETV6* deletion with *ETV6-RUNX1* fusion. Normal Karyotype. At relapse: *RUNX1* x 4-5, *ETV6* deletion, *ETV6-RUNX1* fusion. Karyotype: 46,XY,der(21)add(21)(q22)[25]	EFS: 28 months	ALL-BFM'95/ ALL-REZ-BFM 2002	Case #1 Haltrich, 2013 [12]
5	11/M	0.7	NA	Karyotype: 46,XY,add(21)(q22)	NA	NA	Case #528 Harrison, 2014 [7]
6	13/M	NA	NA	Karyotype: 44,XY,del(1)(p33),-4,i(9)(q10),-17, t(19;?)(q13.3;?),dup(21)(q?),+1 ~ 2mar[cp16]	NA	NA	Case #530 Harrison, 2014 [7]
7	18/M	2.0	54	At diagnosis: *ETV6-RUNX1* fusion. No Karyotype. At relapse: *RUNX1* amplification (5 copies)/ *ETV6-RUNX1* in 27% cells. Complex karyotype.	OS: 26 months	Chemo ASCT[d]	Current Study

[a]*NA* not available
[b]*EFS* event-free survival
[c]*OS* overall survival
[d]*ASCT* allogeneic stem cell transplantation

presumably better prognosis associated with *ETV6-RUNX1* in B-ALL.

In the literature, B-ALL associated with iAMP21 is more frequent than cases of B-ALL with concomitant iAMP21 and *ETV6-RUNX1* fusion. Using an arbitrary age range for adolescents, we summarized 22 cases of B-ALL with iAMP21 for comparison. All these 22 patients had a median age of 15 years at time of diagnosis (range, 13–20) (Table 4) [8, 11, 12, 15, 16] and the male-to-female ratio was 1.75. Most patients had a low WBC count with a median of $3.4\times^9$/L (range, 1–15.8). Three (13.6%) patients had *RUNX1* amplification with a normal karyotype; five (22.7%) patients showed a deletion of chromosome 7 as an additional abnormality. Clinical follow up data were available in 20 (90.9%) patients showing a median OS of 29.5 months (range, 9–86 months). Comparing B-ALL with iAMP21 versus B-ALL patients with coexistent iAMP21 and *ETV6-RUNX1*, the iAMP21 only patients had a younger age at disease onset; 9 years old for iAMP21 versus 15 years old for coexistent

iAMP21 and *ETV6-RUNX1*, *p = 0.00*. Patients with B-ALL and iAMP21 only also had a higher WBC count; 25×10^9/L for iAMP21 only patients versus 5×10^9/L for patients with both iAMP21 and *ETV6-RUNX1*, *p = 0.01*. However, OS was insignificant between these two groups. Although, the clinical data are limited, we believe that patients with B-ALL associated with iAMP21 and *ETV6-RUNX1* can be included in the cytogenetic subgroup of "iAMP21".

In addition to the co-existing of *ETV6-RUNX1* fusion and iAMP21, our patient also showed *TP53* deletion with a concomitant *TP53* mutation. *TP53* deletion is frequently observed in B-ALL, particularly in those with hypodiploidy or familial Li Fraumeni syndrome or cancer predisposition syndrome [17]. Sequencing methods allow identification and better characterization of *TP53* mutation in 90% hypodiploid childhood ALL that is important for prognostic assessment [18, 19]. The concomitant *TP53* mutation with deletion could result in "two hits" for *TP53* loss of function and could result in poorer prognosis in

Table 4 Clinicopathologic features of iAMP21 positive adolescent B-ALL without *ETV6-RUNX1* fusion

Cases	Age(Yr)/ Gender	WBC Count $(10^9$/L)	Additional Abnormalities	*RUNX1* Copies/ Cell	Outcome	References
1	15/M	3.1	−8,der(16)t(1;16),−21	5–6	CR[b]1 × 9 months	Johnson, 2015 [11]
2	17/M	2.4	Normal Karyotype	>5	Relapsed 58 months after diagnosis following SCT, CR2 × 3 y	Johnson, 2015 [11]
3	20/M	2.2	−13,−14,+21	6–7	CR1 × 30 months	Johnson, 2015 [11]
4	19/M	5.3	del(7)(q11.2)	5–9	CR alive for 2 years	Knez, 2015 [15]
5	13/M	3.7	None	5–10	Unknown	Knez, 2015 [15]
6	15/M	2.1	None	4–8	Relapsed after 7 years of CR	Knez, 2015 [15]
7	13/F	3.0	+X	>5	CR and alive for 3 years	Knez, 2015 [15]
8	15/M	15.8	del(7)(q31)	8	Relapse 2.5 y from diagnosis, CR2 at last chemo block	Haltrich, 2013 [12]
9	14/M	2.2	None	5–10	CR 29 months	Reichard, 2011 [8]
10	15/M	2.0	Not Done	6–8	CR 51 months	Reichard, 2011 [8]
11	13/F	2.8	None	5–10	CR 18 months	Soulier, 2003 [16]
12	17/M	1.0	add(1)(q25)	8	CR 19 months	Soulier, 2003 [16]
13	19/F	10.1	del(7)(p14p21)	6–8	CR 21 months	Soulier, 2003 [16]
14	14/M	2.2	inv(7)(p?15q?21)	5–7	CR 23 months	Soulier, 2003 [16]
15	13/F	3.8	del(7)(q22q35),del(11)(p12)	5	CR 61 months	Soulier, 2003 [16]
16	15/F	9.9	None	4	CR 86 months	Soulier, 2003 [16]
17	15/M	4.3	-Y	4–5	CR 32 months	Soulier, 2003 [16]
18	15/F	NA[a]	add(1)(p?),del(6)(q25)	>4	CR 13 months	Soulier, 2003 [16]
19	13/M	7.6	i(9)(q10),−16	4	CR 18 months	Soulier, 2003 [16]
20	13/F	6.6	add(4)(q31),del(7)(q3?2)	5	CR 10 months	Soulier, 2003 [16]
21	14/M	14.5	Normal Karyotype	6–15	CR 48 months	Soulier, 2003 [16]
22	15/F	NA	Normal Karyotype	15–20	Relapsed	Soulier, 2003 [16]

[a]*NA* not available
[b]*CR* complete remission

our patient [20]. In addition, the null-function of *TP53* or other tumor suppressor gene, such as the homozygous *CDKN2A* deletions observed in our patient, can also promote the chromothripsis of 21q at the genomic level [21]. Hetero- or homozygous deletions of *CDKN2A* are recurrent findings in pediatric ALL. However, they are often considered as secondary events in childhood ALL and increase the likelihood of relapse [22, 23]. In our patient, the *CDKN2A* homozygous deletions were likely following the *ETV6-RUNX1* fusions, to drive disease progression together with the iAMP21.

iAMP21 is also a chromothripsis phenomenal, resulted in the remodeling chromosome 21 in a nonrandom fashion, leading to a stable derivative of chromosome 21 with leukemic potential [6]. Recent studies have provided new insight about the mechanistic events and consequences of chromothripsis [4, 24, 25]. These nonrandom genomic instabilities of chromosome 21q could be an initial leukemic event [26] in B-ALL pathogenesis, although it was a secondary event in our patient. The additional segmental copy number aberrations involving other parts of the genome, often reflected by complex karyotypes, are likely a secondary event in pathogenesis. High-resolution microarray based testing integrated with traditional chromosome/FISH analysis, particularly the metaphase FISH as performed in our patient, would allow the refinement of the heterogeneous karyotypic findings in iAMP21 B-ALL cases. The clinically critical regions of iAMP21 likely within the 21q22.2-22q22.3 region encoding for 19 to 32 Mb [26–31] in size. These genomic complexities likely contribute to the tumor progression and the poor response to therapy in this subset of the B-ALL patients.

Conclusions

Our results suggest that the coexistence of iAMP21 and *ETV6-RUNX1* fusion B-ALL is associated with relatively older age, male predominance, and a very poor prognosis. The presence of *ETV6-RUNX1* does not appear to modify the poor prognosis imparted by iAMP21 in B-ALL. Older children with an *ETV6-RUNX1* fusion positive B-ALL should be monitored closely for the development of iAMP21, particularly when a relapse of B-ALL is suspected. Patients with B-ALL associated with both iAMP21 and *ETV6-RUNX1* fit best in the poor prognosis cytogenetic subgroup of "iAMP21". Integrated genomic testing including high-resolution microarray and metaphase FISH is needed to refine the extremely complex genomic rearrangements.

Methods

Flow-cytometry immunophenotypic analyses

Eight- color flow cytometric immunophenotypic analysis was performed according to standard procedures. The panel included antibodies directed against: CD3, CD4, CD5, CD7, CD9, CD10, CD13, CD19, CD20, CD22, CD25, CD33, CD34, CD38, CD52, CD79a, CD117, BCL-2, HLA-DR, myeloperoxidase, IgM (cytoplasmic), kappa and lambda light chains (Becton-Dickinson Biosciences, San Jose, CA, USA), TdT (Supertechs Inc, Bethesda, MD, USA).

Cytogenetic and FISH analysis

Twenty-four and/or forty-eight hour unstimulated bone marrow cultures were setup for conventional cytogenetic analysis. Using a Leica-microscope imaging system (Leica Microsystems Inc., Chicago, IL) 20 metaphases were examined and karyotypes were prepared according to International System for Human Cytogenetic Nomenclature (ISCN 2013).

FISH studies were performed on cultured bone marrow metaphases and interphases using the probe sets targeting *ETV6/RUNX1*, *BCR/ABL1(ES)*, *MLL*, *CDKN2A /CEP9*, D5S23/D5S721/*EGR1*, *TP53/CEP17*, D20S108 (Abbott Molecular, Inc. Abbott Park, IL); and *CSF1R* break-apart (5q32), WCP17, WCP22 (Cytocell Ltd, OGT, UK). A G-banded slide was destained in methanol and hybridized with all the FISH probes above subsequently, according to standard lab procedures. FISH images were then captured in Cytovision and 200 cells were scored by two technologists when applicable.

SNP microarrays

SNP microarray study was performed using the Affymetrix CytoScan HD array (Affymetrix, Inc. Santa Clara, CA) which contains 2.5 million markers, including 750,000 SNPs and 1.7 million non-polymorphic probes, with extensive coverage over 18,500 RefSeq genes, known cancer genes and 12,000 OMIM genes. In brief, 250 ng of genomic DNA for each NK cell line were hybridized to a CytoScan HD array according to the manufacturer's protocols. Array data for copy number alterations (CNAs) and copy-neutral loss of heterozygosity (cnLOH) were analyzed using Affymetrix Chromosome Analysis Suite v.3.1 (ChAS) software and the Nexus copy number 7.5 (BioDiscovery Inc, El Segundo, CA) with a reference framework of NA33 (hg19). Regions of copy number alterations larger than 50 markers/400 kb for gain or 20 markers/100 kb for loss and copy neutral loss of heterozygosity (LOH) larger than 3 Mb are recorded. All CNAs were compared with known public databases of normal genomic variants (DGV).

Molecular study

Nanofluidics-based qualitative multi-parametric reverse-transcriptase polymerase chain reaction (PCR) was performed for the detection of *ETV6-RUNX1* fusion transcripts. PCR-based DNA sequencing was performed to assess for mutations in exons 4 to 9 (codons 33 to 331) of *TP53*.

Abbreviations

ASCT: Allogeneic stem cell transplant; B-ALL: B cell acute lymphoblastic leukemia; CNAs: Copy number alterations; cnLOH: Copy-neutral loss of heterozygosity; CNS: Central nervous system; CR: Complete remission; DGV: Databases of normal genomic variants; EFS: Event-free survival; FISH: Fluorescence in situ hybridization; iAMP21: Intrachromosomal amplification of chromosome 21; OS: Overall survival; PCR: Polymerase chain reaction; SNP array: Single nucleotide polymorphism microarray; WBC: White blood cell counts; WHO: World Health Organization

Acknowledgements

Not applicable.

Funding

No funding was needed for this project.

Authors' contributions

XL designed the study. JG, AR, and XL analyzed and reviewed data. AR collected clinical data and performed SNP array analysis. PL, LF and LJM reviewed the clinical data. KP reviewed the molecular data; CD and KS assisted the literature review. JG, AR, LJM and XL wrote the manuscript and all authors read and approved the final manuscript.

Competing interests

The authors declare that they have no competing interests.

Author details

[1]School of Health Professions, The University of Texas MD Anderson Cancer Center, 1515 Holcombe Blvd. Unit 0002, Houston, TX 77030, USA. [2]Department of Hematopathology, The University of Texas MD Anderson Cancer Center, 1515 Holcombe Blvd. Unit 0350, Houston, TX 77030, USA. [3]Department of Hematopathology, The University of Texas MD Anderson Cancer Center, 1515 Holcombe Blvd. Unit 0149, Houston, TX 77030, USA. [4]Department of Oncology, Jiangsu Hospital of Traditional Chinese Medicine, Nanjing, Jiangsu, China. [5]Department of Hematopathology, The University of Texas MD Anderson Cancer Center, 1515 Holcombe Blvd. Unit 0072, Houston, TX 77030, USA. [6]Department of Pathology, Northwestern University Feinberg School of Medicine, 303 East Chicago Avenue, Tarry 7-723, Chicago, IL 60611, USA.

References

1. Arber DA, Orazi A, Hasserjian R, Thiele J, Borowitz MJ, Le Beau MM, et al. The 2016 revision to the World Health Organization classification of myeloid neoplasms and acute leukemia. Blood. 2016;127(20):2391–405.
2. Li Y, Schwab C, Ryan SL, Papaemmanuil E, Robinson HM, Jacobs P, et al. Constitutional and somatic rearrangement of chromosome 21 in acute lymphoblastic leukaemia. Nature. 2014;508(7494):98–102.
3. Stephens PJ, Greenman CD, Fu B, Yang F, Bignell GR, Mudie LJ, et al. Massive genomic rearrangement acquired in a single catastrophic event during cancer development. Cell. 2011;144(1):27–40.
4. Mardin BR, Drainas AP, Waszak SM, Weischenfeldt J, Isokane M, Stutz AM, et al. A cell-based model system links chromothripsis with hyperploidy. Mol Syst Biol. 2015;11(9):828.
5. Moorman AV, Richards SM, Robinson HM, Strefford JC, Gibson BE, Kinsey SE, et al. Prognosis of children with acute lymphoblastic leukemia (ALL) and intrachromosomal amplification of chromosome 21 (iAMP21). Blood. 2007; 109(6):2327–30.
6. Harrison CJ. Blood Spotlight on iAMP21 acute lymphoblastic leukemia (ALL), a high-risk pediatric disease. Blood. 2015;125(9):1383–6.
7. Harrison CJ, Moorman AV, Schwab C, Carroll AJ, Raetz EA, Devidas M, et al. An international study of intrachromosomal amplification of chromosome 21 (iAMP21): cytogenetic characterization and outcome. Leukemia. 2014; 28(5):1015–21.
8. Reichard KK, Kang H, Robinett S. Pediatric B-lymphoblastic leukemia with RUNX1 amplification: clinicopathologic study of eight cases. Mod Pathol. 2011;24(12):1606–11.
9. Moricke A, Zimmermann M, Reiter A, Gadner H, Odenwald E, Harbott J, et al. Prognostic impact of age in children and adolescents with acute lymphoblastic leukemia: data from the trials ALL-BFM 86, 90, and 95. Klin Padiatr. 2005;217(6):310–20.
10. Moorman AV, Ensor HM, Richards SM, Chilton L, Schwab C, Kinsey SE, et al. Prognostic effect of chromosomal abnormalities in childhood B-cell precursor acute lymphoblastic leukaemia: results from the UK Medical Research Council ALL97/99 randomised trial. Lancet Oncol. 2010;11(5):429–38.
11. Johnson RC, Weinberg OK, Cascio MJ, Dahl GV, Mitton BA, Silverman LB, et al. Cytogenetic variation of B-Lymphoblastic leukemia with intrachromosomal amplification of chromosome 21 (iAMP21): a multi-institutional series review. Am J Clin Pathol. 2015;144(1):103–12.
12. Haltrich I, Csoka M, Kovacs G, Torok D, Alpar D, Ottoffy G, et al. Six cases of rare gene amplifications and multiple copy of fusion gene in childhood acute lymphoblastic leukemia. Pathol Oncol Res. 2013;19(1):123–8.
13. Mikhail FM, Serry KA, Hatem N, Mourad ZI, Farawela HM, El Kaffash DM, et al. AML1 gene over-expression in childhood acute lymphoblastic leukemia. Leukemia. 2002;16(4):658–68.
14. Ma SK, Wan TS, Cheuk AT, Fung LF, Chan GC, Chan SY, et al. Characterization of additional genetic events in childhood acute lymphoblastic leukemia with TEL/AML1 gene fusion: a molecular cytogenetics study. Leukemia. 2001;15(9):1442–7.
15. Knez VM, Carstens BJ, Swisshelm KL, McGranahan AN, Liang X. Heterogeneity of Abnormal RUNX1 Leading to Clinicopathologic Variations in Childhood B-Lymphoblastic Leukemia. Am J Clin Pathol. 2015;144(2):305–14.
16. Soulier J, Trakhtenbrot L, Najfeld V, Lipton JM, Mathew S, Avet-Loiseau H, et al. Amplification of band q22 of chromosome 21, including AML1, in older children with acute lymphoblastic leukemia: an emerging molecular cytogenetic subgroup. Leukemia. 2003;17(8):1679–82.
17. Holmfeldt L, Wei L, Diaz-Flores E, Walsh M, Zhang J, Ding L, et al. The genomic landscape of hypodiploid acute lymphoblastic leukemia. Nat Genet. 2013;45(3):242–52.
18. Muhlbacher V, Zenger M, Schnittger S, Weissmann S, Kunze F, Kohlmann A, et al. Acute lymphoblastic leukemia with low hypodiploid/near triploid karyotype is a specific clinical entity and exhibits a very high TP53 mutation frequency of 93%. Genes Chromosomes Cancer. 2014;53(6):524–36.
19. Hof J, Krentz S, van Schewick C, Korner G, Shalapour S, Rhein P, et al. Mutations and deletions of the TP53 gene predict nonresponse to treatment and poor outcome in first relapse of childhood acute lymphoblastic leukemia. J Clin Oncol. 2011;29(23):3185–93.
20. Hong M, Hao S, Patel KP, Kantarjian HM, Garcia-Manero G, Yin CC, et al. Whole-arm translocation of der(5;17)(p10;q10) with concurrent TP53 mutations in acute myeloid leukemia (AML) and myelodysplastic syndrome (MDS): A unique molecular-cytogenetic subgroup. Cancer Genet. 2016;209(5):205–14.
21. Rausch T, Jones DT, Zapatka M, Stutz AM, Zichner T, Weischenfeldt J, et al. Genome sequencing of pediatric medulloblastoma links catastrophic DNA rearrangements with TP53 mutations. Cell. 2012;148(1-2):59–71.
22. Vijayakrishnan J, Henrion M, Moorman AV, Fiege B, Kumar R, da Silva Filho MI, et al. The 9p21.3 risk of childhood acute lymphoblastic leukaemia is explained by a rare high-impact variant in CDKN2A. Sci Rep. 2015;5:15065.
23. Zack TI, Schumacher SE, Carter SL, Cherniack AD, Saksena G, Tabak B, et al. Pan-cancer patterns of somatic copy number alteration. Nat Genet. 2013; 45(10):1134–40.
24. Leibowitz ML, Zhang CZ, Pellman D. Chromothripsis: a new mechanism for rapid karyotype evolution. Annu Rev Genet. 2015;49:183–211.

25. Storchova Z, Kloosterman WP. The genomic characteristics and cellular origin of chromothripsis. Curr Opin Cell Biol. 2016;40:106–13.
26. Robinson HM, Harrison CJ, Moorman AV, Chudoba I, Strefford JC. Intrachromosomal amplification of chromosome 21 (iAMP21) may arise from a breakage-fusion-bridge cycle. Genes Chromosomes Cancer. 2007;46(4):318–26.
27. Baughn LB, Biegel JA, South ST, Smolarek TA, Volkert S, Carroll AJ, et al. Integration of cytogenomic data for furthering the characterization of pediatric B-cell acute lymphoblastic leukemia: a multi-institution, multi-platform microarray study. Cancer Genet. 2015;208(1-2):1–18.
28. Duployez N, Boudry-Labis E, Decool G, Grzych G, Grardel N, Abou Chahla W, et al. Diagnosis of intrachromosomal amplification of chromosome 21 (iAMP21) by molecular cytogenetics in pediatric acute lymphoblastic leukemia. Clin Case Rep. 2015;3(10):814–6.
29. Rand V, Parker H, Russell LJ, Schwab C, Ensor H, Irving J, et al. Genomic characterization implicates iAMP21 as a likely primary genetic event in childhood B-cell precursor acute lymphoblastic leukemia. Blood. 2011;117(25):6848–55.
30. Sinclair PB, Parker H, An Q, Rand V, Ensor H, Harrison CJ, et al. Analysis of a breakpoint cluster reveals insight into the mechanism of intrachromosomal amplification in a lymphoid malignancy. Hum Mol Genet. 2011;20(13):2591–602.
31. Strefford JC, van Delft FW, Robinson HM, Worley H, Yiannikouris O, Selzer R, et al. Complex genomic alterations and gene expression in acute lymphoblastic leukemia with intrachromosomal amplification of chromosome 21. Proc Natl Acad Sci U S A. 2006;103(21):8167–72.

16

Immunofluorescent staining reveals hypermethylation of microchromosomes in the central bearded dragon, *Pogona vitticeps*

Renae Domaschenz[1,2], Alexandra M. Livernois[1], Sudha Rao[3], Tariq Ezaz[1†] and Janine E. Deakin[1*†]

Abstract

Background: Studies of model organisms have demonstrated that DNA cytosine methylation and histone modifications are key regulators of gene expression in biological processes. Comparatively little is known about the presence and distribution of epigenetic marks in non-model amniotes such as non-avian reptiles whose genomes are typically packaged into chromosomes of distinct size classes. Studies of chicken karyotypes have associated the gene-richness and high GC content of microchromosomes with a distinct epigenetic landscape. To determine whether this is likely to be a common feature of amniote microchromosomes, we have analysed the distribution of epigenetic marks using immunofluorescence on metaphase chromosomes of the central bearded dragon (*Pogona vitticeps*). This study is the first to study the distribution of epigenetic marks on non-avian reptile chromosomes.

Results: We observed an enrichment of DNA cytosine methylation, active modifications H3K4me2 and H3K4me3, as well as the repressive mark H3K27me3 in telomeric regions on macro and microchromosomes. Microchromosomes were hypermethylated compared to macrochromosomes, as they are in chicken. However, differences between macro- and microchromosomes for histone modifications associated with actively transcribed or repressed DNA were either less distinct or not detectable.

Conclusions: Hypermethylation of microchromosomes compared to macrochromosomes is a shared feature between *P. vitticeps* and avian species. The lack of the clear distinction between macro- and microchromosome staining patterns for active and repressive histone modifications makes it difficult to determine at this stage whether microchrosome hypermethylation is correlated with greater gene density as it is in aves, or associated with the greater GC content of *P. vitticeps* microchromosomes compared to macrochromosomes.

Keywords: Reptiles, Methylation, Histone modifications, Epigenetics

Background

Epigenetic marks, such as DNA methylation and histone modifications, change the accessibility of DNA to the transcription machinery, thereby regulating gene expression. Most of our understanding of the role of epigenetic marks in vertebrates has been learnt from the study of model species such as mice, with far fewer studies having been carried out on non-model and non-mammalian species [1]. However, non-model species have genomic features that make them interesting to study from an epigenetic perspective [1]. For instance, the genome organisation of reptiles is quite different to that of mammals, with most species possessing several macrochromosomes and a varying number of microchromosomes [reviewed in 2]. This type of genome arrangement was most likely present in the ancestral amniote, and even in the tetrapod ancestor which diverged over 400 million years ago [3]. The conservation of this division between macro- and microchromosomes over a long evolutionary timescale makes it interesting to characterize the similarities and

* Correspondence: janine.deakin@canberra.edu.au
†Equal contributors
1Institute for Applied Ecology, University of Canberra, ACT 2601, Australia
Full list of author information is available at the end of the article

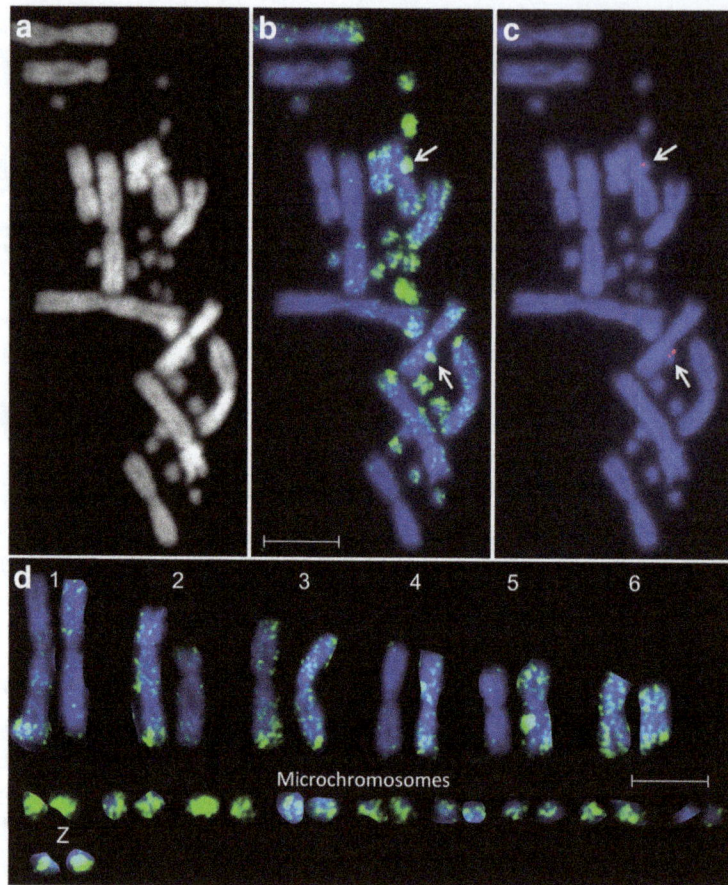

Fig. 1 Methylation patterns on male *Pogona vitticeps* metaphase chromosomes. Images for (**a**) DAPI, (**b**) DNA methylation (5-meC), and (**c**) identification of the Z chromosomes by mapping of BAC 150H19 specific to the sex chromosomes. **d** Karyotype of chromosomes depicted in images a-c. Scalebars represent 10 μm

differences between the two types of chromosomes, including the distribution of epigenetic marks.

Our general understanding of microchromosomes in vertebrates is rather limited considering the number of species in which they are found. Cross-species chromosome painting and gene mapping amongst avian species demonstrate, in most cases, that a microchromosome in one species is conserved as a microchromosome in another [4–7], indicating that microchromosomes are fairly conserved amongst aves. Whole genome sequencing has enabled detailed sequence analysis of chicken microchromosomes and comparisons of genomic features between macro- and microchromosomes. Chicken microchromosomes are early replicating [8], higher in gene density [9, 10], GC and CpG content [11, 12], recombination rate [9] and rate of synonymous substitutions [13] but are lower in repeat content than macrochromosomes [9]. In keeping with the higher CpG content, DNA methylation is enriched on microchromosomes of chicken, quail, pheasant, emu and American rhea [4].

Histone modifications H4K5ac and H4K8ac, associated with actively transcribed DNA, are also enriched on chicken microchromosomes and thought to correlate with the high gene density [8, 14].

Although genes from some chicken microchromosomes are located on macrochromosomes in reptiles [15–17], the smaller number of microchromosomes present in non-avian reptiles display conserved synteny with avian microchromosomes [17]. This has been demonstrated by whole genome sequencing of the green anole lizard genome [17] and comparative gene mapping in other species [3, 15, 16, 18, 19], dating these microchromosomes back to at least the amniote ancestor [3]. However, it appears that the characteristics of chicken microchromosomes may not be conserved across all reptiles. For instance, there is no difference in GC content between anole lizard macrochromosomes and six of the 12 pairs of microchromosomes for which sequence has been assigned [17], although the central bearded dragon [20, 21], tuatara [22] Japanese four-striped rat snake [18] and

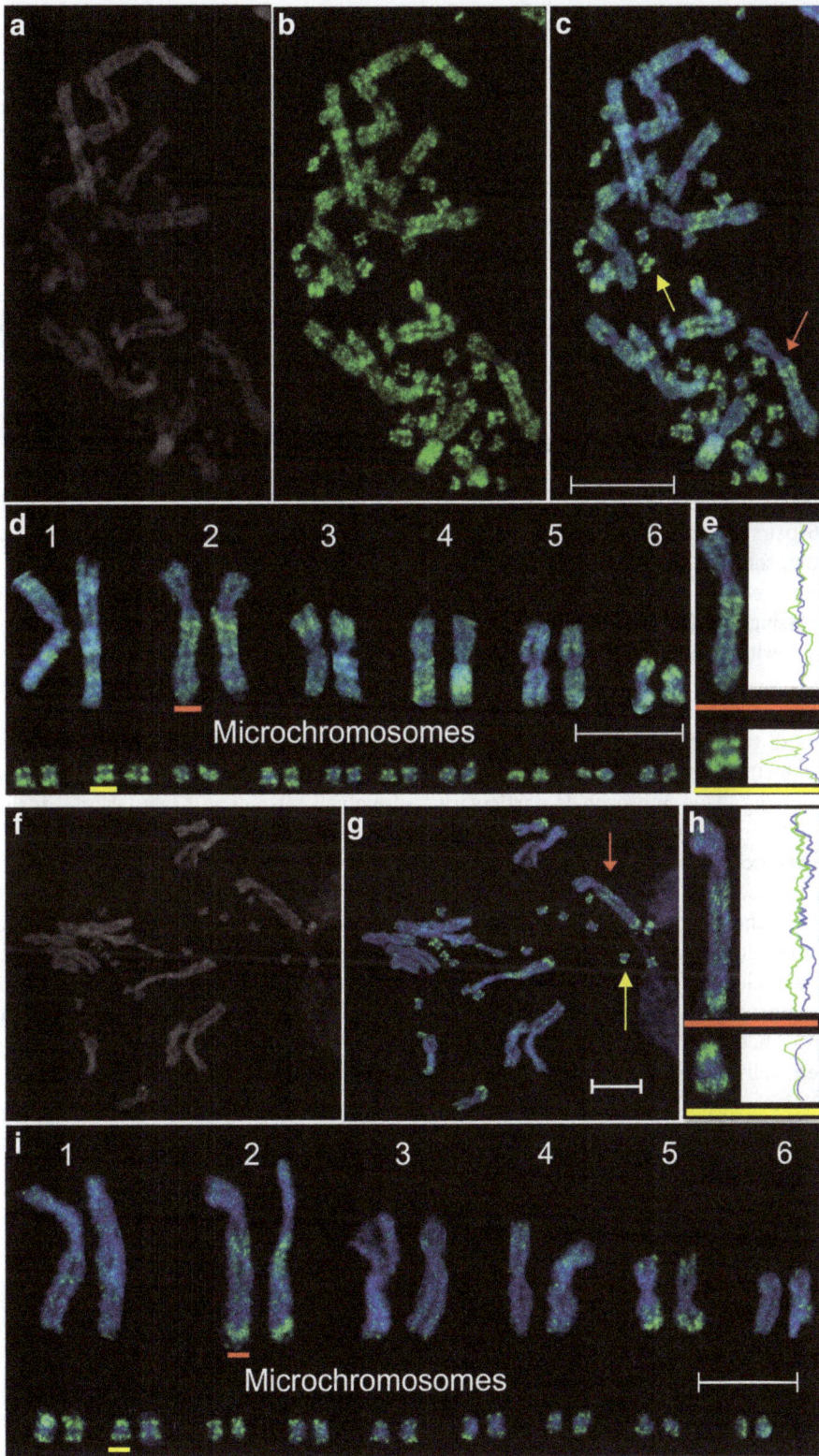

Fig. 2 (See legend on next page.)

(See figure on previous page.)
Fig. 2 Immunofluorescent staining of active marks H3K4me2 and H3K4me3 on *Pogona vitticeps* metaphase chromosomes. Distribution of H3K4me2: (**a**) DAPI stained chromosomes, (**b**) H3K4me2 staining and (**c**) merged image, (**d**) karyotype of chromosomes depicted in image c. **e** Representative line scans of staining on a macrochromosome (red) and microchromosome (yellow). The blue curves correspond to the DAPI staining along the length of the chromosomes. The green curves show the distribution of each epigenetic mark. Distribution of H3K4me3: (**f**) DAPI stained chromosomes, (**g**) merged image showing H3K4me3 staining in green and DAPI staining in blue. **h** Representative line scans of staining on a macrochromosome (red) and microchromosome (yellow). **i** Karyotype of chromosomes depicted in image g. Scalebars represent 10 μm

soft shelled turtle microchromosomes are more GC rich than macrochromosomes [23]. This raises questions whether the epigenetic differences observed between macro- and microchromosomes in chicken would also be observed in non-avian reptiles.

The central bearded dragon (*Pogona vitticeps*) is an Australian lizard species for which there are considerable genetic and genomic resources available, including a molecular cytogenetic map [24] and genome sequence [21]. This species has a diploid chromosome number of 32, consisting of 6 pairs of macrochromosomes and 10 pairs of microchromosomes [25]. A pair of microchromosomes were discovered to be the sex chromosomes in this species, possessing a ZZ male:ZW female sex chromosome system with a highly heterochromatic W chromosome [20].

Here we report the occurrence of DNA methylation as well as two active and two repressive histone modifications on *P.vitticeps* metaphase chromosomes using immunofluorescent staining. This approach is particularly valuable for non-model species where genome sequences lack adequate sequence coverage for a high quality genome assembly to be used as a reference genome for sequence-based approaches like ChIP-seq or bisulfite sequencing. In addition, although these sequencing-based techniques provide valuable, fine-scale information, these data typically represent the mean occurrence of an epigenetic mark from heterogeneous cells, with possible differences between cells arising from them being at different stages of the cell cycle [26]. Immunofluorescent staining of epigenetic modifications on metaphase chromosomes allows the distribution of epigenetic marks along individual chromosomes, including the difficult to sequence repetitive regions, to be examined within a single cell.

The active histone modifications we have chosen are histone H3 di-methylated at lysine 4 (H3K4me2) and H3 tri-methylated at lysine 4 (H3K4me3), which are epigenetic marks typically associated with euchromatin and are closely associated with gene-rich regions of the genome, CpG islands and SINE elements on human chromosomes [26]. In contrast, histone H3 tri-methylated at lysine 27 (H3K27me3) is a repressive epigenetic mark associated with facultative heterochromatin and the repression of gene transcription. The other repressive mark we used is histone H3 di-methylated at lysine 9 (H3K9me2) which is associated with constitutive heterochromatin formation as well as being involved in gene regulation during development (reviewed in [27]).

Results and discussion

We compared the distribution of epigenetic marks between macro- and microchromosomes, using immunofluorescent staining to determine if there is an epigenetic distinction between the two different categories of chromosomes. Despite this technique being a valuable tool to study the epigenetic state of chromosomes

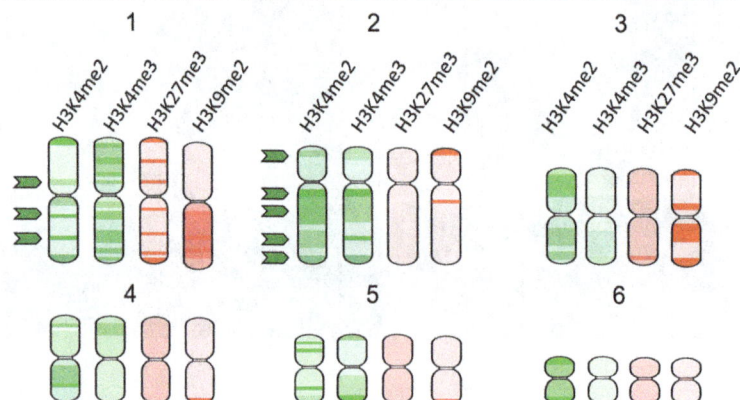

Fig. 3 Ideograms depicting the distribution of active marks (green) H3K4me2 and H3K4me3 and repressive marks (red) H3K27me3 and H3K9me2 on *Pogona vitticeps* macrochromosomes. Arrows indicate regions of overlap between the two active marks

for non-model species, there have been very few studies that have employed this approach for non-model vertebrates. Using this approach, we detected obvious staining differences between macro- and microchromosomes for 5-methylcytosine staining but not for active or repressive histone modifications.

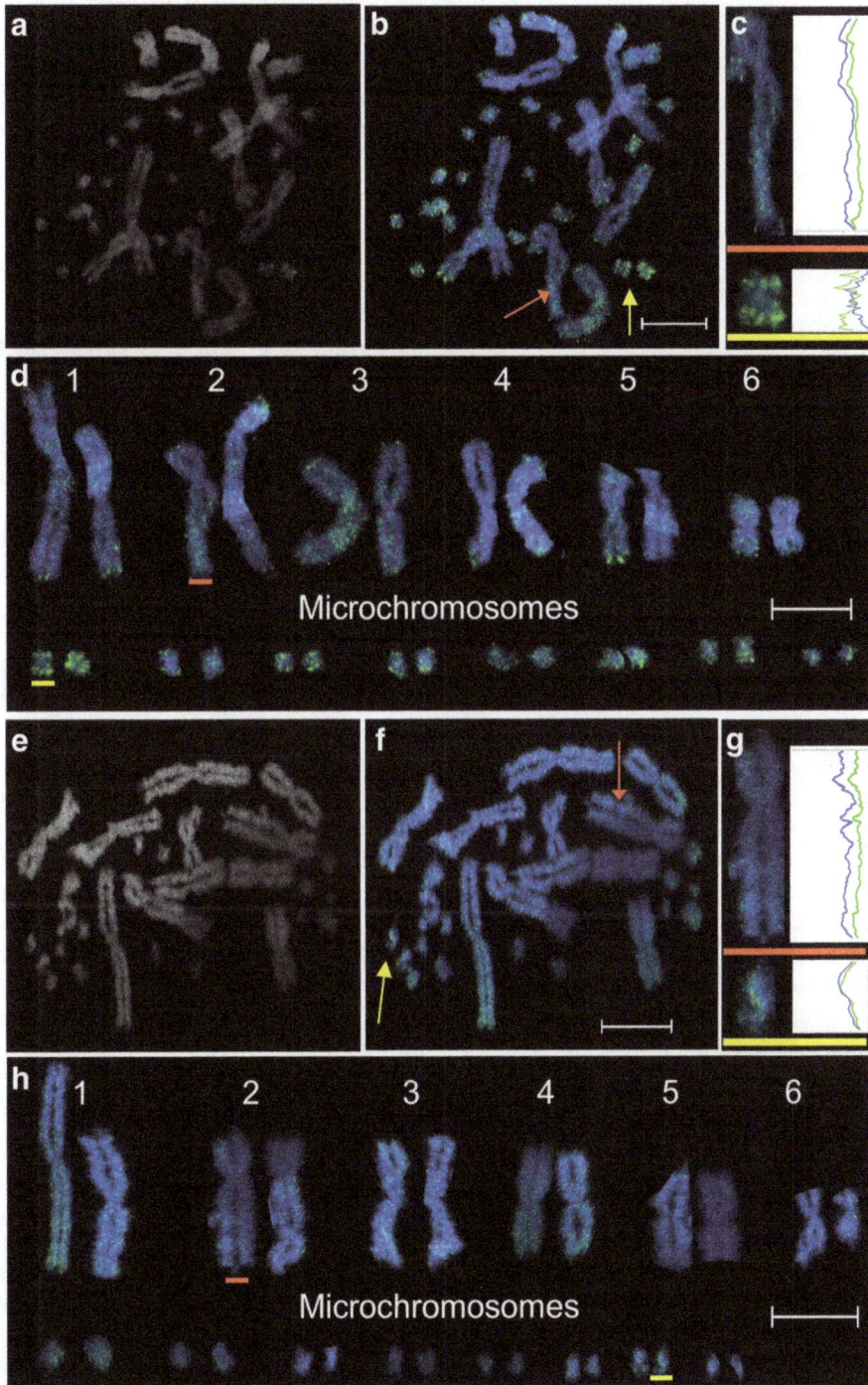

Fig. 4 Distribution of repressive epigenetic marks across *Pogona vitticeps* metaphase chromosomes. Distribution of H3K27me3: (**a**) DAPI stained chromosomes, (**b**) merged image with H3K27me3 staining in green and DAPI in blue, (**c**) Representative line scans of staining on a macrochromosome (red) and microchromosome (yellow). The blue curves correspond to the DAPI staining along the length of the chromosomes. The green curves show the distribution of H3K27me3. **d** Karyotype of chromosomes depicted in image b. Distribution of H3K4me3: (**e**) DAPI stained chromosomes, (**f**) merged image showing H3K9me2 staining in green and DAPI staining in blue. **g** Representative line scans of staining on a macrochromosome (red) and microchromosome (yellow). **h** Karyotype of chromosomes depicted in image g. Scalebars represent 10 µm

Table 1 Primary and secondary antibodies used for immunofluorescence

Antibodies	Raised/type	Source	Catalog no.
Anti-5-methylcytosine (5meC) (Clone 10G4)	Mouse monoclonal	Zymo	A3001
Anti-H3K4me2	Rabbit polyclonal	Upstate (Millipore)	07–030
Anti-H3K27me3	Rabbit polyclonal	Upstate (Millipore)	07–449
Anti-H3K9me2	Rabbit polyclonal	Upstate (Millipore)	07–441
Anti-H3K4me3	Mouse monoclonal	Abcam	ab–1012
Anti-Cy3 anti-mouse	Donkey polyclonal	Jackson Immunoresearch Laboratories	715–165–151
Anti-FITC anti-rabbit	Donkey polyclonal		711–095–152

DNA methylation status

Immunostaining with a 5-methylcytosine (meC) antibody was used to visualize the global DNA methylation state of metaphase chromosomes. Telomeric regions of most *P.vitticeps* chromosomes showed stronger methylation staining than the rest of the chromosome, a pattern that has been observed in a range of species such as human [28], Tasmanian devil [29], platypus [30] and even plants [31]. The telomeric repeat sequence (TTAGGG)n in vertebrates does not contain the CG dinucleotide required for methylation to occur. However, adjacent subtelomeric regions in mammals are GC rich and heavily methylated [32], with methylation of these regions implicated in repressing DNA recombination at telomeres and indirectly regulating telomere length [33]. With the important role telomeres play in protecting the ends of chromosomes from eroding, it is not surprising that methylation of telomeric/subtelomeric regions may not be restricted to mammals.

All observed metaphase spreads from both cell lines examined showed a more intense staining of microchromosomes than macrochromosomes (Fig. 1). This is consistent with the observation that *P. vitticeps* microchromosomes are GC rich [20], as well as the methylation pattern observed in avian species, suggesting that, like birds, *P. vitticeps* microchromosomes are gene rich. Grützner et al. [4] proposed that, given the known role of methylation in gene silencing, higher levels of methylation on the gene-dense avian microchromosomes may indicate that most genes are inactive in any given cell. This may be true if DNA methylation was solely associated with gene silencing, but hypermethylation of gene bodies is associated with gene activity [34, 35]. Thus, hypermethylation of

microchromosomes may be correlated with gene activity of these gene rich chromosomes. Alternatively, the seemingly more intense staining of microchromosomes may simply be attributed to the closeness of the telomeric regions on these tiny chromosomes and DNA methylation may not be an indicator of their gene activity. A sequencing-based approach could prove useful for distinguishing between these alternative explanations for hypermethylation of *P. vitticeps* microchromosomes.

In mammals, inactivation of one X chromosome in females compensates for the differences in dosage of X-borne genes between XX females and XY males. In marsupials and humans, the inactive X in females is hypomethylated compared to the active X and autosomes, most likely as a result of gene-body methylation which is associated with gene activity [30, 35, 36]. As the sex chromosomes in *P. vitticeps* are microchromosomes, we carefully examined male metaphase spreads for a hypomethylated Z chromosome. However, both copies of the Z chromosome were consistently hypermethylated in males (Fig. 1). This suggests that if there is a mechanism in *P. vitticeps* to compensate for the difference in Z gene dosage between ZZ males and ZW females, it is unlikely to be similar to the chromosome-wide mechanism observed in therian (marsupial and eutherians) mammals.

Active modifications

In *P. vitticeps*, distribution of H3K4me2 (Fig. 2a-e) and H3K4me3 (Fig. 2f-i) staining across telomeric regions and on both arms of macrochromosomes was seen with a distinct pattern for each macrochromosome. Although the distributions of these two active marks are different, there is some overlap of intensely stained regions on chromosomes 1 and 2 (Fig. 3). These regions are likely to represent particularly gene-rich regions of the genome. In humans, H3K4me3 enriched regions on chromosomes have been shown to correspond with gene-rich regions [26].

Although the fragile nature of the unfixed chromosomes [37] from primary fibroblast cell lines made karyotyping of all microchromosomes in a metaphase spread challenging, the majority of microchromosomes were consistently detected to gain a general impression of the distribution of these active marks. The line scans (Fig. 2e and h) demonstrate enrichment for H3K4me2 and H3K4me3 in telomeric regions and an absence from the centromeric/pericentric regions of microchromosomes. Like the pattern observed for DNA methylation, it is unclear whether the enrichment for these marks is correlated with gene activity on potentially gene rich microchromosomes or due to the proximity of the telomeres on the tiny chromosomes. Telomeric enrichment of these marks, also observed for human telomeres, may be associated with RNA polymerase II transcription reported at mammalian telomeres [38–40]. In contrast, centromeric chromatin on *P.vitticeps* chromosomes was consistently unstained for H3K4me2 and H3K4me3, which is expected given the heterochromatic nature of centromeres.

Repressive modifications

The modification H3K27me3, associated with gene silencing, showed a distinctive regional distribution along the arms of macrochromosomes, with intense staining detected in 70–80 % of the metaphase spreads in telomeric regions (Fig. 4a-d). H3K27me3 was also strongly enriched at telomeric regions of microchromosomes, a staining pattern we also observed with active modifications H3K4me2 and H3K4me3 as earlier described. Enrichment for H3K27me3 staining at telomeric regions has also been observed on human metaphase chromosomes [26]. Like macrochromosomes, centromeric chromatin was unstained for H3K27me3 on microchromosomes. Also associated with gene silencing, H3K9me2 showed an evenly distributed and much less defined staining pattern along the arms of both macro- and microchromosomes than H3K27me3. (Figure 4e-h). Antibodies for these two histone modifications have shown a similar pattern of staining on tammar wallaby (*Macropus eugenii*) metaphase chromosomes [41]. There is a lack of overlap of regions enriched for these two repressive marks (Fig. 3), which is not surprising given that one is associated with facultative heterochromatin (H3K27me3) and the other with constitutive heterochromatin.

Conclusions

We show a characteristic distribution of various histone modifications across the metaphase genome of *P. vitticeps*, with some modifications showing distinctive regional localisation. DNA cytosine methylation, active modifications H3K4me2 and H3K4me3, as well as the repressive mark H3K27me3 are enriched in telomeric regions. The most notable epigenetic difference between macro- and microchromosomes is the hypermethylation of microchromosomes, a feature shared with birds. None of the histone modifications examined showed as distinct a difference between macro- and microchromosomes as DNA cytosine methylation. The lack of difference between macro- and microchromosomes for histone modifications associated with gene activity makes it unclear whether this difference is correlated with increased gene density, as it is in avian species, or simply a reflection of the increased GC content or closeness of the methylation staining associated with telomeric regions of *P. vitticeps* microchromosomes. With the sequencing of more reptile genomes, including that of *P. vitticeps*, it will be interesting to compare the genomic features of macro- and microchromsomes to their epigenetic signature.

Methods
Cell culture

Primary adult *P.vittceps* fibroblast cell lines were derived as previously described [42] from samples collected under approval from the University of Canberra Committee for Ethics in Animal Experimentation (CE-04-04). Cultured cells were maintained in Gibco AmnioMax medium (Life Technologies Australia Pty Ltd, Mulgrave, VIC, Australia), supplemented with 10 % fetal bovine serum (Autogene Bioclear, Calne, Wiltshire, UK), 1 mM L-glutamine (Gibco-BRL, Life Technologies), 50 U/ml penicillin (Gibco-BRL, Life Technolgies), and 50 µg/ml of streptomycin (Gibco-BRL, Life Technologies). Cells were grown at 28 °C in an atmosphere containing 5 % CO_2.

Immunostaining for DNA methylation

Metaphase slides were prepared using standard protocols [43]. The slides were dehydrated through 70 %, – 90 % - 100 % (v/v) ethanol series (3 min each) and air dried before denaturing in 70 % (v/v) formamide at 70 °C for 1 min and 40 s. The slides were immediately transferred to ice-cold 70 % (v/v) ethanol for 5 min and then continued through 90 and 100 % (v/v) ethanol series (3 min in each). The slides were allowed to air dry before rehydrating in Phosphate Buffered Saline with Tween 20 (PBST: 137 mM NaCl, 2.7 mM KCl, 10 mM NA_2HPO_4, 2 mM 2.4 KH_2PO_4, 0.03 % v/v Polysorbate 20) for 3 min. The slides were blocked in PBST + 1 %(w/v) Bovine Serum Albumin (BSA) for 20 min, after which the primary anti-5-methylcytosine antibody (5meC), diluted 1:200 in PBST, was added to the slides and incubated for 60 min in a humidified chamber at 37 °C. Subsequently, the slides were washed twice for 5 min each in PBST. The area was then covered with the secondary antibody (anti-mouse Cy3) diluted 1:500 in PBST, and incubated for 60 min in a humidified chamber at 37 °C. The slides were then fixed in 4 % (w/v) paraformaldehyde in PBS for 15 min, washed in PBST 3 times for 3 min each, air dried and mounted in Vectashield with 4′-6-diamidino-2-phenylindole (DAPI) (Vector Laboratories Inc., Burlingame, CA, USA). Fluorescent staining was visualized using a Zeiss Axio Scope A1 epifluorescence microscope and captured on an AxioCam Mrm Rev.3 CCD (charge-coupled device) camera (Carl Zeiss Ltd) using Isis FISH Imaging System version 5.4.11 software (MetaSystems, Newton, MA, USA). At least ten metaphase spreads were captured for each cell line. Line scans of DAPI and methylation staining intensities were obtained using Image-Pro Plus software (MediaCybernectics).

Fluorescent in situ hydridisation (FISH)

To identify the sex chromosomes, fluorescent in situ hybridization (FISH) was performed on the same slides as the 5meC staining using a BAC clone known to map to the sex chromosomes. The slide was prepared for FISH by rinsing in 2 × saline sodium citrate (SSC) buffer (0.3 M NaCl, 0.03 M sodium citrate, pH7) and dehydrating it through a 70 % (v/v), 90 % (v/v), 100 % (v/v) ethanol series. DNA for BAC clone Pv_150H19 known to map to the sex chromosomes was extracted using the WIZARD SV Minipreps DNA Purification System (Promega, Alexandria, NSW, Australia). The DNA was fluorescently labelled by nick translation with SpectrumOrange dUTP (Abbott Molecular Inc., Des Plaines, IL, USA) and hybridised as previously described [43]. Unbound probe was removed as described by Deakin et al. [44] and fluorescent signals visualised and captured using the same microscope, camera and software as that used for the detection of 5meC staining.

Immunofluorescence detection of histone modifications

Colcemid (Roche, Castle Hill, Australia) was added to the cell cultures at a final concentration of 0.1 μg/ml before harvesting metaphase chromosomes. Cells were harvested by trypsinization, collected in culture medium, and hypotonized in 0.0375 M KCl for 10 min at room temperature. Samples (0.15 ml) of the hypotonic cell suspension were cytospun onto clean glass slides in the presence of 10 % Tween 20 (3ul) at 800–1,200 rpm for 6 min. The slides were treated with KCM buffer (120 mM KCl, 20 mM NaCl, 10 mM Tris/HCl pH 8.0, 0.5 mM EDTA, 0.1 % Triton X-100) plus 1 % bovine serum albumin for 5 min at room temperature and rinsed in KCM buffer twice before immunostaining. The slides were incubated in a humidified chamber at room temperature with primary antibodies for 2 h, and secondary antibodies for 1 h. Primary and secondary antibodies are listed in Table 1. Each incubation with antibodies was accompanied by washing in KCM buffer (3 × 5 min). After the last washing, the slides were counterstained with DAPI, fixed in 4 % paraformaldehyde (w/v) for 10 min at room temperature, and mounted in Vectashield mounting medium (Vector Laboratories). The chromosomes were visualized using a Nikon Eclipse Ti fluorescence microscope and NIS Elements AR software. For each chromatin modification, at least 10 metaphases of the primary culture were analyzed. The line scans of DAPI and histone modification intensities were obtained using Image-Pro Plus software (MediaCybernectics).

Abbreviations

CCD: Charge-coupled device; DAPI: 4′–6-diamidino-2-phenylindole; FISH: Fluorescent in situ hybridization; H3K4me2: Histone H3 di-methylated at lysine 4; H3K4me3: H3 tri-methylated at lysine 4; H3K27me3: Histone H3 tri-methylation at lysine 27; H3K9me2: Histone H3 di-methylation of lysine 9; meC: 5-methylcytosine; PBST: Phosphate buffered saline with Tween 20.

Competing interests

The authors declare that they have no competing interests.

Authors' contributions

TE performed preliminary experiments and designed the study in discussion with RD, SR and JED. RD and AML performed experiments. RD analysed data with assistance from JED. RD, AML and JED drafted the manuscript. All authors commented on a draft, and read and approved the final manuscript.

Acknowledgements

This work was supported by a University of Canberra postdoctoral fellowship (awarded to TE, SR, Stephen Sarre, JED, Kris Hardy and Arthur Georges, and supporting RD and AL). TE is supported by an Australian Research Council Future Fellowship (FT110100733).

Author details

[1]Institute for Applied Ecology, University of Canberra, Canberra, ACT 2601, Australia. [2]Present address: John Curtin School of Medical Research, The Australian National University, Canberra, ACT, Australia. [3]Discipline of Biomedical Sciences, Faculty of Education, Science, Technology and Mathematics, University of Canberra, Canberra, ACT 2601, Australia.

References

1. Deakin JE, Domaschenz R, Siew Lim P, Ezaz T, Rao S. Comparative epigenomics: an emerging field with breakthrough potential to understand evolution of epigenetic regulation. AIMS Genet. 2014;1:34–54.
2. Deakin JE, Ezaz T. Tracing the evolution of amniote chromosomes. Chromosoma. 2014;123:201–16.
3. Uno Y, Nishida C, Tarui H, Ishishita S, Takagi C, Nishimura O, et al. Inference of the protokaryotypes of amniotes and tetrapods and the evolutionary processes of microchromosomes from comparative gene mapping. PLoS One. 2012;7:e53027.
4. Grützner F, Zend-Ajusch E, Stout K, Munsche S, Niveleau A, Nanda I, et al. Chicken microchromosomes are hypermethylated and can be identified by specific painting probes. Cytogenet Cell Genet. 2001;93:265–9.
5. Griffin DK, Haberman F, Masabanda J, O'Brien P, Bagga M, Sazanov A, et al. Micro- and macrochromosome paints generated by flow cytometry and microdissection: tools for mapping the chicken genome. Cytogenet Cell Genet. 1999;87:278–81.
6. Griffin DK, Robertson LB, Tempest HG, Vignal A, Fillon V, Crooijmans RPMA, et al. Whole genome comparative studies between chicken and turkey and their implications for avian genome evolution. BMC Genomics. 2008;9:168.
7. Derjusheva S, Kurganova A, Habermann F, Gaginskaya E. High chromosome conservation detected by comparative chromosome painting in chicken, pigeon and passerine birds. Chromosom Res. 2004;12:715–23.
8. McQueen HA, Siriaco G, Bird AP. Chicken microchromosomes are hyperacetylated, early replicating, and gene rich. Genome Res. 1998;8:621–30.
9. International Chicken Genome Sequencing Consortium. Sequence and comparative analysis of the chicken genome provide unique perspectives on vertebrate evolution. Nature. 2004;432:695–716.
10. Smith J, Bruley CK, Paton IR, Dunn I, Jones CT, Windsor D, et al. Differences in gene density on chicken macrochromosomes and microchromosomes. Anim Genet. 2000;31:96–103.
11. Auer H, Mayr B, Lambrou M, Schleger W. An extended chicken karyotype, including the NOR chromosome. Cytogenet Cell Genet. 1987;45:218–21.
12. McQueen HA, Fantes J, Cross SH, Clark VH, Archibald AL, Bird AP. CpG islands of chicken are concentrated on microchromosomes. Nat Genet. 1996;12:321–4.
13. Axelsson E, Webster MT, Smith NGC, Burt DW, Ellegren H. Comparison of the chicken and turkey genomes reveals a higher rate of nucleotide divergence on microchromosomes than macrochromosomes. Genome Res. 2005;15:120–5.
14. Bisoni L, Batlle-morera L, Bird AP, Suzuki M, Mcqueen HA. Female-specific hyperacetylation of histone H4 in the chicken Z chromosome. Chromosom Res. 2005;5:205–14.

15. Srikulnath K, Nishida C, Matsubara K, Uno Y, Thongpan A, Suputtitada S, et al. Karyotypic evolution in squamate reptiles: comparative gene mapping revealed highly conserved linkage homology between the butterfly lizard (*Leiolepis reevesii rubritaeniata*, Agamidae, Lacertilia) and the Japanese four-striped rat snake (*Elaphe quadrivirgata*, Colubridae, Serpentes). Chromosome Res. 2009;17:975–86.

16. Srikulnath K, Uno Y, Nishida C, Matsuda Y. Karyotype evolution in monitor lizards: cross-species chromosome mapping of cDNA reveals highly conserved synteny and gene order in the toxicofera clade. Chromosom Res. 2013;21:805–19.

17. Alföldi J, Di Palma F, Grabherr M, Williams C, Kong L, Mauceli E, et al. The genome of the green anole lizard and a comparative analysis with birds and mammals. Nature. 2011;477:587–91.

18. Matsubara K, Kuraku S, Tarui H, Nishimura O, Nishida C, Agata K, et al. Intra-genomic GC heterogeneity in sauropsids: evolutionary insights from cDNA mapping and GC(3) profiling in snake. BMC Genomics. 2012;13:604.

19. Matsubara K, Tarui H, Toriba M, Yamada K, Nishida-Umehara C, Agata K, et al. Evidence for different origin of sex chromosomes in snakes, birds, and mammals and step-wise differentiation of snake sex chromosomes. Proc Natl Acad Sci U S A. 2006;103:18190–5.

20. Ezaz T, Quinn AE, Miura I, Sarre SD, Georges A, Marshall Graves JA. The dragon lizard *Pogona vitticeps* has ZZ/ZW micro-sex chromosomes. Chromosom Res. 2005;13:763–76.

21. Georges A, Li Q, Lian J, Meally DO, Deakin J, Wang Z, et al. High-coverage sequencing and annotated assembly of the genome of the Australian dragon lizard *Pogona vitticeps*. Gigascience. 2015;4:45.

22. O'Meally D, Miller H, Patel HR, Graves JAM, Ezaz T. The first cytogenetic map of the tuatara, Sphenodon punctatus. Cytogenet Genome Res. 2009;127:213–23.

23. Kuraku S, Ishijima J, Nishida-Umehara C, Agata K, Kuratani S, Matsuda Y. cDNA-based gene mapping and GC3 profiling in the soft-shelled turtle suggest a chromosomal size-dependent GC bias shared by sauropsids. Chromosom Res. 2006;14:187–202.

24. Young MJ, Meally DO, Sarre SD. Molecular cytogenetic map of the central bearded dragon, Pogona vitticeps (Squamata : Agamidae). Chromosom Res. 2013;21:361–74.

25. Witten G. Some Karyotypes of Australian Agamids (Reptilia : Lacertilia). Aust J Zool. 1983;31:533–40.

26. Terrenoire E, McRonald F, Halsall JA, Page P, Illingworth RS, Taylor AMR, et al. Immunostaining of modified histones defines high-level features of the human metaphase epigenome. Genome Biol. 2010;11:R110.

27. Zhang T, Cooper S, Brockdorff N, Ash L, Dot L. The interplay of histone modifications – writers that read. EMBO Rep. 2015;16:1467–81.

28. Barbin A, Montpellier C, Kokalj-Vokac N, Gibaud A, Niveleau A, Malfoy B, et al. New sites of methylcytosine-rich DNA detected on metaphase chromosomes. Hum Genet. 1994;94:684–92.

29. Ingles ED, Deakin JE. Global DNA Methylation patterns on marsupial and devil facial tumour chromosomes. Mol Cytogenet. 2015;8:74.

30. Rens W, Wallduck MS, Lovell FL, Ferguson-Smith MA, Ferguson-Smith AC. Epigenetic modifications on X chromosomes in marsupial and monotreme mammals and implications for evolution of dosage compensation. Proc Natl Acad Sci U S A. 2010;107:17657–62.

31. Frediani M, Giraldi E, Ruffini Castiglione M. Distribution of 5-methylcytosine-rich regions in the metaphase chromosomes of Vicia faba. Chromosom Res. 1996;4:141–6.

32. Brock GJR, Charlton J, Bird A. Densely methylated sequences that are preferentially localized at telomere-proximal regions of human chromosomes. Gene. 1999;240:269–77.

33. Gonzalo S, Jaco I, Fraga MF, Chen T, Li E, Esteller M, et al. DNA methyltransferases control telomere length and telomere recombination in mammalian cells. Nat Cell Biol. 2006;8:416–24.

34. Zilberman D, Gehring M, Tran RK, Ballinger T, Henikoff S. Genome-wide analysis of *Arabidopsis thaliana* DNA methylation uncovers an interdependence between methylation and transcription. Nat Genet. 2007;39:61–9.

35. Hellman A, Chess A. Gene body-specific methylation on the active X chromosome. Science. 2007;315:1141–3.

36. Loebel DA, Johnston PG. Analysis of DNase 1 sensitivity and methylation of active and inactive X chromosomes of kangaroos (*Macropus robustus*) by in situ nick translation. 1993;102:81–87.

37. Terrenoire E, Halsall JA, Turner BM. Immunolabelling of human metaphase chromosomes reveals the same banded distribution of histone H3 isoforms

methylated at lysine 4 in primary lymphocytes and cultured cell lines. BMC Genet. 2015;16:1–7.

38. Rosenfeld JA, Wang Z, Schones DE, Zhao K, DeSalle R, Zhang MQ. Determination of enriched histone modifications in non-genic portions of the human genome. BMC Genomics. 2009;10:143.

39. Azzalin CM, Reichenbach P, Khoriauli L, Giulotto E, Lingner J. Telomeric repeat containing RNA and RNA surveillance factors at mammalian chromosome ends. Science. 2007;318:798–801.

40. Schoeftner S, Blasco MA. Developmentally regulated transcription of mammalian telomeres by DNA-dependent RNA polymerase II. Nat Cell Biol. 2008;10:228–36.

41. Koina E, Chaumeil J, Greaves IK, Tremethick DJ, Graves JAM. Specific patterns of histone marks accompany X chromosome inactivation in a marsupial. Chromosome Res. 2009;17:115–26.

42. Ezaz T, O'Meally D, Quinn AE, Sarre SD, Georges A, Marshall Graves JA. A simple non-invasive protocol to establish primary cell lines from tail and toe explants for cytogenetic studies in Australian dragon lizards (Squamata: Agamidae). Cytotechnology. 2008;58:135–9.

43. Alsop AE, Miethke P, Rofe R, Koina E, Sankovic N, Deakin JE, et al. Characterizing the chromosomes of the Australian model marsupial *Macropus eugenii* (tammar wallaby). Chromosom Res. 2005;13:627–36.

44. Deakin JE, Bender HS, Pearse AM, Rens W, O'Brien PCM, Ferguson-Smith MA, et al. Genomic restructuring in the tasmanian devil facial tumour: Chromosome painting and gene mapping provide clues to evolution of a transmissible tumour. PLoS Genet. 2012;8:e1002483.

17

Is cancer progression caused by gradual or simultaneous acquisitions of new chromosomes?

Mathew Bloomfield[1,2] and Peter Duesberg[1*]

Abstract

Background: Foulds defined, "Tumor progression (as a) permanent, irreversible qualitative change in one or more of its characters" (Cancer Res. 1954). Accordingly progressions, such as metastases and acquired drug-resistance, were since found to be subspecies of cancers with conserved and numerous new chromosomes. Here we ask whether cancers acquire numerous new chromosomes gradually or simultaneously in progressions. The currently prevailing theory of Nowell (Science, 1976) holds that unexplained "genetic instability" generates "variant sublines (with) changes in chromosome number" and that "clonal" progressions arise by "stepwise selection of more aggressive sublines". The literature, however, contains many examples of "immediate" selections of progressions with numerous new chromosomes - notably experimentally initiated fusions between cancers and heterologous cells. Furthermore, the stepwise progression theory predicts intermediate sublines of cancers with multiple non-clonal additions of new chromosomes. However, the literature does not describe such intermediates.

Results: In view of these inconsistencies with stepwise progression we test here a saltational theory, in which the inherent variability of cancer-specific aneuploidy generates "immediate" progressions with individual clonal karyotypes, transcriptomes and phenotypes in single steps. Using cell fusion as an established controllable model of "immediate" progression, we generated seven immortal murine hybridomas by fusing immortal murine myeloma cells and normal antibody-producing B-cells with polyethylene glycol within a few minutes. These immortal hybridomas contained individual sets of 71 to 105 clonal chromosomes, compared to the 52 chromosomes of the parental myeloma. Thus the myeloma had gained 19 to 53 new clonal chromosomes in seven individual hybridomas in a single step. Furthermore, no stable intermediates were found, as would be predicted by a saltational process.

Conclusions: We conclude that random fusions between myelomas and normal B-cells generate clonal hybridomas with multiple, individual chromosomes in single steps. Similar single-step mechanisms may also generate the "late" clonal progressions of cancers with gains of numerous new chromosomes and thus explain the absence of intermediates. Latency would reflect the low probability of rare stochastic progressions. In conclusion, the karyotypic clonality of hybridomas and spontaneous progressions suggests karyotypic alterations as proximate causes of neoplastic progressions. Since cancer-specific aneuploidy catalyzes karyotypic variation, the degree of aneuploidy predicts the clinical risk of neoplastic progression, confirming classical predictions based on DNA content.

Keywords: Saltational progression, Metastasis, Cancer drug-resistance, Cell fusion, Hybridoma, Aneuploidy-catalyzed karyotype variation

* Correspondence: duesberg@berkeley.edu
[1]Department of Molecular and Cell Biology, Donner Laboratory, University of California at Berkeley, Berkeley, CA 94720, USA
Full list of author information is available at the end of the article

Background

Foulds defined, "Tumor progression (as a) permanent, irreversible qualitative change in one or more of its characters" [1]. Accordingly several labs including ours have recently shown that progressions such as metastases and drug-resistant variants are actually clonal subspecies of cancers with parental and typically numerous new chromosomes [2–13].

Here we ask whether multiple new chromosomes of progressions are acquired gradually or simultaneously in one-off events.

The currently prevailing theory of Nowell (Science, 1976) holds that unexplained "genetic instability" generates "variant sublines (with) changes in chromosome number" and that "clonal" progressions arise by "stepwise selection of more aggressive sublines" [14]. The literature, however, contains numerous examples of selections of "immediate" progressions [14] with multiple new chromosomes [7, 15–18] - notably experimentally initiated fusions between cancers and heterologous cells [18–26]. Furthermore, the prevailing stepwise theory predicts stable intermediate sublines of cancers with multiple non-clonal additions of new chromosomes. However, the literature does not support the existence of non-clonal intermediates [14, 26, 27].

Alternative single-step theory of progression

In view of these inconsistencies with stepwise progression we test here a single-step or saltational theory of progression, in which the inherent instability of cancer-specific aneuploidy catalyzes steady karyotypic variations in single steps automatically by unbalancing thousands of balance-sensitive genes. Most of these variants alter parental cancer karyotypes within clonal margins of cancer-specific autonomy, typically by the gain or loss of single copies of chromosomes, while others lose autonomy and thus perish [9, 28–31].

A small minority of these random karyotypic variations would however, acquire new autonomous clonal karyotypes, transcriptomes and phenotypes, which are still related to, but distinct from parental predecessors [9–13, 32]. These new subspecies or progressions are also clonally stabilized by selections for cancer-specific autonomy, just like parental cancers are [9–12, 28, 29, 33, 34].

Using cell fusion as an established controllable model of "immediate" progression, we generated seven individual murine hybridomas of immortal murine myeloma cells and normal antibody-producing B-cells by fusing these cells with polyethylene glycol in a virtually immediate fusion process of minutes [21, 23, 25, 35]. Such progressions would thus be new clonal subspecies of parental cancers.

A saltational mechanism of progression would make three testable predictions: (1) Time-independent progressions with unpredictable numbers of chromosomes at low stochastic rates – just like de novo carcinogenesis [9]. (2) As per definition the saltational mechanism would also predict the absence of stable intermediates [9, 11, 30]. (3) The theory would also predict spontaneous progressions of progressions on the same principles as primary progressions.

In an effort to distinguish between a single step and multi-step theories, we tested an established experimental system of "immediate" progression [14], namely the immortalization of antibody-producing murine B-cells by fusion (or cell hybridization) with immortal murine myeloma cells to "hybridomas" [21, 23, 35] (Fig. 1). In this system, fusions of immortal myeloma cells convert normal B-cells to immortal clonal hybridomas in a few minutes in the presence of inactivated Sendai virus or polyethylene glycol- at rates of 10^{-4} to 10^{-5} hybridoma per myelolma cells [23, 35–37]. This short reaction time effectively limits fusion events to a single step process [21, 23, 35]. The resulting hybridoma clones are indeed already known to have new hybrid karyotypes [23, 26, 38] (Fig. 1). To test the predictions of our theory that simultaneous acquisitions of multiple new chromosomes may generate clonal progressions or subspecies in single steps, we prepared and analyzed the chromosomes and phenotypes of seven new immortal hybridomas.

In short we found that all seven hybridomas were individual subspecies of the parental myeloma with numerous new clonal chromosomes and that there were no karyotypic intermediates. These results support a saltational process of cancer progression.

Results

In the following we describe: (a) The preparation of seven hybridomas as models of immediate saltational progressions by experimental fusions of immortal murine myeloma Ag8 cells and normal B-cells (Fig. 1 and Methods). (b) Evidence for individual phenotypes of these hybridomas, which the saltational theory postulates based on selection of random recombinations of chromosomes of two or more cells hybridized by fusion. (c) Evidence for the clonality and individuality of the karyotypes of hybridomas, which the saltational theory postulates based on the low probability that random fusions of chromosomes of two types of cells generate a new immortal hybridoma species.

Preparation of hybridomas

Our colleagues Jennifer Zeitler and Robert Beatty kindly offered to us seven hybridomas from their undergraduate course in immunology here at UC Berkeley. Following published procedures, these hybridomas were prepared by fusions of immortal mouse myeloma Ag8 cells without functional thymidine kinase genes with equal amounts of normal thymidine kinase-positive B-cells and selections for immortal thymidine-dependent hybridoma clones in the presence of aminopterin, an

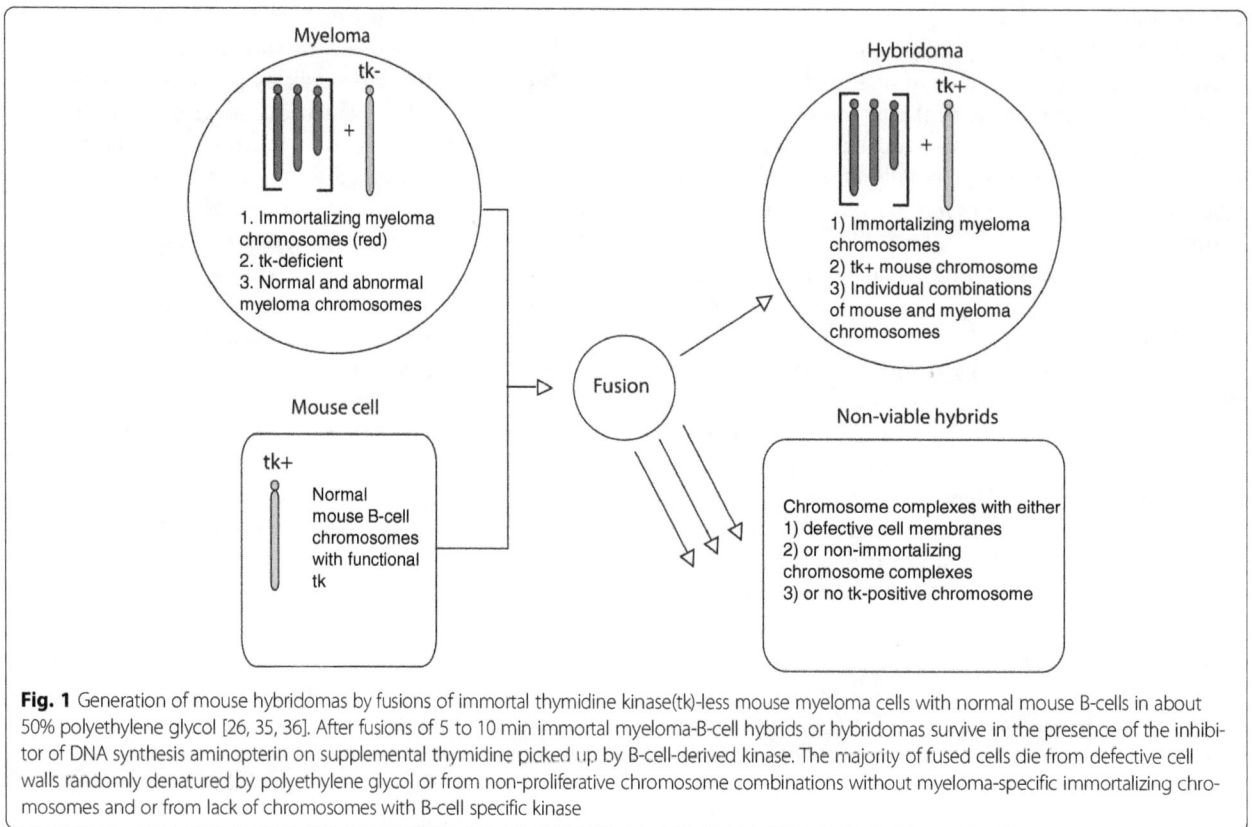

Fig. 1 Generation of mouse hybridomas by fusions of immortal thymidine kinase(tk)-less mouse myeloma cells with normal mouse B-cells in about 50% polyethylene glycol [26, 35, 36]. After fusions of 5 to 10 min immortal myeloma-B-cell hybrids or hybridomas survive in the presence of the inhibitor of DNA synthesis aminopterin on supplemental thymidine picked up by B-cell-derived kinase. The majority of fused cells die from defective cell walls randomly denatured by polyethylene glycol or from non-proliferative chromosome combinations without myeloma-specific immortalizing chromosomes and or from lack of chromosomes with B-cell specific kinase

inhibitor of de novo thymidine synthesis [21, 23, 26, 35, 36] (Fig. 1, Methods). Based on these procedures our myeloma and B-cells were fused with polyethylene glycol for several minutes, then washed and incubated in selective medium containing aminopterin and thymidine. As shown graphically in Fig. 1, under these conditions only cell hybrids between myeloma-specific immortalizing chromosomes (defined below) and B-cell-derived thymidine kinase-positive chromosomes survive. By contrast un-fused myeloma cells perish, because de novo DNA synthesis is inhibited by aminopterin or because cells are damaged by polyethylene glycol [35, 38]. At the same time un-fused B-cells perish spontaneously in cell culture in a few cell generations.

As described previously, only about one in $10^4 - 5$ myeloma Ag8 cells is converted to an immortal hybridoma cell by fusion with equal amounts of B-cells under these conditions [23, 35–37]. These low yields of progressions or subspeciation from myeloma to hybridoma are consistent with the low probabilities to generate new autonomous subspecies by random variation of the chromosomes of an existing species [9–11, 28, 33, 34] (Background).

Within one to two weeks after fusion we first detected hybridoma clones emerging in this selective medium as microscopic clones. Seven of such hybridoma clones were then grown to about 10^6 cells for karyotypic and phenotypic analyzes, typically about a month after fusion or later [23, 26, 36].

As shown in Table 1, three of these seven hybridomas were confirmed to produce antibodies against the specific antigens used to immunize the mice from which the B-cells derived by our colleagues Zeitler and Beatty, and hence termed Hyb CN-13 ab+, Hyb cl-12 ab + and Hyb cl-9 ab+. Table 1 also lists the remaining four hybridomas that were not tested for the production of antibodies against inducing antigens and thus labeled Hyb H12 ab-, Hyb F3 ab-, and Hyb 94 and Hyb 1-5 for reasons described below.

Clonal phenotypes of hybridomas

To test our theory that hybridomas are individual, clonal subspecies of myelomas with individual phenotypes [10, 11], we first looked at cell morphologies. As shown in Fig. 2a-c the cells of the myeloma Ag8 and of the two hybridomas Hyb H12 ab- and Hyb CN-13 ab + were spherical, like all other hybridomas (not shown) and thus hard to distinguish from each other morphologically - in contrast to the distinct 2-dimensional morphologies of cells from solid cancers attached to culture dishes as described by us elsewhere [11]. Nevertheless, both myeloma Ag8 and hybridoma Hyb H12 ab- differed from Hyb CN-13 ab + in forming 3-dimensional aggregates of cells in suspension, in which

Table 1 Average clonal chromosome numbers of the mouse, of murine myeloma Ag8 and of seven myeloma-mouse B-cell hybridomas

Myeloma and Hybridoma clones	Clonal chromosome number ± SD	Gains of chromosomes compared to the 52 of myeloma	Gains / losses of chromosomes compared to the 92 of a theoretical myeloma-B-cell hybrid
Mouse	40	–	–
Myeloma Ag8	52 ± 1	–	–
Hyb CN-13 ab+	85 ± 2	33	- 7
Hyb cl-12 ab+	86 ± 9	34	- 6
Hyb cl-9 ab+	105 ± 11	53	+ 13
Hyb H12 ab-	71 ± 2.5	19	- 21
Hyb F3 ab-	79 ± 2	27	- 13
Hyb 94	74 ± 5	22	- 18
Hyb 1-5	99 ± 7.5	47	+ 7

they are attached to each other. The non-attached cells settled at the bottom of the dish. In contrast all Hyb CN-13 ab + cells formed a dense layer of loose cells at the bottom of the dish. In addition Hyb CN-13 ab + cells were on average a bit larger than Hyb H12 ab- and myeloma cells.

Furthermore, Table 1 shows that some hybridomas differed from others in the production of specific antibodies, e.g. Hyb CN-13 ab+, Hyb cl-12 ab+, Hyb cl-9 ab+. By contrast, Hyb H12 ab- and Hyb F3 ab- are probably antibody-negative, although they were not directly tested, for two reasons: 1) As shown below in Fig. 6, they both lacked intact copies of murine chromosome 12, which encodes the heavy chain of mouse antibodies [39], and 2) The parental myeloma Ag8 of the hybridomas studied here also lacks functional antibody genes [40]. It would follow that both of these clones are antibody-negative.

Moreover the seven hybridomas could be distinguished by individual growth rates (data not shown). For example, hybridomas Hyb H12 ab-, Hyb F3 ab- and Hyb 94 grew about twice as fast as the three anti-body-producing hybridomas Hyb CN-13 ab+, Hyb cl-12 ab+, Hyb cl-9 ab + and the hybridoma Hyb 1-5 (Table 1). These individualities of our hybridomas confirmed and extended earlier observations by Kohler and Milstein [23].

In sum, we conclude that the seven hybridomas have descriptively and functionally distinct clonal phenotypes.

Next we set out to determine whether the chromosomes of our hybridomas were indeed individual and clonal as predicted by the saltational theory.

Are the chromosomes of hybridomas individual and clonal as predicted by the saltational theory?

The saltational theory of the origin of progressions predicts that each progression of a clonal cancer is a new, individual sub-clone with clonal parental and new progression-specific chromosomes. To test this prediction of the saltational theory of progression, we asked

whether the seven hybridomas each contained individual sets of clonal chromosomes.

To answer this question chromosome numbers of individual hybridoma cells were determined from karyotypes prepared from metaphase chromosomes. Owing to the inherent clonal heterogeneity of the chromosome numbers of cancer karyotypes, generated by cancer-specific aneuploidy (see Background, Alternative single-step theory of progression), we used averages of the primary chromosome numbers of five individual cells as standards of clonality.

Examples of individual karyotypes of three hybridomas, namely hybridomas Hyb CN-13 ab+, Hyb H12 ab- and Hyb F3 ab-, and of the parental myeloma Ag8 are shown in Fig. 3a-d. As can be seen in this figure, each immortal hybridoma contained individual chromosome numbers, as predicted by the theory that hybridomas are individual subspecies of the myeloma. Moreover the individual numbers of chromosomes of these karyotypes already indicated that each hybridoma apparently contained considerably more chromosomes than the parental myeloma, although clonality had yet to be determined.

To determine clonality the chromosome numbers, five individual cells of each hybridoma and parental myeloma were compared in 3-dimensional tables, termed 'karyotype arrays' [11]. Such arrays list the numbers of all intact and marker chromosomes on the x-axis, the copy numbers of the chromosomes on the y-axis, and the numbers of karyotypes (K) analyzed on the z-axis. The resulting 3-dimensional arrays show clonality as parallel lines, which are formed by chromosomes from distinct cells with the same copy numbers. At the same time, non-clonal chromosomes show up as readily detectable non-parallel lines in karyotype arrays.

In the following we show the karyotype arrays of our seven hybridomas and of the parental myeloma in pairwise comparisons in Figs. 4, 5, 6 and 7 and the resulting average clonal chromosome numbers in Table 1 and primary numbers in Tables 2 and 3:

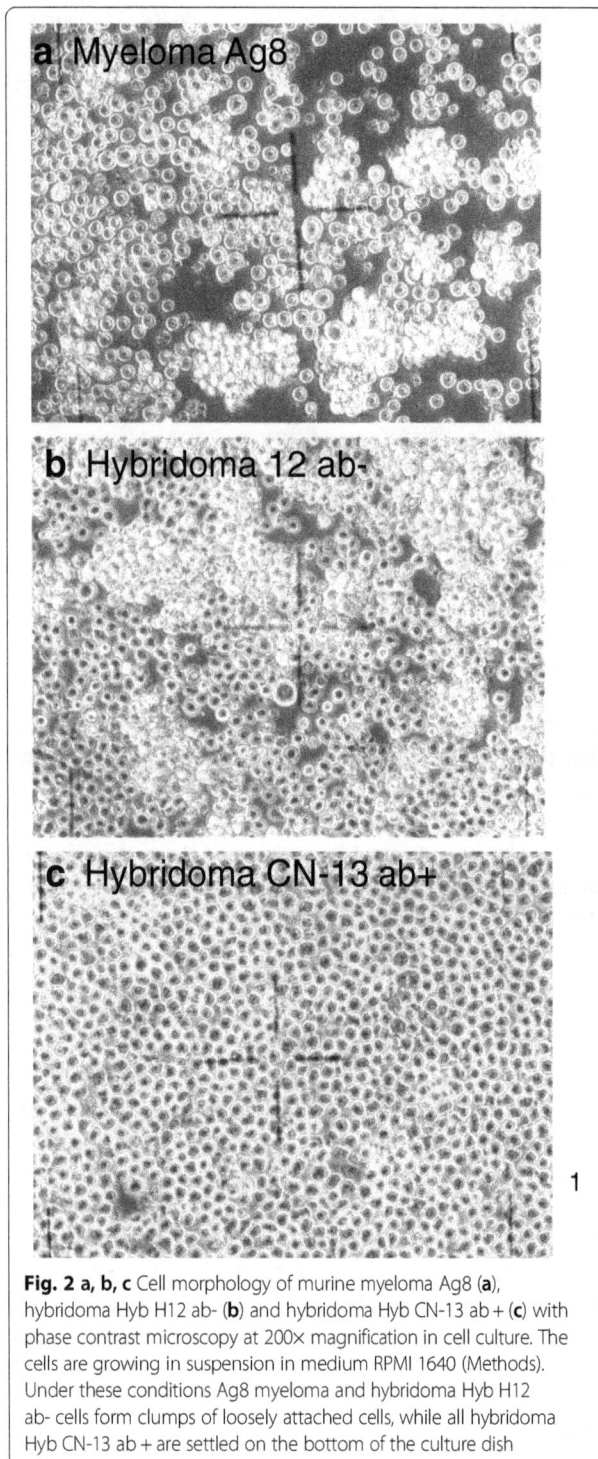

Fig. 2 a, b, c Cell morphology of murine myeloma Ag8 (**a**), hybridoma Hyb H12 ab- (**b**) and hybridoma Hyb CN-13 ab + (**c**) with phase contrast microscopy at 200× magnification in cell culture. The cells are growing in suspension in medium RPMI 1640 (Methods). Under these conditions Ag8 myeloma and hybridoma Hyb H12 ab- cells form clumps of loosely attached cells, while all hybridoma Hyb CN-13 ab + are settled on the bottom of the culture dish

Karyotype-arrays of myeloma Ag8 and hybridoma Hyb CN-13 ab + (Fig. 4a, b). As can be seen in Fig. 4a and in Tables 1 and 2 most chromosomes of five karyotypes of myeloma Ag8 arrayed in panel (a) and of hybridoma CN-13 ab + arrayed in panel (b) formed parallel lines and are thus clonal. The resulting percentages of clonalities are listed on the x-axis of the arrays, above the

respective chromosome numbers. With few exceptions they were predominantly 80 to 100% clonal. At the same time minorities of some chromosomes were non-clonal, differing from the majority of clonal counterparts mostly in the gains or losses of single chromosomes as shown in Fig. 4 and listed in Table 2.

Moreover the comparison of the two arrays shows the individualities of the two clones, and also their similarities. These similarities consisted primarily of 31 highly clonal and highly abnormal marker chromosomes shared by myeloma Ag8 and hybridoma CN-13 ab+. Further, the myeloma lacked several normal mouse chromosomes and shared all of its normal murine chromosomes with the hybridoma CN-13 ab+, although at lower copy numbers than in the hybridoma. The individualities and commonalities of the two karyotype-arrays thus confirmed the preliminary results of the single karyotypes of these clones shown above in Fig. 3a, b., namely that the myeloma had gained 33 new clonal chromosomes in its conversion to hybridoma CN-13 ab + (Table 1). The relatively high numerical gain of chromosomes by the hybridoma compared to the parental myeloma in the short times of fusion thus supports the single-step theory of progression.

Karyotype-arrays of hybridomas Hyb cl-12 ab + and Hyb cl-9 ab + (Fig. 5a, b). As can be seen in Fig. 5 (and Table 2), the copy numbers of most chromosomes of the karyotypes of Hyb cl-12 ab + and of Hyb cl-9 ab + formed parallel lines and are thus quasi-clonal. The prevailing 60 to 100% clonalities of the chromosomes are listed on the x-axis of the arrays, above the respective chromosome numbers. At the same time the copy number of the remaining non-clonal minorities of certain chromosomes typically differed from the majority of clonal counterparts mostly in the gains or losses of single chromosomes as shown in Fig. 5 and in Table 2.

Moreover comparison of the two arrays shows the individualities of the two clones and also their similarities. These similarities consisted again primarily of the 31 highly clonal, myeloma-specific marker chromosomes, which are also shared with the hybridoma shown in Fig. 4. This is further correlative evidence that the 31 myeloma-specific marker chromosomes encode the common, myeloma-specific immortality [30].

Further, the two hybridomas Hyb cl-12 ab + and Hyb cl-9 ab + shared with each other and with hybridoma CN-13 ab + all normal murine chromosomes, but mostly at hyper-diploid copy numbers. This suggests that probably more than one mouse B-cells were fused with the myeloma parent in the formation of these hybridomas.

With regard to the mechanism of progression, we emphasize again that the average clonal chromosome copy number of hybridoma cl-12ab + was 86 and that of hybridoma cl-9 ab + was 105. These hybridomas thus differ from the parental myeloma in 34 and 53 additional

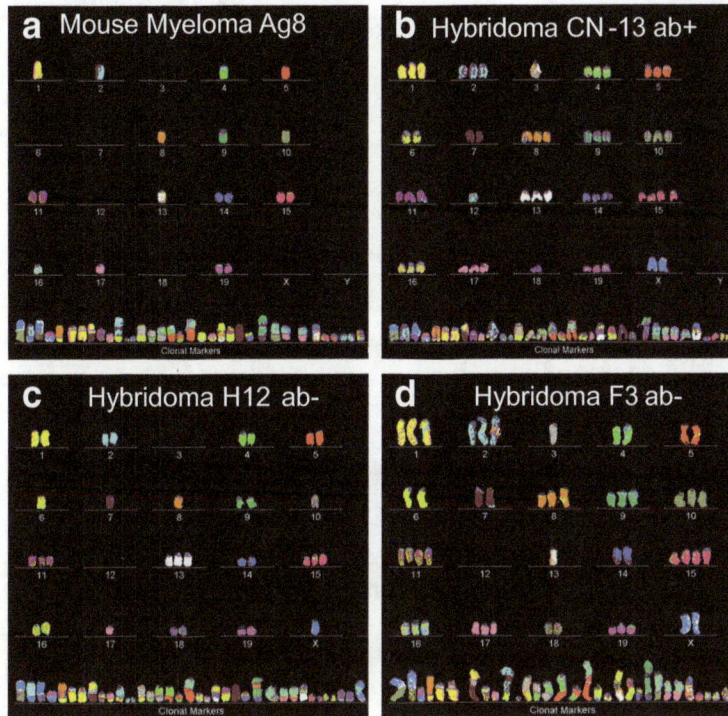

Fig. 3 a, b, c, d Karyotypes of murine myeloma Ag8 (**a**), and three hybridoma subspecies of myeloma Ag8, Hyb CN-13 ab + (**b**), Hyb H12 ab- (**c**) and Hyb F ab- (**d**). It can be seen that all four immortal clones shared the myeloma-specific set of about 31 marker chromosomes, which define the karyotype of the immortal myeloma clone, from which the hybridomas were derived

chromosomes respectively (Tables 1 and 2). These relatively high numerical gains of chromosomes by the hybridomas compared to the parental myeloma in the short times of fusions again support the single-step theory of progression.

Karyotype-arrays of hybridomas Hyb H12 ab- and Hyb F3 ab- (Fig. 6a, b). As can be seen in Fig. 6, the copy numbers of most chromosomes of the karyotypes of hybridomas Hyb H12 ab- and Hyb F3 ab- formed parallel lines. The exact percentages of the clonalities of the chromosomes ranged between 60 to 100% as listed on the x-axis of the arrays above the respective chromosome numbers. The corresponding chromosomes are thus quasi-clonal. At the same time the copy number of non-clonal minorities of these chromosomes typically differed from the majority of clonal counterparts mostly in the gains or losses of single chromosomes, as shown in Fig. 6 and listed in Table 3.

Moreover comparison of the two arrays shows the individualities of the two clones and also their similarities. Again these similarities consisted primarily of the 31 highly clonal, myeloma-specific marker chromosomes, which are also shared with the three hybridomas shown in Figs. 4 and 5 (and those shown in Fig. 7 below). This confirms again the view that the 31 myeloma-specific marker chromosomes encode the common, myeloma-specific neoplastic immortality

[30]. Further, the two antibody-negative (ab-) hybridomas H12 ab- and F3 ab- both lacked mouse chromosome 12. Notably chromosome 12 is also missing in the parental myeloma (Fig. 4a) and is known to encode the heavy chain of moues antibodies [36, 39, 40]. In view of this, we pointed out above that the absence of intact chromosome 12 in Hyb H12 ab- and Hyb F3 ab- and the lack of functional antibody in the parental myeloma Ag8 indicate that these two hybridomas must both be antibody-negative (see Results, Clonal phenotypes of hybridoma). As expected, the individual and common chromosomes of Hyb H12 ab- and Hyb F3 ab- shown above in the karyotypes of Fig. 3c, d. confirmed and extended the patterns of the two arrays shown here, namely that hybridomas contained numerous new chromosomes compared to the parental myeloma.

With regard to the mechanism of progression, we emphasize again that the numbers of clonal chromosomes of the hybridoma H12 ab- are 71 and those of F3 ab- are 79 (Tables 1 and 3) and are thus significantly higher than the 52 chromosomes of the parental myeloma Ag8. They differed from the parental myeloma in 19 and 27 additional, clonal chromosomes (Tables 1 and 3). These relatively high numerical gains of chromosomes by the hybridomas compared to the parental myeloma in the short times of fusions thus support again the single-step theory of progression.

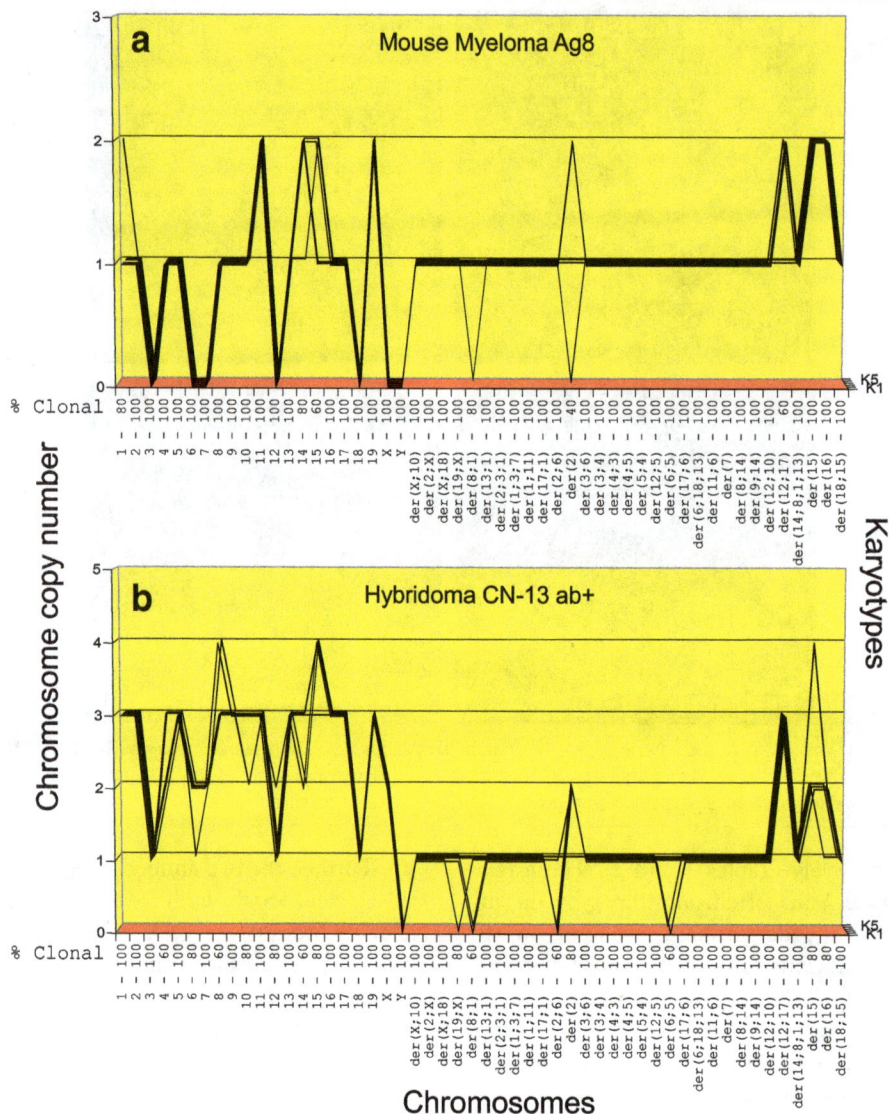

Fig. 4 a, b Karyotype-arrays of mouse myeloma Ag8 (**a**) and the corresponding hybridoma subspecies Hyb CN-13 ab + (**b**). Karyotype-arrays compare the copy numbers of individual chromosomes of multiple karyotypes of a potential cell clone in three-dimensional tables. The tables list the chromosome numbers of arrayed karyotypes, K1 to K5, on the x-axis, the copy numbers of each chromosome on the y-axis, and the number of the five karyotypes arrayed on the z-axis, as described by us [9, 11] and others [12]. Since chromosomes with the same copy numbers form parallel lines in 3-dimensonal karyotype arrays they visually identify clonality. The clonality of each chromosome in percent is listed on the abscissa of each array. Here we compared the karyotype array of myeloma Ag8 (**a**) to that of an antibody-producing (ab+) hybridoma subspecies Hyb CN-13 ab + (**b**). As can be seen in Fig. 4 and Table 2, hybridoma Hyb CN-13 ab + shared with the parental myeloma about 31 highly clonal, myeloma-specific marker chromosomes. In addition the hybridoma shared with the parental myeloma clonal copies of all myeloma-specific normal mouse chromosomes, although the copy numbers of shared mouse chromosomes were 2-3-fold higher in the hybridoma than in the myeloma. By contrast the myeloma lacked several normal mouse chromosomes. Based on the shared clonal myeloma-specific marker and normal mouse chromosomes, the hybridoma Hyb CN-13 ab + is a subspecies of the myeloma and the murine B-cell. It is consistent with the complete set of normal mouse B-cell chromosomes of this hybridoma that it produced antibodies

Karyotype-arrays of hybridomas Hyb 94 and Hyb 1-5 (Fig. 7a, b). As can be seen in Fig. 7a (and Table 3) the individual chromosome numbers of the five hybridoma Hyb 94 cells analyzed formed several non-parallel lines and accordingly ranged from 71 to 82 chromosomes per cell - for a clonal average of 74 (Table 1). This hybridoma is thus clonally heterogeneous. Nevertheless, all five

Hyb 94 karyotypes shared two Hyb 94-specific marker chromosomes and all but three of the 31 myeloma-specific chromosomes (Table 3). The Hyb 94 karyotypes are thus quasi-clonal, with copy numbers ranging from 40 to 100% clonality (Fig. 7a). The simplest explanation for the relatively high clonal heterogeneity of Hyb 94 suggests that this clone is a sub-clonal precursor of a

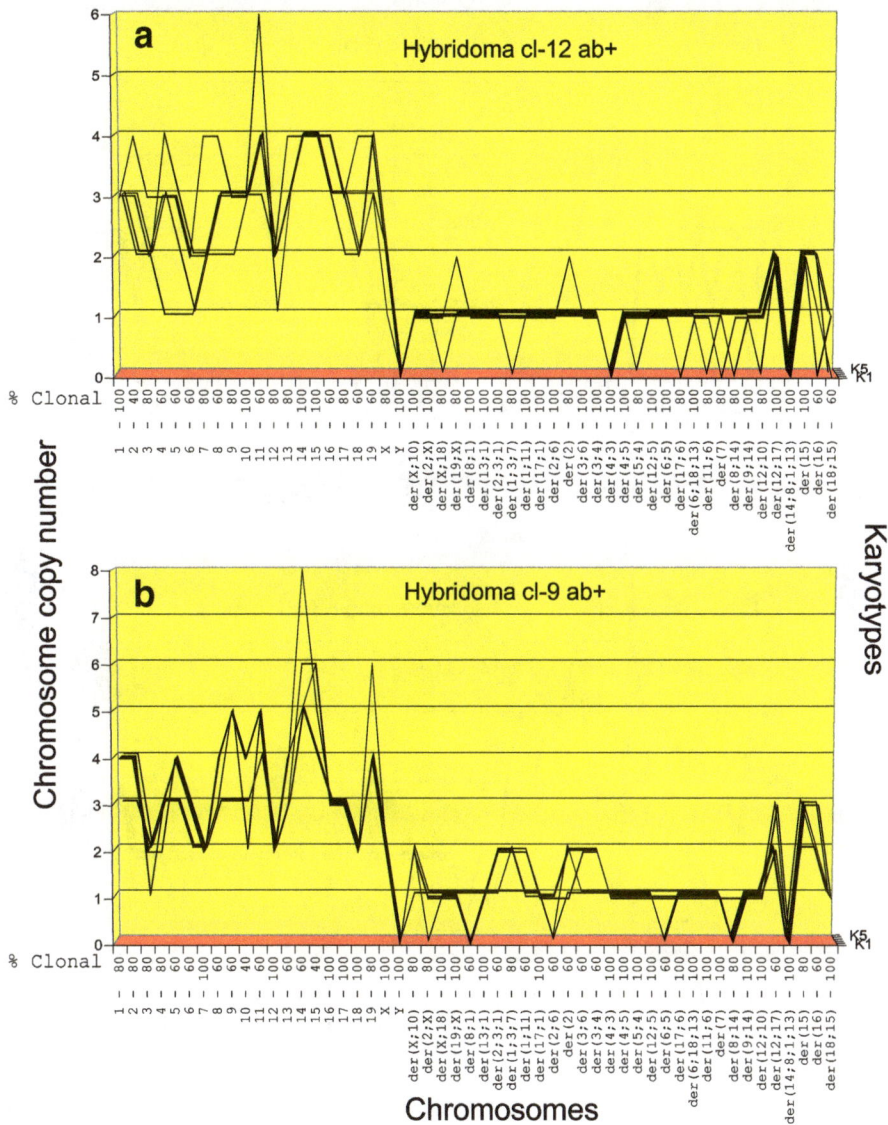

Fig. 5 a, b Karyotype-arrays of five cells (K1 to K5) of hybridoma Hyb cl-12 ab + (**a**) and hybridoma Hyb cl-9 ab + (**b**). As described in Fig. 4 karyotype-arrays reveal the clonality of cancer-specific chromosomes based on the percentage of cells with chromosomes that form parallel lines and thus have identical copy numbers. The arrays of hybridoma Hyb CN-13 ab + and of hybridoma Hyb cl-9 ab + shared highly clonal copies of all 31 myeloma-specific, abnormal marker chromosomes described in Fig. 4a and Table 2. They also share highly clonal copies of all normal mouse chromosomes from the parental B-cell, although at individually distinct copy numbers. Based on the shared clonal myeloma-specific and clonal normal mouse chromosomes shown in Table 2, the two hybridomas are individually distinct clonal subspecies of the myeloma and normal B-cell. The presence of complete sets of normal mouse chromosomes in both hybridomas is consistent with their production of mouse anti-bodies

hybridoma that is losing non-clonogenic chromosomes after it originated from a fusion of myeloma with B-cells. Such clonal heterogeneity has also been observed previously in metastases of solid cancers [11].

As shown in Fig. 7b, the karyotype array of Hyb 1-5 was also relatively heterogeneous. The clonality of chromosome numbers ranged from 40 to 100% and averaged at about 60% (Fig. 7b). Nevertheless, all five Hyb 1-5 karyotypes shared all but one of the 31 myeloma-specific chromosomes (Table 3). The simplest explanation for the high

clonal heterogeneity of Hyb 1-5 suggests again that this clone, like Hyb 94 above, is a heterogeneous precursor of a prospective hybridoma that is losing non-clonogenic chromosomes after it originated from an unstable fusion of myeloma with B-cells.

With regard to the mechanism of progression, we emphasize again that the average numbers of quasi-clonal chromosomes of hybridoma Hyb 94, namely 74, and of Hyb 1-5, namely 99, differed from the parental set of myeloma chromosomes by 22 and 47 additional chromosomes

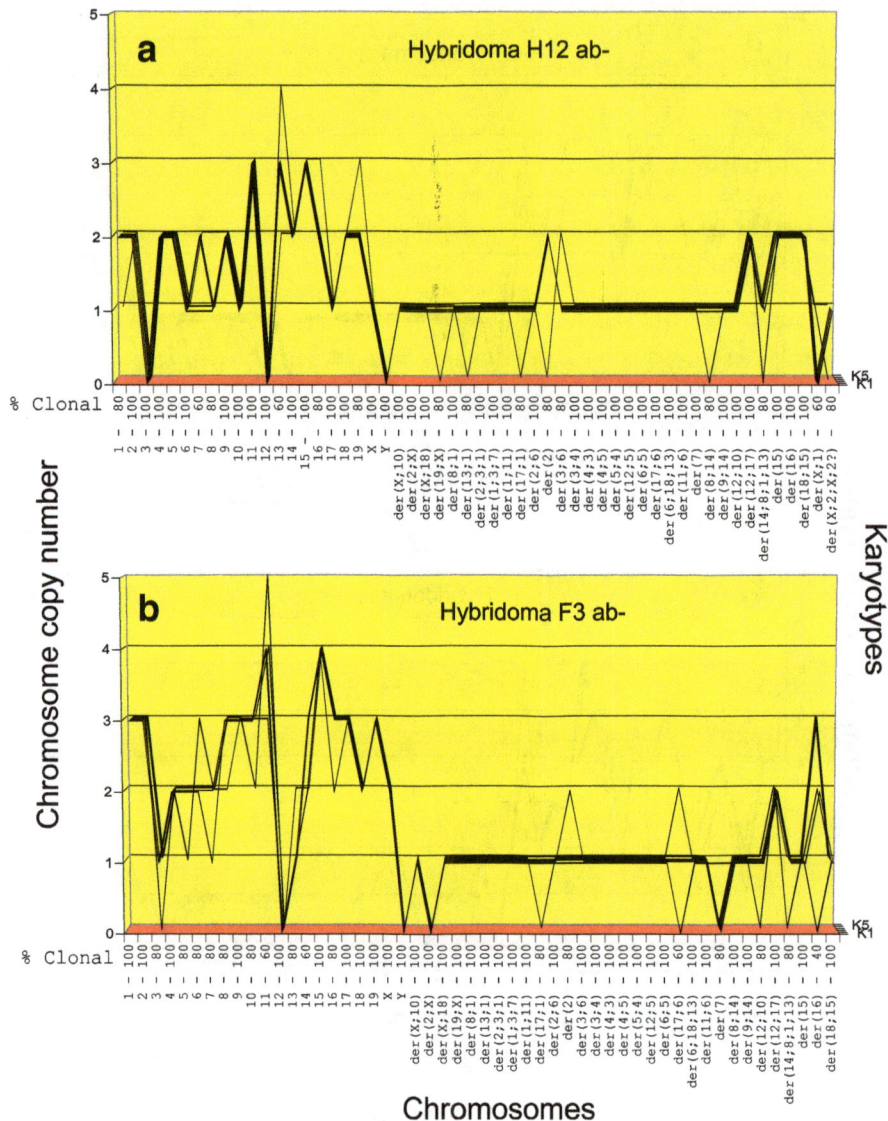

Fig. 6 a, **b** Karyotype-arrays of five cells of hybridoma Hyb 12 ab- (**a**) and hybridoma Hyb F3 ab- (**b**). The arrays of hybridoma Hyb 12 ab- and of hybridoma Hyb F3 ab- shared highly clonal copies of the 31 myeloma-specific marker chromosomes described in Fig. 4. They also shared highly clonal copies of all normal mouse chromosomes from the parental B-cell, although at individually distinct copy numbers. Based on the shared clonal myeloma-specific and normal mouse chromosomes (see Table 3), the two hybridomas are individually distinct, clonal subspecies of the myeloma and normal B-cells. The absence of normal mouse chromosome 12, which encodes the heavy chain of mouse antibodies in both hybridomas explains their failure to produce of mouse antibodies (see text, Are the chromosomes of hybridomas individual and clonal as predicted by the saltational theory?)

respectively (Table 1). This multiplicity of newly acquired chromosomes during the short fusion events again supports a single step model of fusion-mediated neoplastic progression, which continued to evolve after fusion.

Discussion

Multiple studies including ours have found "late" but also "immediate" progressions of cancers with numerous new, progression-specific chromosomes [14, 25, 41]. However no intermediates or prospective progressions with subsets of new progression-specific chromosomes were reported. In view of this and the existence of "immediate"

progressions with numerous new chromosomes we have advanced here the theory that neoplastic progressions are saltational events, in which all chromosomes of progressions are united in single steps. To test this saltational theory, we asked here, whether the numerous new chromosomes of most neoplastic progressions are acquired gradually or simultaneously in single steps.

Simultaneous acquisitions of numerous new chromosomes convert myelomas to immortal hybridomas in single steps

In view of evidence that neoplastic progressions of certain cancers, notably immortal hybridomas from myelomas

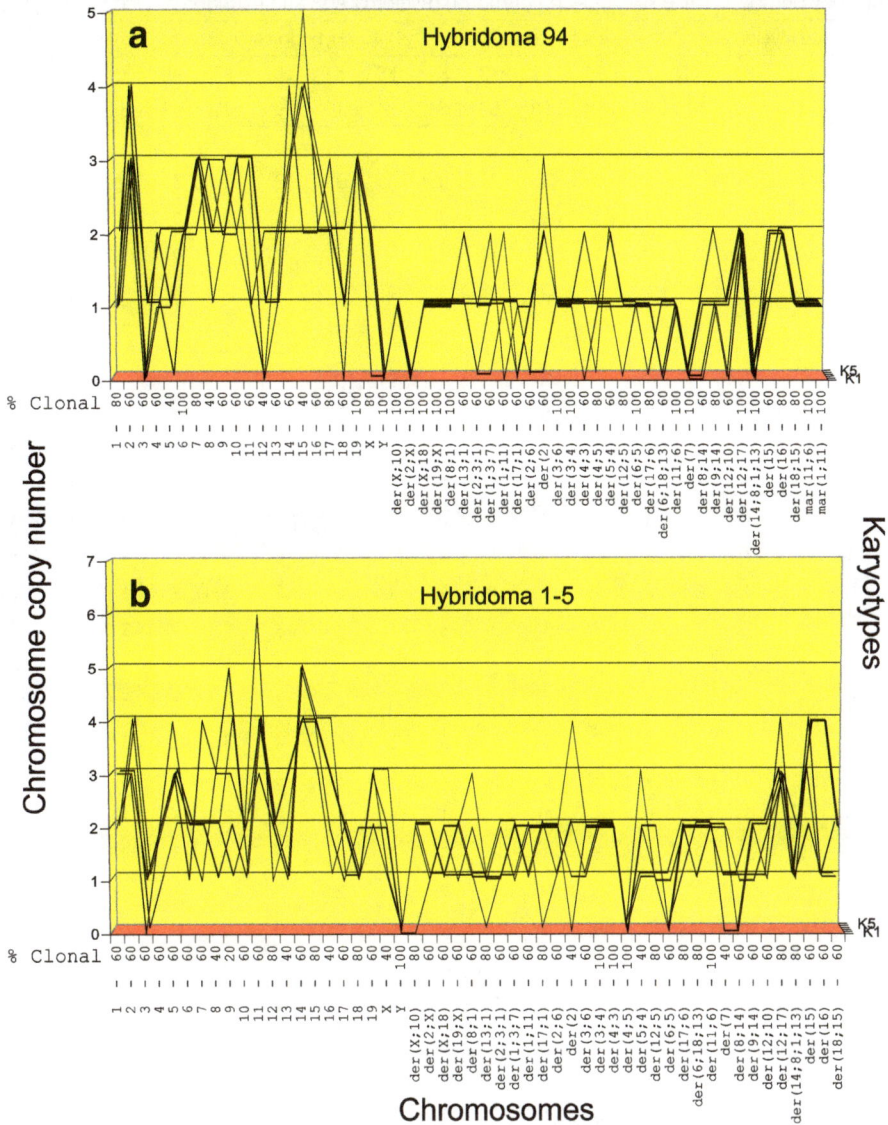

Fig. 7 a, b Karyotype-arrays of five cells of hybridoma Hyb 94 (**a**) and hybridoma Hyb 1-5 (**b**). Both hybridomas are clonally heterogeneous with chromosomal clonalities ranging from 40 to 100%. For example, the individual chromosome numbers of the five hybridoma Hyb 94 cells analyzed range from 71 to 82 for a clonal average of 74 (Tables 1 and 3). Nevertheless, all five Hyb 94 karyotypes shared 28 of the 31 myeloma-specific marker chromosomes and two Hyb 94-specific marker chromosomes (Table 3). The karyotype array of Hyb 1-5 was also relatively heterogeneous. Nevertheless, all five Hyb 1-5 karyotypes shared 30 of the 31 myeloma-specific marker chromosomes with the parental myeloma. In addition they shared all normal murine chromosomes with the parental mouse B-cell and some also with the parental myeloma. The simplest explanation for the high clonal heterogeneity of Hyb 94 and Hyb 105 suggests that these clones are still evolving precursor clones that are losing non-stabilizing chromosomes

can be generated within a few minutes by fusions of heterologous cells, we tested our saltational theory by analyses of the chromosomes of seven hybridomas for new hybridoma-specific chromosomes and for the absence of detectable intermediates.

As shown in Table 1, our experiments demonstrated that seven individual and immortal hybridomas had indeed gained from 19 to 53 chromosomes from fusions with B-cells within a few minutes – and that there were no detectable intermediates. We also show in Table 1 that these seven hybridomas differed from a theoretical parental hybrid of 92 chromosomes (52 myeloma and 40 B-cell chromosomes) in gains of 13 to losses of 21 chromosomes. These discrepancies between the experimental and theoretical sums of chromosome numbers confirmed original observations of Kohler and Milstein and subsequent studies by Wollweber et al. [23, 26].

In view of these results, we conclude that hybridomas are generated by haphazard combinations of the chromosomes of fused cells in single steps. This conclusion explains the fast kinetics of hybridomagenesis, the absence of karyotypic intermediates, the low yields of only

Table 2 Chromosome copy numbers of five kayotypes (K) of mouse myeloma Ag8 and hybridomas Hyb cl-12, Hyb CN-13 and Hyb cl-9

Clone	Mouse Myeloma					Hybridoma CN-13					Hybridoma cl-12					Hybridoma cl-9				
Karyotypes	K1	K2	K3	K4	K5	K1	K2	K3	K4	K5	K1	K2	K3	K4	K5	K1	K2	K3	K4	K5
Chromosome Copy #	53	53	51	51	49	84	88	87	84	84	101	90	75	89	87	113	115	111	90	95
Chromosomes																				
1	1	1	2	1	1	3	3	3	3	3	3	3	3	3	3	4	4	4	3	4
2	1	1	1	1	1	3	3	3	3	3	4	3	2	3	2	4	4	4	3	4
3	0	0	0	0	0	1	1	1	1	1	3	2	2	2	2	2	2	1	2	2
4	1	1	1	1	1	2	2	3	3	2	3	3	1	4	3	2	3	3	3	3
5	1	1	1	1	1	3	3	3	3	3	3	3	1	3	2	4	4	4	3	3
6	0	0	0	0	0	2	2	2	1	2	2	2	1	2	1	3	3	3	2	2
7	0	0	0	0	0	2	2	2	2	2	4	2	2	2	2	2	2	2	2	2
8	1	1	1	1	1	4	3	3	3	4	4	3	2	3	3	3	4	4	3	3
9	1	1	1	1	1	3	3	3	3	3	3	3	2	3	3	5	5	5	3	3
10	1	1	1	1	1	3	3	3	2	3	3	3	3	3	3	4	4	2	3	3
11	2	2	2	2	2	3	3	3	3	3	6	4	3	4	4	5	5	5	4	4
12	0	0	0	0	0	1	2	1	1	1	2	2	2	2	1	2	2	2	2	2
13	1	1	1	1	1	3	3	3	3	3	4	3	3	3	3	4	3	4	3	3
14	2	2	2	2	1	2	3	3	3	2	4	4	4	4	4	5	6	8	5	5
15	2	1	1	2	2	4	3	4	4	4	4	4	4	4	4	6	6	5	4	4
16	1	1	1	1	1	3	3	3	3	3	4	4	3	3	3	3	3	3	3	3
17	1	1	1	1	1	3	3	3	3	3	3	3	2	3	3	3	3	3	3	3
18	0	0	0	0	0	1	1	1	1	1	4	2	2	3	2	2	2	2	2	2
19	2	2	2	2	2	3	3	3	3	3	4	4	3	3	4	4	6	4	4	4
X	0	0	0	0	0	2	2	2	2	2	2	2	1	2	2	2	2	2	2	2
Y	0	0	0	0	0	0	0	0	0	0	0	0	0	0	0	0	0	0	0	0
der(X;10)	1	1	1	1	1	1	1	1	1	1	1	1	1	1	1	2	2	2	1	2
der(2;X)	1	1	1	1	1	1	1	1	1	1	1	1	1	1	1	1	1	0	1	1
der(X;18)	1	1	1	1	1	1	1	1	1	1	1	1	1	0	1	1	1	1	1	1
der(19;X)	1	1	1	1	1	1	0	1	1	1	2	1	1	1	1	1	1	1	1	1
der(8;1)	1	1	1	1	0	0	1	1	1	0	1	1	1	1	1	0	0	0	1	1
der(13;1)	1	1	1	1	1	1	1	1	1	1	1	1	1	1	1	1	1	1	1	1
der(2;3;1)	1	1	1	1	1	1	1	1	1	1	1	1	1	1	1	2	2	2	1	1
der(1;3;7)	1	1	1	1	1	1	1	1	1	1	1	1	0	1	1	2	2	2	2	1
der(1;11)	1	1	1	1	1	1	1	1	1	1	1	1	1	1	1	2	1	2	1	1
der(17;1)	1	1	1	1	1	1	1	1	1	1	1	1	1	1	1	1	1	1	1	1
der(2;6)	1	1	1	1	1	0	1	0	1	0	1	1	1	1	1	1	1	1	0	0
der(2)	2	2	1	0	1	2	2	2	1	2	2	1	1	1	1	1	2	2	1	2
der(3;6)	1	1	1	1	1	1	1	1	1	1	1	1	1	1	1	2	2	2	1	1
der(3;4)	1	1	1	1	1	1	1	1	1	1	1	1	1	1	1	2	2	2	1	1
der(4;3)	1	1	1	1	1	1	1	1	1	1	0	0	0	0	0	1	1	1	1	1
der(4;5)	1	1	1	1	1	1	1	1	1	1	1	1	1	1	1	1	1	1	1	1
der(5;4)	1	1	1	1	1	1	1	1	1	1	1	1	1	1	0	1	1	1	1	1
der(12;5)	1	1	1	1	1	1	1	1	1	1	1	1	1	1	1	1	1	1	1	1
der(6;5)	1	1	1	1	1	0	1	1	1	0	1	1	1	1	1	1	1	0	0	1
der(17;6)	1	1	1	1	1	1	1	1	1	1	0	1	1	1	1	1	1	1	1	1

Table 2 Chromosome copy numbers of five kayotypes (K) of mouse myeloma Ag8 and hybridomas Hyb cl-12, Hyb CN-13 and Hyb cl-9 *(Continued)*

Clone	Mouse Myeloma					Hybridoma CN-13					Hybridoma cl-12					Hybridoma cl-9				
Karyotypes	K1	K2	K3	K4	K5	K1	K2	K3	K4	K5	K1	K2	K3	K4	K5	K1	K2	K3	K4	K5
Chromosome Copy #	53	53	51	51	49	84	88	87	84	84	101	90	75	89	87	113	115	111	90	95
der(6;18;13)	1	1	1	1	1	1	1	1	1	1	1	1	1	1	1	1	1	1	1	1
der(11;6)	1	1	1	1	1	1	1	1	1	1	1	1	0	1	1	1	1	1	1	1
der(7)	1	1	1	1	1	1	1	1	1	1	0	1	1	1	1	1	1	1	1	1
der(8;14)	1	1	1	1	1	1	1	1	1	1	1	0	1	1	1	1	0	0	0	0
der(9;14)	1	1	1	1	1	1	1	1	1	1	1	1	1	1	1	1	1	1	1	1
der(12;10)	1	1	1	1	1	1	1	1	1	1	1	1	0	1	1	1	1	1	1	1
der(12;17)	2	2	1	2	1	3	3	3	3	3	2	2	2	2	2	3	2	3	2	2
der(14;8;1;13)	1	1	1	1	1	1	1	1	1	1	0	0	0	0	0	0	0	0	0	0
der(15)	2	2	2	2	2	2	4	2	2	2	2	2	2	2	2	3	3	3	2	3
der(16)	2	2	2	2	2	2	2	2	1	2	1	0	2	2	2	3	2	3	2	2
der(18;15)	1	1	1	1	1	1	1	1	1	1	0	1	1	0	1	1	1	1	1	1
Non-Clonal Markers	0	1	0	0	0	0	0	0	0	0	2	2	0	0	2	3	4	2	0	0

about one viable hybridoma per 10^4-5 fused cells (Background), and the individuality of the resulting hybridomas described here and previously (Background and references [9, 11, 23, 26, 30]).

Are saltational single-step mechanisms also generating spontaneous, late neoplastic progressions?

The following rare observations on the origin of spontaneous neoplastic progressions also support the saltational theory of neoplastic progressions:

1) Distinguishing between paternal and maternal chromosomes by restriction length polymorphisms Onodera et al. found in 1992 highly symmetric distributions of paternal and maternal chromosomes in hyperdiploid leukemias. The authors concluded that, "These results suggest that the hyperdiploid karyotype usually arises by simultaneous gain of chromosomes from a diploid karyotype during a single abnormal cell division" [42]. This study was confirmed and extended by Paulsson et al. in 2005 [43].

2) Studying progression of prostate cancers in 2013 Baca et al. detected "considerable genomic derangement over relatively few events in prostate cancer and other neoplasms, supporting a model of punctuated cancer evolution." [44].

3) Stepanenko et al. observed in 2015 that, "Transfection of either the empty vector pcDNA3.1 or pcDNA3.1 CHI3L1 (a growth factor) into 293-cells (a human embryo kidney cell line) initiated the punctuated genome changes" of simultaneous gains and losses of chromosomes [12].

4) Studying the progression of breast cancers Gao et al. observed by whole genome sequencing in 2016, "Despite profiling hundreds of single cells from many spatial regions, we did not detect any intermediate copy number profiles, indicative of gradual evolution," and concluded, "our data challenge the paradigm of gradual evolution" [45].

5) In a comparison of single with multi-hit or "linear" theories of metastatic progressions in 2016 Turajlic and Swanton conclude, "It is conceivable that macroevolutionary leaps (large-scale genomic alterations) could catalyze all the steps to metastases, especially in narrow time frames" [46] – much as those studied by us here.

Further we have shown previously that spontaneous metastatic and drug-resistant progressions have individual clonal karyotypes with numerous progression-specific chomosomes [11, 34], just as the hybridomas studied here. The individuality, complexity and clonality of the karyotypes [9–11] and transcriptomes [10, 32] of spontneous progressions indicate, however, a saltational, speciation-type of event [9, 47, 48] – much like the saltational events we found here for hybridomas.

It would appear then that saltational, single step mechanisms could generate rare progressions "early" and "late" by spontaneous karyotypic rearrangements (see Background, Alternative single-step theory of progression), independent of cell fusions. Accordingly the typically long latencies between cancers and progressions would simply reflect the low probabilities of speciation by random karyotypic variations.

Nevertheless, there is also sporadic evidence for a role of cell fusions in spontaneous progressions based on

Table 3 Chromosome copy numbers of five karyotypes (K) of mouse hybridomas Hyb H12, Hyb F3, Hyb 94 and Hyb 1-5

Clone	Hybridoma H12					Hybridoma F3					Hybridoma 94					Hybridoma 1-5				
Karyotypes	K1	K2	K3	K4	K5	K1	K2	K3	K4	K5	K1	K2	K3	K4	K5	K1	K2	K3	K4	K5
Chromosome Copy #	71	70	71	68	75	77	78	80	81	81	71	77	71	71	82	107	105	93	89	99
Chromosomes																				
1	2	2	2	1	2	3	3	3	3	3	1	1	1	2	1	2	3	2	3	2
2	2	2	2	2	2	3	3	3	3	3	3	4	3	4	3	3	3	4	3	4
3	0	0	0	0	0	1	1	0	1	1	0	0	0	1	1	0	1	1	0	1
4	2	2	2	2	2	2	2	2	2	2	1	2	1	1	2	2	2	2	1	2
5	2	2	2	2	2	2	2	1	2	2	1	1	2	0	2	4	3	3	2	3
6	1	1	1	1	1	2	2	3	2	2	2	2	2	2	2	2	1	2	2	2
7	1	2	2	1	2	1	2	2	2	2	2	3	3	3	3	1	4	2	2	2
8	1	1	1	1	2	3	3	2	3	3	3	3	2	1	2	3	3	1	2	2
9	2	2	2	2	2	3	3	3	3	3	2	3	2	2	3	5	3	2	1	4
10	1	1	1	1	1	3	3	3	2	3	2	2	3	3	3	2	2	1	2	1
11	3	3	3	3	3	4	4	3	5	4	3	1	1	3	3	6	3	4	4	4
12	0	0	0	0	0	0	0	0	0	0	0	0	2	1	1	1	2	2	2	2
13	3	3	3	2	4	1	1	1	2	1	2	1	2	1	2	2	1	3	1	3
14	2	2	2	2	2	2	2	3	2	3	3	4	2	3	3	4	5	4	5	4
15	3	3	3	3	3	4	4	4	4	4	4	2	2	5	4	4	4	4	4	3
16	2	2	2	2	3	2	3	3	3	3	3	2	2	2	3	2	3	3	4	1
17	1	1	1	1	1	3	3	3	3	3	2	3	2	2	2	1	2	2	1	2
18	2	2	2	2	2	2	2	2	2	2	0	1	1	1	2	2	1	1	1	1
19	2	2	2	2	3	3	3	3	3	3	3	3	3	3	3	2	3	2	3	3
X	1	1	1	1	1	2	2	2	2	2	2	2	0	2	2	2	2	1	1	3
Y	0	0	0	0	0	0	0	0	0	0	0	0	0	0	0	0	0	0	0	0
der(X;10)	1	1	1	1	1	1	1	1	1	1	1	1	1	1	1	0	2	2	2	2
der(2;X)	1	1	1	1	1	0	0	0	0	0	0	0	0	0	0	1	1	2	2	1
der(X;18)	1	1	1	1	1	1	1	1	1	1	1	1	1	1	1	2	2	1	1	1
der(19;X)	1	1	0	1	1	1	1	1	1	1	1	1	1	1	1	1	2	2	1	2
der(8;1)	1	1	1	1	1	1	1	1	1	1	1	1	1	1	1	2	3	1	1	1
der(13;1)	1	1	1	1	0	1	1	1	1	1	2	2	1	1	1	1	1	1	0	1
der(2;3;1)	1	1	1	1	1	1	1	1	1	1	1	1	1	0	0	2	1	1	1	2
der(1;3;7)	1	1	1	1	1	1	1	1	1	1	2	1	1	0	1	1	2	2	1	2
der(1;11)	1	1	1	1	1	1	1	1	1	1	0	2	1	1	1	2	2	1	2	1
der(17;1)	1	1	1	1	0	1	1	1	0	1	1	0	0	1	1	2	2	2	0	2
der(2;6)	1	1	1	1	1	1	1	1	1	1	1	1	1	0	0	2	2	2	1	1
der(2)	2	2	2	2	0	1	2	1	1	1	2	2	2	3	0	4	0	1	2	2
der(3;6)	1	1	1	1	2	1	1	1	1	1	1	1	1	1	1	2	2	1	2	1
der(3;4)	1	1	1	1	1	1	1	1	1	1	1	1	1	1	1	2	2	2	2	2
der(4;3)	1	1	1	1	1	1	1	1	1	1	0	2	1	1	1	2	2	2	2	2
der(4;5)	1	1	1	1	1	1	1	1	1	1	1	1	1	1	0	0	0	0	0	0
der(5;4)	1	1	1	1	1	1	1	1	1	1	1	2	1	1	2	2	2	1	3	1
der(12;5)	1	1	1	1	1	1	1	1	1	1	1	1	0	1	1	1	2	1	1	1
der(6;5)	1	1	1	1	1	1	1	1	1	1	1	1	1	1	1	1	0	0	0	1
der(17;6)	1	1	1	1	1	0	1	1	2	1	1	1	1	0	1	2	2	2	1	2

Table 3 Chromosome copy numbers of five karyotypes (K) of mouse hybridomas Hyb H12, Hyb F3, Hyb 94 and Hyb 1-5 (Continued)

Clone	Hybridoma H12					Hybridoma F3					Hybridoma 94					Hybridoma 1-5				
Karyotypes	K1	K2	K3	K4	K5	K1	K2	K3	K4	K5	K1	K2	K3	K4	K5	K1	K2	K3	K4	K5
Chromosome Copy #	71	70	71	68	75	77	78	80	81	81	71	77	71	71	82	107	105	93	89	99
der(6;18;13)	1	1	1	1	1	1	1	1	1	1	0	1	0	1	1	2	2	1	2	2
der(11;6)	1	1	1	1	1	1	1	1	1	1	1	1	1	1	1	2	2	2	2	2
der(7)	1	1	1	1	1	1	0	0	0	0	0	0	0	0	0	2	0	2	1	1
der(8;14)	1	0	1	1	1	1	1	1	1	1	0	1	0	1	1	1	0	0	1	1
der(9;14)	1	1	1	1	1	1	1	1	1	1	1	1	1	1	2	1	2	2	1	2
der(12;10)	1	1	1	1	1	1	1	1	0	1	0	1	0	1	1	2	1	2	1	2
der(12;17)	2	2	2	2	2	2	2	2	2	2	2	2	2	2	2	3	3	3	4	3
der(14;8;1;13)	1	0	1	1	1	1	1	1	0	1	0	0	0	0	0	2	1	1	1	1
der(15)	2	2	2	2	2	1	1	1	1	1	2	1	2	1	1	4	4	2	4	3
der(16)	2	2	2	2	2	2	0	2	3	3	2	2	2	1	2	4	4	1	1	1
der(18;15)	2	2	2	2	2	1	1	1	1	1	1	1	1	1	2	2	2	1	2	1
der(X;1)	0	0	0	1	1															
der(X;2;X;2?)	1	1	1	0	1															
mar(11;6)											1	1	1	1	1					
mar(1;11)											1	1	1	1	1					
Non-Clonal Markers	1	1	1	0	2	0	0	3	2	0	1	1	6	0	4	0	1	3	0	3

several independent studies that were recently reviewed by Lazebnick [49].

Finally, it did not escape our attention that the single-step theory of progression or subspeciation of cancers advanced here and previously [7, 10, 11, 33, 34, 48] derives independent support from chromosomal theories postulating that conventional speciations or subspeciations also occur in single saltational steps - without stable intermediates [47, 50–53].

Conclusions

We conclude that the evidence from the hybridoma model tested here and the independent observations of others including us about spontaneous clonal progressions are based on saltational recombinations of cancer chromosomes or of cancer chromosomes with chromosomes of heterologous cells. This model encourages the following clinically relevant conclusions:

1) Our analysis of the karyotypic basis of progressions here and previously [9–11] indicates that the progressions of cancers are clonal and thus probably the proximate causes of neoplastic progressions. This conclusion confirms and extends a prior prediction of Heng et al. [54].

2) The inherent karyotypic variability of cancer- and progression-specific aneuploidy (Background) thus explains and supports Foulds' rule, that "progression does not always reach an end-point within the life-span of the host" [1], and Nowell's similar

observation, "that the process is a continuing one" [41]. Therefore, we conclude that progressions of progressions are a lasting concern [1, 12], particularly since progressions are responsible for 90% of the mortality of cancers [55, 56].

3) Further we propose that the degree of cancer-specific aneuploidy predicts the clinical risk of neoplastic progression, because cancer-specific aneuploidy catalyzes karyotypic variation. This view thus confirms and extends classical predictions based on DNA content [57–61].

Methods

Preparation of hybridomas

Thymidine-kinase deficient myeloma Ag8 cells and B-cells from mice, induced to produce antibodies with specific antigens, were fused at equal numbers for about 5-10 min in about 50% polyethylene glycol following established methods of Zeitler and Beatty (UC Berkeley, above) and of the literature [26, 35, 36]. After fusions the cells were washed and incubated at 37 C for one to 2 days in selective medium containing aminopterin, which inhibits natural thymidine synthesis and thymidine, which substitutes lacking thymidine after fusion with B-cells (Sigma Co, St Louis, MO or ATCC, Rockville, MD). In these conditions fused Ag8 myeloma cells survive from added thymidine picked up by B-cell-derived thymidine kinase. Within a few days after fusion, un-fused myeloma cells die out due to lack of thymidine and toxicity of aminopterin, and un-fused B-cells perish spontaneously within several generations in culture. At that time normal medium was used for the propagation of surviving hybridoma cells. One to 2 weeks later microscopic clones appeared, which were then sub-cultured in conventional RPMI 1640 medium supplemented with 10% fetal calf serum following published procedures [23, 26, 35, 36]. Clonal cultures of immortalized myeloma-B-cell hybrids arose from fusions at rates of about one hybridoma per 10^4 to 5 myeloma cells. Hybridoma cells were then propagated in suspension cultures in RPMI 1640 medium supplemented with 10% to 20% fetal calf serum and 1% of 100× *Antibiotic Antimycotic* (Sigma Co, St Louis, USA).

Karyotypic analyses myeloma and hybridoma cells

One to 2 days before karyotyping, cells were seeded at about 50% confluence in a 5-cm culture dish with 3 ml of the medium described above. After reaching ~75% quasi-confluence, 250–300 ng colcemid in 25–30 µl solution (KaryoMax, Gibco) was added to 3 ml medium. The culture was then incubated at 37 °C for 4–8 h. Subsequently cells were washed twice with 3 ml of physiological saline and then incubated in 0.075 M KCl at 37 °C for 15 min. The cell suspension was then cooled in ice-water, mixed ('prefixed') with 0.1 volume of the freshly mixed glacial acetic acid-methanol (1:3, vol. per vol.) and centrifuged at 800 g for 6 min at room temperature. The cell pellet was then suspended in about 100 µl supernatant and mixed drop-wise with 5 ml of the ice-cold acetic acid-methanol solution and then incubated at room temperature for 15–30 min or overnight at 5C. This cell suspension was then pelleted and was then either once more re-suspended in fixative and pelleted, or was directly re-suspended in a small volume of the acetic acid-methanol solution for microscopic examination. For this purpose an aliquot of a visually turbid suspension was transferred with a micropipette tip to a glass microscope slide, allowed to evaporate at room temperature and inspected under the microscope at 200× for an adequate, non-overlapping density of metaphase chromosomes. Metaphase chromosomes attached to glass slides were then hybridized to color-coded, mouse chromosome-specific DNA probes as described by the manufacturer, *MetaSystems* (Newton, MA 02458). Chromosomes were then sorted into conventional karyotypes with a computerized Zeiss Imager M1 microscope, programmed by *MetaSystems* (Newton, MA 02458) following published procedures [11, 33, 34, 61].

Acknowledgments

We thank Karen Davies (Lawrence Berkeley Lab and UC Berkeley, Donner Lab); Yuri Lazebnik, Yale Cardiovascular Research Center; New Haven, CT USA; Mark Vincent, University of Western Ontario Oncology, Ontario, Canada and Peter Walian (Lawrence Berkeley National Laboratory, Donner Lab, Berkeley CA) for critical reviews of this manuscript and for stimulating discussions and ideas. David Raulet (UCB) is thanked for valuable advice and discussions. We thank especially Jennifer Zeitler and Robert Beatty for the gifts of hybridomas and myeloma and for the preparation and testing these cells. Bong-Gyoon Han (Lawrence Berkeley National Laboratory, Donner Lab at UC Berkeley) is specifically thanked for drafting and designing Fig. 1. In addition we are grateful to two UC Berkeley interns Ankit Hirpara and Nicholas Brady, and also Kelly Yang (Head Royce High School) for karyotyping hybridoma and myeloma cells and for stimulating questions and ideas. P.D. thanks Sigrid Duesberg for asking new questions about several drafts of this paper. Our study would not have been possible without the generous support of the philanthropists Robert Leppo (San Francisco CA, USA), Christian Fiala (Gynmed Ambulatorium, Mariahilferguertel 37, Vienna, Austria), Peter Rozsa (Taubert Memorial Foundation, Cottage Grove OR 97424), Richard Fischer (Alexandria VA) and the support of the Vice Provost for the Faculty Benjamin Hermalin by two very timely grants at $4000 per year from the *Berkeley Excellence Accounts for Research*.

Funding

Private sources (see Acknowledgments).

Authors' contributions

MB and PD equally participated in planning and conducting experiments and writing of the manuscript. Both authors read and approved the final manuscript.

Competing interests

The authors declare that they have no competing interests.

Author details

[1]Department of Molecular and Cell Biology, Donner Laboratory, University of California at Berkeley, Berkeley, CA 94720, USA. [2]Present address: Department of Natural Sciences and Mathematics, Dominican University of California, San Rafael, CA, USA.

References

1. Foulds L. Tumor progression: a review. Cancer Res. 1954;14:327–39.
2. Kovacs G. Papillary renal cell carcinoma. A morphologic and cytogenetic study of 11 cases. Am J Pathol. 1989;134(1):27–34.
3. Nishizaki T, DeVries S, Chew K, Goodson WH 3rd, Ljung BM, Thor A, Waldman FM. Genetic alterations in primary breast cancers and their metastases: direct comparison using modified comparative genomic hybridization. Gen Chrom Canc. 1997;19(4):267–72.
4. Bissig H, Richter J, Desper R, Meier V, Schraml P, Schaffer AA, Sauter G, Mihatsch MJ, Moch H. Evaluation of the clonal relationship between primary and metastatic renal cell carcinoma by comparative genomic hybridization. Am J Pathol. 1999;155(1):267–74.
5. Achuthan R, Bell SM, Roberts P, Leek JP, Horgan K, Markham AF, MacLennan KA, Speirs V. Genetic events during the transformation of a tamoxifen-sensitive human breast cancer cell line into a drug-resistant clone. Cancer Genet Cytogenet. 2001;130(2):166–72.
6. Tonnies H, Poland J, Sinha P, Lage H. Association of genomic imbalances with drug resistance and thermoresistance in human gastric carcinoma cells. Int J Cancer. 2003;103(6):752–8.

7. Li R, Hehlmann R, Sachs R, Duesberg P. Chromosomal alterations cause the high rates and wide ranges of drug resistance in cancer cells. Cancer Genet Cytogenet. 2005;163(1):44–56.

8. Duesberg P, Li R, Sachs R, Fabarius A, Upender MB, Hehlmann R. Cancer drug resistance: the central role of the karyotype. Drug Resist Updat. 2007; 10(1-2):51–8.

9. Duesberg P, Mandrioli D, McCormack A, Nicholson JM. Is carcinogenesis a form of speciation? Cell Cycle. 2011;10(13):2100–14.

10. Duesberg P, Iacobuzio-Donahue C, Brosnan JA, McCormack A, Mandrioli D, Chen L. Origin of metastases: subspecies of cancers generated by intrinsic karyotypic variations. Cell Cycle. 2012;11(6):1151–66.

11. Bloomfield M, Duesberg P. Inherent variability of cancer-specific aneuploidy generates metastases. Mol Cytogenet. 2016;9:90.

12. Stepanenko A, Andreieva S, Korets K, Mykytenko D, Huleyuk N, Vassetzky Y, Kavsan V. Step-wise and punctuated genome evolution drive phenotype changes of tumor cells. Mutat Res. 2015;771:56–69.

13. Gao C, Su Y, Koeman J, Haak E, Dykema K, Essenberg C, Hudson E, Petillo D, Khoo SK, Vande Woude GF. Chromosome instability drives phenotypic switching to metastasis. Proc Natl Acad Sci U S A. 2016;113(51):14793–8.

14. Nowell PC. The clonal evolution of tumor cell populations. Science. 1976; 194(4260):23–8.

15. Granzow C, Nielsen K. A genome mutation in three related sublines of the Ehrlich-lettre mouse ascites tumor. Hereditas. 1984;100(1):93–110.

16. Duesberg P, Stindl R, Hehlmann R. Origin of multidrug resistance in cells with and without multidrug resistance genes: chromosome reassortments catalyzed by aneuploidy. Proc Natl Acad Sci U S A. 2001;98(20):11283–8.

17. Kerbel RS, Dennis JW, Largarde AE, Frost P. Tumor progression in metastasis: an experimental approach using lectin resistant tumor variants. Cancer Metastasis Rev. 1982;1(2):99–140.

18. Lagarde AE, Donaghue TP, Dennis JW, Kerbel RS. Genotypic and phenotypic evolution of a murine tumor during its progression in vivo toward metastasis. J Natl Cancer Inst. 1983;71(1):183–91.

19. Barski G, Cornefert F. Charactersitics of "hybrid"-type clonal cell lines obtained from mixed cultures in vitro. J Natl Cancer Inst. 1962;28:801–21.

20. Ephrussi B, Sorieul S. New observations on the in vitro hybridization of mouse cells. C R Hebd Seances Acad Sci. 1962;254:181–2.

21. Littlefield JW. Selection of hybrids from Matings of fibroblasts in vitro and their presumed recombinants. Science. 1964;145(3633):709–10.

22. Wiener F, Cochran A, Klein G, Harris H. Genetic determinants of morphological differentiation in hybrid tumors. J Natl Cancer Inst. 1972;48(2):465–86.

23. Kohler G, Milstein C. Continuous cultures of fused cells secreting antibody of predefined specificity. Nature. 1975;256(5517):495–7.

24. Stanbridge EJ, Flandermeyer RR, Daniels DW, Nelson-Rees WA. Specific chromosome loss associated with the expression of tumorigenicity in human cell hybrids. Somatic Cell Genet. 1981;7(6):699–712.

25. Benedict WF, Weissman BE, Mark C, Stanbridge EJ. Tumorigenicity of human HT1080 fibrosarcoma X normal fibroblast hybrids: chromosome dosage dependency. Cancer Res. 1984;44(8):3471–9.

26. Wollweber L, Munster H, Hoffmann S, Siller K, Greulich KO. Early phase karyotype analysis of chromosome segregation after formation of mouse-mouse hybridomas with chromosome painting probes. Chromosom Res. 2000;8(1):37–44.

27. Vogelstein B, Papadopoulos N, Velculescu VE, Zhou S, Diaz LA Jr, Kinzler KW. Cancer genome landscapes. Science. 2013;339(6127):1546–58.

28. Li L, McCormack AA, Nicholson JM, Fabarius A, Hehlmann R, Sachs RK, Duesberg PH. Cancer-causing karyotypes: chromosomal equilibria between destabilizing aneuploidy and stabilizing selection for oncogenic function. Cancer Genet Cytogenet. 2009;188(1):1–25.

29. Nicholson JM, Duesberg P. On the karyotypic origin and evolution of cancer cells. Cancer Genet Cytogenet. 2009;194(2):96–110.

30. Duesberg P, McCormack A. Immortality of cancers: a consequence of inherent karyotypic variations and selections for autonomy. Cell Cycle. 2013; 12(5):783–802.

31. Duesberg PH. Does aneuploidy destabilize karyotypes automatically? Proc Natl Acad Sci U S A. 2014;111(11):E974.

32. Chen X, Cheung ST, So S, Fan ST, Barry C, Higgins J, Lai KM, Ji J, Dudoit S, Ng IO et al: Gene expression patterns in human liver cancers. Mol Biol Cell. 2002;13(6):1929–939.

33. Bloomfield M, McCormack A, Mandrioli D, Fiala C, Aldaz CM, Duesberg P. Karyotypic evolutions of cancer species in rats during the long latent periods after injection of nitrosourea. Mol Cytogenet. 2014;7(1):71.

34. Bloomfield M, Duesberg P. Karyotype alteration generates the neoplastic phenotypes of SV40-infected human and rodent cells. Mol Cytogenet. 2015;8:79.

35. Gefter ML, Margulies DH, Scharff MD. A simple method for polyethylene glycol-promoted hybridization of mouse myeloma cells. Somatic Cell Genet. 1977;3(2):231–6.

36. Davis JM, Pennington JE, Kubler AM, Conscience JF. A simple, single-step technique for selecting and cloning hybridomas for the production of monoclonal antibodies. J Immunol Methods. 1982;50(2):161–71.

37. Oshimura M, Koi M, Ozawa N, Sugawara O, Lamb PW, Barrett JC. Role of chromosome loss in ras/myc-induced Syrian hamster tumors. Cancer Res. 1988;48(6):1623–32.

38. Karpas A, Dremucheva A, Czepulkowski BH. A human myeloma cell line suitable for the generation of human monoclonal antibodies. Proc Natl Acad Sci U S A. 2001;98(4):1799–804.

39. Ohno S, Babonits M, Wiener F, Spira J, Klein G, Potter M. Nonrandom chromosome changes involving the Ig gene-carrying chromosomes 12 and 6 in pristane-induced mouse plasmacytomas. Cell. 1979;18(4):1001–7.

40. Kearney JF, Radbruch A, Liesegang B, Rajewsky K. A new mouse myeloma cell line that has lost immunoglobulin expression but permits the construction of antibody-secreting hybrid cell lines. J Immunol. 1979;123(4):1548–50.

41. Nowell PC. Mechanisms of tumor progression. Cancer Res. 1986;46(5):2203–7.

42. Onodera N, McCabe NR, Rubin CM. Formation of a hyperdiploid karyotype in childhood acute lymphoblastic leukemia. Blood. 1992;80(1):203–8.

43. Paulsson K, Morse H, Fioretos T, Behrendtz M, Strombeck B, Johansson B. Evidence for a single-step mechanism in the origin of hyperdiploid childhood acute lymphoblastic leukemia. Genes Chromosomes Cancer. 2005;44(2):113–22.

44. Baca SC, Prandi D, Lawrence MS, Mosquera JM, Romanel A, Drier Y, Park K, Kitabayashi N, MacDonald TY, Ghandi M, et al. Punctuated evolution of prostate cancer genomes. Cell. 2013;153(3):666–77.

45. Gao R, Davis A, Mcdonald TO, Sei E, Shi X, Wang Y, Tsai PC, Casasent A, Waters J, Zhang H, et al. Punctuated copy number evolution and clonal stasis in triple-negative breast cancer. Nat Genet. 2016;48(10):1119–30.

46. Turajlic S, Swanton C. Metastasis as an evolutionary process. Science. 2016; 352(6282):169–75.

47. Forsdyke DR. Speciation: Goldschmidt's heresy, once supported by Gould and Dawkins, is again reinstated. Biol Theory. 2017;12:4–12.

48. Vincent MD. Cancer: beyond speciation. Adv Cancer Res. 2011;112:283–350.

49. Lazebnik Y. The shock of being united and symphiliosis. Another lesson from plants? Cell Cycle. 2014;13(15):2323–9.

50. Goldschmidt RB. The material basis of evolution. New Haven: Yale University Press; 1940.

51. White MJD. Modes of speciation. San Francisco: W H Freeman and Co.; 1978.

52. King M. Species evolution: the role of chromosome change. Cambridge: Cambridge University Press; 1993.

53. O'Brien S, Menotti-Raymond M, Murphy W, Nash W, Wirnberg J, Stanyon R, Copeland N, Jenkins N, Womack J, Marshall Graves J. The promise of comparative genomics in mammals. Science. 1999;286:458–81.

54. Heng HH, Bremer SW, Stevens J, Ye KJ, Miller F, Liu G, Ye CJ. Cancer progression by non-clonal chromosome aberrations. J Cell Biochem. 2006; 98(6):1424–435.

55. Weinberg RA. The biology of cancer. Second ed. New York; London: Garland Science; 2014.

56. Alberts B, Johnson A, Lewis J, Raff M, Roberts K, Walter P. Molecular biology of the cell. New York: Garland Publishing, Inc.; 2014.

57. Mellors RC, Keane JF Jr, Papanicolaou GN. Nucleic acid content of the squamous cancer cell. Science. 1952;116(3011):265–9.

58. Atkin NB, Kay R. Prognostic significance of modal DNA value and other factors in malignant tumours, based on 1465 cases. Br J Cancer. 1979;40(2):210–21.

59. Bocking A, Auffermann W, Vogel H, Schlondorff G, Goebbels R. Diagnosis and grading of malignancy in squamous epithelial lesions of the larynx with DNA cytophotometry. Cancer. 1985;56(7):1600–4.

60. Forsslund G, Esposti PL, Nilsson B, Zetterberg A. The prognostic significance of nuclear DNA content in prostatic carcinoma. Cancer. 1992;69(6):1432–9.

61. McCormack A, Fan JL, Duesberg M, Bloomfield M, Fiala C, Duesberg P. Individual karyotypes at the origins of cervical carcinomas. Mol Cytogenet. 2013;6(1):44.

18

Application of chromosomal microarray to investigate genetic causes of isolated fetal growth restriction

Gang An[1,2], Yuan Lin[2], Liang Pu Xu[2], Hai Long Huang[2], Si Ping Liu[1], Yan Hong Yu[1*] and Fang Yang[1*]

Abstract

Background: Application of chromosomal microarray analysis (CMA) to investigate the genetic characteristics of fetal growth restriction (FGR) without ultrasonic structural anomalies at 18–32 weeks.

Methods: This study includes singleton fetuses with the estimated fetal weight (EFW) using the formula of Hadlock C below the 10th percentile for gestational age. FGRs without structural anomalies were selected, and the ones at high risk of noninvasive prenatal testing for trisomy 13, 18 and 21 would be excluded. The cases were divided into two groups: early-onset group (< 24^{+0} weeks) and late-onset group (24–33 weeks). All patients were offered invasive prenatal testing with CMA and karyotype analysis.

Results: CMA detected 10 pathogenic copy number variants and 2 variant of uncertain significance case. CMA has a 5.5% (7/127) incremental yield of pathogenic chromosomal abnormalities over karyotyping. The positive detected rate was 9.6% (5/52) in early-onset group and 9.3% (7/75) in late-onset group respectively.

Conclusions: When FGR without structural anomaly is diagnosed before 33 weeks, an invasive prenatal procedure is strongly recommended. CMA can identify a 5.5% (7/127) incremental detection rate of pathogenic chromosomal abnormalities, which would impact clinical management for FGR.

Keywords: Fetal growth restriction, Prenatal diagnosis, Chromosomal microarray, Karyotype analysis, Uniparental disomy

Background

Fetal growth restriction (FGR) is a common complication of pregnancy that has been associated with a variety of adverse perinatal outcomes [1]. Although many factors have been implicated in the process of fetal growth, the precise molecular and cellular mechanisms by which normal fetal growth occurs are still not well understood [2].There is a strong association between FGR and chromosome aberrations. Fetuses with chromosome disorders, including aneuploidy, duplication and deletion, are frequently growth restricted [3].

Although conventional karyotyping is the current gold standard for prenatal cytogenetic analysis for several decades, chromosomal microarray analysis (CMA) has been introduced into clinical practice, due to its high-resolution and whole-genome screening feature. Single-nucleotide polymorphism (SNP) array, a CMA platform used in prenatal diagnosis, can detect almost all genomic imbalances recognized by karyotyping, as well as smaller deletions and duplications in the kilobase (Kb) range, termed copy-number variants (CNV) [4]. It has further facilitated the detection of uniparental disomy (UPD) [5], which could also be a potential cause of FGR [6].

CMA can detect a potentially pathogenic CNV in an additional 6–7% of cases with fetal structural abnormalities detected by ultrasound [7].The American Congress of Obstetricians and Gynecologists (ACOG) and the Society for Maternal-fetal Medicine (SMFM) recommend that CMA as a first-line test is recommended when genetic analysis is performed in cases with fetal structural anomalies [8]. For those FGR fetuses without ultrasonic structural anomaly, also defined as isolated FGR,

* Correspondence: yuyh1010@hotmail.com; fangfangy@hotmail.com
[1]Nanfang Hospital, Southern Medical University, Guangzhou 510515, Guangdong, China
Full list of author information is available at the end of the article

whether to implement CMA is still under consideration. In this study, we sought to investigate the genetic causes of isolate FGR by SNP array and karyotype.

Results

A total of 155 cases with isolate FGR met the inclusion criteria. 28 cases refused to accept an invasive procedure and 127 cases were consented to participate in the study. 52 prenatal samples were obtained by amniocentesis and 75 were obtained by cordocentesis. The clinical characteristics of pregnant women included in this study were summarized in Table1.Early-onset group and late-onset one were similar regarding maternal age, height, BMI and nulliparity (Table 1).

Among the 127 cases, 9.4% (12/127) chromosomal abnormalities were detected totally and the clinical characteristic and related syndromes or phenotype were listed (Table 2). Taking into accounting the diagnosed gestation, the positive detected rate was 9.6% (5/52) in early-onset group and 9.3% (7/75) in late-onset group respectively. The difference between early-onset group and late-onset group is no significant ($P = 1.00$). Karyotype analysis identified 4 cases including 3 imbalanced genomes and 1 pericentric inversion. CMA detected 10 pathogenic CNV and 2 VOUS case. Compared to karyotype analysis, CMA has a 5.5% (7/127) incremental yield of pathogenic chromosomal abnormalities and a 1.6% (2/127) VOUS detected rate.

In Case 1-Case 10, there were ten pathogenetic CNVs de novo detected by CMA with parent-offspring analysis. In Case 1, due to an indication of isolated FGR, the patient requested a diagnosis of CMA to get more genetic information about the fetus and reduce the waiting time. CMA revealed an abnormal female chromosome complement, including the loss of one complete X chromosome. This finding is consistent with 45,X. Karyotype analysis of cultured amniocytes confirmed the CMA result. The fetus was delivered at 36^{+4} weeks, the birth weights of the infant were 2300 g. In Case 2, the pregnant woman experienced an amniocentesis because NIPT indicated a high risk of trisomy 22. Cultured

amniocytes showed a normal 46,XY karyotype, and no trisomy 22 or small markers were observed after counting 70 metaphase cells. Interphase FISH was not selected by the patient in the prenatal testing. SNP array showed a mosaic of trisomy 22 in the uncultured samples, which was discordant with the normal result of karyotype. At present, the pregnancy is still going on. The other 8 (Case 3–10) pathogenic CNV cases were terminated with the parents' request after the genetic counseling. Case 3 was revealed a four-copy fragment of 68 Mb in 9p24.3q13, and karyotyping demonstrated a marker chromosome with 47, XX,+mar[39]/46,XX [11]. Case 4 was shown a loss of 35.1 Mb of chromosome 4p16.3p15.1 overlapping the Wolf-Hirschhorn syndrome region. Case 5 was revealed a loss of 2.8 Mb of chromosome 15p11.2. The fetus was diagnosed as Prader-willi syndrome because of a paternal loss confirmed by trios analysis. A loss of 3.1 Mb of chromosome 22q11.21 related to DiGeorge syndrome was found in Case 6. In Case 7,CMA revealed a loss of 1.5 Mb of chromosome 7q11.23. This deletion is termed the "Willianms-Beuren syndrome". In Case 8 and Case 9, CMA showed pathogenic CNVs related to delayed development and mental retardation according to the Decipher database. In Case 10,CMA showed a copy neutral loss of heterozygosity (LOH) of 19.2 Mb of chromosome 15q14q21.3.After trios analysis with UPD tool, a maternal UPD(15) was confirmed and the fetus was diagnosed as Prader-willi syndrome. Case 11 was confirmed a karyotype of 46, XX, inv.(4)(p14;q28),which inherited from the paternity, and CMA revealed a gain of four copies of 670 Kb in chromosome 5p15.31. No information was available for its pathogenesis. The parents refused to have further CMA trios testing. The clinical significance of this duplication is not known. Fetal death in uterus was diagnosed by ultrasound at 34 weeks. In Case 12, SNP array revealed a gain of 493 Kb of chromosome 22q11.21. This segment highly varied according to the database. The origin of the gained copy was unclear due to the parents' decline. A male infant was delivered with a 2300 g birth weight at 37^{+4} weeks and following up to 10 months was

Table 1 Clinical characteristics of the pregnant women

Group	Early-onset ($n = 52$)	Late-onset ($n = 75$)
maternal age (years)	33.6(19.9–43.5)	32.4(20.5–41.5)
height(cm)	160.1(154.5–171.5)	161.2(149.5–169.3)
BMI[a]	23.3(19.2-26.8)	24.1(18.5–27.4)
Nullipara	(62.4%)	(65.3%)
gestational age at diagnosis(weeks)	22.5(19.0–23.8)[b]	28.2(24.0-32.5)[b]

[a]BMI based on the weight and height at the visit of the first trimester;
[b]$P < 0.05$

Table 2 Karyotype and SNP array abnormal results

Case NO.	Gestational age (weeks)	Ultrasound findings	Karyotype results	SNP array results	Length	Inheritance	Syndrome/phenotype	Pregnancy outcome
Case 1	23[+1]	None	45,X	arr[hg19] Xp22.33q28(168,546–155,233,731)×1	155 Mb	de novo	Turner syndrome	preterm birth
Case 2	21[+2]	None	46,XY	array[h19](22)x2–3[a]	WC	de novo	Mosaic trisomy 22	In pregnancy
Case 3	23[+3]	None	47,XX,+mar[39]/46,XX [11]	arr[hg19] 9p24.3q13(208,454–68,216,577)×4	68 Mb	de novo	mosaic tetrasomy 9p	TOP
Case 4	28[+2]	Hypoplastic Nasal Bone	46,XX,del(4)(p15)	arr[hg19] 4p16.3p15.1(68,345–35,252,743) × 1	35.1 Mb	de novo	Wolf-Hirschhorn syndrome	TOP
Case 5	22[+4]	None	46,XX	arr[hg19] 15q11.2(22,770,421–25,626,665) × 1	2.8 Mb	de novo	Prader-Willi syndrome	TOP
Case 6	24[+3]	None	46,XY	arr[hg19] 22q11.21(18,648,855–21,800,471) × 1	3.1 Mb	de novo	DiGeorge syndrome	TOP
Case 7	27[+6]	None	46,XY	arr[hg19] 7q11.23(72,624,203–74,143,240) × 1	1.5 MB	de novo	Willianms-Beuren syndrome	TOP
Case 8	24[+2]	Oligohydramnios	46,XX	arr[hg19] 14q32.33(104,856,497–107,281,980)×1,19p13.3(260,912–4,226,075)× 3	2.4 Mb / 4.0 Mb	de novo	delayed development,mental retardation	TOP
Case 9	22[+4]	None	46,XY	arr[hg19] 3q26.33q27.2(182,374,672–185,041,523)×1	2.6 Mb	de novo	delayed development,mental retardation	TOP
Case 10	31[+3]	Polyhydramnios	46,XX	arr[hg19] 15q14q21.3(35,077,111–54,347,324) hmz[b]	19.2 Mb	de novo	Prader-Willi syndrome	TOP
Case 11	24[+3]	Tricuspid Regurgitation	46,XX, inv.(4)(p14;q28)pat	arr[hg19] 5p15.31(6,752,756–7,429,552) × 4	670 Kb	unknown	VOUS	Intrauterine death
Case 12	25[+4]	Echogenic intracardiac focus	46,XY	arr[hg19] 22q11.21(18,512,066–19,004,772)×3	493 Kb	unknown	VOUS	Term birth

TOP termination of pregnancy, *WC* whole chromosome, *VOUS* variant of uncertain significance
[a] the detected sample was uncultured amniocyte
[b] a maternal UPD(15) was diagnosed by UPD tool

normal. The rest cases with negative results had no identifiable phenotype at birth.

Discussion

Several organizations recommend that CMA should be applied to detect genetic abnormalities in fetus with structural anomalies. Significant fetal growth restriction is often seen with trisomy 13 and trisomy 18, which are usually confirmed multiple malformations by ultrasound. But, it is ambiguous that whether a pregnant woman should accepted the invasive prenatal procedures when a FGR is diagnosed with a normal ultrasound scanning. In this study, we determined the incidence and patterns of chromosomal abnormalities in a cohort of 127 FGR without structural anomalies. The overall detection rate of chromosomal abnormalities were 9.4% (12/127).We explored the genetic abnormalities of FGR diagnosed at different gestational ages, However, there was no statistical difference between the early-onset group and late-onset one (9.6% vs. 9.3%, $P = 1.00$).The reason may due to limited sample size. We still recommended that it was reasonable to discuss the probability of an invasive prenatal procedure with pregnant woman in case of isolate FGR diagnosed before 33 weeks. Although Merel recommends that testing for chromosomal anomalies should be offered in case of FGR between 18 and 24 weeks gestation [9].

Frequently, FGR is a major and only manifestation in the prenatal diagnosis of some micro-duplication/deletion syndromes, and intellect disability or delayed development was solely clinical presentation after birth. Due to the limited resolution of karyotype analysis, many well-characterized disease-causing genetic variants could not be detected. This study demonstrated 5 pathogenic CNV de novo (Case5–9), which only detected by CMA, because the genetically material imbalance was less than 5 Mb in length. After genetic diagnosis, each case was re-evaluated by ultrasound. Just like in Case 6, DiGeorge syndrome was found by CMA in the isolated FGR fetus and confirmed by FISH. Common ultrasound anomalies included palatal anomalies, cardiovascular anomalies and scoliosis [10] were easy to confirm, however, this case was just an isolated FGR without any structural anomaly. At 27 weeks, a smaller thymus gland was confirmed by Ultrasound before termination of pregnancy with the parent's request.

Uniparental disomy (UPD) is another genetic cause of FGR. The concept of UPD was first introduced by Eric Engel, owing to the fact that both members of such a pair of chromosomes from only one parent [11]. The pathogenesis of UPD is determined by both epigenetic imprinting as well as demasking of autosomal-recessive diseases (homozygosity by isodisomy). It is striking that many UPDs are associated with disturbed intrauterine

growth [12]. A maternal uniparental disomy (mUPD) in which two copies of chromosome 15 of maternal origin accounts for 20–25% of Prader-Willi syndrome (PWS) [13]. A study from the UK supports that the changing genetic subtype proportions of PWS are due to an increase in the numbers of mUPD babies because of the increasing proportions of older mothers [14]. The incidence of UPD is estimated to be approximately 1:3500 live births and growing numbers of patients will be detected with the advent of the whole-genome techniques [15]. As in Case 10, a 41-year-old woman accepted cordocentesis procedure with Indication of isolated FGR and decreased fetal movement at 31^{+3} weeks of gestation. Finally, a UPD(15)mat has been confirmed by trios analysis with UPD tool [16], and the fetus was diagnosed with PWS. So UPD should deserve more attention in FGR cases especially with advanced-aged pregnant women.

In the prenatal setting, it may be difficult to interpret the significance of a CNV due to the limitations of fetal imaging and the limited information currently available correlating prenatal CNV findings with postnatal phenotype [17]. VOUS may cause considerable stress and anxiety as the parents may not obtain a satisfied expectation. The parents refused to have further testing. Case 11 exhibited a chromosome complement with the gain of 670 Kb in chromosome 5p15.31 involved two genes: PAPD7 and ADCY2. Four copies were detected and the breakpoints occurred in PAPD7 and ADCY2 respectively, revealed by CMA. So far, both of the genes whether cause disorders has not been reported. Parental DNA was not available for further analysis and the fetus died in uterus at 34 weeks. We were unable to determine whether the duplication had occurred de novo. Similarly, a VOUS was defined in Case 12. Finally, the VOUS detected rate was 1.6%, similar to the literature [18].

CMA does not provide information about the chromosomal mechanism of a genetic imbalance. For example, the fetus of Case 8 was diagnosed as mosaic tetrasomy 9p with the combination of CMA and karyotype analysis. The components of the prenatal sample would change following the culture process, which increased the uncertainty of diagnosis results. In Case 2, the result of CMA indicated a mosaic of trisomy 22 and the karyotype was normal. Maybe, the direct detection of uncultured samples by CMA can more fully represent the genetic characteristics of the fetus.The ACOG and SMFM recommend that providers discuss the benefits and limitations of CMA and conventional karyotype with patients, and that both options are available to women who choose to undergo prenatal diagnostic testing [19]. QF-PCR or FISH analysis would be an alternative in the rapid prenatal test for trisomy 13, 18, 21and sex chromosome aneuploidies. But CMA could detect micro-deletion/duplication with a high-resolution view of the whole genome and copy neutral LOH with platforms incorporating SNP probes. More pregnant women are willing to choose CMA in the prenatal setting.

Inevitably, a limitation of the prospective study is that the postnatal follow-up is still pending, in order to acquire the long-term growth and development aspects of born cases. How to select a proper criterion to define FGR is another puzzle [20]. The ultrasound limit for FGR is fetal weight (EFW) or abdominal circumference (AC) under the 3rd, 5th, 10th percentile or below 2 Standard Deviation (SD) from the population standard or reference [21]. We choose the 10th percentile as a cut-off to avoid omitting the so-called "mildly growth restricted" which are at increased risk for complications between the 3th and 10th percentile [22]. This fact may result in a selection bias leading to underestimated incremental yield of CMA.

Conclusion

In summary, as underlying factors in case of FGR, aneuploidy, submicroscopic abnormality and UPD should be considered comprehensively. An invasive prenatal procedure is strongly recommended when FGR is diagnosed before 33 weeks. CMA detected all the chromosomal aberration detected by karyotyping, and has a 5.5% (7/127) incremental detection rate of genetic cause of isolated FGR, which could impact the clinical decision. CMA as the first-line test plus karyotyping is effective and feasible as a joined prenatal testing for suspected FGR cases.

Methods

Ethics and cases selection

The study was approved by the ethics review boards of Nanfang Hospital (No.NFEC-2016-093) and Fujian Provincial Maternity and Children's Hospital (No.12). Written informed consent was obtained in all cases.

This prospective multi-centers cohort study consisted of singleton FGR cases underwent invasive prenatal diagnostic testing at Fujian Provincial Maternity and Children's Hospital (FPMCH) and Nanfang Hospital (NFH) of Southern Medical University from July 2015 to February 2018. These two hospitals are tertiary referral prenatal diagnosis center in each province. Gestational age (GA) was assessed according to last menstrual period (LMP) and crown-rump length (CRL) at 11 to 13^{+6} weeks. Inclusion criteria was FGR without structural anomalies diagnosed by ultrasound when the EFW is less than the 10th percentile for gestational age based on the formula of Hadlock C [23]. At high risk of noninvasive prenatal testing for trisomy 13, 18 and 21, multiple gestation, chronic nephropathy, preeclampsia, antiphospholipid syndrome, TORCH infection,

substance use and abuse were excluded. All the morphology scan were performed by experienced operators according to the practice guidelines for performance of the routine fetal ultrasonic scan released by the International Society of Ultrasound in Obstetrics and Gynecology(ISUOG). Based on the gestational age at diagnosis, the cases were divided into two groups: early-onset group ($< 24^{+0}$ weeks) and late-onset group (24–33 weeks). All women received pre-test counseling regarding the procedure-related risks and benefits from karyotype and microarray. Women with positive results were offered fully counseling by the fetal medicine specialists. All the prenatal samples obtained by amniocentesis or cordocentesis were processed in parallel using both SNP array and G-banding for conventional karyotyping.

Karyotype analysis

Amniotic Fluid or fetal cord blood samples were obtained according to the prenatal procedure protocol [24]. The cultured amniocytes or lymphocytes were analyzed by routine cytogenetic analysis using G-banding techniques at a resolution of 400–500 bands. The number of cells examined varied between 20 and 30.The results of cultured amniocytes are available within 14 to 20 days and the ones of lymphocytes within 5 to 7 days.

SNP array and data interpretation

A CytoScan 750 K array (Affymetrix Inc., Santa Clara, CA, USA) was used for assessing the prenatal samples, which covered over 750,000 markers distributed across the entire human genome, including 200,000 probes for single nucleotide polymorphisms (SNPs) and 550,000 probes for copy number variations (CNVs). Hybridization, data extraction and analysis were performed as per the manufacturer's protocol. A resolution was generally applied: gains or losses ≥400 kb and loss of heterozygosity (LOH) ≥ 10 Mb [25]. The results were analyzed with Chromosome Analysis Suite (ChAS) software (Affymetrix, USA), using annotations of the genome version GRCH37 (hg19). The Database of Genomic Variants (DGV), the Database of Chromosome Imbalance and Phenotype in Humans Using Ensemble Resources (DECIPHER), the International Standards for Cytogenomic Arrays Consortium (ISCA), OMIM genes and the local database were used to evaluate the CNVs identified in this study. The CNVs were classified as benign, pathogenic, or variants of uncertain significance(VOUS) according to the American College of Medical Genetics (ACMG) guideline [26]. Blood samples were collected from both parents and were analyzed if variants of uncertain significance (VOUS) were detected in the fetal sample by CMA.

Statistical analysis

SPSS software v20.0 (SPSS Inc., Chicago, IL, USA) was used for statistical analysis of the data. Statistical comparisons were performed using the chi-square test and Fisher exact test was used in cases where a table cell contained < 5 observations. Differences were considered as statistically when $P < 0.05$.

Funding

This study were supported by Fujian Provincial Science and Technology Major Project (No.2013YZ0002–1) and Fujian Provincial Natural Science Foundation (No.2017 J01238).

Authors' contributions

GA has analyzed and interpreted the array data and was a major contributor in writing the manuscript. LX, HH and SL have partly interpreted the data. YL has diagnosed the patients, supervised the sample drawing and revised the draft of the paper. YY and FY have supervised the study, and prepared the paper. All authors read and approved the final manuscript.

Competing interests

The authors declare that they have no competing interests.

Author details

[1]Nanfang Hospital, Southern Medical University, Guangzhou 510515, Guangdong, China. [2]Fujian Provincial Key Laboratory for Prenatal diagnosis and Birth Defect, Fujian Provincial Maternity and Children's Hospital of Fujian Medical University, Fuzhou, Fujian, China.

References

1. Fetal growth restriction. Practice Bulletin No. 134. American College of Obstetricians and Gynecologists. Obstet Gynecol. 2013;121:1122–33.
2. Monk D, Moore GE. Intrauterine growth restriction–genetic causes and consequences. Semin Fetal Neonatal Med. 2004;9(5):371–8.
3. Shaffer LG, Rosenfeld JA, Dabell MP, Coppinger J, Bandholz AM, Ellison JW, Ravnan JB, Torchia BS, Ballif BC, Fisher AJ. Detection rates of clinically significant genomic alterations by microarray analysis for specific anomalies detected by ultrasound. Prenat Diagn. 2012;32(10):986–95.
4. Karampetsou E, Morrogh D, Chitty L. Microarray Technology for the Diagnosis of fetal chromosomal aberrations: which platform should we use? J Clin Med. 2014;3(2):663–78.
5. Chantot-Bastaraud S, Stratmann S, Brioude F, Begemann M, Elbracht M, Graul-Neumann L, Harbison M, Netchine I, Eggermann T. Formation of upd(7)mat by trisomic rescue: SNP array typing provides new insights in chromosomal nondisjunction. Mol Cytogenet. 2017;10:28.
6. Martin CL, Kirkpatrick BE, Ledbetter DH. Copy number variants, aneuploidies, and human disease. Clin Perinatol. 2015;42(2):227–42. vii
7. Reddy UM, Page GP, Saade GR, Silver RM, Thorsten VR, Parker CB, Pinar H, Willinger M, Stoll BJ, Heim-Hall J, Varner MW, Goldenberg RL, Bukowski R, Wapner RJ, Drews-Botsch CD, O'Brien BM, Dudley DJ, Levy B, Network NSCR. Karyotype versus microarray testing for genetic abnormalities after stillbirth. N Engl J Med. 2012;367(23):2185–93.
8. Dugoff L, Norton ME, Kuller JA. The use of chromosomal microarray for prenatal diagnosis. Am J Obstet Gynecol. 2016;215(4):B2–9.
9. de Wit MC, Srebniak MI, Joosten M, Govaerts LC, Kornelisse RF, Papatsonis DN, de Graaff K, Knapen MF, Bruggenwirth HT, de Vries FA, Van Veen S, Van Opstal D, Galjaard RJ, Go AT. Prenatal and postnatal findings in small-for-gestational-age fetuses without structural ultrasound anomalies at 18-24 weeks. Ultrasound Obstet Gynecol. 2017;49(3):342–8.
10. Bassett AS, Chow EW, Husted J, Weksberg R, Caluseriu O, Webb GD, Gatzoulis MA. Clinical features of 78 adults with 22q11 deletion syndrome. Am J Med Genet A. 2005;138(4):307–13.
11. Eric Engel MD. A new genetic concept: uniparental disomy and its potential effect, isodisomy. Am J Med Genet B Neuropsychiatr Genet. 1980;6(2):137–43.
12. Eggermann T, Zerres K, Eggermann K, Moore G, Wollmann HA. Uniparental disomy: clinical indications for testing in growth retardation. Eur J Pediatr. 2002;161(6):305–12.
13. Dudley O, Muscatelli F. Clinical evidence of intrauterine disturbance in Prader-Willi syndrome, a genetically imprinted neurodevelopmental disorder. Early Hum Dev. 2007;83(7):471–8.
14. Whittington JE, Butler JV, Holland AJ. Changing rates of genetic subtypes of Prader-Willi syndrome in the UK. Eur J Hum Genet. 2007;15(1):127–30.
15. Liu W, Zhang H, Wang J, Yu G, Qiu W, Li Z, Chen M, Choy KW, Sun X. Prenatal diagnosis of complete maternal uniparental isodisomy of chromosome 4 in a fetus without congenital abnormality or inherited disease-associated variations. Mol Cytogenet. 2015;8:85.
16. Schroeder C, Sturm M, Dufke A, Mau-Holzmann U, Eggermann T, Poths S, Riess O, Bonin M. UPDtool: a tool for detection of iso- and heterodisomy in parent-child trios using SNP microarrays. Bioinformatics. 2013;29(12):1562–4.
17. McGillivray G, Rosenfeld JA, Gardner MK, Gillam LH. Genetic counselling and ethical issues with chromosome microarray analysis in prenatal testing. Prenat Diagn. 2012;32(4):389–95.
18. Hillman SC, McMullan DJ, Hall G, Togneri FS, James N, Maher EJ, Meller CH, Williams D, Wapner RJ, Maher ER. Use of prenatal chromosomal microarray: prospective cohort study and systematic review and meta-analysis. Ultrasound Obstetrics Gynecol the Official J International Society of Ultrasound in Obstetrics & Gynecology. 2013;41(6):610–20.
19. American College of O, Gynecologists Committee on G. Committee opinion no. 581: the use of chromosomal microarray analysis in prenatal diagnosis. Obstet Gynecol. 2013;122(6):1374–7.
20. Figueras F, Gratacós E. Update on the diagnosis and classification of fetal growth restriction and proposal of a stage-based management protocol. Fetal Diagnosis Therapy. 2014;30(11):86–98.
21. Unterscheider J, Daly S, Geary MP, Kennelly MM, McAuliffe FM, O'Donoghue K, Hunter A, Morrison JJ, Burke G, Dicker P. Optimizing the definition of intrauterine growth restriction: the multicenter prospective PORTO Study. Am J Obstetrics Gynecol. 2013;208(4):290.e291.
22. Clausson B, Gardosi J, Francis A, Cnattingius S. Perinatal outcome in SGA births defined by customised versus population-based birthweight standards. BJOG Int J Obstet Gynaecol. 2001;108(8):830–4.
23. Hadlock FP, Harrist RB, Sharman RS, Deter RL, Park SK. Estimation of fetal weight with the use of head, body, and femur measurements–a prospective study. Am J Obstetrics Gynecol. 1985;151(3):333.
24. Ghi T, Sotiriadis A, Calda P, Da Silva Costa F, Raine-Fenning N, Alfirevic Z, McGillivray G. ISUOG Practice Guidelines: invasive procedures for prenatal diagnosis. Ultrasound Obstet Gynecol. 2016;48(2):256–68.
25. Miller DT, Adam MP, Aradhya S, Biesecker LG, Brothman AR, Carter NP, Church DM, Crolla JA, Eichler EE, Epstein CJ, Faucett WA, Feuk L, Friedman JM, Hamosh A, Jackson L, Kaminsky EB, Kok K, Krantz ID, Kuhn RM, Lee C, Ostell JM, Rosenberg C, Scherer SW, Spinner NB, Stavropoulos DJ, Tepperberg JH, Thorland EC, Vermeesch JR, Waggoner DJ, Watson MS, Martin CL, Ledbetter DH. Consensus statement: chromosomal microarray is a first-tier clinical diagnostic test for individuals with developmental disabilities or congenital anomalies. Am J Hum Genet. 2010;86(5):749–64.
26. South ST, Lee C, Lamb AN, Higgins AW, Kearney HM. Working Group for the American College of medical G, genomics laboratory quality assurance C: ACMG standards and guidelines for constitutional cytogenomic microarray analysis, including postnatal and prenatal applications: revision 2013. Genet Med. 2013;15(11):901–9.

19

Identification of novel genomic imbalances in Saudi patients with congenital heart disease

Zuhair N. Al-Hassnan[1,2,7], Waad Albawardi[2†], Faten Almutairi[2†], Rawan AlMass[2], Albandary AlBakheet[2], Osama M. Mustafa[2], Laila AlQuait[2], Zarghuna M. A. Shinwari[2], Salma Wakil[2], Mustafa A. Salih[3], Majid Al-Fayyadh[4], Saeed M. Hassan[3], Mansour Aljoufan[4], Osima Al-Nakhli[2], Brynn Levy[5], Balsam AlMaarik[2], Hana A. Al-Hakami[2], Maysoon Alsagob[2], Dilek Colak[6] and Namik Kaya[2*] ⓘ

Abstract

Background: Quick genetic diagnosis of a patient with congenital heart disease (CHD) is quite important for proper health care and management. Copy number variations (CNV), chromosomal imbalances and rearrangements have been frequently associated with CHD. Previously, due to limitations of microscope based standard karyotyping techniques copious CNVs and submicroscopic imbalances could not be detected in numerous CHD patients. The aim of our study is to identify cytogenetic abnormalities among the selected CHD cases (n = 17) of the cohort using high density oligo arrays.

Results: Our screening study indicated that six patients (~35%) have various cytogenetic abnormalities. Among the patients, only patient 2 had a duplication whereas the rest carried various deletions. The patients 1, 4 and 6 have only single large deletions throughout their genome; a 3.2 Mb deletion on chromosome 7, a 3.35 Mb deletion on chromosome 3, and a 2.78 Mb a deletion on chromosome 2, respectively. Patients 3 and 5 have two deletions on different chromosomes. Patient 3 has deletions on chromosome 2 (2q24.1; 249 kb) and 16 (16q22.2; 1.8 Mb). Patient 4 has a 3.35 Mb an interstitial deletion on chromosome 3 (3q13.2q13.31).

Based on our search on the latest available literature, our study is the first inclusive array CGH evaluation on Saudi cohort of CHD patients.

Conclusions: This study emphasizes the importance of the arrays in genetic diagnosis of CHD. Based on our results the high resolution arrays should be utilized as first-tier diagnostic tool in clinical care as suggested before by others. Moreover, previously evaluated negative CHD cases (based on standard karyotyping methods) should be re-examined by microarray based cytogenetic methods.

Keywords: Congenital heart disease, Cervical ankylosis, Hypoplastic thumb, Osteopenia, Fused central vertebrae

Background

Congenital heart disease (CHD) is the most common anomaly affecting newborns and also leading cause of mortality and morbidity among neonates [1–4]. This group of disorders is predicted to have an incidence rate of 8–9 in every 1000 live birth [4, 5] and leads to ~10% of spontaneous miscarriages [5]. Despite the still largely ambiguous pathophysiology of CHD, genetic factors were found to contribute to the etiology in many cases. In addition, numerous incidents of CHD were found to have chromosomal abnormalities; particularly among cases with associated multiple organ malformations, developmental delays, and growth abnormalities [6, 7]. Interestingly enough such cases are prone to harbor morbidities of additional chromosomal syndromes such as Williams-Beuren and DiGeorge or even monogenic hereditary disorders such as Noonan [6].

* Correspondence: nkaya@kfshrc.edu.sa; namikkaya@gmail.com
†Equal contributors
2Department of Genetics, King Faisal Specialist Hospital and Research Centre, MBC: 03, Riyadh 11211, Kingdom of Saudi Arabia
Full list of author information is available at the end of the article

Advances in molecular and cytogenetic techniques in the recent years gave rise to tools of higher sensitivity such as single nucleotide polymorphism (SNP) based microarrays [8], array comparative genomic hybridization (aCGH) platforms [9–11] and nextgen sequencing [12] techniques, which are enabling the detection of chromosomal aberrations and sub-microscopic copy number variations (CNVs) on an unprecedented resolution that was not possible with standard and high-resolution karyotyping techniques. This facilitated the discovery of novel pathogenic copy number variations, genes and mutations, and the establishment of genotype-phenotype correlations for various diseases [10, 13–15] including heart defects [16]. The dense coverage of the microarray probes can also be quite helpful in refining breakpoints of novel genomic imbalances as well as further characterization and fine mapping of already known gains and losses in different human chromosomes [15, 17].

It has been well-established that standard microscope based chromosome analysis misses quite many gains and losses due to its low resolution. Hence, aCGH and/or similar array platforms have been proposed to be utilized as a first-tier diagnostic tool for various disorders including autism, intellectual disability and more recently for newborn screenings of CHD patients [18–21]. In this study we screened Saudi CHD patients using high density oligo arrays to identify likely chromosomal imbalances.

Methods

Patients

We ascertained 223 patients inflicted with one or more of the following clinical problems: autism spectrum disorder, intellectual disability, heart defects, developmental delay, language delay, and dysmorphic features of unknown origin evaluated at the Kind Faisal Specialist Hospital and Research Center using the institutionally approved IRB protocols (RAC# 2040042, 2,030,046, 2,120,022, 2,080,032). Before the sample collection, the patients and parents were signed the written informed consents. All the patients were clinically examined and underwent a consistent study protocol for with perinatal history, and neurological assessment. The patients also underwent aCGH testing as a first-tier approach and then tested with one of the followings; FISH, standard cytogenetics, and targeted sequencing.

DNA isolation

Blood samples were collected from all participants. DNA was isolated using PureGene DNA Purification Kit (Gentra Systems, Inc. Minneapolis, MN, US).

Affymetrix microarrays and analysis

Affymetrix's Cytogenetics Whole-Genome 2.7 M arrays (Affymetrix Inc., Santa Clara, CA, US) and CytoScan HD arrays were used in the study. Both assays have over

2 million probes that interrogate polymorphic and non-polymorphic genomic sequences. The assay preparation, scanning, image processing, genotyping, and preliminary data analysis were all done according to manufacturer's protocols and guidelines. CNV detection was done using Affymetrix's in-house developed software called "Chromosome Analysis Software" otherwise known as ChAS using the software's default detection settings for high resolution. Previously reported benign CNVs were excluded from the analysis.

Cytogenetic banding analysis

The microscope based standard karyotype analysis was performed onTrypsin-Wright (GTW) banded metaphase spreads (at least 20 metaphases were analyzed and 2 were karyotyped using cultured peripheral blood lymphocytes according to standard protocols. Karyotypes were interpreted according to the International System for Human Cytogenetic Nomenclature.

Array CGH

A custom designed oligonucleotide microarray assay from Agilent (Agilent Technologies, Santa Clara, CA, USA) was utilized for CNV assessment [22]. The assay was developed and tested through an academic laboratory consortium [22]. Human male or female DNA (Promega Corp., Nepean, Canada) was used as a reference control. After DNA GC check, good quality DNA was digested, labelled, and then hybridized onto the custom arrays. Then, the slides were washed and scanned with either Agilent DNA Microarray Scanner (Agilent Technologies) or GenePix 4000B (Molecular Devices, Sunnyvale, CA). The images were processed using Agilent Feature Extraction software (v10.0), and transferred to Agilent Genomic Workbench software for data analysis, CNV visualization, and detection. During the analysis, softwares defaults were not changed and the analysis was based on human genome build hg19/GRCh37. All the assays protocols were performed according to the manufacturer's instructions (Agilent Inc.).

Fish

Confirmatory Fluorescence in situ hybridization (FISH) analysis was performed using p-arm and q-arm specific probes for the all chromosomes using standard protocols (Abbott Laboratories, Abbott Parl, IL, USA). In the absence of ready probes, custom FISH probes were designed and used. The experiments were carried out standard protocols.

Results

Case 1

The patient is now a 13 year old male who was initially admitted to the hospital for percutaneous valve implantation.

He was born with pulmonary atresia with ventricular septal defect (VSD) that was completely repaired with RV to PA conduit in July 2003. He did not suffer any significant cardiac complications, and the follow-up examination reported no cardiac symptoms but the patient had speech delays. Cardiovascular examination showed S1 and S2 were normal with systolic murmur in the left lower sternal border. Echocardiogram revealed normal biventricular systolic function. Right-sided ventricular chambers were mild to moderately dilated but the dilatation has improved post-PPVI. Respiratory and gastrointestinal examinations were insignificant. The patient had speech and developmental delays and brain malformation was suspected. He is mentally retarded. An MRI examination revealed a nonspecific right frontal centrum semiovale hyperintense lesion.

Molecular cytogenetic analysis indicated that he has a novel 3.2 Mb deletion extending on 7q33-q34 (Fig. 1). The deletion begins at 137,917,363 bp genomic position and ends at 141,131,675 bp. The deleted region contains 44 genes including 12 uncharacterized genes, 20 pseudogenes, and one miRNA according to Mapviewer Human Annotation Release 107.

Case 2

The patient is a 13-years old female referred to our center for evaluation of dysmorphic features and congenital heart disease. She was born at term with uneventful prenatal and peripartum period. She was noticed after birth to have hypoplastic right thumb. Her parents, who are not related, have 4 other normal children. When she was initially evaluated in our center at the age of 6 and ½ years, her examination showed a head circumference of 45 cm (4.7 SD below the mean), a weight of 14.6 kg (4 SD below the mean) and a height of 100.5 cm (3 SD below the mean). She had upslanting palpebral fissures, bulbous nose, malformed right ear, retrognathia, low posterior hairline, webbed neck, and widely spaced nipples. The chest and abdominal examination was unremarkable. The cardiovascular examination revealed normal first heart sound, fixed split of second heart sound, and a systolic murmur grade 3/6 over the left upper sternal border. She had normal tone, power and deep tendon reflexes. The musculoskeletal examination revealed right thumb hypoplasia with absent thenar muscles, absent extensor pollicis longus, and thumb extensors. There was significant instability of the metacarpophalangeal joints of the right thumb. Skeletal survey revealed ankylosis between C3, C4 and C5 spine. The thoraacolumbar spine and the long tubular bones of both upper limbs were osteopenic. The right fifth metacarpal bone was short with hypoplasia of the first right metacarpal bone. The epiphysis of the first metacarpal bone was absent bilaterally. There was mild bilateral subluxation of the hip joints. The tibia and fibula were normal bilaterally. Hallux valgus at the interphalangeal joint was seen bilaterally. There was coning of the epiphysis of the second to fourth toes bilaterally. Echocardiogram revealed large secundum atrial septal defect measuring 12 mm with left to right shunt. Ultrasound of abdomen and pelvis indicated that the left kidney was rotated and ectopic lying down into the pelvis.

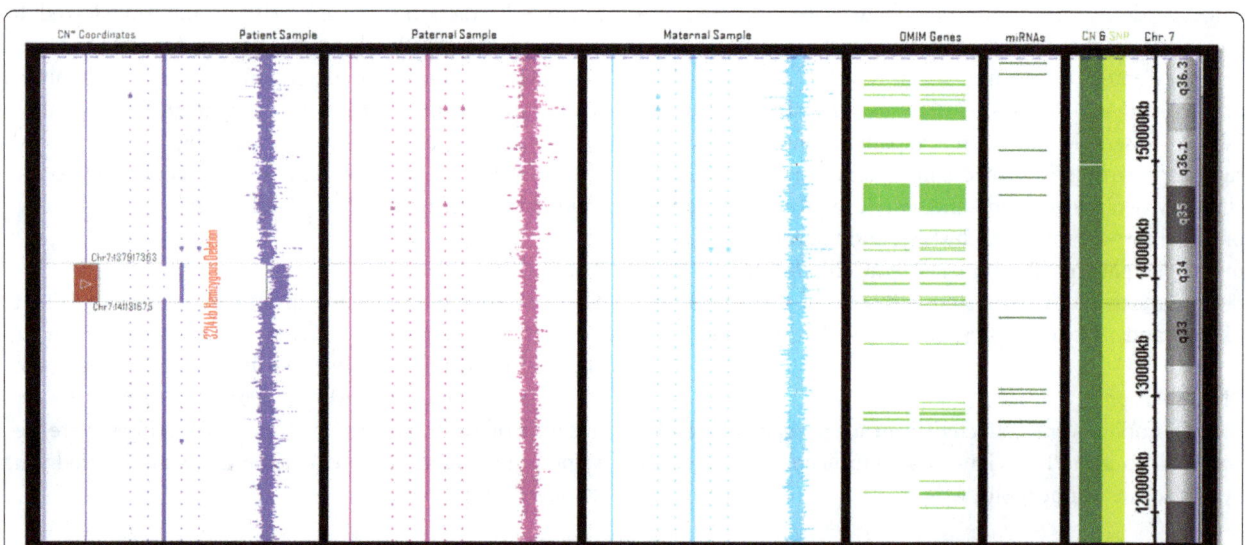

Fig. 1 The visual diagram is adopted from Chromosome Analysis Suite (Affymetrix Inc.,). From right to left the diagram presents copy number coordinates, the patient's probe distribution, paternal and maternal probes distributions, OMIM genes, miRNAs, all SNP and copy number probes in the region, and chromosomal coordinates. The patient has 3214 kb deletion (presented in blue color) while father and mother are normal

As part of routine diagnostic procedures a high-resolution GTW-banding study was carried on the patient's sample. No gross abnormality was detected. Then, an aCGH experiment was performed as a further clinical screening and indicated an interstitial duplication pointed by 33 oligonucleotide probes on 5q35.2-q35.3. An interphase FISH using a probe (CTD-2301A4) within the duplicated interval re-confirmed the findings. To better characterize the duplication a high-resolution array (Cytogenetics Whole-Genome 2.7 M) from Affymetrix Inc. (Affymetrix Inc., San Paolo, CA, US) was utilized to further delineate the gain missed during the initial standard microscope based-karyotyping. This particular chip array utilizes 2.7 million markers including 400,000 SNP probes that provide whole-genome coverage with the one of the highest density coverage among the present platforms. Based on Affymetrix's cytogenetic assay results, the duplication extends from 175,349,728 to 177,347,753 bp (hg19) and comprises 58 genes targeted by more than 600 SNP and copy number (CN) probes covering approximately 2.0 Mb (Fig. 2). In comparison to the previously published duplications this duplication seems novel and does not share breakpoints with the compared cases.

Case 3

A 5- year-old Saudi male, the first child of non-consanguineous healthy parents, was born at term following in-vitro fertilization (IVF) pregnancy via cesarean section. His birth weight was 3.5 Kg. He was admitted to the neonatal intensive care unit for 1 week because of Jaundice, treated with phototherapy, and was discovered to have congenital heart disease (patent ductus arteriosus [PDA]). Since early infancy, he was noted to have slow psychomotor development, sitting at 10 months and starting to walk independently at 2 years of age. He had significant delay in initiation of language which he developed. At age 1 month, he was admitted to the hospital with febrile illness and treatment as a case of sepsis. When he was 2 years of age, he underwent surgery to place testes (bilateral orchidopexy). There is no previous history of convulsion; however, recently he developed one episode of unprovoked convulsion with semiology of cyanosis and jerky movements of the limbs. Mother had history of two abortions following IVF pregnancy, and there is no family history of epilepsy or neurological problems. Examination at the age of 4 ½ years revealed no dysmorphic features and no neurocutaneuos marks apart from a single hypo pigmented patch at the right forearm. His growth parameters were: weight 18.2 Kg (75th centile), height 110 cm (75th centile), and head circumference 50 cm (50th centile). Vision and hearing were normal. Cardiovascular examination showed apex beat in the fifth intercostal space within the midclavicular line. There were no thrills, no left parasternal heave or palpable P2. Auscultation revealed no murmurs. Neurological examination revealed no gross abnormalities. Laboratory investigations (including complete blood count [CBC], renal function tests, bone profile, liver function tests [LFT], thyroid function tests, and serum lactate and

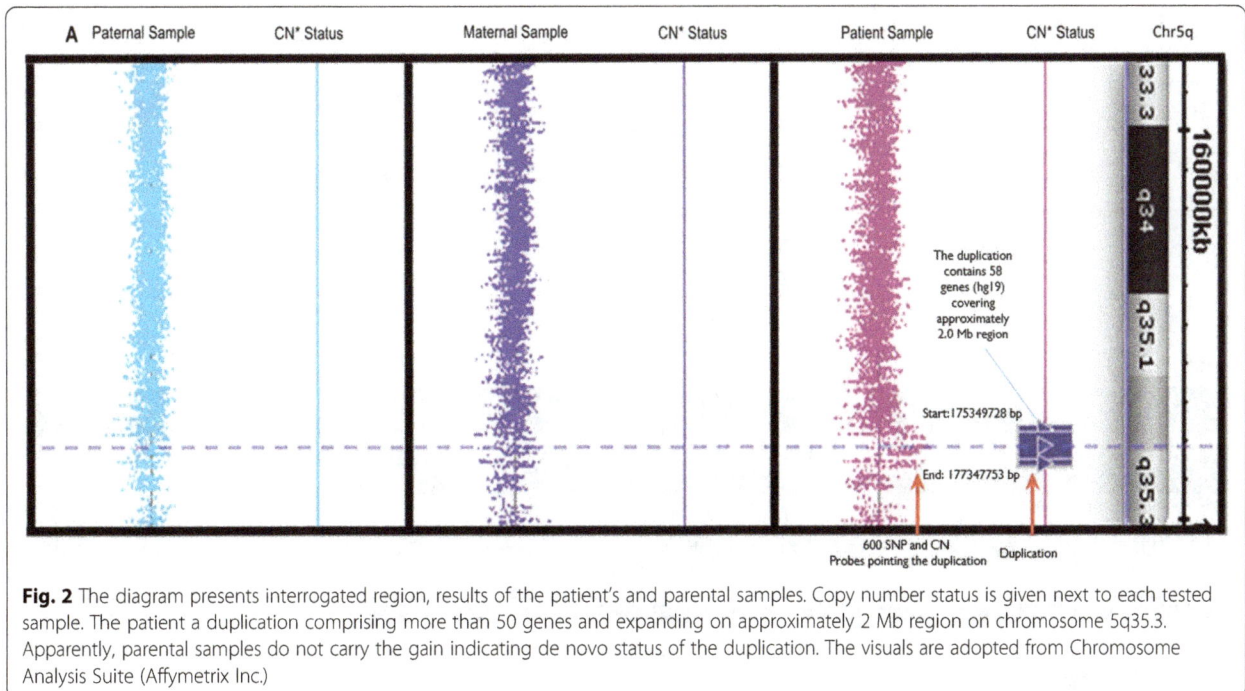

Fig. 2 The diagram presents interrogated region, results of the patient's and parental samples. Copy number status is given next to each tested sample. The patient a duplication comprising more than 50 genes and expanding on approximately 2 Mb region on chromosome 5q35.3. Apparently, parental samples do not carry the gain indicating de novo status of the duplication. The visuals are adopted from Chromosome Analysis Suite (Affymetrix Inc.)

ammonia) were all normal. Brain magnetic resonance imaging (MRI) and magnetic resonance angiography (MRA) were unremarkable. Electroencephalography (EEG) showed normal findings. Recently, the patient had psychometry with IQ score of 57. He was also evaluated by a cardiologist and echocardiogram revealed a small PDA (1.5 mm) with good cardiac functions.

Whole genome screening of chromosomal aberrations using Affymetrix's cytogenetic microarrays revealed presence of two large hemizygous deletions at chromosomes 2 (2q24.1 Size: 249 kb) and 16 (16q22.2 Size:1819 kb). Genomic locations of the deletions are chromosome 2, positions: 159,140,953–159,390,141 bp, and chromosome 16 positions: 71,589,375–73,408,685 according hg19 (Figs. 3 and 4). The deleted region in chromosome 2 contains 2 genes and chromosome 16 comprises 18 genes, 5 of which are OMIM-annotated and associated with Tyrosinemia type II (OMIM#: 613,018), Anhaptoglobinemia (OMIM#: 140,100), Hypohaptoglobinemia (OMIM#: 140,100), Prostate cancer susceptibility (OMIM#: 104,155). The patient's mother was also tested and found negative for above mentioned deletions. Unfortunately, paternal DNA sample was not available for testing and we were unable to recruit the father for further investigation.

Case 4

This is a 7-year-old boy who was the product of full normal spontaneous vaginal delivery with a birthweight of 3.5 kg. He was well until the age of 8 months when he was noticed to have flexion swinging movements in the hands and wrists that were spontaneous and exaggerated by irritability. There were no other abnormal movements or seizures. He was delayed in attaining milestones with severely impaired cognitive, linguistics and social skills. He was also diagnosed with atrial septal defect. His parents are first-cousins. They have 2 other children who are alive and well. There was no family history of a similar disease. On examination, his head circumference was around 50th percentile, weight was at the 97th percentile, and height was just above the 97th percentile. He had low-set ears and prominent philtrum. His tone, power and reflexes were normal. There were no neurocutaneous manifestations. Skeletal survey, brain MRI and ultrasound of abdomen were normal.

Molecular cytogenetic studies identified a 3.35 Mb interstitial deletion on the long arm of chromosome 3 from 112,146,815 bp to 115,496,750 bp (3q13.2q13.31) (hg19). This region contains over 27 genes, one of which is an annotated OMIM disease gene (*DRD3*). All remaining regions did not show any significant DNA copy number gains or losses.

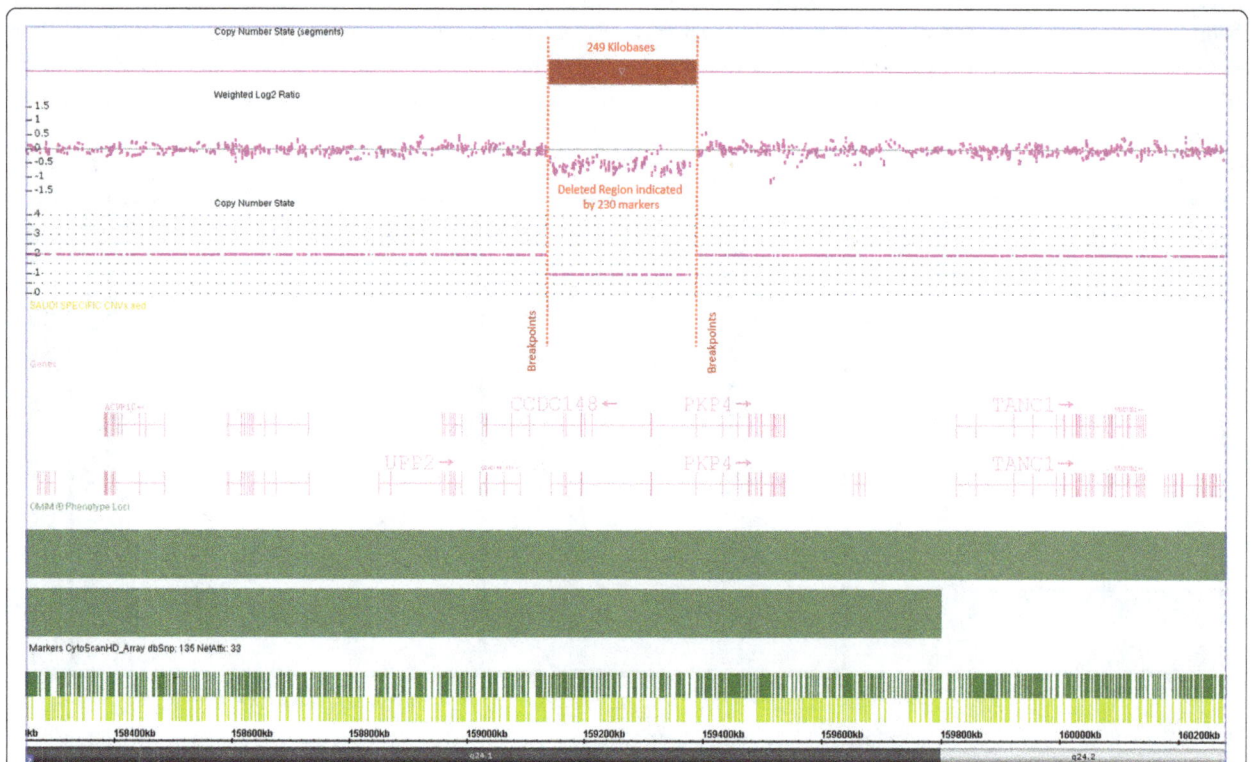

Fig. 3 Microarray results are displayed for chromosome 2q23.3–24.3 bands. A deletion is seen on 2q24.1 cytoband expanding over more than 249 kb genomic region

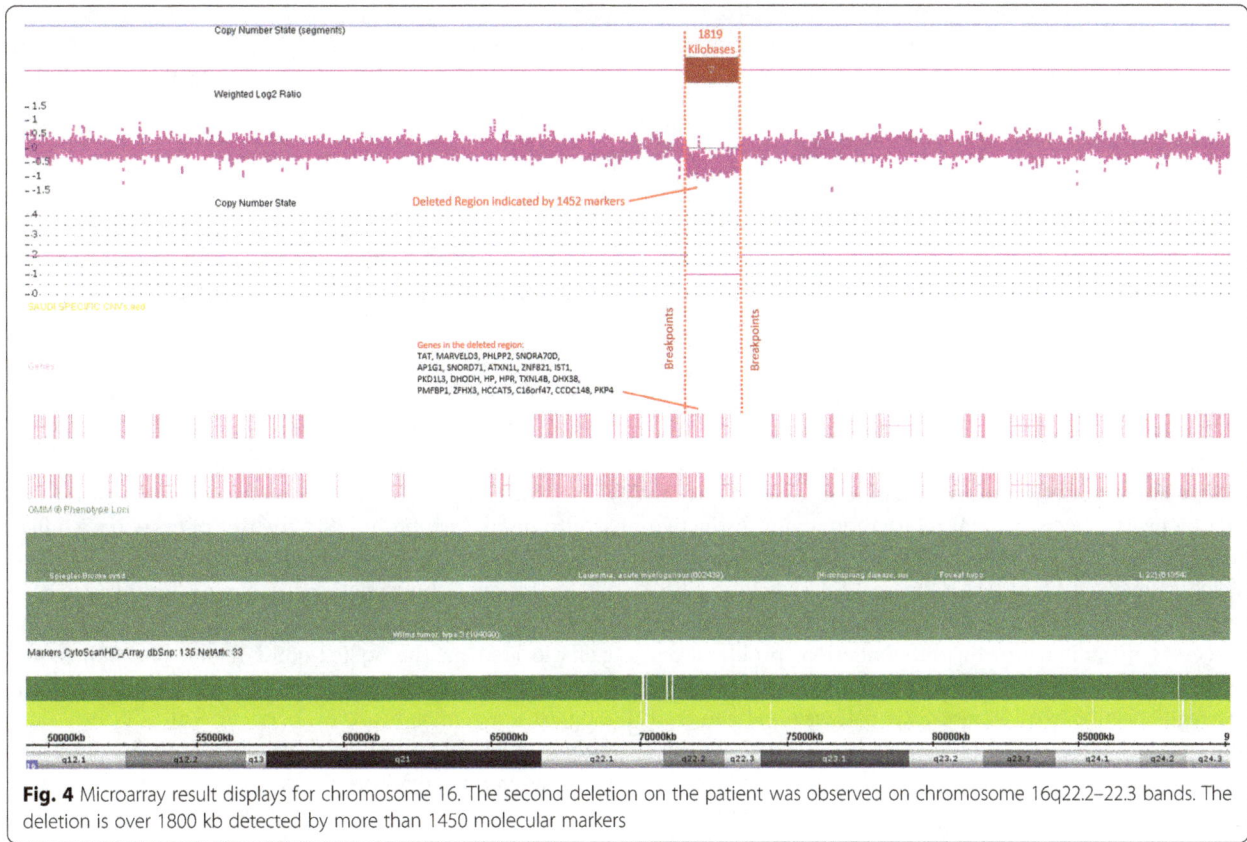

Fig. 4 Microarray result displays for chromosome 16. The second deletion on the patient was observed on chromosome 16q22.2–22.3 bands. The deletion is over 1800 kb detected by more than 1450 molecular markers

Case 5

This is a three-year-old girl who was a product of an in vitro fertilization delivered at 34 weeks of gestation to consanguineous parents with negative family history. She was noticed to have dysmorphic features with low set ears, depressed nasal bridge, and long philtrum. Ophthalmological examination revealed left choroidal coloboma involving the macula and optic disc. Echocardiogram showed large atrial septal defect, large, perimembranous ventricular septal defect, hypoplastic right upper pulmonary vein. She had surgical intervention with ASD and VSD closure and repair of upper pulmonary vein stenosis. She has had global developmental delay and growth failure with all the parameters below the 5th percentile (head circumference – 2.7 SD, weight -6SD, height -4SD). Brain MRI and ultrasound abdomen were normal.

Based on 20 metaphase cells, standard g-banding karyotyping at 425 band resolution indicated an apparently balanced translocation between the q-arm of chromosome 10 and the q arm of chromosome 12 (46,XX,t(10;12)(q22;q22)) was found in all the cells; however, loss of chromosomal material cannot be ruled out based on the low band resolution seen. Although this translocation could be de-novo most likely one of the parents is a carrier for the translocation. Follow-up aCGH study indicated presence of two deletions; one on

chromosome 12 (12p12.1p11.21; 25,320,816–31,285,151; ~5.96 Mb) and the other on the chromosome 16 (16p11.2; 29,567,295–30,321,320; ~754 Kb), (hg19). The deletion on chromosome 16 is paternally inherited. The larger deletion (chromosome 12) observed in this patient is not present in either parent and therefore appears to be a de novo event.

Case 6

This is a 4-year-old female who was the product of full normal spontaneous vaginal delivery with a birthweight of 1.45. She stayed in the NICU for 2 months and was diagnosed with perimembranous ventricular septal defect. She was noticed to have global developmental delay and poor growth. There was no history of seizures. The parents are not consanguineous. There is no family history of a similar problem. Her physical examination was notable for microcephaly (7 SD below the mean). Her weight was -5SD and height was -3SD. She had low anterior hair line, squint, broad nasal bridge, short philtrum, and micrognathia. The muscle tone was mildly increased in the upper and lower extremities. Ultrasound of abdomen showed mild right upper pole caliectasis.

Molecular cytogenetic analysis revealed presence of 2.78 Mb interstitial deletion in the short arm of chromosome 2 (extending between 59,170,950 bp and 61, 946,

784 bp over chromosome 2p16.1 deletion syndrome region) (Fig. 5). Although the region is large in size, it is relatively gene-poor region with a total of only 27 genes, six of which are OMIM-annotated. Among these *PEX13* is known to associate with Zellweger syndrome.

Discussion
Case 1

Deletions in the 7q33-q34 region are rarely reported in the scientific literature. Reported deletions in this region are mostly associated with developmental delay, intellectual disability, microcephaly, and significant morphological and developmental phenotypes. The deleted region in this case contains 50 genes including the *BRAF*; the mutation of which is known to be associated with cardiofaciocutaneous (CFC) syndrome [23], a disease characterized by heart defects, mental retardation and a distinctive facial appearance. *BRAF* encodes for the BRAF protein, which is involved in the MAP kinase/ERK signalling pathway; an important pathway that implicates various cell processes including growth, differentiation, proliferation, senescence and apoptosis [24]. Mutations in *BRAF* disrupt the regulation of MAP kinase/ERK pathway and can lead to a range of complications including various types of cancers as well as developmental disorders such as Noonan syndrome (NS), Costello syndrome, LEOPARD syndrome, and Cardiofaciocutaneous syndrome (CFC). Interestingly,

only one of the previously described cases shared a deletion in the genomic region constituting the *BRAF* gene [25]. This makes it a likely candidate to explain the clinical features in these cases.

Case 2

Chromosome 5q35.2-q35.3 deletions are well-known mainly due to Sotos syndrome. Altogether, these genomic alterations reach to a significant number [26–28]. Compared to deletions [27, 29–33] duplications in the region are rare and not well-characterized [34–37]. Moreover, there is no well-established genotype-phenotype correlation for these gains currently since they are in variable sizes and lack precise breakpoints. Interestingly among these cases only singleton have been reported to have Sotos syndrome-like symptom [38]. The rest of cases have different phenotypic findings mostly in the form of developmental delay and short stature. Among these cases, two duplications exceed nearly twice the size of the rest of the gains located on the 5q35.2-q35.3 region [34, 38]. In the present study we describe a patient with a duplication leading to congenital heart disease, cervical ankylosis, and thumb hypoplasia in addition to microcephaly, short stature, and various dysmorphic features. Intriguingly, among the duplication carrying patients, beside our case, there are only three patients who have heart defects [38, 39].

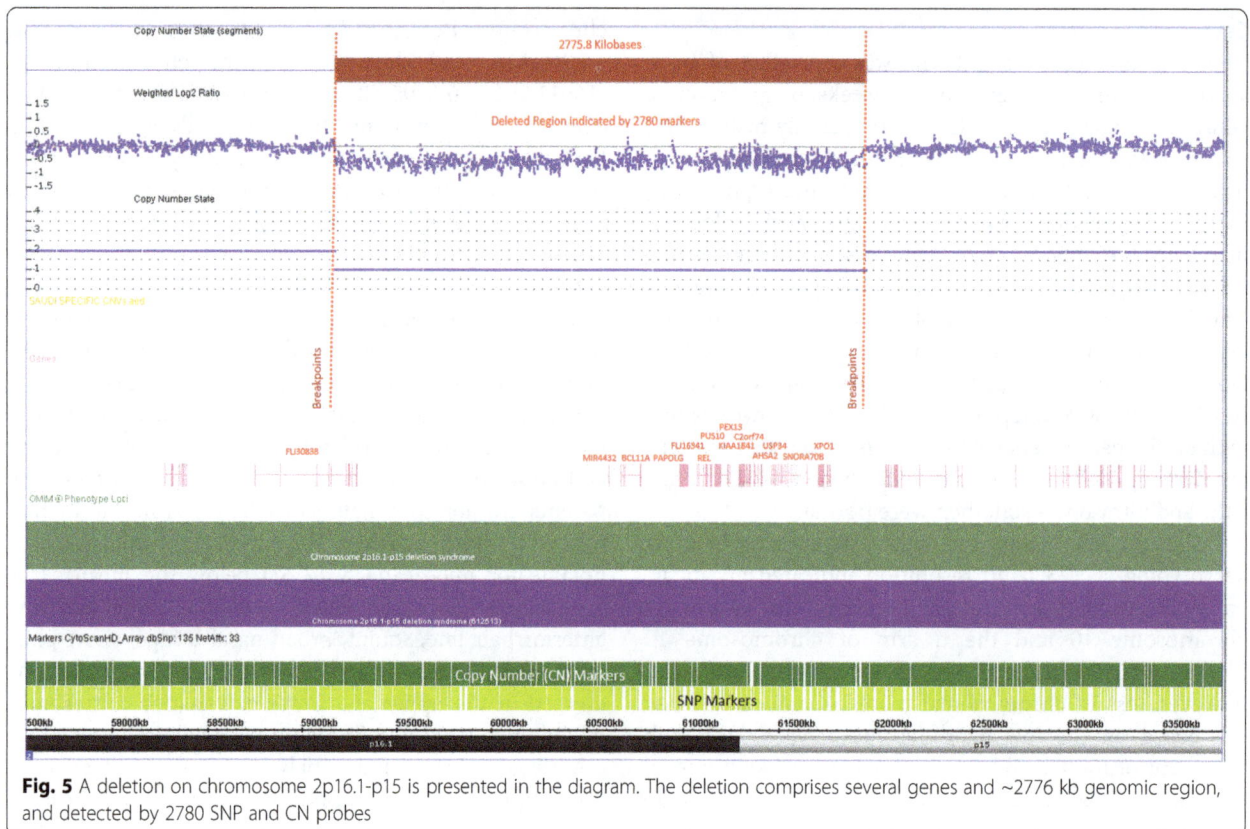

Fig. 5 A deletion on chromosome 2p16.1-p15 is presented in the diagram. The deletion comprises several genes and ~2776 kb genomic region, and detected by 2780 SNP and CN probes

In their study Jamsheer et al. [38] pointed out likely involvement of *MSX2* in radial agenesis as well as complex heart defect, and *FGFR4* as causative factor of limb formation. Although *FGFR4* is shared by both gains (ours and that of Jamsheer et al. [38]), *MSX2* is located outside the boundaries of our duplication. Deletions of both genes, *NSD1* and *FGFR4*, were previously reported with congenital heart anomalies [40]. However, interestingly, *FGFR4* is not a shared gene between all four cases having heart defects. In other words it is not in the shared region of the patients reported in Rosenfeld et al.'s study [39]. Hence, involvement of this gene in the reported heart defects is less likely. Relatedly Rosenfeld et al. raised the likely contribution of another candidate gene *PDLIM7* which is shared among all the cases with the heart defect including ours according to recent human assembly (hg38, 39). *PDLIM7* is a scaffold protein that regulates *Tbx5* which has critical roles in heart and limb development. Moreover, suppressed expression of *Pdlim7* in zebrafish led to the development of heart abnormalities in the animals.

Case 3

The deletion is large (1.8 Mb) and comprises 18 genes (*TAT, MARVELD3, PHLPP2, SNORA70D, AP1G1, SNORD71, ATXN1L, ZNF821, IST1, PKD1L3, DHODH, HP, HPR, TXNL4B, DHX38, PMFBP1, ZFHX3, HCCAT5, C16orf47*) located in 16q22.1-q24 cytogenetic region. Such deletions are frequently seen among breast cancer patients [41]. Moreover, two different cases having cytogenetic abnormalities in the long arm of chromosome 16, were previously described with ventricular septal defect [42, 43]. However, these abnormalities are not overlapping with 16q22.2 cytogenetic band.

The partial deletion of 16q is implicated in the rare 16q22 deletion syndrome (OMIM #614541) characterized by failure to thrive, growth retardation, dysmorphic facial features, and hypotonia. *DHODH* is one of the implicated genes that encodes for dihydroorotate dehydrogenase which catalyzes the oxidation of dihydroorotate to orotate, thereby facilitating the biosynthesis of pyrimidine blocks. Moreover, the mutations in *DHODH* lead to Miller syndrome, also known as postaxial acrofacial dysostosis [44]. Interestingly, it was also found that DHODH is involved in the transcriptional elongation of *BRAF* [45] that is a well-known oncogene, a member of the Raf kinase family, and an important molecule for RAS/MAPK signaling pathway. Mutations in this gene cause different hereditary disorders such as cardiofaciocutaneous syndrome, multiple lentigines syndrome, and Noonan syndrome as well as the development of birth defects.

Small deletions in the 2q24.1q24.2 region are quite rare [46]. A female patient was screened with SNP arrays and found to carry de novo deletion of 2q24.1q24.2 region. The patient had mental retardation and generalized hypotonia but lacking any cardiovascular problem [46]. The deleted region on chromosome 2 in our patient harbors two genes: *CCDC148* and *PKP4*. *PKP4* has been speculated to be a modifier gene for *LMNA* in which a splicing mutation caused sudden death, ventricular arrhythmia, cardiomyopathy, and heart failure in a 63-year-old male with a family history of individuals (>10) with similar problems [47].

It is also noteworthy to mention that paternal DNA sample was not available for cytogenetic testing. Hence, we were unable to confirm the de novo status of the deletions in our patient.

Case 4

Our molecular cytogenetic studies identified an interstitial microdeletion on 3q13.2q13.31 cytobands. Such deletions are rare [48] and only few cases have been reported by now. There are more cases of larger deletions in the region (3q11q23) with a range of various phenotypic features such as developmental delay, facial dysmorphisms, and musculoskeletal abnormalities [49–54]. A recent study summarized most of these cases excluding few recently reported patients [55–57]. The study narrowed down all the deletions to a shared region that harbors expectedly significantly lesser genes than those of the larger region from the previous 3q deletion studies [58]. In this study the smallest deletion was nearly 0.6 Megabases of size and located on 3q13.31. This region contains over 27 genes, one of which is an annotated OMIM disease gene (*DRD3*). Genotype-phenotype comparison of more than 20 patients shared 3q13.31 deletion and all shared some common phenotypic features developmental delay, muscular hypotonia, a high arched palate, and recognizable facial features including short philtrum and protruding lips. Heart related abnormalities were not among the listed characteristics. The authors speculated that developmental delay seen in these patients is related to *DRD3* and *ZBTB20*. Intriguingly none of these cases of 3q13.31 deletion have heart related abnormality. Moreover, considering that the parents are closely related, the phenotype is likely to originate from the consanginuity. However, this needs further investigations.

Case 5

Chromosome 12p (12p12.1p11.21) and chromosome 16p (16p11.2) deletions are not commonly co-occurring. There are reports for deletions for 12p and 16 p regions [59, 60]. There is only a single report of an interesting patient, who harbors two-hits, maternally inherited 16p13.11-p12.3 duplication and a de novo 12p12.1 deletion [61] whereas our patient has a paternally inherited 16p11.2 deletion and a de novo 12p12.1p11.21 deletion. However, considering the gain type and affected cytogenetic bands our patient is unique and will add to literature of two-hits patients. Deletions of 16p11.2 have been associated with the highly variable phenotype ranging from intellectual disability autism and congenital abnormalities to mildly affected or unaffected cases [62]. In such cases a child may be on one and of the conical spectrum. A recent comprehensive study revisits deletions and duplications in this region in 246 patients. The interesting difference between carriers of the 16p11.2 deletions and duplications is the frequent encounter of macrocephaly among the deletion cases [63]. However, the larger deletion (Chromosome 12) observed in this patient is not present in either parents and therefore appears to be a de novo event as such it is likely to be a significant contributor to the patient's phenotype. Chromosome 12p12.1 deletions harboring SOX5 have been previously reported [64–66]. Among these few patients were reported to have heart related problems such as ventricular septal defect, slight arrhythmia, secundumatrial septal defect, and atrioventricular canal [66]. Phenotypic consequences of these patients were linked to SOX5 haploinsufficiency.

Case 6

2p16.1p15 deletion harbors 27 genes including *PEX13*. While compound heterozygous and homozygous mutations in *PEX13* are associated with Zellweger syndrome (Type PDB11A (OMIM#614883). Haploinsufficiency of this gene due to a heterozygous deletion has not been reported to be a cause of the disease. A *PEX13* sequence based mutation on the non-deleted chromosome could conceivably give rise to a clinical phenotype that differs from Zellweger syndrome and sequencing of this gene is considered. However, the plasma very long chain fatty acids assay was normal in the patient; hence, the sequencing of *PEX13* was not performed. Until recently, microdeletions of 2p15–16.1 were identified in 15 patients with a recognizable syndrome of dysmorphic features, microcephaly and intellectual disability [67] in addition to the patients deposited to the public databases such as DECIPHER and ISCA. Among the cases, no patient has a report of heart related defect. Hence, the relationship of this deletion to our patient's phenotype needs further delineation. Moreover, parental studies would be useful in order to determine whether this alteration represents a familial variant or a de novo change. De novo changes are more likely to be clinically significant.

Conclusions

In conclusion, we present the first chromosomal imbalances associated with congenital heart abnormalities among Saudi patients. Such information, combined with further delineation of similar cases and relatedly collection of Saudi Specific CNVs, will allow better understanding of the pathobiology as well as management of the CHD patients in Saudi Arabia.

Acknowledgements

We gratefully thank to the patients and the parents for their kind participation to the study. We also thank KFSHRC Core Facilities at Genetics Department, Research Advisory Council Committees and Purchasing Departments, especially Mr. Faisal Al-Otaibi and his team, for facilitating and expediting our requests.

Funding

This study was supported by King Faisal Specialist Hospital and Research center's seed grants (KFSHRC-RAC# 2120022) and funds King Abdulaziz City for Science and Technology (KACST# 11-MED1439–20, KACST#14-MED2007–20, KACST#14-BIO2221–20, and KACST#11-BIO2072–20) and King Salman Center for Disability Research (Project#: 02-R-0029-NE-02-AU-1). M. A. S. was supported by the Deanship of Scientific Research, King Saud University, Riyadh, Saudi Arabia through research group no RGP-VPP- 301.

Declaration

We have obtained consents from the studied patients for the study. The patients were evaluated at the Kind Faisal Specialist Hospital and Research Center using the institutionally approved IRB protocols (RAC# 2040042, 2030046, 2120022, 2080032).

Authors' contributions

NK conceived and designed the experiments, drafted manuscript, reviewed the data analyses. DC involved in experimental design, reviewed the data analyses, involved in drafting the manuscript, ZA involved in experimental designed, reviewed the charts, evaluated the patients, undertook patient care and management, collected clinical data, delineated the patients' phenotype and drafted the manuscript. WA involved in drafting the manuscript, analyzed the data. FA, RA, AA performed the experiments. OMM reviewed the charts and involved in drafting and revising the manuscript. ZS, SW involved in performing experiments, MAS, MA, SMH, MAJ reviewed the charts, evaluated the patients, undertook patient care and management, and collected clinical data, OA, BL, BA involved in data analyses, read and revise the manuscript. All authors read and approved the final manuscript.

Competing interests

The authors declare that they have no competing interests.

Author details
[1]Department of Medical Genetics, King Faisal Specialist Hospital and Research Centre, Riyadh, Kingdom of Saudi Arabia. [2]Department of Genetics, King Faisal Specialist Hospital and Research Centre, MBC: 03, Riyadh 11211, Kingdom of Saudi Arabia. [3]Division of Pediatric Neurology, Department of Pediatrics, College of Medicine, King Saud University, Riyadh, Kingdom of Saudi Arabia. [4]Heart Center, King Faisal Specialist Hospital and Research Centre, Riyadh, Kingdom of Saudi Arabia. [5]Department of Pathology and Cell Biology, Columbia University, New York, NY, USA. [6]Department of Biostatistics, Epidemiology and Scientific Computing, King Faisal Specialist Hospital and Research Centre, Riyadh, Kingdom of Saudi Arabia. [7]College of Medicine, Alfaisal University, Riyadh, Saudi Arabia.

References

1. Bernier PL, Stefanescu A, Samoukovic G, Tchervenkov CI. The challenge of congenital heart disease worldwide: epidemiologic and demographic facts. Semin Thorac Cardiovasc Surg Pediatr Card Surg Ann. 2010;13(1):26–34.

2. Hoffman JI, Kaplan S. The incidence of congenital heart disease. J Am Coll Cardiol. 2002;39(12):1890–900.

3. Dolk H, Loane M, Garne E, European Surveillance of Congenital Anomalies Working G. Congenital heart defects in Europe: prevalence and perinatal mortality, 2000 to 2005. Circulation. 2011;123(8):841–9.

4. van der Linde D, Konings EE, Slager MA, Witsenburg M, Helbing WA, Takkenberg JJ, Roos-Hesselink JW. Birth prevalence of congenital heart disease worldwide: a systematic review and meta-analysis. J Am Coll Cardiol. 2011;58(21):2241–7.

5. Yan Y, Wu Q, Zhang L, Wang X, Dan S, Deng D, Sun L, Yao L, Ma Y, Wang L. Detection of submicroscopic chromosomal aberrations by array-based comparative genomic hybridization in fetuses with congenital heart disease. Ultrasound Obstet Gynecol. 2014;43(4):404–12.

6. Pierpont ME, Basson CT, Benson DW Jr, Gelb BD, Giglia TM, Goldmuntz E, McGee G, Sable CA, Srivastava D, Webb CL, et al. Genetic basis for congenital heart defects: current knowledge: a scientific statement from the American Heart Association congenital cardiac defects committee, council on cardiovascular disease in the young: endorsed by the American Academy of Pediatrics. Circulation. 2007;115(23):3015–38.

7. Thienpont B, Mertens L, de Ravel T, Eyskens B, Boshoff D, Maas N, Fryns JP, Gewillig M, Vermeesch JR, Devriendt K. Submicroscopic chromosomal imbalances detected by array-CGH are a frequent cause of congenital heart defects in selected patients. Eur Heart J. 2007;28(22):2778–84.

8. Colak D, Al-Dhalaan H, Nester M, Albakheet A, Al-Younes B, Al-Hassnan Z, Al-Dosari A, Chedrawi A, Al-Owain M, Abudheim N, et al. Genomic and transcriptomic analyses distinguish classic Rett and Rett-like syndrome and reveals shared altered pathways. Genomics. 2011;97(1):19–28.

9. Kaya N, Al-Owain M, Albakheet A, Colak D, Al-Odaib A, Imtiaz F, Coskun S, Al-Sayed M, Al-Hassnan Z, Al-Zaidan H, et al. Array comparative genomic hybridization (aCGH) reveals the largest novel deletion in PCCA found in a Saudi family with propionic acidemia. Eur J Med Genet. 2008;51(6):558–65.

10. Kaya N, Colak D, Albakheet A, Al-Owain M, Abu-Dheim N, Al-Younes B, Al-Zahrani J, Mukaddes NM, Dervent A, Al-Dosari N, et al. A novel X-linked disorder with developmental delay and autistic features. Ann Neurol. 2012;71(4):498–508.

11. Kaya N, Imtiaz F, Colak D, Al-Sayed M, Al-Odaib A, Al-Zahrani F, Al-Mubarak BR, Al-Owain M, Al-Dhalaan H, Chedrawi A, et al. Genome-wide gene expression profiling and mutation analysis of Saudi patients with Canavan disease. Genet Med. 2008;10(9):675–84.

12. Redin C, Brand H, Collins RL, Kammin T, Mitchell E, Hodge JC, Hanscom C, Pillalamarri V, Seabra CM, Abbott MA, et al. The genomic landscape of balanced cytogenetic abnormalities associated with human congenital anomalies. Nat Genet. 2016;

13. Bonnet C, Andrieux J, Beri-Dexheimer M, Leheup B, Boute O, Manouvrier S, Delobel B, Copin H, Receveur A, Mathieu M, et al. Microdeletion at chromosome 4q21 defines a new emerging syndrome with marked growth restriction, mental retardation and absent or severely delayed speech. J Med Genet. 2010;47(6):377–84.

14. Shaffer LG, Theisen A, Bejjani BA, Ballif BC, Aylsworth AS, Lim C, McDonald M, Ellison JW, Kostiner D, Saitta S, et al. The discovery of microdeletion syndromes in the post-genomic era: review of the methodology and characterization of a new 1q41q42 microdeletion syndrome. Genet Med. 2007;9(9):607–16.

15. Sharp AJ, Mefford HC, Li K, Baker C, Skinner C, Stevenson RE, Schroer RJ, Novara F, De Gregori M, Ciccone R, et al. A recurrent 15q13.3 microdeletion syndrome associated with mental retardation and seizures. Nat Genet. 2008; 40(3):322–8.

16. Ballif BC, Theisen A, Rosenfeld JA, Traylor RN, Gastier-Foster J, Thrush DL, Astbury C, Bartholomew D, McBride KL, Pyatt RE, et al. Identification of a recurrent microdeletion at 17q23.1q23.2 flanked by segmental duplications associated with heart defects and limb abnormalities. Am J Hum Genet. 2010;86(3):454–61.

17. Rosenfeld JA, Stephens LE, Coppinger J, Ballif BC, Hoo JJ, French BN, Banks VC, Smith WE, Manchester D, Tsai AC, et al. Deletions flanked by breakpoints 3 and 4 on 15q13 may contribute to abnormal phenotypes. Eur J Hum Genet. 2011;19(5):547–54.

18. Miller DT, Adam MP, Aradhya S, Biesecker LG, Brothman AR, Carter NP, Church DM, Crolla JA, Eichler EE, Epstein CJ, et al. Consensus statement: chromosomal microarray is a first-tier clinical diagnostic test for individuals with developmental disabilities or congenital anomalies. Am J Hum Genet. 2010;86(5):749–64.

19. Battaglia A, Doccini V, Bernardini L, Novelli A, Loddo S, Capalbo A, Filippi T, Carey JC. Confirmation of chromosomal microarray as a first-tier clinical diagnostic test for individuals with developmental delay, intellectual disability, autism spectrum disorders and dysmorphic features. Eur J Paediatr Neurol. 2013;17(6):589–99.

20. Connor JA, Hinton RB, Miller EM, Sund KL, Ruschman JG, Ware SM. Genetic testing practices in infants with congenital heart disease. Congenit Heart Dis. 2014;9(2):158–67.

21. Bachman KK, DeWard SJ, Chrysostomou C, Munoz R, Madan-Khetarpal S. Array CGH as a first-tier test for neonates with congenital heart disease. Cardiol Young. 2015;25(1):115–22.

22. Baldwin EL, Lee JY, Blake DM, Bunke BP, Alexander CR, Kogan AL, Ledbetter DH, Martin CL. Enhanced detection of clinically relevant genomic imbalances using a targeted plus whole genome oligonucleotide microarray. Genet Med. 2008;10(6):415–29.

23. Niihori T, Aoki Y, Narumi Y, Neri G, Cave H, Verloes A, Okamoto N, Hennekam RC, Gillessen-Kaesbach G, Wieczorek D, et al. Germline KRAS and BRAF mutations in cardio-facio-cutaneous syndrome. Nat Genet. 2006;38(3):294–6.

24. Hussain MR, Baig M, Mohamoud HS, Ulhaq Z, Hoessli DC, Khogeer GS, Al-Sayed RR, Al-Aama JY. BRAF gene: from human cancers to developmental syndromes. Saudi J Biol Sci. 2015;22(4):359–73.

25. Kaminsky EB, Kaul V, Paschall J, Church DM, Bunke B, Kunig D, Moreno-De-Luca D, Moreno-De-Luca A, Mulle JG, Warren ST, et al. An evidence-based approach to establish the functional and clinical significance of copy number variants in intellectual and developmental disabilities. Genet Med. 2011;13(9):777–84.

26. Dikow N, Maas B, Gaspar H, Kreiss-Nachtsheim M, Engels H, Kuechler A, Garbes L, Netzer C, Neuhann TM, Koehler U, et al. The phenotypic spectrum of duplication 5q35.2-q35.3 encompassing NSD1: is it really a reversed Sotos syndrome? Am J Med Genet A. 2013;161(9):2158–66.

27. Kurotaki N, Harada N, Shimokawa O, Miyake N, Kawame H, Uetake K, Makita Y, Kondoh T, Ogata T, Hasegawa T, et al. Fifty microdeletions among 112 cases of Sotos syndrome: low copy repeats possibly mediate the common deletion. Hum Mutat. 2003;22(5):378–87.

28. Mochizuki J, Saitsu H, Mizuguchi T, Nishimura A, Visser R, Kurotaki N, Miyake N, Unno N, Matsumoto N. Alu-related 5q35 microdeletions in Sotos syndrome. Clin Genet. 2008;74(4):384–91.

29. Fickie MR, Lapunzina P, Gentile JK, Tolkoff-Rubin N, Kroshinsky D, Galan E, Gean E, Martorell L, Romanelli V, Toral JF, et al. Adults with Sotos syndrome: review of 21 adults with molecularly confirmed NSD1 alterations, including a detailed case report of the oldest person. Am J Med Genet A. 2011; 155A(9):2105–11.

30. Hoglund P, Kurotaki N, Kytola S, Miyake N, Somer M, Matsumoto N. Familial Sotos syndrome is caused by a novel 1 bp deletion of the NSD1 gene. J Med Genet. 2003;40(1):51–4.

31. Miyake N, Kurotaki N, Sugawara H, Shimokawa O, Harada N, Kondoh T, Tsukahara M, Ishikiriyama S, Sonoda T, Miyoshi Y, et al. Preferential paternal origin of microdeletions caused by prezygotic chromosome or chromatid rearrangements in Sotos syndrome. Am J Hum Genet. 2003;72(5):1331–7.

32. Peredo J, Quintero-Rivera F, Bradley JP, Tu M, Dipple KM. Cleft lip and palate in a patient with 5q35.2-q35.3 microdeletion: the importance of chromosomal microarray testing in the craniofacial clinic. Cleft Palate Craniofac J. 2013;50(5):618–22.

33. Sohn Y, Lee C, Ko J, Yang JA, Yun JN, Jung EJ, Jin HS, Park SJ, Jeong S. Clinical and genetic spectrum of 18 unrelated Korean patients with Sotos syndrome: frequent 5q35 microdeletion and identification of four novel NSD1 mutations. J Hum Genet. 2013;58(2):73–7.

34. Chen CP, Lin SP, Lin CC, Chen YJ, Chern SR, Li YC, Hsieh LJ, Lee CC, Pan CW, Wang W. Molecular cytogenetic analysis of de novo dup(5)(q35.2q35.3) and review of the literature of pure partial trisomy 5q. Am J Med Genet A. 2006; 140(14):1594–600.

35. Franco LM, de Ravel T, Graham BH, Frenkel SM, Van Driessche J, Stankiewicz P, Lupski JR, Vermeesch JR, Cheung SW. A syndrome of short stature, microcephaly and speech delay is associated with duplications reciprocal to the common Sotos syndrome deletion. Eur J Hum Genet. 2010;18(2):258–61.

36. Kasnauskiene J, Cimbalistiene L, Ciuladaite Z, Preiksaitiene E, Kucinskiene ZA, Hettinger JA, Sismani C, Patsalis PC, Kucinskas V. De novo 5q35.5 duplication with clinical presentation of Sotos syndrome. Am J Med Genet A. 2011; 155A(10):2501–7.

37. Kirchhoff M, Bisgaard AM, Bryndorf T, Gerdes T. MLPA analysis for a panel of syndromes with mental retardation reveals imbalances in 5.8% of patients with mental retardation and dysmorphic features, including duplications of the Sotos syndrome and Williams-Beuren syndrome regions. Eur J Med Genet. 2007;50(1):33–42.

38. Jamsheer A, Sowinska A, Simon D, Jamsheer-Bratkowska M, Trzeciak T, Latos-Bielenska A. Bilateral radial agenesis with absent thumbs, complex heart defect, short stature, and facial dysmorphism in a patient with pure distal microduplication of 5q35.2-5q35.3. BMC Med Genet. 2013;14:13.

39. Rosenfeld JA, Kim KH, Angle B, Troxell R, Gorski JL, Westemeyer M, Frydman M, Senturias Y, Earl D, Torchia B, et al. Further evidence of contrasting phenotypes caused by reciprocal deletions and duplications: duplication of NSD1 causes growth retardation and Microcephaly. Mol Syndromol. 2013;3(6):247–54.

40. Fagali C, Kok F, Nicola P, Kim C, Bertola D, Albano L, Koiffmann CP. MLPA analysis in 30 Sotos syndrome patients revealed one total NSD1 deletion and two partial deletions not previously reported. Eur J Med Genet. 2009; 52(5):333–6.

41. Driouch K, Dorion-Bonnet F, Briffod M, Champeme MH, Longy M, Lidereau R. Loss of heterozygosity on chromosome arm 16q in breast cancer metastases. Genes Chromosom Cancer. 1997;19(3):185–91.

42. Fryns JP, Melchoir S, Jaeken J, van den Berghe H. Partial monosomy of the long arm of chromosome 16 in a malformed newborn: karyotype 46,XX,del(16)(q21). Hum Genet. 1977;38(3):343–6.

43. Stratakis CA, Lafferty A, Taymans SE, Gafni RI, Meck JM, Blancato J. Anisomastia associated with interstitial duplication of chromosome 16, mental retardation, obesity, dysmorphic facies, and digital anomalies: molecular mapping of a new syndrome by fluorescent in situ hybridization and microsatellites to 16q13 (D16S419-D16S503). J Clin Endocrinol Metab. 2000;85(9):3396–401.

44. Ng SB, Buckingham KJ, Lee C, Bigham AW, Tabor HK, Dent KM, Huff CD, Shannon PT, Jabs EW, Nickerson DA, et al. Exome sequencing identifies the cause of a mendelian disorder. Nat Genet. 2010;42(1):30–5.

45. White RM, Cech J, Ratanasirintrawoot S, Lin CY, Rahl PB, Burke CJ, Langdon E, Tomlinson ML, Mosher J, Kaufman C, et al. DHODH modulates transcriptional elongation in the neural crest and melanoma. Nature. 2011;471(7339):518–22.

46. Palumbo O, Palumbo P, Palladino T, Stallone R, Zelante L, Carella M. A novel deletion in 2q24.1q24.2 in a girl with mental retardation and generalized hypotonia: a case report. Mol Cytogenet. 2012;5(1):1.

47. Zaragoza MV, Fung L, Jensen E, Oh F, Cung K, LA MC, Tran CK, Hoang V, Hakim SA, Grosberg A. Exome sequencing identifies a novel LMNA splice-site mutation and Multigenic Heterozygosity of potential modifiers in a family with sick sinus syndrome, dilated Cardiomyopathy, and sudden cardiac death. PLoS One. 2016;11(5):e0155421.

48. Lowther C, Costain G, Melvin R, Stavropoulos DJ, Lionel AC, Marshall CR, Scherer SW, Bassett AS. Adult expression of a 3q13.31 microdeletion. Mol Cytogenet. 2014;7(1):23.

49. Jenkins MB, Stang HJ, Davis E, Boyd L. Deletion of the proximal long arm of chromosome 3 in an infant with features of turner syndrome. Ann Genet. 1985;28(1):42–4.

50. Okada N, Hasegawa T, Osawa M, Fukuyama Y. A case of de novo interstitial deletion 3q. J Med Genet. 1987;24(5):305–8.

51. Fujita H, Meng J, Kawamura M, Tozuka N, Ishii F, Tanaka N. Boy with a chromosome del (3)(q12q23) and blepharophimosis syndrome. Am J Med Genet. 1992;44(4):434–6.

52. Genuardi M, Calvieri F, Tozzi C, Coslovi R, Neri G. A new case of interstitial deletion of chromosome 3q, del(3q)(q13.12q21.3), with agenesis of the corpus callosum. Clin Dysmorphol. 1994;3(4):292–6.

53. Mackie Ogilvie C, Rooney SC, Hodgson SV, Berry AC. Deletion of chromosome 3q proximal region gives rise to a variable phenotype. Clin Genet. 1998;53(3):220–2.

54. Lawson-Yuen A, Berend SA, Soul JS, Irons M. Patient with novel interstitial deletion of chromosome 3q13.1q13.3 and agenesis of the corpus callosum. Clin Dysmorphol. 2006;15(4):217–20.

55. Gimelli S, Leoni M, Di Rocco M, Caridi G, Porta S, Cuoco C, Gimelli G, Tassano E. A rare 3q13.31 microdeletion including GAP43 and LSAMP genes. Mol Cytogenet. 2013;6(1):52.

56. Vuillaume ML, Delrue MA, Naudion S, Toutain J, Fergelot P, Arveiler B, Lacombe D, Rooryck C. Expanding the clinical phenotype at the 3q13.31 locus with a new case of microdeletion and first characterization of the reciprocal duplication. Mol Genet Metab. 2013;110(1–2):90–7.

57. Herve B, Fauvert D, Dard R, Roume J, Cognard S, Goidin D, Lozach F, Molina-Gomes D, Vialard F. The emerging microduplication 3q13.31: expanding the genotype-phenotype correlations of the reciprocal microdeletion 3q13.31 syndrome. Eur J Med Genet. 2016;59(9):463–9.

58. Molin AM, Andrieux J, Koolen DA, Malan V, Carella M, Colleaux L, Cormier-Daire V, David A, de Leeuw N, Delobel B, et al. A novel microdeletion syndrome at 3q13.31 characterised by developmental delay, postnatal overgrowth, hypoplastic male genitals, and characteristic facial features. J Med Genet. 2012;49(2):104–9.

59. Leyser M, Dias BL, Coelho AL, Vasconcelos M, Nascimento OJ. 12p deletion spectrum syndrome: a new case report reinforces the evidence regarding the potential relationship to autism spectrum disorder and related developmental impairments. Mol Cytogenet. 2016;9:75.

60. Iourov IY, Vorsanova SG, Kurinnaia OS, Zelenova MA, Silvanovich AP, Yurov YB. Molecular karyotyping by array CGH in a Russian cohort of children with intellectual disability, autism, epilepsy and congenital anomalies. Mol Cytogenet. 2012;5(1):46.

61. Quintela I, Barros F, Lago-Leston R, Castro-Gago M, Carracedo A, Eiris J. A maternally inherited 16p13.11-p12.3 duplication concomitant with a de novo SOX5 deletion in a male patient with global developmental delay, disruptive and obsessive behaviors and minor dysmorphic features. Am J Med Genet A. 2015;167(6):1315–22.

62. Cooper GM, Coe BP, Girirajan S, Rosenfeld JA, TH V, Baker C, Williams C, Stalker H, Hamid R, Hannig V, et al. A copy number variation morbidity map of developmental delay. Nat Genet. 2011;43(9):838–46.

63. Steinman KJ, Spence SJ, Ramocki MB, Proud MB, Kessler SK, Marco EJ, Green Snyder L, D'Angelo D, Chen Q, Chung WK, et al. 16p11.2 deletion and duplication: characterizing neurologic phenotypes in a large clinically ascertained cohort. Am J Med Genet A. 2016;170(11):2943–55.

64. Lee RW, Bodurtha J, Cohen J, Fatemi A, Batista D. Deletion 12p12 involving SOX5 in two children with developmental delay and dysmorphic features. Pediatr Neurol. 2013;48(4):317–20.

65. Schanze I, Schanze D, Bacino CA, Douzgou S, Kerr B, Zenker M. Haploinsufficiency of SOX5, a member of the SOX (SRY-related HMG-box) family of transcription factors is a cause of intellectual disability. Eur J Med Genet. 2013;56(2):108–13.

66. Lamb AN, Rosenfeld JA, Neill NJ, Talkowski ME, Blumenthal I, Girirajan S, Keelean-Fuller D, Fan Z, Pouncey J, Stevens C, et al. Haploinsufficiency of SOX5 at 12p12.1 is associated with developmental delays with prominent language delay, behavior problems, and mild dysmorphic features. Hum Mutat. 2012;33(4):728–40.

67. Balci TB, Sawyer SL, Davila J, Humphreys P, Dyment DA. Brain malformations in a patient with deletion 2p16.1: a refinement of the phenotype to BCL11A. Eur J Med Genet. 2015;58(6–7):351–4.

20

Copy number variation and regions of homozygosity analysis in patients with MÜLLERIAN aplasia

Durkadin Demir Eksi[1†], Yiping Shen[2,3,4,5†], Munire Erman[6], Lynn P. Chorich[7,8], Megan E. Sullivan[7,8], Meric Bilekdemir[6], Elanur Yılmaz[9], Guven Luleci[9], Hyung-Goo Kim[7,8], Ozgul M. Alper[9*] and Lawrence C. Layman[7,8*]

Abstract

Background: Little is known about the genetic contribution to Müllerian aplasia, better known to patients as Mayer-Rokitansky-Küster-Hauser (MRKH) syndrome. Mutations in two genes (*WNT4* and *HNF1B*) account for a small number of patients, but heterozygous copy number variants (CNVs) have been described. However, the significance of these CNVs in the pathogenesis of MRKH is unknown, but suggests possible autosomal dominant inheritance. We are not aware of CNV studies in consanguineous patients, which could pinpoint genes important in autosomal recessive MRKH. We therefore utilized SNP/CGH microarrays to identify CNVs and define regions of homozygosity (ROH) in Anatolian Turkish MRKH patients.

Result(s): Five different CNVs were detected in 4/19 patients (21%), one of which is a previously reported 16p11.2 deletion containing 32 genes, while four involved smaller regions each containing only one gene. Fourteen of 19 (74%) of patients had parents that were third degree relatives or closer. There were 42 regions of homozygosity shared by at least two MRKH patients which was spread throughout most chromosomes. Of interest, eight candidate genes suggested by human or animal studies (*RBM8A*, *CMTM7*, *CCR4*, *TRIM71*, *CNOT10*, *TP63*, *EMX2*, and *CFTR*) reside within these ROH.

Conclusion(s): CNVs were found in about 20% of Turkish MRKH patients, and as in other studies, proof of causation is lacking. The 16p11.2 deletion seen in mixed populations is also identified in Turkish MRKH patients. Turkish MRKH patients have a higher likelihood of being consanguineous than the general Anatolian Turkish population. Although identified single gene mutations and heterozygous CNVs suggest autosomal dominant inheritance for MRKH in much of the western world, regions of homozygosity, which could contain shared mutant alleles, make it more likely that autosomal recessively inherited causes will be manifested in Turkish women with MRKH.

Keywords: Müllerian aplasia, Mayer-Rokitansky-Küster-Hauser syndrome, MRKH, Congenital absence of the uterus and vagina, Copy number variant, CNV, Candidate gene, Regions of homozygosity, ROH

* Correspondence: oalper@akdeniz.edu.tr; oalper8@yahoo.com; lalayman@augusta.edu
†Equal contributors
9Department of Medical Biology and Genetics, Akdeniz University, Faculty of Medicine, 07058 Antalya, Turkey
7Section of Reproductive Endocrinology, Infertility, & Genetics, Department of Obstetrics & Gynecology Medical College of Georgia at Augusta University, Augusta, GA, USA
Full list of author information is available at the end of the article

Introduction

Approximately 7–10% of women have uterovaginal anomalies [1], but perhaps the most severe is Müllerian aplasia, which is also known as Mayer-Rokitansky-Küster-Hauser (MRKH) syndrome—the name patients prefer [2]. These patients have congenital absence of the uterus and vagina (type I; MIM# 277000), or they may also have associated anomalies such as renal agenesis, skeletal abnormalities, cardiac anomalies, or deafness (type II; MIM# 601076) [3]. Additionally, emotional issues as well as concerns regarding family planning are prevalent for these patients [4]. Although MRKH affects ~ 1/4500–1/5000 females, it accounts for about 10% of the causes of primary amenorrhea in females [5].

There is evidence for genetic transmission, as there are some families with more than one affected MRKH individual [6, 7]. In our recent characterization of both North American and Turkish families ($n = 147$ probands), no family had more than one affected individual, but some had another person with one or more of the associated anomalies [2]. Vertical transmission is challenging to confirm unless the MRKH woman conceive with IVF and use a gestational carrier. Consequently, the genetic etiology of MRKH is largely unknown. To date, only two genes—WNT4 [8–11] and HNF1B [12]—have confirmed, causative mutations in a handful of MRKH patients. A total of four translocations have been identified in MRKH [13–15], but in only one were the breakpoints mapped [15]. Although no gene was directly disrupted, this valuable patient with a translocation involving chromosomes 3p22.3 and 16p13.3 can help pinpoint potential candidate genes that could be affected by a position effect [15].

A number of investigators have utilized chromosomal microarrays (CMAs) in MRKH either by comparative genomic hybridization (CGH) and/or single nucleotide polymorphism (SNP) techniques [16–21]. Reported copy number variants (CNVs) identified are abundant, but several have been found repetitively including deletions of 17q12, 16p11, and 22q11 [19]. Deletions and duplications of 1q21.1 have also been described by multiple investigators [16, 20, 22, 23]. These chromosomal regions contain numerous genes, and although they contain promising candidate genes, their role in causation is currently unknown. To date, all of the CNV studies in MRKH have been in mixed, nonconsanguineous, non-autosomal recessive populations. In the present study, we sought to use CMAs to identify CNVs and regions of homozygosity (ROH) in a suspected consanguineous Turkish population to provide additional clues to important candidate genes which might cause autosomal recessive MRKH.

Methods

Patients

Nineteen Anatolian Turkish patients with a normal 46,XX karyotype were diagnosed with MRKH in the Department of Obstetrics and Gynecology at Akdeniz University Hospital, Turkey and the study took place there and at the Medical College of Georgia at Augusta University, USA. The study was approved by the Institutional Review Boards at both locations, and each person signed a consent form. All patients had normal breast development and an absent vagina by exam supported by imaging studies. Of these 19, three had renal agenesis and two had hypoplastic ovaries (Table 1). Consanguinity was ascertained by family history when the patient was enrolled in the study. Genomic DNA was extracted from peripheral blood samples of patients and available family members by a non-enzymatic salt-precipitation method as described previously [24].

Copy number variation (CNV) analysis

Copy number variant analysis was performed on all 19 patients and available family members (if a CNV was identified) with the use of an Affymetrix Cytoscan HD array (Affymetrix, Inc., Santa Clara, CA), which contains 750,000 single-nucleotide polymorphism probes and 1.9 million oligonucleotide probes. The lower limit of detection for CNVs was 50 kilobases (kb). One hundred nanograms of genomic DNA was labeled and used along with the Cytoscan reagent kit according to the manufacturer's instructions. The array data were analyzed with Chromosome Analysis Suite software as described previously [25]. Human genome hg19 assembly was used to map genomic coordinates. The identified CNVs were compared with Database of Genomic Variants (DGV, http://projects.tcag.ca/cgi-bin/variation/gbrowse/hg19/) to determine if they were unique or previously identified. The CNVs were also investigated for potential pathogenicity using Decipher (https://decipher.sanger.ac.uk/).

Analysis of parental consanguinity and regions of homozygosity

Patient history was used to ascertain degree of consanguinity in the parents of the MRKH subject. Regions of homozygosity (ROH) analysis was performed on all 19 Turkish patients tested using the Affymetrix Cytoscan

Table 1 The associated clinical findings in the MRKH cohort

Patient	Finding
3	Hypoplastic ovary
10	Unilateral Renal agenesis
14	Hypoplastic ovary
16	Unilateral Renal agenesis
17	Unilateral Renal agenesis

HD platform. The degree of parental consanguinity was assessed according to the percentage of homozygosity (F_{ROH}), which is also known as a coefficient of consanguinity. F_{ROH} was calculated by summing autosomal homozygous DNA basepairs (> 5 Mb includes at least 100 consecutive probes) and dividing by total basepair of autosomal genome DNA [25]. The percentage of autosome/genome homozygosity (CHP Summary) determined by F_{ROH} was analyzed using Chromosome Analysis Suite (ChAS) 1.2 software (Affymetrix Data Analysis Software). The thresholds of the percentage of ROH to predict the degree of consanguinity were taken from Sund et al. [25]. Overlapping homozygous genomic regions in at least two patients were determined by comparing the length of shared sequence.

Results

Five different likely pathogenic CNVs were identified in four of 19 (21%) Turkish patients by CMA (Table 2), all of whom had isolated (type I) MRKH. One was the previously described 16p11.2 in MRKH, which was a 746 kb deletion, for which a similar sized CNV was seen in DGV six times, but not in Decipher. Note that when any sized CNV that overlaps the 16p11.2 region is considered, this was seen 125 times in DGV and 10 times in Decipher. This patient also had an Xq25 deletion of 768 kb present once in DGV, but not Decipher (any sized CNV 17 times in DGV; none in Decipher). Within the Xq25 deletion, there was only one gene. One patient had 16p13.3 deletion, which was present multiple times in both DGV and Decipher. The other two MRKH patients had duplications of 13q14.11 (once in DGV; not in Decipher) and 1p31.1 (not in DGV or Decipher) (Table 2). Except for the 16p11.2 deletion, which contained 39 genes, the other CNVs each only had 1–3 genes (Table 2). Family members for these four MRKH patients were not able to be studied, so it is not known if they are de novo.

By history, 11 of the 19 Turkish patients did not know if consanguinity was present, while eight stated that their parents were first cousins. First cousins

should share 1/16 (6.25%) of sequence. When ROH were analyzed, the degree of consanguinity was greater than the patient previously reported (Table 3). Instead of parents being third degree relatives, six were found to be second degree relatives with sharing of 8.8–18.3% loci, one was first or second degree (20% shared loci), and one was first degree (23.5% shared loci). For the 11 for whom no history was known, parents were second degree in one and third degree in three, while the others were third or fourth degree relatives. In total, 14 of 19 (~ 74%) MRKH patients had parents that were third degree relatives or closer.

In addition, there were 42 regions across the genome in which at least two MRKH patients had overlapping homozygous genomic regions (Table 4 and Fig. 1). The most frequently shared chromosomes were chromosomes 2, 3, and 4. All chromosomes were represented except 11, 16, 19, and 21. The shared regions contained as few as 10 genes or as many as 354 genes. None of the shared regions included the more common 17q12 or 16p11.2 CNVs, but two shared the 22q11.21 CNV region (Table 4).

Discussion

The pathogenesis of MRKH in humans is largely unknown, but could include genetic (germline or somatic cell mutations), epigenetic, and/or environmental etiologies. There is evidence supporting a genetic etiology, as demonstrated by families with more than one affected proband [7]. Although twin studies in which monozygotic twins show greater concordance vs. dizygotic twins support a genetic component [26], there have been few studies in MRKH. Those small number of monozygotic twins have been discordant for MRKH [27–29]. The genetic basis of MRKH is largely unknown except for occasional heterozygous *WNT4* or *HNF1B* mutations [8, 12]. Many investigators have performed CMA on MRKH patients and have suggested possible pathogenic CNVs [19, 30]. It is interesting to note that these CNVs

Table 2 Shown are five different copy number variants (CNV) that were identified in four Turkish patients with type I MRKH

Patient	CNV Location	Size/Type	Coordinates	# times in DGV	# times in Decipher	Genes in CNV
6	16p11.2	746 kb Del	29,432,212–30,177,916	6 (125)	0 (10)	39
	Xq25	768 kb Del	126,937,856–127,706,114	8 (17)	0 (0)	1 (*ACTRT1*)
7	16p13.3	243 kb Del	6,774,500–7,017,793	Multiple (131)	Multiple [25]	1(*RBFOX1*)*
8	13q14.11	116 kb Dup	41,178,626–41,294,741	1 (12)	0 (0)	1 (*FOXO1*)
9	1p31.1	263 kb Dup	76,357,590–76,620,268	0 (19)	0 (0)	3 (*ST6GALNAC3*, *MSH4*, *ASB17*)

DGV Database of Genomic Variants, *Del* deletion, *Dup* duplication. The number of times a very similar sized CNV is listed for both DGV and Decipher. In parentheses, shown is the number of times a CNV of any size overlapped any portion of our CNV region

*RBFOX1 is a gene known in relation to autism. Only patient number 6 had parents who were not consanguineous (4th degree relatives). Patient numbers 7 and 8 had parents that were 3rd degree relatives, while patient 9 had parents that were 2nd degree relatives

Table 3 Re-defined degree of consanguinity

Patient	Before Analysis	After Analysis	
	Parental Consanguinity (based on patient's interview)	% Autosomal ROH	Parental Consanguinity Degree
1	No Info	3.7%	Fourth degree
2	No Info	2.9%	Fourth degree
3	First Cousins	10.3%	Second degree
4	First Cousins	10.7%	Second degree
5	First Cousins	11.4%	Second degree
6	No Info	4.0%	Fourth degree
7	No Info	6.86%	Third degree
8	No Info	5.8%	Third degree
9	No Info	9.9%	Second degree
10	No Info	4.4%	Third or fourth degree
11	No Info	3.7%	Fourth degree
12	No Info	13.1%	Second degree
13	First Cousins	18.3%	Second degree
14	First Cousins	8.8%	Second degree
15	First Cousins	14.7%	Second degree
16	First Cousins	20%	First or second degree
17	No Info	6.4%	Third Degree
18	First Cousins	23.5%	First degree
19	No Info	20.9%	Second degree

Consanguinity Degree	Theoretic Percentage	Percentage of Homozygosity (Confidence Interval)
First or closer	> 25%	> 28.7%
First	25%	21.3–28.7%
First or second		15.3–21.3%
Second	12.5%	9.7–15.3%
Second or third		8.3–9.7%
Third	6.25%	4.6–8.3%
Third or fourth		4.2–4.6%
Fourth	3.125%	2.6–4.2%
Fourth or fifth		1.6–2.6%
Fifth	1.5625%	0.5–1.6%

may be found in isolated MRKH (type I) or those with associated anomalies (type II) [19, 30]. In the present study, we found five CNVs in four patients with type I MRKH, three of whom were products of consanguineous parents. This is consistent with the overall 75% rate of consanguinity in our study. The 21%

prevalence of CNVs in our largely consanguineous Turkish population does not seem to differ with the prevalence in studies of Europe and North America, which range from 16 to 46% (26% overall in four studies) [17, 19–21].

The previously reported 16p11.2 deletion was observed in one patient. Patients with microdeletions at 16p11.2 may show variable clinical features including autism [31], epilepsy, global developmental delay, dysmorphism, behavioral problems, abnormal head size [32], and obesity [32]. Microdeletions at 16p11.2 are also common in patients with type I and type II MRKH [19, 21]. This region contains more than 30 genes. The T Box 6 (*TBX6*) gene located in this region represents an attractive candidate gene, but to date, no causative mutations have been confirmed. This same patient had an Xq25 deletion, which contains one gene—*ACTRT1* (actin-related protein T1), which has no proven relation to MRKH at this time. Two other type I patients had CNVs containing only one gene—a 16p13.3 deletion (*RBFOX1*) and a 13q14.11 duplication (*FOXO1*). The remaining type I patient had a 1p31.1 duplication containing three genes (*ST6GALNAC3*, *MSH4*, and *ASB17*). The 16p13.3 region and the *RBFOX1* gene have been implicated in autism; *FOXO1* is a transcription factor; and *ST6GALNAC3* is expressed in the reproductive tract. *MSH4* is a member of the DNA mismatch repair mutS family necessary for reciprocal recombination and proper segregation of homologous chromosomes at meiosis I. *ASB17*, which is highly expressed in the testis, is a component of E3 ubiquitin-protein ligase complex that mediates the ubiquitination and subsequent proteasomal degradation of target proteins.

The significance of these CNVs is uncertain at this time, but it is unlikely that the 16p13.3 deletion is involved in the pathogenesis of MRKH because it occurs frequently in both the DGV and Decipher databases. Alternatively, the 16p11.2 CNV has been previously reported in MRKH, and large CNVs similar in size are infrequent in these two databases. The other three are potentially pathogenic CNVs—Xq25, 13q14.11, and 1p31.1.

When the literature is examined, chromosomal regions 17q12, 16p11, 22q11, and 1q21.1 harbor some of the more common CNVs in MRKH [16–21]. Deletions of 17q12 generally range from 1.2–1.8 Mb in size and contain ~ 17–20 genes. Known causative gene and transcription factor *HNF1B* resides within this region and heterozygous mutations result in maturity onset diabetes of the young type 5 (MODY5). Associated findings with this phenotype may include renal cysts and Müllerian aplasia [12]. *LHX1* is another potential causative gene within this region, as the knockout mouse has a phenotype consistent with MRKH. However, there are currently no clear causative human *LHX1* mutations, confirmed by in vitro analyses supported by family studies [2, 33]. We have recently performed Sanger DNA sequencing on 100 North American

Table 4 Overlapping regions of homozygosity

Chromosome	Cytoband Start	Min (Hg19)	Max (Hg19)	Gene Count	Number of patients (n)	Candidate gene
1	p22.3	87,889,117	101,551,513	150	2	
1	q21.1	144,033,938	150,574,441	56	2	*RMB8A*
1	q43	242,177,676	249,198,692	354	2	
2	p16.3	49,466,260	65,782,717	246	3	
2	p14	67,193,897	74,970,256	23	3	
2	q24.3	171,534,387	175,330,938	45	2	
2	q31.1	192,319,867	217,837,588	237	2	
2	q31.1	177,426,525	185,333,874	342	2	*CMTM7, CCR4, TRIM71, CNOT10*
3	p12.3	76,456,413	90,485,635	67	2	
3	p24.3	31,161,056	36,796,647	89	2	
3	q11.1	102,994,376	115,492,735	321	3	
3	q23	139,702,339	150,629,667	234	2	
3	q26.31	187,040,042	190,991,439	65	2	*TP63*
4	p14	40,533,584	45,755,965	76	2	
4	p15.33	11,546,274	16,693,715	34	2	
4	q11	65,736,529	71,893,827	87	3	
4	q22.1	111,799,253	139,609,452	231	3	
5	p15.1	9,998,327	17,326,672	341	2	
5	p15.2	18,320,731	31,181,789	23	2	
6	q16.1	106,018,502	110,701,451	45	2	
6	q25.2	153,345,184	158,377,316	56	2	
7	q21.3	103,575,957	105,632,704	78	2	
7	q31.1	111,645,191	124,187,217	65	3	*CFTR*
7	q35	144,922,849	150,951,819	89	2	
8	q12.1	58,780,480	65,128,132	78	2	
9	p24.2	3,939,996	12,907,793	98	2	
10	q23.31	116,005,494	124,214,355	120	2	*EMX2*
12	p13.32	3,780,336	7,918,460	89	2	
12	q13.13	58,000,215	68,228,170	56	2	
12	q13.3	103,118,607	113,263,934	45	3	
13	q12.13	33,381,720	34,694,189	32	4	
13	q22.3	77,503,539	87,943,460	23	2	
14	q31.3	92,919,833	94,993,744	45	2	
15	q22.2	60,644,347	68,204,581	67	2	
17	q11.1	35,694,046	41,797,254	34	2	
18	p11.22	8,993,423	12,697,711	60	3	
18	q22.1	66,236,242	74,326,105	78	2	
20	q11.21	45,391,728	46,347,251	24	2	
20	q13.12	50,008,791	53,427,207	12	2	
22	q11.21	44,669,027	45,906,107	10	2	
X	q11.1	61,932,503	66,974,524	45	8	
X	q13.1	71,819,690	77,853,204	32	2	

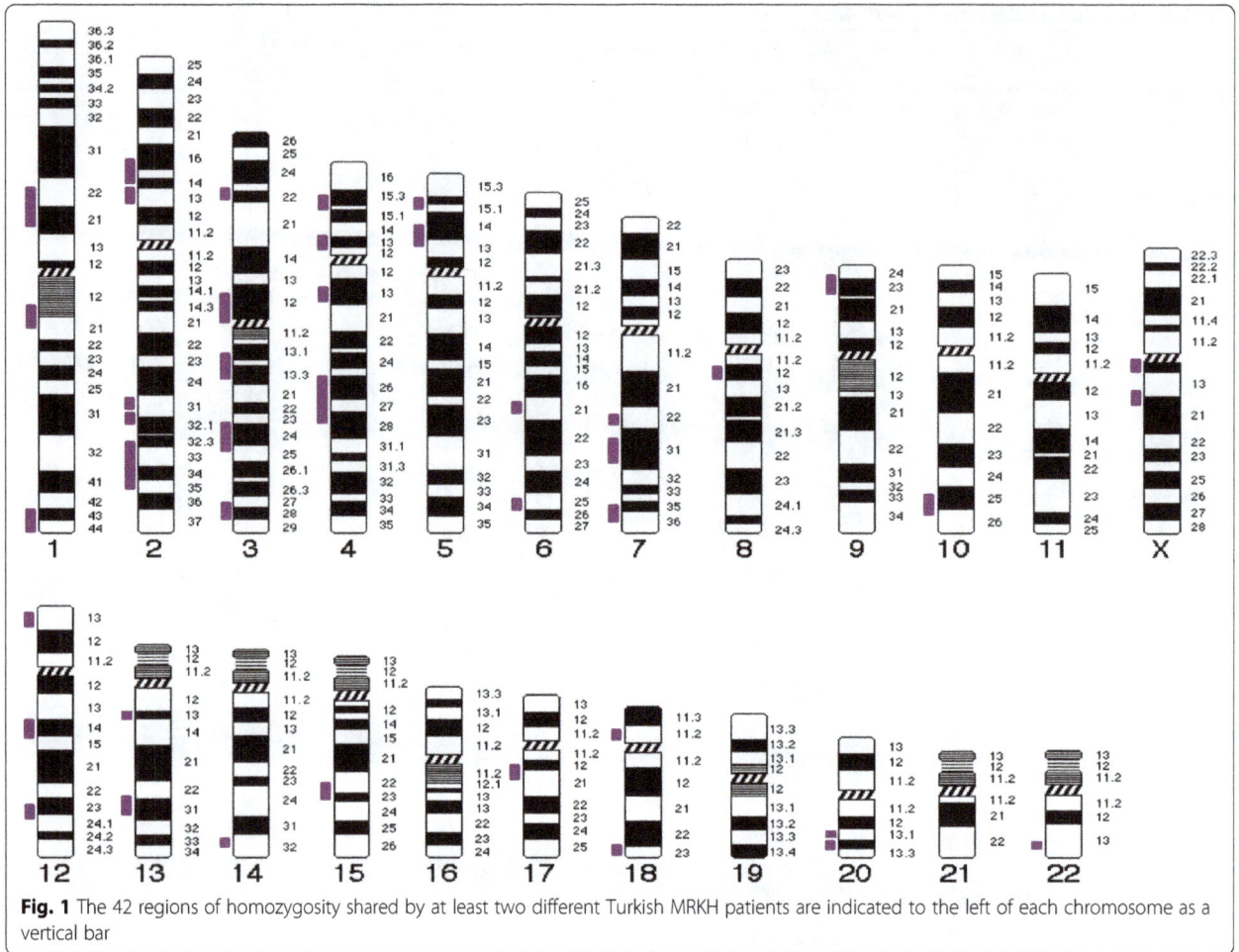

Fig. 1 The 42 regions of homozygosity shared by at least two different Turkish MRKH patients are indicated to the left of each chromosome as a vertical bar

and Turkish MRKH women and none had small insertion/deletions or point mutations in *WNT4*, *LHX1*, or *HNF1B* suggesting variants are rare in these genes [2]. The 22q11 region is involved in the DiGeorge phenotype and other associated disorders, while deletions or duplications of 1q21.1 have been identified in ttype I MRKH. However, their significance to the pathophysiology of MRKH is unknown at this time [30].

Copy number variants are typically heterozygous [2], but since consanguineous marriages are common in Turkey, we sought to determine if MRKH patients had large regions of homozygosity (ROH). Turkish patients in the current study consisted of Anatolian-origin Caucasians, who are predominantly from Antalya, Turkey. As reported by Alper et al. in 2004, the rate of consanguineous marriages in the province of Antalya was found to be 33.9% [34]. People in this region have a greater risk of autosomal recessively inherited genetic diseases. Analysis of ROH may provide a good starting point to determine the genetic basis of disease in the offspring of such consanguineous families. Ours is the first study, to our

knowledge, to examine ROH analysis in consanguineous MRKH families by CMA.

It is interesting that nearly three quarters of our Turkish MRKH patients demonstrated consanguinity, as defined by having parents that were third degree relatives or closer. In all eight of our patients who stated their parents were first cousins, all were second or first degree relatives. For the remaining 11 MRKH patients who did not know whether consanguinity was present, 7/11 had parents that were third or second degree

Table 5 Genes implicated in mullerian development are shown from mouse and human studies, including the 3;16 translocation. Genes in bold reside within regions of homozygosity in ≥ 2 MRKH patients

Mouse studies	*Wnt4*, *Lhx1*, **Emx2**, *Pbx2* *Wnt9b*, *Pax2*, *Wnt5a*, *Rar*, *Rxr*, **Tp63**, *Wnt7a*, *Hoxa9*, *Hoxa10*, *Hoxa11*, *Hoxa12*, *Hoxa13*
Human Studies	*WNT4*, *HNF1B*, *ZNHIT3*, *WT1*, **CFTR**, *WNT7A*, *GALT*, *HOXA7*, *PBX1*, *HOXA10*, *AMH*, *AMHR*, *RARG*, *RXRA*, *CTNNB1*, *PAX2*, *LAMC1*, *DLGH1*, *SHOX*,*MMP14*, *LRP10*, *WNT9B* *PBX1*, *LHX1*, **RBM8A**, *TBX6*
Human Translocation	**CMTM7, CCR4**, *IL32*, *MEFV*, **TRIM71, CNOT10**, *ZNF200*, *OR1F1*, *ZNF213*, *ZNF205*

relatives. Therefore, the chance of consanguinity was greater in MRKH patients than reported for Anatolian people in general, which suggests that autosomal recessive loci could be responsible for some causes of MRKH.

Further supporting consanguinity, there were 42 regions across the genome in which at least two MRKH patients had overlapping homozygous genomic regions, most frequently chromosomes 2, 3, and 4. None of the shared regions included the 17q12 or 16p11.2 CNVs, but did include 22q11.21. When putative candidate genes from the literature are surveyed, either based upon probable function and/or animal models, eight genes (*RBM8A, CMTM7, CCR4, TRIM71, CNOT10, TP63, EMX2,* and *CFTR*) reside within these shared regions, which could suggest a role in MRKH and a possible founder effect if mutations are discovered (Table 5).

The inheritance of MRKH is most likely to be autosomal dominant for most of the world based upon heterozygous single gene mutations and heterozygous CNVs. However, the large percentage of consanguinity and shared regions of homozygosity in Turkish MRKH patients suggest the existence of an autosomal recessive form. Ideally, homozygosity mapping followed by whole exome sequencing to pinpoint the causative genes should be done in more patients and their family members to narrow down candidate genomic regions for MRKH. However, our results provide additional candidate genes to study, and we suggest that there may be autosomal recessive causes of MRKH that could be identified in consanguineous Turkish families.

Conclusion

CNVs were identified in approximately 20% of Turkish MRKH patients, but it is unknown if they are causative. It is interesting that the 16p11.2 deletion CNV seen in other populations was also found in a Turkish MRKH patient. Our findings suggest that Turkish MRKH patients have a greater chance of consanguinity than the general Anatolian Turkish population. In contrast to other reports suggesting autosomal dominant inheritance of MRKH, the extremely high rate of shared regions of homozygosity suggests that inheritance of some cases of MRKH in Turkey could be autosomal recessive.

Acknowledgements
None

Funding
LCL was funded by NIH HD33004 and the Department of Ob/Gyn at Augusta University and OMA was funded by the Research Funds Office of Akdeniz University, Antalya, Turkey (Grant #2012. 03.0122.001).

Authors' contributions
The premise of the paper was conceived by LCL, OMA, GL, HK, and DDE. DDE, OMA, and LCL wrote the paper, and all co-authors contributed revision. Most of the editing of the paper was done by OMA, KH, YS, LCL, MES, LPC, and LCL. ME, MB, and OMA were involved in collecting patient data and blood samples. LPC, MES, DDE and EY received samples, prepared DNA, and collected the data from the CNV analysis. DDE, LPC, MES, and YS performed the CNV analysis (YS oversaw the CNV analysis). LCL oversaw all aspects of the manuscript, funded the project, edited the final manuscript, and is the co-corresponding author with OMA. All authors read and approved the final manuscript.

Competing interests
The authors declare that they have no competing interests.

Author details
[1]Department of Medical Biology, Alanya Alaaddin Keykubat University, Faculty of Medicine, Antalya, Turkey. [2]Guangxi Maternal and Child Health Hospital, Nanning, China. [3]Department of Pathology, Harvard Medical School, Boston, MA 02115, USA. [4]Division of Genetics and Genomics, Boston Children's Hospital, Boston, MA 02115, USA. [5]Shanghai Children's Medical Center, Shanghai Jiaotong University School of Medicine, Shanghai 200127, China. [6]Department of Obstetrics and Gynecology, Akdeniz University, Faculty of Medicine, Antalya, Turkey. [7]Section of Reproductive Endocrinology, Infertility, & Genetics, Department of Obstetrics & Gynecology Medical College of Georgia at Augusta University, Augusta, GA, USA. [8]Department of Neuroscience & Regenerative Medicine, Medical College of Georgia at Augusta University, 1120 15th Street, CA2041, Augusta, GA 30912, USA. [9]Department of Medical Biology and Genetics, Akdeniz University, Faculty of Medicine, 07058 Antalya, Turkey.

References
1. Acien P, Acien M, Sanchez-Ferrer M. Complex malformations of the female genital tract. New types and revision of classification. Hum Reprod. 2004;19:2377–84.
2. Williams LS, Demir Eksi D, Shen Y, Lossie AC, Chorich LP, Sullivan ME, et al. Genetic analysis of Mayer-Rokitansky-Kuster-Hauser syndrome in a large cohort of families. Fertil Steril. 2017;108:145–51. e2
3. Oppelt PG, Lermann J, Strick R, Dittrich R, Strissel P, Rettig I, et al. Malformations in a cohort of 284 women with Mayer-Rokitansky-Kuster-Hauser syndrome (MRKH). Reprod Biol Endocrinol. 2012;10:57.
4. Bean EJ, Mazur T, Robinson AD. Mayer-Rokitansky-Kuster-Hauser syndrome: sexuality, psychological effects, and quality of life. J Pediatr Adolesc Gynecol. 2009;22:339–46.
5. Reindollar RH, Byrd JR, McDonough PG. Delayed sexual development:study of 252 patients. Am J Obstet Gynecol. 1981;140:371–80.
6. Simpson JL. Genetics of female infertility due to anomalies of the ovary and mullerian ducts. Methods Mol Biol. 2014;1154:39–73.
7. Herlin M, Hojland AT, Petersen MB. Familial occurrence of Mayer-Rokitansky-Kuster-Hauser syndrome: a case report and review of the literature. Am J Med Genet A. 2014;164A:2276–86.
8. Biason-Lauber A, De Filippo G, Konrad D, Scarano G, Nazzaro A, Schoenle EJ. WNT4 deficiency–a clinical phenotype distinct from the classic Mayer-Rokitansky-Kuster-Hauser syndrome: a case report. Hum Reprod. 2007;22:224–9.
9. Biason-Lauber A, Konrad D, Navratil F, Schoenle EJ. A WNT4 mutation associated with Mullerian-duct regression and virilization in a 46,XX woman. N Engl J Med. 2004;351:792–8.
10. Philibert P, Biason-Lauber A, Gueorguieva I, Stuckens C, Pienkowski C, Lebon-Labich B, et al. Molecular analysis of WNT4 gene in four adolescent girls with mullerian duct abnormality and hyperandrogenism (atypical Mayer-Rokitansky-Kuster-Hauser syndrome). Fertil Steril. 2011;95:2683–6.
11. Philibert P, Biason-Lauber A, Rouzier R, Pienkowski C, Paris F, Konrad D, et al. Identification and functional analysis of a new WNT4 gene mutation among 28 adolescent girls with primary amenorrhea and mullerian duct abnormalities: a French collaborative study. J Clin Endocrinol Metab. 2008;93:895–900.

12. Lindner TH, Njolstad PR, Horikawa Y, Bostad L, Bell GI, Sovik O. A novel syndrome of diabetes mellitus, renal dysfunction and genital malformation associated with a partial deletion of the pseudo-POU domain of hepatocyte nuclear factor-1beta. Hum Mol Genet. 1999;8:2001–8.

13. Kucheria K, Taneja N, Kinra G. Autosomal translocation of chromosomes 12q & 14q in mullerian duct failure. Indian J Med Res. 1988;87:290–2.

14. Amesse L, Yen FF, Weisskopf B, Hertweck SP. Vaginal uterine agenesis associated with amastia in a phenotypic female with a de novo 46,XX,t(8; 13)(q22.1;q32.1) translocation. Clin Genet. 1999;55:493–5.

15. Williams LS, Kim HG, Kalscheuer VM, Tuck JM, Chorich LP, Sullivan ME, et al. A balanced chromosomal translocation involving chromosomes 3 and 16 in a patient with Mayer-Rokitansky-Kuster-Hauser syndrome reveals new candidate genes at 3p22.3 and 16p13.3. Mol Cytogenet. 2016;9:57.

16. Cheroki C, Krepischi-Santos AC, Rosenberg C, Jehee FS, Mingroni-Netto RC, Pavanello Filho I, et al. Report of a del22q11 in a patient with Mayer-Rokitansky-Kuster-Hauser (MRKH) anomaly and exclusion of WNT-4, RAR-gamma, and RXR-alpha as major genes determining MRKH anomaly in a study of 25 affected women. Am J Med Genet A. 2006;140:1339–42.

17. Cheroki C, Krepischi-Santos AC, Szuhai K, Brenner V, Kim CA, Otto PA, et al. genomic imbalances associated with mullerian aplasia. J Med Genet. 2008;45:228–32.

18. Morcel K, Watrin T, Pasquier L, Rochard L, Le Caignec C, Dubourg C, et al. Utero-vaginal aplasia (Mayer-Rokitansky-Kuster-Hauser syndrome) associated with deletions in known DiGeorge or DiGeorge-like loci. Orphanet J Rare Dis. 2011;6:9.

19. Nik-Zainal S, Strick R, Storer M, Huang N, Rad R, Willatt L, et al. High incidence of recurrent copy number variants in patients with isolated and syndromic Mullerian aplasia. J Med Genet. 2011;48:197–204.

20. Ledig S, Schippert C, Strick R, Beckmann MW, Oppelt PG, Wieacker P. Recurrent aberrations identified by array-CGH in patients with Mayer-Rokitansky-Kuster-Hauser syndrome. Fertil Steril. 2011;95:1589–94.

21. Sandbacka M, Laivuori H, Freitas E, Halttunen M, Jokimaa V, Morin-Papunen L, et al. TBX6, LHX1 and copy number variations in the complex genetics of Mullerian aplasia. Orphanet J Rare Dis. 2013;8:125.

22. McGowan R, Tydeman G, Shapiro D, Craig T, Morrison N, Logan S, et al. DNA copy number variations are important in the complex genetic architecture of mullerian disorders. Fertil Steril. 2015;103:1021–30. e1

23. Chen MJ, Wei SY, Yang WS, Wu TT, Li HY, Ho HN, et al. Concurrent exome-targeted next-generation sequencing and single nucleotide polymorphism array to identify the causative genetic aberrations of isolated Mayer-Rokitansky-Kuster-Hauser syndrome. Hum Reprod. 2015;30:1732–42.

24. Lahiri DK, Nurnberger JI Jr. A rapid non-enzymatic method for the preparation of HMW DNA from blood for RFLP studies. Nucleic Acids Res. 1991;19:5444.

25. Sund KL, Zimmerman SL, Thomas C, Mitchell AL, Prada CE, Grote L, et al. regions of homozygosity identified by SNP microarray analysis aid in the diagnosis of autosomal recessive disease and incidentally detect parental blood relationships. Genetics in medicine : official journal of the American College of Medical Genetics. 2013;15:70–8.

26. Kondo S, Schutte BC, Richardson RJ, Bjork BC, knight AS, Watanabe Y, et al. mutations in IRF6 cause van der Woude and popliteal pterygium syndromes. Nat Genet. 2002;32:285–9.

27. Duru UA, Laufer MR. Discordance in Mayer-von Rokitansky-Kuster-Hauser syndrome noted in monozygotic twins. J Pediatr Adolesc Gynecol. 2009;22:e73–5.

28. Milsom SR, Ogilvie CM, Jefferies C, Cree L. discordant Mayer-Rokitansky-Kuster-Hauser (MRKH) syndrome in identical twins - a case report and implications for reproduction in MRKH women. Gynecological endocrinology : the official journal of the International Society of Gynecological Endocrinology. 2015;31:684–7.

29. Rall K, Eisenbeis S, Barresi G, Ruckner D, Walter M, Poths S, et al. Mayer-Rokitansky-Kuster-Hauser syndrome discordance in monozygotic twins: matrix metalloproteinase 14, low-density lipoprotein receptor-related protein 10, extracellular matrix, and neoangiogenesis genes identified as candidate genes in a tissue-specific mosaicism. Fertil Steril. 2015;103:494–502. e3

30. Layman LC. The genetics of mullerian aplasia. Expert Rev Endocrinol Metab. 2014;9:411–9.

31. Weiss LA, Shen Y, Korn JM, Arking DE, miller DT, Fossdal R et al. association between microdeletion and microduplication at 16p11.2 and autism. N Engl J Med 2008;358:667–675.

32. Walters RG, Jacquemont S, Valsesia A, de Smith AJ, martinet D, Andersson J, et al. a new highly penetrant form of obesity due to deletions on chromosome 16p11.2. Nature. 2010;463:671–5.

33. Zhang W, Zhou X, Liu L, Zhu Y, Liu C, Pan H, et al. Identification and functional analysis of a novel LHX1 mutation associated with congenital absence of the uterus and vagina. Oncotarget. 2017;8:8785–90.

34. Alper OM, Erengin H, Manguoglu AE, Bilgen T, Cetin Z, Dedeoglu N, et al. Consanguineous marriages in the province of Antalya, Turkey. Ann Genet. 2004;47:129–38.

21

Compound phenotype in a girl with r(22), concomitant microdeletion 22q13.32-q13.33 and mosaic monosomy 22

Anna A. Kashevarova[1][*] , Elena O. Belyaeva[1], Aleksandr M. Nikonov[2], Olga V. Plotnikova[2], Nikolay A. Skryabin[1], Tatyana V. Nikitina[1], Stanislav A. Vasilyev[1], Yulia S. Yakovleva[1,3], Nadezda P. Babushkina[1], Ekaterina N. Tolmacheva[1], Mariya E. Lopatkina[1], Renata R. Savchenko[1], Lyudmila P. Nazarenko[1,3] and Igor N. Lebedev[1,3]

Abstract

Background: Ring chromosome instability may influence a patient's phenotype and challenge its interpretation.

Results: Here, we report a 4-year-old girl with a compound phenotype. Cytogenetic analysis revealed her karyotype to be 46,XX,r(22). aCGH identified a 180 kb 22q13.32 duplication, a *de novo* 2.024 Mb subtelomeric 22q13.32-q13.33 deletion, which is associated with Phelan-McDermid syndrome, and a maternal single gene 382-kb *TUSC7* deletion of uncertain clinical significance located in the region of the 3q13.31 deletion syndrome. All chromosomal aberrations were confirmed by real-time PCR in lymphocytes and detected in skin fibroblasts. The deletions were also found in the buccal epithelium. According to FISH analysis, 8% and 24% of the patient's lymphocytes and skin fibroblasts, respectively, had monosomy 22.

Conclusions: We believe that a combination of 22q13.32-q13.33 deletion and monosomy 22 in a portion of cells can better define the clinical phenotype of the patient. Importantly, the *in vivo* presence of monosomic cells indicates ring chromosome instability, which may favor karyotype correction that is significant for the development of chromosomal therapy protocols.

Keywords: Compound phenotype, Phelan-McDermid syndrome, *FAM19A5* gene, Ring chromosome 22, Chromosome 22 monosomy

Background

Terminal deletions at 22q13 are often associated with ring chromosome formation. To date, no more than a hundred patients with r(22) have been described, and their clinical phenotype is similar to those with a terminal 22q deletion [1–7]. Ring chromosomes are known to be unstable during mitotic divisions: the ring may change in size or may be lost, and dicentric and interlocking rings may appear [8, 9]. The loss of the ring chromosome followed by the amplification of the remaining normal homolog in induced pluripotent stem cells (iPSCs) formed the basis of *in vitro* karyotype correction and chromosomal therapy [10–12].

A combination of r(22) and cells with monosomy for chromosome 22 was described previously in one of two mentally retarded monozygotic twins with minor physical abnormalities [13]. In one twin, two of 50 metaphases had a 45,XX,-22 karyotype. Significantly, two cells of the 50 metaphases of the second twin had an apparently normal chromosome number, and one cell had 46 chromosomes with a dicentric ring. The remaining cells in both patients were 46,XX,r(22).

Heterozygous contiguous gene deletion at 22q13 or mutations in the *SHANK3* gene (OMIM 606230), located within the minimum critical region, cause Phelan-McDermid syndrome (PHMDS, OMIM 606232). The frequent clinical findings are intrauterine and postnatal growth retardation, intellectual disability, speech delay, delayed motor development, microcephaly, large and misshapen ears, mild hypertelorism, strabismus, epicanthic

* Correspondence: kashevarova.anna@gmail.com
[1]Research Institute of Medical Genetics, Tomsk NRMC, Tomsk, Russia
Full list of author information is available at the end of the article

folds, ptosis of the upper lips, bushy eyebrows and synophrys, a depressed and broad nasal bridge, short mandible, malocclusion and irregular position of the teeth, high palate, clinodactyly of the little fingers, partial syndactyly between the 2nd and 3rd toes, hypotonia, seizures and behavior problems.

Here, for the first time, we report a patient with a compound phenotype who exhibits ring chromosome 22, mosaic monosomy for chromosome 22 in lymphocytes and skin fibroblasts, and a microdeletion at 3q13.31 of maternal origin. Both microdeletions, del3q13.31 and del22q13.32-q13.33, were also detected by real-time PCR in the buccal epithelium.

The single-gene deletion of *TUSC7* at 3q13.31 in the index patient is located in the region of the 3q13.31 deletion syndrome (OMIM 615433). Although the *TUSC7* gene encodes the long non-coding RNA associated with various types of cancer [14], its expression has been shown to be closely related to the expression of the *LSAMP* gene [15], which is involved in neurodevelopmental impairments [16, 17].

Clinical report

The patient (Fig. 1), a 4-year-old girl, was referred to the clinical geneticist for the first time when she was one year and eight months old because of development delay, hyperexcitability, mood swings, and sleep disturbance. The girl did not walk alone, did not speak, and her head circumference did not increase. She is an only child of non-consanguineous healthy parents. Her father's nephew is intellectually disabled and receives education at home.

The patient was born at the 34th week of gestation via Cesarean section. Her birth weight was 1422 g (< 3rd centile); birth length was 48 cm (25th centile); head circumference was 25 cm (< 3rd centile); and chest circumference was 24 cm (< 3rd centile). Her Apgar score was 6. She was able to sit at the age of 8 months and walk independently at the age of 2 years.

The patient had neonatal hypotonia and hyporeflexia. Anticonvulsant therapy was prescribed at the age of 2 months because of seizures. At the age of 3 months, the seizures stopped, and the drugs were discontinued. After birth, the girl was placed on artificial feeding and had trouble gaining weight.

Currently, the patient is regularly observed by a neurologist, with diagnoses of cerebral palsy, atonic-astatic form, psychomotor and speech development delay, and by a psychiatrist due to mental disorder and decreased intelligence to the level of pronounced debility, psychomotor disinhibition syndrome, and unformed control functions for physiological sentiments.

At the age of 4 years, the girl's weight was 14.5 kg (25th centile); height was 108 cm (95th centile); and head circumference was 45.5 cm (<2th centile). She exhibited plagiocephaly, flat occiput, high anterior hairline, broad forehead, micrognathia, epicanthus, widely spaced eyes, upslanted palpebral fissure, upper eyelid fullness, straight eyebrows, prominent ears, wide and depressed nasal bridge, bulbous nose, smooth and short philtrum, thin vermillion of the upper lip, widely spaced teeth, high palate, clinodactyly (radial, F5, bilateral), proximally placed thumb (bilateral), thickening of the distal phalanx of the thumb (bilateral), pes planus, sandal gap, cutaneous syndactyly of the toes (T2-3, bilateral), short toes (T3-5, bilateral), dysplastic nails of the feet, asthenic body, wide umbilical ring, and a sacral dimple. The patient demonstrated aggression, signs of autism, attention deficit hyperactivity disorder (ADHD), and enuresis.

When the girl was 6 months old, echoencephalography showed ventriculomegaly. At the age of 1 year and 6 months, magnetic resonance imaging of the brain revealed a Dandy-Walker variant: hypoplasia of the cerebellar tonsils. Echocardiography revealed small heart anomalies, including an open oval window with a minimal left-right discharge, an enlarged coronary sinus, and a diagonal false chord of the left ventricle.

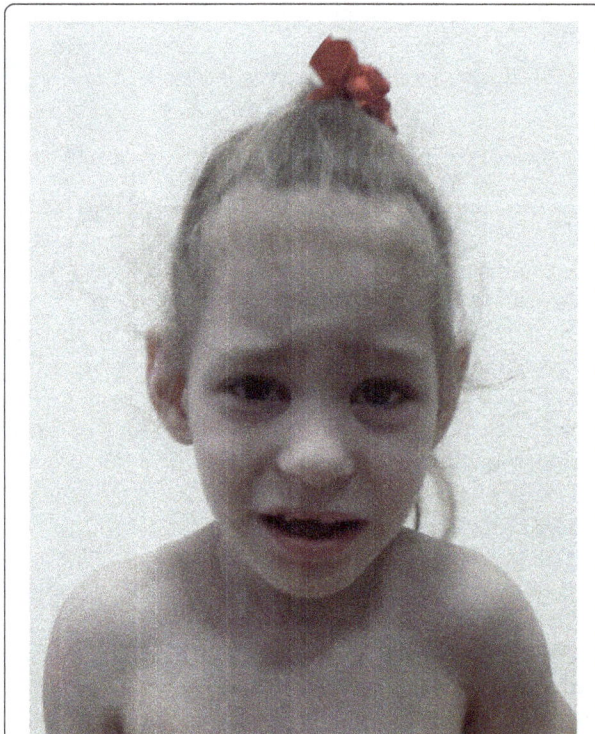

Fig. 1 The patient at 4 years of age (note plagiocephaly, high anterior hairline, broad forehead, epicanthus, widely spaced eyes, upslanted palpebral fissure, upper eyelid fullness, straight eyebrows, prominent ears, wide and depressed nasal bridge, bulbous nose, smooth and short philtrum, and thin vermillion of the upper lip)

Methods

The patient was subject to aCGH analysis due to her compound phenotype and r(22), as determined by conventional cytogenetic analysis of her blood lymphocytes. The aCGH findings were confirmed by real-time PCR in three different tissues: lymphocytes, skin fibroblasts, and buccal epithelium. FISH analysis was used to confirm the ring form of chromosome 22 and to determine the level of cells with monosomy 22 among lymphocytes and skin fibroblasts. SNP analyses identified the maternal origin of the ring chromosome. All techniques were performed by using equipment of the Center "Medical Genomics" of Research Institute of Medical Genetics, Tomsk NRMC.

Materials

For molecular genetic analyses, peripheral blood was collected in tubes containing EDTA. A primary culture of the patient's skin fibroblasts was obtained from two full-thickness skin biopsies. A buccal smear was collected with a cotton swab, which was transported in a dry tube for further DNA extraction.

Cytogenetic analyses

Conventional cytogenetic analysis was performed based on GTG-banded metaphases from peripheral blood lymphocytes from the patient at a 400-band resolution.

Fibroblast culture

The biopsies of fibroblasts were washed twice with Hank's solution containing antibiotics and antifungal agents and then treated with 0.2% collagenase in culture medium for 3 h at 37°C. The suspension was subsequently cultured in AminoMax culture medium. A confluent monolayer formed in one day.

Array-based Comparative Genomic Hybridization (aCGH) analyses

aCGH was performed using the SurePrint G3 Human CGH Microarray Kit (8×60K) (Agilent Technologies, Santa Clara, CA USA), according to the manufacturer's recommendations. Labeling and hybridization of patient and reference DNA (#5190-3796, Human Reference DNA, Agilent Technologies, Santa Clara, CA USA) were performed using enzymatic labeling and hybridization protocols (v. 7.5 Agilent Technologies, Santa Clara, CA USA). Array images were acquired with an Agilent SureScan Microarray Scanner (Agilent Technologies, Santa Clara, CA USA). Data analysis was performed using Cytogenomics Software (v. 3.0.6.6) (Agilent Technologies), the publicly available Database of Genomic Variants (DGV), and the Database of Chromosomal Imbalance and Phenotype in Humans employing Ensembl Resources (DECIPHER). Annotations of the genes located within the

region of genomic imbalance were retrieved from the NCBI Gene Database, OMIM, and the literature.

Confirmation of copy number variation using quantitative real-time PCR

Target sequences within and outside the deleted chromosomal regions and specific amplification primers for quantitative real-time PCR assays were selected using Primer 3 software (Additional file 1). The presence of 3q13.31 microdeletion, 22q13.32 microduplication and 22q13.32-q13.33 microdeletion was tested using genomic DNA from peripheral blood lymphocytes from the patient, her parents, and maternal mother (maternal father was not available for the analysis) as well as in cultured skin fibroblasts and a buccal smear from the patient and using the AriaMX Real-Time PCR System (Agilent Technologies, Santa Clara, CA USA). Control genomic DNA was obtained from the peripheral blood lymphocytes, skin fibroblasts and a buccal smear of a healthy donor. The control gene was *HEXB*, which encodes the beta subunit of hexosaminidase and is located at 5q13 (Additional file 1).

Fluorescent *In Situ* Hybridization (FISH)

FISH was performed using PCR-based probes for the centromeres of chromosomes 14 and 22 and the *TBC1D22A* gene located close to del22q13.32-q13.33 in lymphocytes and cultured skin fibroblasts from the proband following the standard protocol. *E. coli* clones carrying plasmids with inserts of centromere-specific alpha-satellite DNA sequences as well as the BAC clone RP11-569D9 were kindly provided by Professor M. Rocchi (Resources for Molecular Cytogenetics, Institute of Genetics, Bari, Italy). The probe for the *TBC1D22A* gene was generated using a long-range PCR kit (BioLabMix, Novosibirsk, Russia) (Additional file 1). Probes 14/22 and TBC1D22A were labeled with TAMRA-dUTP and Fluorescein-dUTP (BioSan, Russia), respectively.

The results of the aCGH and FISH analyses are described further according to the International System for Human Cytogenomic Nomenclature (ISCN 2016).

SNP analyses

Nine SNPs (rs11541025, rs2272837, rs8238, rs11703226, rs6010218, rs28637964, rs11547734, rs28379706, rs5771206) located at 22q13.32-q13.33 were selected to determine the parental origin of chromosome 22 with deletion. SNP investigation was performed via SNaPshot analysis.

Results

Metaphase analysis of the G-banded chromosomes from peripheral blood lymphocytes showed a karyotype 46,XX,r(22) [11] (Fig. 2a). FISH analysis detected 8% of monosomic cells (Table 1). aCGH using an Agilent 60K

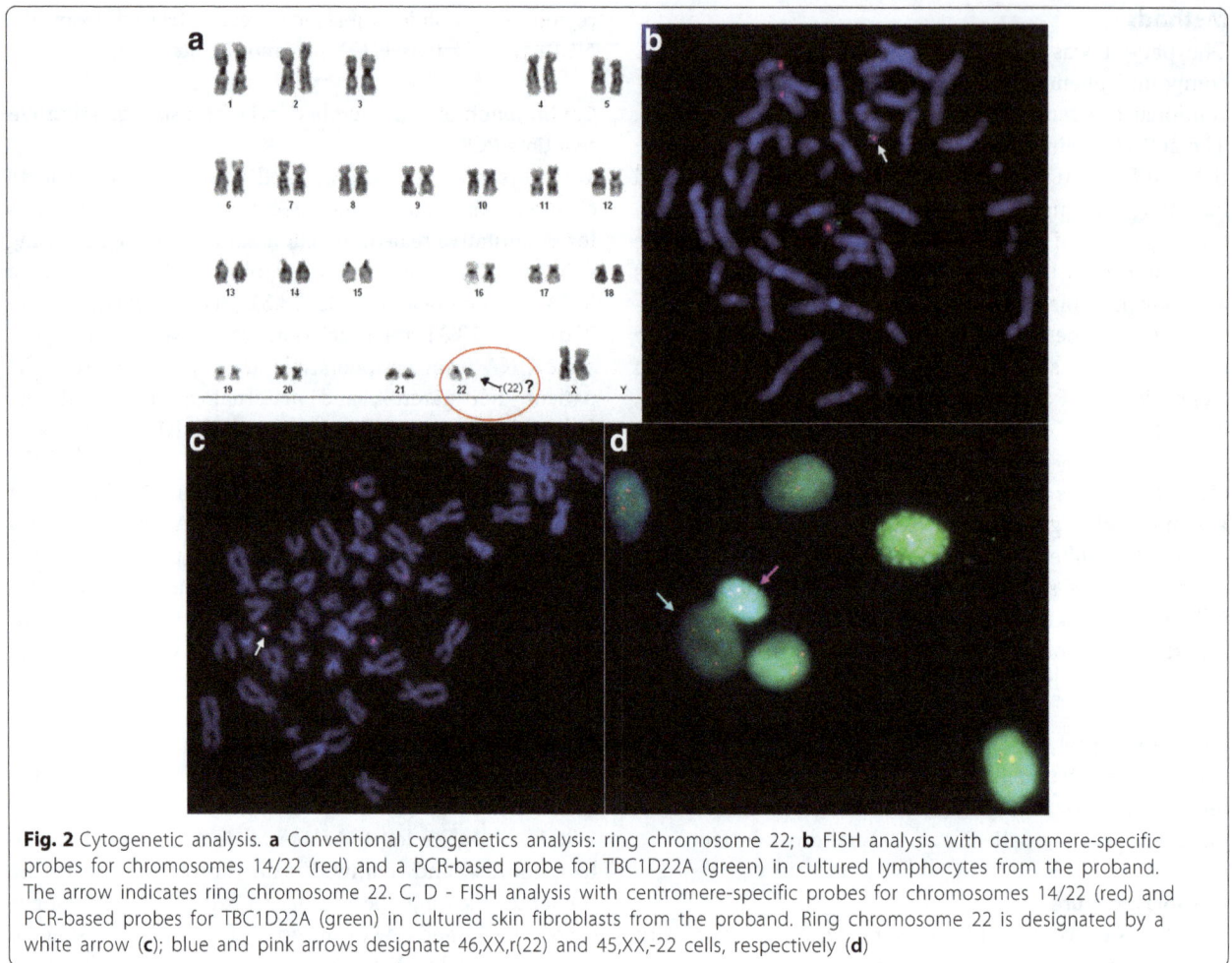

Fig. 2 Cytogenetic analysis. **a** Conventional cytogenetics analysis: ring chromosome 22; **b** FISH analysis with centromere-specific probes for chromosomes 14/22 (red) and a PCR-based probe for TBC1D22A (green) in cultured lymphocytes from the proband. The arrow indicates ring chromosome 22. C, D - FISH analysis with centromere-specific probes for chromosomes 14/22 (red) and PCR-based probes for TBC1D22A (green) in cultured skin fibroblasts from the proband. Ring chromosome 22 is designated by a white arrow (**c**); blue and pink arrows designate 46,XX,r(22) and 45,XX,-22 cells, respectively (**d**)

microarray revealed del3q13.31, dup22q13.32, and del22q13.32-q13.33 of 382 kb, 180 kb, and 2.024 Mb, in size, respectively: arr[hg19] 3q13.31(116233164_116615500)×1,22q13.32(48886812_49059015)×3, 22q13.32-q13.33(49115584_51178264)×1 (Fig. 3a). The distal breakpoint of dup22q13.32 is located within intron 2 of the *FAM19A5* gene, i.e., exons 1-2 are duplicated, and the proximal breakpoint of del22q13.32-q13.33 is located within intron 3 of the *FAM19A5* gene, i.e., exon 4 is deleted. The 3q13.31 microdeletion involved the single *TUSC7* gene. The microdeletion was confirmed via

quantitative real-time PCR analysis and was shown to be inherited from the intellectually normal mother and grandmother (Fig. 3c). *TUSC7* is known to be regulated together with the neighboring *LSAMP* [15], which is associated with neuropsychiatric disorders in patients with 3q13.31 deletion syndrome (OMIM615433). We also investigated the number of copies of the latter gene, which appeared to be normal (Fig. 3c). Similar microdeletions and reciprocal microduplications were present in DGV in one and two reports, respectively, and in DECIPHER (nos. 264508 and 299972). However,

Table 1 Cytogenetic results for lymphocytes and skin fibroblasts from the index patient

Cell type/duration of culturing or passage number	FISH			
	D14Z1/D22Z1×3	D14Z1/D22Z1×4	Total	% of cells with monosomy 22
Lymphocytes/72 h	41	438	479	8.56
Fibroblasts/P1	27	86	113	23.89
		Metaphase analysis		
Cell type/duration of culturing	45,XX,-22	46,XX,r(22)	46,XX,+mar	Total	% of cells with monosomy 22
Lymphocytes/72 h	-	11	-	11	0

Footnotes. D14Z1/D22Z1×3 – monosomy 14 or 22; D14Z1/D22Z1×4 – two chromosomes 14 and 22; P1 – first passage

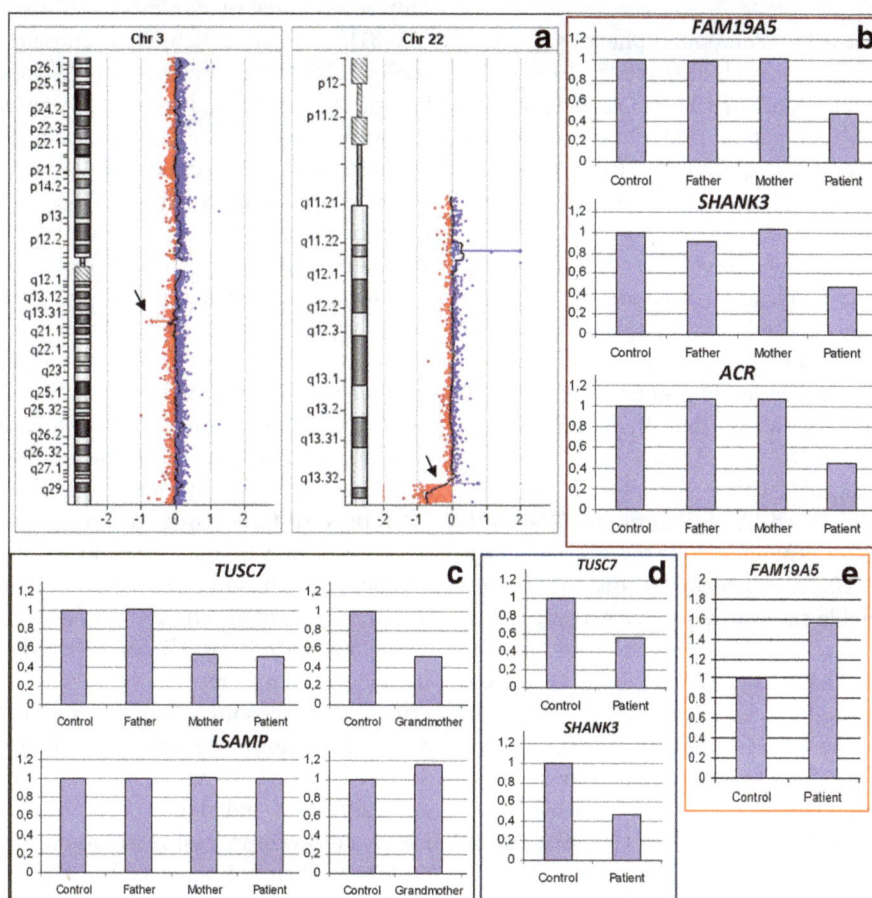

Fig. 3 Molecular genetic analysis. **a** An aCGH image of chromosomes 3 and 22 in the lymphocytes of the patient. Deletions are designated by arrows. **b** Confirmation of the deletion at 22q13.32-q13.33 by quantitative real-time PCR analysis. **c** Confirmation of the deletion at 3q13.31 by quantitative real-time PCR analysis. **d** Identification of the deletions at 3q13.31 and 22q13.32-q13.33 in the buccal epithelium by quantitative real-time PCR analysis. **e** Confirmation of the duplication at 22q13.32 by quantitative real-time PCR analysis

the gene located within this region in DECIPHER is *LSAMP*, with the coordinates - chr3:115521235-117716095 (hg19) vs. chr3:115521210-116164385 (hg19) in DGV. The deletion in the index patient (chr3:116233164-116615500 (hg19)) is within the DECIPHER region.

The 22q13.32-q13.33 microdeletion overlaps with the region of PHMDS and includes 43 RefSeq genes. The main candidate gene within this region is *SHANK3* (606230) [18]. Real-time PCR confirmed the presence of the microdeletion with primers for the *FAM19A5*, *SHANK3*, and *ACR* genes (Fig. 3b). According to the SNP analysis, the 22q13.32-q13.33 microdeletion originated *de novo* on the maternal chromosome.

The ring chromosome 22 was confirmed via FISH using centromere-specific DNA probes for chromosomes 14 and 22 and for the *TBC1D22A* gene located in the intact part of chromosome 22 close to del22q13.32-q13.33 (Fig. 2b). In addition, 8% of lymphocytes were

observed to exhibit monosomy for chromosome 22 (nuc ish(D14Z1/D22Z1×3)[41/479],(TBC1D22A×1)[41/479]).

Skin fibroblasts of the patient were investigated using the Agilent 60K microarray as well. The 22q13.32-q13.33 microdeletion (arr[hg19]22q13.32-q13.33(49084185_51043490) ×1) was found and further confirmed via real-time PCR, while the 3q13.31 deletion and 22q13.32 duplication were not revealed by aCGH but were also determined by real-time PCR (Fig. 3e). aCGH demonstrated the shift of chromosomal profiles at 3q13.31 and 22q13.32 towards the deletion and duplication, respectively, which, however, did not reach the significance level due to the high variance of the fluorescence intensity over the chromosomes. FISH analysis showed that 24% of the fibroblasts initially had monosomy of chromosome 22 (Fig. 2c and d): nuc ish(D14Z1/D22Z1×3)[27/113], (TBC1D22A×1)[27/113].

The buccal epithelium was investigated via real-time PCR. Both 3q13.31 and 22q13.32-q13.33 deletions were confirmed (Fig. 3d).

Discussion

We present a patient with a compound phenotype and a combination of chromosomal abnormalities: del3q13.31 (single *TUSC7* gene), dup22q13.32 (LOC284933 and exons 1-2 of *FAM19A5* gene), ring chromosome 22 associated with del22q13.32-q13.33 (43 RefSeq genes), and mosaic chromosome 22 monosomy in 8% of lymphocytes and 24% of fibroblasts. Both microdeletions were present in lymphocytes, fibroblasts, and the buccal epithelium. The microduplication was present in lymphocytes and fibroblasts; the buccal epithelium was not investigated. The del3q13.31 was inherited from the apparently healthy mother and grandmother and is located within the region of the 3q13.31 deletion syndrome (OMIM 615433).

The only gene located within the deleted 3q13.31 region is *TUSC7*, also called LSAMP antisense RNA3. It is a putative suppressor gene in various tumors, including glioma [19]. Low *TUSC7* expression is associated with significantly unfavorable survival and may be a risk factor for distant metastases [20]. Frequent deletions in the 3q13.31, including *LSAMP* and *TUSC7*, have also been identified in patients with osteosarcomas [14]. Although the copy number of the *LSAMP* gene is preserved in our patient, *LSAMP* and *TUSC7* expression are known to be closely related [15]. The authors also showed that, although the patient with acute myeloid leukemia had a 250-kb deletion in 3q13.31, which included the *TUSC7* gene but not *LSAMP*, the expression of both genes was increased by an unknown mechanism. *LSAMP*, implicated in the regulation of emotional and social behavior in mice [21] and associated with major depressive disorder and schizophrenia in humans [16, 17], is also one of the candidate genes for the 3q13.31 deletion syndrome.

Del22q13.32-q13.33 in our patient originated *de novo* on the maternal chromosome. This deletion is associated with the origin of the ring chromosome and includes part of the minimal critical region of PHMDS ([hg19] 22q13.33(51045516_51187844)) with the *MAPK8IP2*, *ARSA*, *SHANK3*, and *ACR* genes. PHMDS is a developmental disorder (OMIM 606232). The symptoms of the index proband commonly associated with PHMDS are listed in Table 2.

The most important contributing factor to PHMDS is *SHANK3* haploinsufficiency [22]. Mutations in this gene have also been associated with schizophrenia [23]. Analysis of human neurons differentiated from the induced pluripotent cells of patients with PHMDS showed impaired synaptic transmission and increased input resistance [24].

The instability of r(22) in the index patient led to the loss of chromosome 22 in a portion of cells, resulting in monosomy for chromosome 22. Non-mosaic monosomy for chromosome 22 is incompatible with life. To date,

only seven cases of monosomy 22 have been published [25–31], four of which were mosaic. The oldest described child was three years old. None of the patients had r(22), which could somehow, during the early stages of the development before its elimination from the cell, compensate for the phenotype. The symptoms of our proband are similar to those described in patients with mosaicism for monosomy 22 and are listed in Table 2. In addition, the index patient exhibits some symptoms that have not been described in any patient with either of the anomalies discussed above.

How can the clinical phenotype of our patient be interpreted? To our knowledge, two explanations may exist: phenotypic variability and a combined effect of del22q13.32-q13.33 and mosaic monosomy for chromosome 22. Phenotypic variability is typical for the manifestation of most CNV-associated syndromes. Variability can be associated with the variability of the breakpoints. In addition, the phenotype of a patient may also result from a combination of genetic and non-genetic modifiers.

The heterogeneous clinical phenotype in carriers of the ring chromosome 22 was first explained by mosaicism with monosomy 22 by Lejeune in 1968 [32]. Later, Stoll and Roth described a family with 46,XX/ 46,XX,r(22) and 46,XY/46,XY,r(22) karyotypes in three generations of individuals with both normal development and severe mental retardation. In these individuals, 40-50% of their lymphocytes had a ring chromosome 22, and a few cells were observed to carry two ring chromosomes. Skin biopsies were refused [33]. In 2014, a patient with a developmental delay and dysmorphic features was described, from whom 12% of lymphocytes and 40-48% of fibroblasts had r(22), and the remaining cells had a normal karyotype - 46,XX/46,XX,r(22). In some metaphase cells of a patient, the ring chromosome was duplicated or lost [23]. In our patient, the initial metaphase analysis revealed only cells with the 46,XX,r(22) karyotype. Using FISH, we performed a search for mosaicism of the ring chromosome 22 in interphase nuclei of peripheral blood lymphocytes and skin fibroblasts of the index patient. Approximately 8% of lymphocytes and 24% of fibroblasts had monosomy 22 in combination with 46,XX,r(22) cells. The discrepancy between the results of these two analyses can be due to the low level of monosomic cells among lymphocytes detected by FISH, which was not revealed by metaphase analysis, as well as to the potential inability of monosomic cells to proliferate in vitro.

To the best of our knowledge, only four live-born infants with mosaicism for monosomy of chromosome 22 have been described. The first one is a 2-year-old male child with moderate psychomotor retardation, generalized hypotonia, large ears, epicanthus, synophrys, and cutaneous syndactyly between all the fingers [28].

Table 2 Symptoms in the index patient common to Phelan-McDermid syndrome and mosaic monosomy for chromosome 22 as well as atypical symptoms

Index patient	Phelan-McDermid syndrome	Mosaic monosomy 22
Developmental delay	+	+
Sleep disturbance	+	
Neonatal hypotonia[a]		+
Seizures	+	
Speech delay	+	
Low weight[a]		+
Accelerated growth	+	
Microcephaly	+	+
Plagiocephaly		
Flat occiput		
High anterior hairline		
Broad forehead[a]		+
Micrognathia[a]		+
Epicanthus	+	+
Widely spaced eyes[a]		+
Upslanted palpebral fissure		
Upper eyelid fullness		
Straight eyebrows		
Prominent ears	+	+
Wide and depressed nasal bridge[a]		+
Bulbous nose	+	
Smooth and short philtrum	+	
Thin vermillion of the upper lip[a]		+
Widely spaced teeth	+	
High palate[a]		+
Clinodactyly (radial, F5, bilateral)[a]		+
Proximally placed thumb (bilateral)		
Thickening of distal phalanx of thumb (bilateral)		
Pes planus		
Sandal gap		
Cutaneous syndactyly of the toes (T2-3, bilateral)[a]		+
Short toes (T3-5, bilateral)		
Dysplastic nails of the feet	+	
Asthenic body		
Wide umbilical ring		
Sacral dimple	+	
Aggression	+	
Signs of autism	+	
Attention deficit hyperactivity disorder	+	
Enuresis		
Dandy-Walker variant[b]	+	
Ventriculomegaly	+	
Small heart anomalies[a]		+

Footnotes. Symptoms of the index proband never before described in patients with Phelan-McDermid syndrome or mosaic monosomy for chromosome 22 are shown in bold. [a]-symptoms specific to monosomy 22. [b] - patient P60 from [37] had Dandy-Walker malformation.

The patient's karyotype was 45,XY,-22/46,XY [12/50], i.e., 24% of lymphocytes were monosomic. The second case was published by Verloes et al. [31], who observed a slightly dysmorphic and mentally defective three-year-old child with a 45,XY,-22/46,XY karyotype. Chromosome 22 was absent in 10.5% of lymphocytes and 8.3% of fibroblasts. The third case was a newborn with gastroschisis and absent cerebral diastolic flow. The baby died on its second day of life. The karyotype was 45,XY,-22/46,XY [3/50] [26]. The fourth child was an abnormal premature male infant with a 45,XY,-22/46,XY [15/100] karyotype [29]. He had a unique facial appearance, similar to those with DiGeorge syndrome (OMIM 188400), hypertonicity, limitation of extension at the major joints, and flexion contractures of all fingers. However, the direct comparison of the phenotypes of these patients with the symptoms of our proband seem to be incorrect because, in addition to monosomy for chromosome 22, she also has a deletion at 22q13.32-q13.33.

For the index patient, among 43 identified symptoms, 18 have previously been described in other patients with PHMDS and 15 in patients with mosaic monosomy 22, while 14 symptoms have never been observed in any of the mentioned cases (Table 2). These symptoms include skeletal abnormalities, facial dysmorphism, wide umbilical ring, and enuresis. Significantly, two important papers concerning the *FAM19A5* gene, which is disrupted by the CNV breakpoints in the index patient, have been recently published. The first paper demonstrates that the gene is a crucial candidate for modulating osteoclast formation and bone disorders [34], i.e., we can assume that the skeletal abnormalities are due to FAM19A5 protein deficiency. In addition, the second paper is the first to show that FAM19A5 is highly expressed and secreted by adipocytes and adipose tissue protein [35]. Thus, its deficiency can probably be related to the low weight and asthenic body of the proband. Moreover, *FAM19A5* is also expressed in the brain and acts as a modulator of immune response in nervous cells, which can make it responsible for neuropsychiatric processes [36].

Conclusions

In conclusion, we present the first patient with a compound phenotype and a combination of a 382-kb deletion at 3q13.31, encompassing the single *TUSC7* gene, a 180-kb duplication at 22q13.32, a 2.024-Mb deletion at 22q11.32-q11.33, including part of the PHMDS critical region, and monosomy for chromosome 22 in 8% of lymphocytes and 24% of fibroblasts. The presence of deletions was detected by real-time PCR in the buccal epithelium. The clinical significance of the 3q13.31 deletion is unclear, though the *TUSC7* gene is associated with various types of tumors. Special attention should thus be paid to the early prevention and diagnosis of cancer in a carrier. In addition, only the combination of the 22q13.32-q13.33 deletion and monosomy for chromosome 22 allowed us to explain most of the clinical features of the patient. Therefore, in cases with a compound phenotype, it is important to use a combination of different methods and sometimes to investigate more than one tissue. The presence of monosomic cells in patients with a ring chromosome indicates ring chromosome instability. A monosomic karyotype can be the intermediate step in the process of chromosomal defect correction, which can underlie the chromosomal therapy of genetic diseases.

Abbreviations

aCGH: Array comparative genomic hybridization; CNV: Copy number variation; DECIPHER: Database of Chromosomal Imbalance and Phenotype in Humans Using Ensembl Resources; iPSC: Induced pluripotent stem cell; OMIM: Online Mendelian Inheritance in Man; PCR: Polymerase chain reaction; PHMDS: Phelan-McDermid syndrome; SNP: Single-nucleotide polymorphism

Acknowledgements

This study used data generated by the DECIPHER Consortium. A full list of the centers that helped to generate the data is available at http://decipher.sanger.ac.uk and can be obtained via e-mail from decipher@sanger.ac.uk. Funding for the DECIPHER project was provided by the Wellcome Trust.
We would like to thank the family of our patient for their assistance with the clinical evaluation.

Funding

This study was supported by the Russian Science Foundation (project 16-15-10231).

Authors' contributions

The patient was examined clinically by AMN, LPN, AAK, and EOB. Cytogenetic analysis was performed by OVP and Yu.S.Ya. Array CGH analysis was performed by NAS. Primer design and real-time PCR assays were performed by AAK, MEL, and RRS. FISH probes were created and the analysis was performed by ENT and SAV. Fibroblasts were obtained and cultured by TVN. The buccal epithelium was analyzed by ENT. SNP analysis was performed by NPB. The manuscript was written by AAK and INL. All authors read and approved the final manuscript.

Competing interests

The authors declare that they have no competing interests.

Author details

[1]Research Institute of Medical Genetics, Tomsk NRMC, Tomsk, Russia. [2]Diagnostic Center of the Altai Region, Barnaul, Russia. [3]Siberian State Medical University, Tomsk, Russia.

References

1. De Mas P, Chassaing N, Chaix Y, Vincent MC, Julia S, Bourrouillou G, et al. Molecular characterisation of a ring chromosome 22 in a patient with severe language delay: a contribution to the refinement of the subtelomeric 22q deletion syndrome. J Med Genet. 2002;39:e17.
2. Guilherme RS, Soares KC, Simioni M, Vieira TP, Gil-da-Silva-Lopes VL, Kim C, et al. Clinical, cytogenetic, and molecular characterization of six patients with ring chromosomes 22, including one with concomitant 22q11.2 deletion. Am J Med Genet A. 2014;164A:1659–65.
3. Ishmael HA, Cataldi D, Begleiter ML, Pasztor LM, Dasouki MJ, Butler MG. Five new subjects with ring chromosome 22. Clin Genet. 2003;63:410–4.
4. Jeffries AR, Curran S, Elmslie F, Sharma A, Wenger S, Hummel M, et al. Molecular and phenotypic characterization of ring chromosome 22. Am J Med Genet A. 2005;137:139–47.
5. MacLean JE, Teshima IE, Szatmari P, Nowaczyk MJ. Ring chromosome 22 and autism: report and review. Am J Med Genet. 2000;90:382–5.
6. Schinzel A. Catalogue of unbalanced chromosome aberrations in man. 2. Berlin, Germany: Walter de Gruyter; 2001.7.
7. Kurtas N, Arrigoni F, Errichiello E, Zucca C, Maghini C, D'Angelo MG, Beri S, Giorda R, Bertuzzo S, Delledonne M, Xumerle L, Rossato M, Zuffardi O, Bonaglia MC. Chromothripsis and ring chromosome 22: a paradigm of genomic complexity in the Phelan-McDermid syndrome (22q13 deletion syndrome). J Med Genet. 2018;55:269–77.
8. Pristyazhnyuk IE, Menzorov AG. Ring chromosomes: from formation to clinical potential. Protoplasma. 2018;255:439-49.
9. Yip MY. Autosomal ring chromosomes in human genetic disorders. Transl Pediatr. 2015;4:164–74.
10. Kim T, Bershteyn M, Wynshaw-Boris A. Chromosome therapy. Correction of large chromosomal aberrations by inducing ring chromosomes in induced pluripotent stem cells (iPSCs). Nucleus. 2014;5:391–5.
11. Kim T, Plona K, Wynshaw-Boris A. A novel system for correcting large-scale chromosomal aberrations: Ring chromosome correction via reprogramming into induced pluripotent stem cell (iPSC). Chromosoma. 2017;126:457–63.
12. Plona K, Kim T, Halloran K, Wynshaw-Boris A. Chromosome therapy: potential strategies for the correction of severe chromosome aberrations. Am J Med Genet C Semin Med Genet. 2016;172:422–30.
13. Lindenbaum RH, Bobrow M, Barber L. Monozygotic twins with ring chromosome 22. J Med Genet. 1973;10:85–9.
14. Kresse SH, Ohnstad HO, Paulsen EB, Bjerkehagen B, Szuhai K, Serra M, et al. LSAMP, a novel candidate tumor suppressor gene in human osteosarcomas, identified by array comparative genomic hybridization. Genes Chromosomes Cancer. 2009;48:679–93.
15. Coccaro N, Zagaria A, Tota G, Anelli L, Orsini P, Casieri P, et al. Overexpression of the LSAMP and TUSC7 genes in acute myeloid leukemia following microdeletion/duplication of chromosome 3. Cancer Genet. 2015;208:517–22.
16. Innos J, Koido K, Philips MA, Vasar E. Limbic system associated membrane protein as a potential target for neuropsychiatric disorders. Front Pharmacol. 2013;4:32.
17. Koido K, Janno S, Traks T, Parksepp M, Ljubajev Ü, Veiksaar P, et al. Associations between polymorphisms of LSAMP gene and schizophrenia. Psychiatry Res. 2014;215:797–8.
18. Mitz AR, Philyaw TJ, Boccuto L, Shcheglovitov A, Sarasua SM, Kaufmann WE, Thurm A. Identification of 22q13 genes most likely to contribute to Phelan McDermid syndrome. Eur J Hum Genet. 2018;3:293–302.
19. Shang C, Guo Y, Hong Y, Xue YX. Long non-coding RNA TUSC7, a target of miR-23b, plays tumor-suppressing roles in human gliomas. Front Cell Neurosci. 2016;10:235.
20. Li N, Yang M, Shi K, Li W. Prognostic value of decreased long non-coding RNA TUSC7 expression in some solid tumors: A systematic review and meta-analysis. Oncotarget. 2017;8:59518–26.
21. Philips MA, Lilleväli K, Heinla I, Luuk H, Hundahl CA, Kongi K, et al. Lsamp is implicated in the regulation of emotional and social behavior by use of alternative promoters in the brain. Brain Struct Funct. 2015;220:1381–93.
22. Betancur C, Buxbaum JD. SHANK3 haploinsufficiency: A "common" but underdiagnosed highly penetrant monogeniccause of autism spectrum disorders. Mol Autism. 2013;4:17.
23. Guilmatre A, Huguet G, Delorme R, Bourgeron T. The emerging role of SHANK genes in neuropsychiatric disorders. Dev Neurobiol. 2014;74:113–22.

Compound phenotype in a girl with r(22), concomitant microdeletion 22q13.32-q13.33 and mosaic...

219

24. Shcheglovitov A, Shcheglovitova O, Yazawa M, Portmann T, Shu R, Sebastiano V, et al. SHANK3 and IGF1 restore synaptic deficits in neurons from 22q13 deletion syndrome patients. Nature. 2013;503:267–71.

25. DeCicco F, Steele MW, Pan S, Park SC. Monosomy of chromosome No. 22. A case report. J Pediatr. 1973;83:836–8.

26. Lewinsky RM, Johnson JM, Lao TT, Winsor EJ, Cohen H. Fetal gastroschisis associated with monosomy 22 mosaicism and absent cerebral diastolic flow. Prenat Diagn. 1990;10:605–8.

27. Merino A, De Perdigo A, Nomballais F, Yvinec M, Lopes P. Digeorge syndrome with total monosomy 22 diagnosed prenatally. Prenat Diagn. 1995;15:189–92.

28. Moghe MS, Patel ZM, Peter JJ, Ambani LM. Monosomy 22 with mosaicism. J Med Genet. 1981;18:71–3.

29. Pinto-Escalante D, Ceballos-Quintal JM, Castillo-Zapata I, Canto-Herrera J. Full mosaic monosomy 22 in a child with DiGeorge syndrome facial appearance. Am J Med Genet. 1998;76:150–3.

30. Rosenthal IM, Bocian M, Krmpottik E. Multiple anomalies including thymic aplasia associated with monosomy-22. Pediatr Res. 1972;6:358.

31. Verloes A, Herens C, Lambotte C, Frederic J. Chromosome 22 mosaic monosomy (46,XY/45,XY,-22). Ann Genet. 1987;30:178–9.

32. Lejeune J. On the duplication of circular structures. Ann Genet. 1968;11:71–7.

33. Stoll C, Roth MP. Segregation of a 22 ring chromosome in three generations. Hum Genet. 1983;63:294–6.

34. Park MY, Kim HS, Lee M, Park B, Lee HY, Cho EB, et al. FAM19A5, a brain-specific chemokine, inhibits RANKL-induced osteoclast formation through formyl peptide receptor 2. Sci Rep. 2017;7:15575.

35. Wang Y, Chen D, Zhang Y, Wang P, Zheng C, Zhang S, et al. A Novel Adipokine, FAM19A5, Inhibits Postinjury Neointima Formation through Sphingosine-1-Phosphate Receptor 2. Circulation. 2018; https://doi.org/10.1161/CIRCULATIONAHA.117.032398.

36. Tom Tang Y, Emtage P, Funk WD, Hu T, Arterburn M, Park EE, Rupp F. TAFA: a novel secreted family with conserved cysteine residues and restricted expression in the brain. Genomics. 2004;83:727–34.

37. Tabet AC, Rolland T, Ducloy M, Lévy J, Buratti J, Mathieu A, et al. A framework to identify contributing genes in patients with Phelan-McDermid syndrome. NPJ Genom Med. 2017;2:32.

22

Bone marrow failure may be caused by chromosome anomalies exerting effects on *RUNX1T1* gene

R. Valli[1], L. Vinti[2], A. Frattini[1,3], M. Fabbri[1,4], G. Montalbano[1], C. Olivieri[5], A. Minelli[5], F. Locatelli[2], F. Pasquali[1] and E. Maserati[1*] ⓘ

Abstract

Background: The majority of the cases of bone marrow failure syndromes/aplastic anaemias (BMFS/AA) are non-hereditary and considered idiopathic (80–85%). The peripheral blood picture is variable, with anaemia, neutropenia and/or thrombocytopenia, and the patients with idiopathic BMFS/AA may have a risk of transformation into a myelodysplastic syndrome (MDS) and/or an acute myeloid leukaemia (AML), as ascertained for all inherited BMFS. We already reported four patients with different forms of BMFS/AA with chromosome anomalies as primary etiologic event: the chromosome changes exerted an effect on specific genes, namely *RUNX1*, *MPL*, and *FLI1*, leading to the disease.

Results: We report two further patients with non-hereditary BM failure, with diagnosis of severe aplastic anaemia and pancytopenia caused by two different constitutional structural anomalies involving chromosome 8, and possibly leading to the disorder due to effects on the *RUNX1T1* gene, which was hypo-expressed and hyper-expressed, respectively, in the two patients. The chromosome change was unbalanced in one patient, and balanced in the other one.

Conclusions: We analyzed the sequence of events in the pathogenesis of the disease in the two patients, including a number of non-haematological signs present in the one with the unbalanced anomaly. We demonstrated that in these two patients the primary event causing BMFS/AA was the constitutional chromosome anomaly. If we take into account the cohort of 219 patients with a similar diagnosis in whom we made cytogenetic studies in the years 2003–2017, we conclude that cytogenetic investigations were instrumental to reach a diagnosis in 52 of them. We postulate that a chromosome change is the primary cause of BMFS/AA in a not negligible proportion of cases, as it was ascertained in 6 of these patients.

Keywords: Severe aplastic anaemia, Pancytopenia, Chromosome structural anomalies, Chromosome 8, Chromosome 2, *RUNX1T1* gene

Background

Bone marrow failure syndromes/aplastic anaemias (BMFS/AA) are a heterogeneous group of disorders characterized by the inability of the bone marrow (BM) to produce an adequate number of blood cells. The consequence is peripheral blood (PB) cytopenia, which may be uni-, bi-, or trilinear, resulting in anaemia, neutropenia and/or thrombocytopenia.

The BMFS/AA are inherited with a Mendelian pattern in about 15–20% of the patients: in these inherited BMFS (IBMFS) a number of extra-haematological signs are present, and many causative gene mutations have been identified [1]. The majority of the non-hereditary cases are considered idiopathic because their etiology is not known [2]. A risk of transformation into myelodysplastic syndrome (MDS) and/or acute myeloid leukaemia (AML) is ascertained for all IBMFS [3], and it may affect also patients with idiopathic BMFS/AA. This risk is well established for long-term survivors of acquired idiopathic AA [4], and it may be present also in different conditions belonging to the group defined

* Correspondence: emanuela.maserati@uninsubria.it
[1]Genetica Umana e Medica, Dipartimento di Medicina e Chirurgia, Università dell'Insubria, Varese, Italy
Full list of author information is available at the end of the article

above of BMFS/AA, which share almost all the haematological and clinical characteristics of IBMFS except the monogenic etiology.

We have already reported four patients with different forms of BMFS/AA with chromosome anomalies as primary etiologic event. They were two patients with complex structural rearrangements of chromosome 21, constitutional in one of them and acquired in BM in the other one, causing the disruption or the loss of the gene *RUNX1*, which was therefore hypo-expressed and lead to a Severe AA (SAA) in one patient, and to a congenital thrombocytopenia in the other one [5]. Another patient showed a paracentric inversion of a chromosome 1 as acquired clonal anomaly in the BM: we postulated that it caused AA due to a position effect acting on the gene *MPL*, severely hypo-expressed, with a final diagnosis of Congenital Amegakaryocytic Thrombocytopenia (CAMT) [5]. The clonal anomaly in the BM of one further patient was a complex unbalanced translocation with partial monosomy of the long arm of chromosome 11 implying the loss of the *FLI1* gene, consequently hypo-expressed and leading to diagnosis of Paris-Trousseau type thrombocytopenia [6].

We report here two further patients with non-hereditary BM failure, with diagnosis of SAA and pancytopenia, respectively, caused by two different constitutional structural anomalies involving chromosome 8, and leading to the disorder due to effects on the *RUNX1T1* gene. We postulate that a chromosome change is the primary cause of BMFS/AA in a not negligible proportion of cases.

Clinical reports
Patient 1
Female child, born in 2009 from non-consanguineous healthy parents; her birthweight was Kg 3.200. Two elder sibs were healthy. No relevant perinatal problems were present, but an ostium secundum atrial septal defect was diagnosed at 1 month of life: the right heart overload led then to surgical treatment, in January 2015.

She was admitted to hospital firstly at 8 months due to growth delay (weight, height, and cranium circumference < 3rd centile), psychomotor retardation, and facial dysmorphisms. In July 2012 she was hospitalized due to seizure episodes, and a severe non-haemolitic anaemia was noticed (Hb 4.7 g/dL). BM smear had a normal appearance, but the biopsy showed a hypoplastic marrow with slight dysplastic signs. BM cell cultures showed relevant reduction of all haemopoietic progenitors. The Diepoxybutane (DEB) test excluded Fanconi Anaemia (FA), and also Blackfan Diamond Anaemia was excluded. Her spleen was enlarged at echo-scan. Her radii were normal at Rx-scan, as normal were metabolic tests and a magnetic resonance tomography of her head. A diagnosis of AA was made, and therapy required monthly transfusions.

BM morphology was checked in November 2012 and in May 2013: it was hypocellular, with signs of trilinear dysplasia that worsened slightly in time, although the erythroid series showed some signs of recovery. In May 2014 the BM picture was substantially unchanged, with a hypocellular marrow and some dysplastic signs that did not reach the criteria to change the diagnosis to Refractory Cytopenia. Blood test in April 2016 showed: Hb 10.6 g/dL, WBC 3.9×10^9/L, platelets 173×10^9/L.

In November 2013 an echo-scan revealed a left kidney reduced (< 3rd centile) and a duplex kidney at the right (mass > 97th centile).

Epileptic seizures were observed three times from 2012 to 2014. Some epileptic anomalies were present at EEG, the last in October 2015, but no episodes took place after 2014. A neuropsychological examination in 2014 showed a border-line cognitive level, with normal speech, but under logopaedic treatment.

Patient 2
Female child, born in 2013 by Caesarian section from non-consanguineous healthy parents; her birthweight was Kg 2.900. Prenatal diagnosis performed through amniocentesis had shown the presence of a constitutional chromosome anomaly, interpreted as a balanced translocation involving the short arm of chromosome 2 and the long arm of chromosome 8. She has a healthy elder sister.

At 7 months of age she was admitted to hospital due to fever, and pancytopenia was diagnosed: the blood count showed Hb 5 g/dL, WBC 4.8×10^9/L with 0.180×10^9/L neutrophils, platelets 74×10^9/L. A panel of virological tests gave negative results. BM examination showed arrested maturation with dyserythropoiesis. In November 2013 her general conditions were good, her growth was normal both as to weight and height, repeated microbiological and virological tests were negative. BM cell cultures failed to show any abnormal results, whereas the trilinear cytopenia persisted. The DEB test excluded FA. Transfusions were given, and the administration of Ig led to increase the platelet number, which varied variously in the following months. In December 2013, her blood count showed Hb 9.8 g/dL, WBC 4.210×10^9/L with 0.210×10^9/L neutrophils, platelets 102×10^9/L. Ig administration and RBC transfusions were periodically given in the following months, Hb and platelets increased while neutropenia persisted. A blood count in May 2014 showed Hb 10.9 g/dL, WBC 4.3×10^9/L with 0.390×10^9/L neutrophils, platelets 94×10^9/L, and in March 2015 Hb 12.2 g/dL, WBC 5.7×10^9/L with 1.830×10^9/L neutrophils, platelets 176×10^9/L.

Results
Patient 1
Chromosome analysis performed with QFQ-banding technique on PB stimulated cultures (in 2012 and 2014), on

BM (in 2013 and 2014), and on the lymphoblastoid cell line consistently showed a normal karyotype. The a-CGH performed on DNA from PB revealed two imbalances: a duplication of the short arms of chromosome 1 of 4.304 Mb, from 92,091,957 to 96,396,550 bp (genome assembly hg19) (Fig. 1a), and a deletion of the long arms of chromosome 8 of 2.045 Mb, from 92,249,936 to 94,294,548 bp (Fig. 1b). Fluorescent In Situ Hybridization (FISH) with a commercial probe designed to detect the translocation t(8;21) (Table 1) showed that the signal of the *RUNX1T1* gene (alias *ETO*) was absent from the deleted chromosome 8 in mitoses from PB. On the same material the painting with a whole chromosome 1 library covered entirely the duplicated chromosome 1, without any signal elsewhere. The expression of *RUNX1T1*, evaluated by real-time on BM drawn in 2014, was significantly lower than controls (Fig. 2).

The karyotype of the parents was normal, and the result of a-CGH, performed on mother's vs. father's DNA, showed no significant deviation.

Patient 2

Chromosome analysis performed with QFQ-banding technique on PB stimulated cultures (in 2013 and 2014), on BM (in 2013), and on the lymphoblastoid cell line consistently showed a complex anomaly, already found at prenatal diagnosis performed elsewhere on amniotic fluid, and interpreted as a translocation t(2;8). Painting by FISH with libraries of chromosomes 2 and 8 (Table 1) showed that the anomaly consisted in fact of two separate insertions of material from the short arms of chromosome 2 into two points of the long arms of chromosome 8 (Fig. 3). FISH with a probe recognizing the entire sequence of the *RUNX1T1* gene (Table 1) showed that it was intact and included in the segment of chromosome 8 between the two insertions (Fig. 3e). The a-CGH performed on DNA from BM showed normal results, confirming that the rearrangement did not lead to any imbalances.

We then performed several dual color FISH with the probes of chromosomes 2 and 8 listed in Table 1 in various combinations to define precisely the breakpoints. The results, compared with the morphological appearance of the rearranged chromosomes, permitted to indicate the linear composition of the derivatives der(2) and der(8) as follows: 2pter→2p23.3::2p16.3→2qter; 8pter→8q21.12::2p16.3→2p22.2::8q21.12→8q22.2::2p23.3→2p22.2::8q22.2→8qter (Figures in Additional files 1 and 2).

The expression of *RUNX1T1*, evaluated by real-time on BM drawn in 2014, was significantly higher than controls (Fig. 4).

The karyotype of the parents and of the sister was normal.

Discussion

About 80–85% of BMFS/AA are considered idiopathic as the primary cause remains unknown [2]. We have already reported four patients with an initial diagnosis of idiopathic BMFS/AA, who were shown to bear a chromosome anomaly, either as constitutional change, or clonal in the BM, which led to the disorder through effects on genes localized in the chromosomes involved and their deregulated expression [5, 6]. The final diagnosis became SAA and congenital neutropenia in two patients, in whom the expression of the *RUNX1* gene (and possibly other uninvestigated genes) was reduced: both these conditions are usually not hereditary. In one case the final diagnosis became CAMT, likely due to effects on the *MPL* gene: this disorder is inherited usually as an autosomal recessive trait. Thrombocytopenia of the Paris-Trousseau type (TCPT) was the final diagnosis of another patient, due to the loss of the *FLI1* gene caused by a complex unbalanced translocation: this condition is usually not transmitted as a monogenic trait, but it is due to subtle deletions of the region of chromosome 11 containing the *FLI1* gene. The chromosome change is inherited from a parent in very few reported cases of TCPT [7].

We report here two further patients with a similar pathogenetic pathway, in whom we postulate that a chromosome anomaly was the primary event with subsequent deregulated expression of the *RUNX1T1* gene.

The strategy of analysis that we followed gave the proof that *RUNX1T1* expression dysregulation was the cause of the bone marrow failure in these two patients. We made a list of all genes included in the regions involved in the imbalances of our patient 1, and of genes in regions with proximity to the breakpoints of patient 2 (genome assembly hg19) [8]. These lists included 45 genes in the region duplicated of chromosome 1, and 6 genes in the region of chromosome 8 deleted in patient 1. As to patient 2, the lists included 227 genes in the two inserted regions of chromosome 2, and 139 genes in the region of chromosome 8 left between the two insertions and in the adjacent regions above and below the insertions (bands 8q21.12 – 8q22.2). We selected from these lists the genes known to be relevant in haematopoiesis. Thus, we arrived to the genes *GFI1*, on chromosome 1, and *RUNX1T1*, on chromosome 8, and we analyzed their expression. Data on the function of *RUNX1T1* are scarce in literature: it encodes a member of the myeloid translocation gene family, which interacts with DNA-bound transcription factors and recruit a range of corepressors to facilitate transcriptional repression, playing an important role in haematopoiesis, myogenesis [9], and neuronal differentiation [10]. Most reports on *RUNX1T1* are related to the translocation t(8;21)(q22;q22), which is one of the most frequent

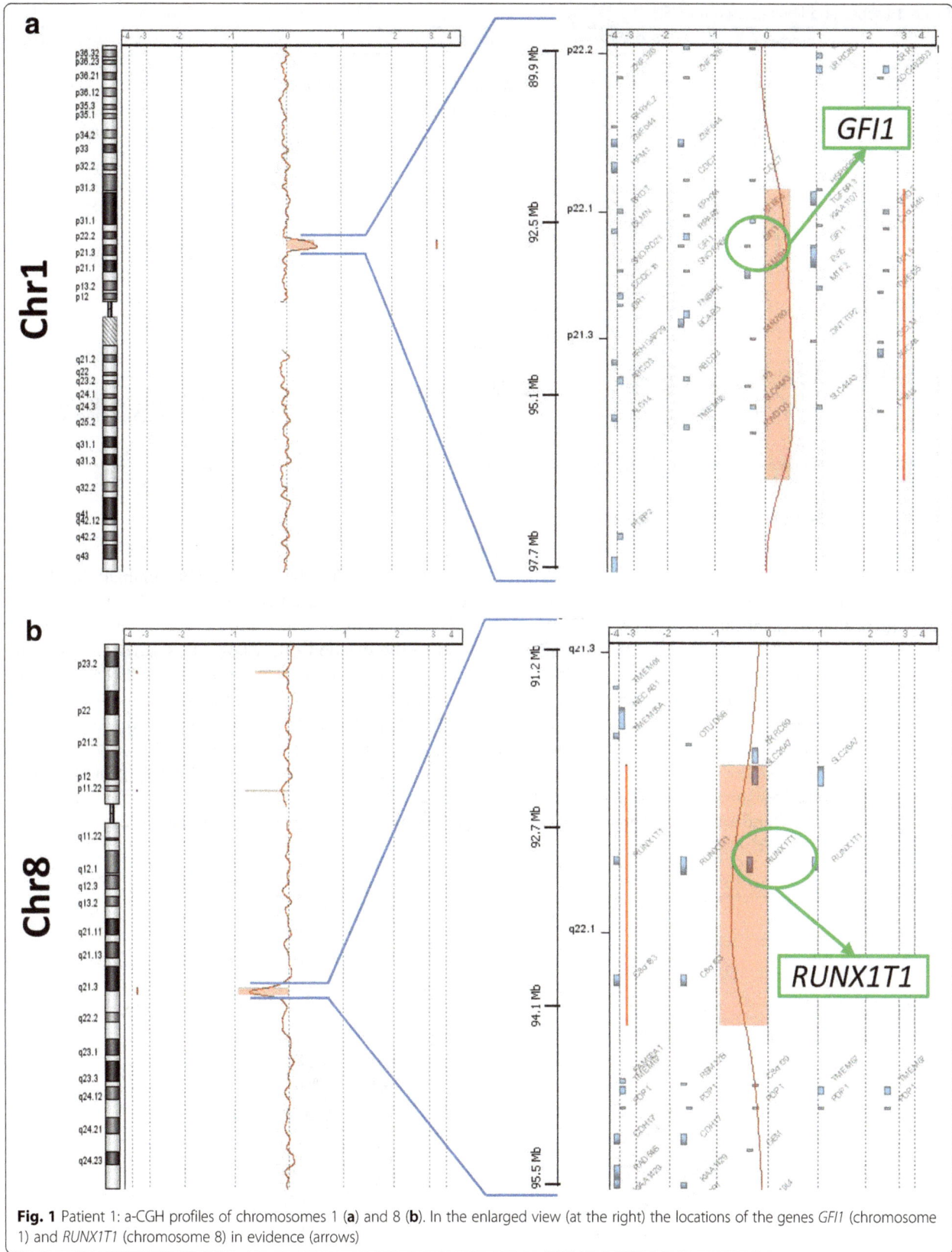

Fig. 1 Patient 1: a-CGH profiles of chromosomes 1 (**a**) and 8 (**b**). In the enlarged view (at the right) the locations of the genes *GFI1* (chromosome 1) and *RUNX1T1* (chromosome 8) in evidence (arrows)

Table 1 Probes and libraries used for FISH

Pt	Chromosome	Probes/libraries	Band localization	Genomic Localization (bp) (hg19)
1	8	AML1/ETO[a]	designed for t(8;21)	–
		WCP 1[b]	Whole chromosome paint library	
2	2	WCP 2[b]	Whole chromosome paint library	27,436,476–27,577,216 bp
		CTD-2314L14[c]	2p23.3	29,678,603–29,819,833 bp
		CTD-2599D22[c]	2p23.2	-
		ALK[d]	2p23.2–23.1	31,532,615–31,667,611 bp
		CTD-3028D11 [c]	2p23.1	36,717,490–36,828,693 bp
		CTD-2232H14[c]	2p22.2	38,563,970–38,725,504 bp
		CTD-2566H13[c]	2p22.2–22.1	42,157,290–42,301,116 bp
		CTD-2532N8[c]	2p21.3	46,582,036–46,715,607 bp
		CTD-2371H10[c]	2p21.1	48,326,711–48,434,143 bp
		CTD-2382F21[c]	2p16.3	61,463,234–61,600,608 bp
		CTD-2052G24[c]	2p15	64,034,477–64,232,972 bp
		CTD-3058K15[c]	2p15–14	
	8	WCP 8[b]	Whole chromosome paint	-
		AML1/ETO[a]	library designed for t(8;21)	83,886,651–83,982,215 bp
		CTD-2341G19[c]	8q21.13	87,885,140–87,980,460 bp
		CTD-2246G22[c]	8q21.3	91,740,722–91,959,017 bp
		CTD-3245G9[c]	8q21.3	92,778,106–92,922,619 bp
		CTD-2330N9[c]	8q21.3	

[a]AML1/ETO translocation, dual fusion probe, Cytocell Technologies, Cambridge, UK
[b]WCP, Cytocell Technologies, Cambridge, UK
[c]BAC probes, Thermo Fisher Scientific, Waltham, MA, USA
[d]ZytoLight SPEC ALK Dual Color Break Apart probe, Zytovision GmbH, Bremerhaven, Germany

acquired chromosome changes in the BM of patients with AML. This translocation gives a chimeric gene made up of the 5′-region of the runt-related transcription factor 1 gene (*RUNX1*) fused to the 3′-region of *RUNX1T1*. The chimeric protein so produced interferes with the expression of a number of genes relevant to normal haematopoiesis [11].

The sequence of pathological events that we postulate for our patient 1 is as follows: constitutional unbalanced chromosome anomaly involving the chromosomes 1 and 8, not detectable at standard chromosome analysis, but precisely identified by a-CGH. This anomaly led to the duplication of a segment of 4.304 Mb in the bands p22.1–p21.3 of the short arm of chromosome 1 (Fig. 1a), and to the deletion of a 2.044 Mb segment in the band q22.1 of the long arm of chromosome 8 (Fig. 1b). The gene *RUNX1T1* is in this region of chromosome 8 (Fig. 1b): its haploinsufficiency led to hypo-expression in BM (Fig. 2), which, in turn, caused the SAA. In the duplicated region of chromosome 1, the only gene known to play a role in haematopoiesis is *GFI1* (Fig. 1a), which functions as a transcription repressor [12]. It would be

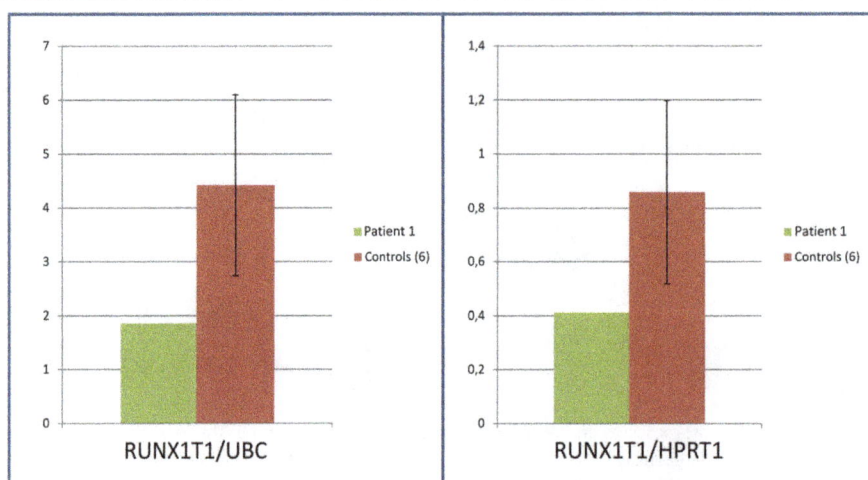

Fig. 2 Relative expression of *RUNX1T1* in the BM of patient 1. The green bars refer to the patient and the red bars to 6 controls' average values: two control housekeeping genes were used, *UBC* (left) and *HPRT1* (right). Standard error is shown for controls

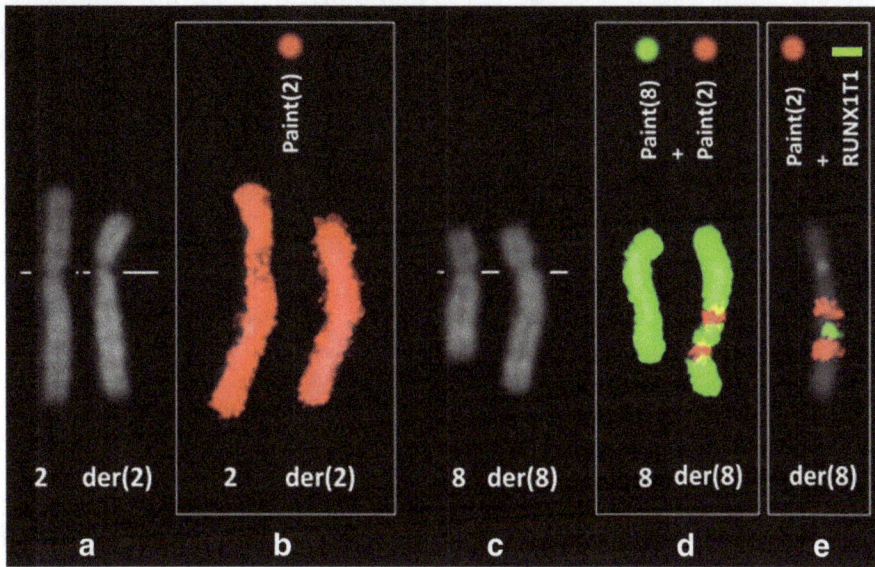

Fig. 3 Cut-out of the chromosomes involved in the rearrangement in patient 2. In **a** and **c** the Q-banded chromosomes (normal 2 and 8 at the left). In **b** the painting result on the normal chromosome 2 (left) and on the rearranged one (right) with the chromosome 2 library. In **d** the result of dual color painting with chromosomes 2 and 8 libraries on the normal chromosome 8 (left) and on the rearranged one (right). In **e** the dual color FISH with the chromosome 2 library (red) and a probe recognizing the entire sequence of the *RUNX1T1* gene, part of the system to detect the AML1/ETO translocation (Table 1) (green)

speculative to link the duplication of *GFI1* with the SAA of our patient, but in any case we analysed its expression and found it normal in comparison with six controls (Figure in Additional file 3). On the contrary, the hypoexpression of *RUNX1T1* is conceivable to deregulate the expression of other genes leading to SAA.

Extra-haematological symptoms of patient 1 include developmental and psychomotor delay, facial dysmorphisms, slight intellectual disability, rare seizures episodes, ostium secundum atrial septal defect, and kidney malformations. They are due to the chromosome imbalances of chromosomes 1 and 8, but a reliable comparison with patients with similar cytogenetic anomalies is not feasible, although some signs of our patient are common to similar reported cases. If we look at literature based on standard cytogenetics, we may compare our patient with cases as those reviewed by Utkus et al. [13] with duplications of at least part of band 1p21 (but with no imbalance of chromosome

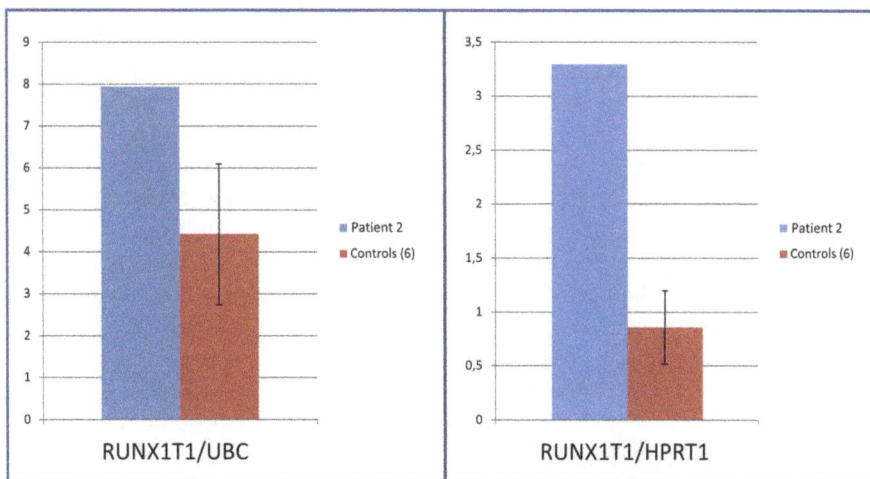

Fig. 4 Relative expression of *RUNX1T1* in the BM of patient 2. The blue bars refer to the patient and the red bars to 6 controls' average values: two control housekeeping genes were used, *UBC* (left) and *HPRT1* (right). Standard error is shown for controls

8). If we take into account cases defined at DNA base-pair level, the DECIPHER web-based database of Chromosome imbalances [14] includes 19 patients with duplications of chromosome 1 at least partially overlapping with the duplication of our patient, and 13 patients with deletions of chromosome 8 at least partially overlapping with the deletion. Some clinical signs of our patient are present in some of these cases, although the clinical definition of the reported patients is often somehow generic: intellectual disability, often moderate (10/32 patients), developmental delay (2/32), congenital heart defects (4/32) (including one case of interatrial, but also interventricular, defect in one patient with deletion of 8q), seizures (2/32), dysmorphisms (6/32). However, the duplication and the deletion of these patients are not identical to the imbalances of our patient, and none had both the imbalances of chromosomes 1 and 8. A number of patients with constitutional deletion of the long arm of chromosome 8 have been reported, with loss of material which included also the *RUNX1T1* gene. In these reports, however, as the ones of Zhang et al. and Allanson et al. [10, 15], the focus is almost exclusively on dysmorphisms/malformations, intellectual disability, and growth problems, no laboratory data at all are given and possible haematological issues may have been overlooked.

The sequence of pathological events that we postulate for our patient 2 is as follows: constitutional complex and balanced chromosome rearrangement involving chromosomes 2 and 8, with two contiguous but separate segments of the short arm of chromosome 2 (p23.3-p22.2, p22.2-p16.3) inserted in two bands of the long arms of chromosome 8 (q21.12, q22.2) (Fig. 3 and in Additional files 1 and 2). No loss or gain of chromosome material was confirmed by a-CGH. The *RUNX1T1* gene was shown to be intact, and it is normally located between the two insertions. It was highly hyper-expressed in the BM (Fig. 4): we believe that this led to BM failure and pancytopenia. Also the hyperexpression of *RUNX1T1* is apt to deregulate the expression of other genes leading to SAA.

We performed also whole transcriptome analysis on BM of both patients, and we found no other genes significantly over- or hypoexpressed (data not shown).

A pathogenetic pathway similar to that of our patients led to Diamond-Blackfan anaemia (DBA) in a reported boy with a de novo constitutional microdeletion of the band q13.2 of chromosome 19, where the gene *RPS19* is located [16]. This gene is known to cause DBA, and also in this patient the primary event leading to the BMFS was the chromosome anomaly, which caused also non-haematological features.

Conclusions

In the period 2003–2017 we performed cytogenetic analyses in a heterogeneous cohort of 219 pediatric patients

with BMF/AA during the evaluations made to reach a diagnosis. We found chromosome lesions in the BM or in the PB of 55 of these patients. The majority of them, 37, were diagnosed as affected by Fanconi Anaemia, as they showed chromosome breaks in PB cultures, in particular with the DEB test. In 9 patients with monosomy 7 or trisomy 8 in BM the final diagnosis was MDS [17, 18]. One patient with acquired trisomy 8 was then diagnosed as affected by Congenital Amegakaryocytic Thrombocytopenia (CAMT, OMIM # 604998) caused by biallelic mutations of the *MPL* gene [19]. One patient with an isochromosome of the long arm of a chromosome 7 was then diagnosed as affected by Shwachman-Diamond syndrome, as he was found to be compound heterozygote for mutations of the *SBDS* gene [20]. One patient with a translocation t(8;17)(p21;q25) acquired in BM, was a case of Diamond-Blackfan anaemia (DBA). Then there are the four patients mentioned above, in whom the primary event leading to BMF/AA was a chromosome constitutional or acquired anomaly, in absence of morphological evidence of frank MDS, acting through effects on the *RUNX1*, *MPL*, or *FLI1* genes and leading to the different final diagnoses already mentioned [5, 6].

With the two patients reported here, the total number of cases with BMF/AA bearing a chromosome lesion is 55 out of 219, and the chromosome anomaly, either constitutional or acquired, was the primary etiologic event in 6 of them. We might add two further patients of our cohort in whom the pattern of etiology and pathogenesis could be again similar, although we were not able to reach a firm conclusion in this sense due to the lack of informative material to analyse. They are the case of DBA mentioned above, with a clonal translocation in BM involving chromosome 8 short arm, where a causative gene not yet identified is localized [21], and a 10-year-old patient with AA who had a normal karyotype when we had the opportunity to study her, but in whom a previous analysis, as far as we were informed, showed an acquired deletion of the long arm of chromosome 8 in the BM, approximately in the region of the *RUNX1T1* gene (personal communication from Dr. Marco Zecca, Pavia, Italy, and Drs. Svetlana Donska, Larysa Peresada and Elena Kreminska, Kyiv, Ukraine).

The considerations above show that cytogenetic analyses may often be instrumental to reach a correct diagnosis in BMFS/AA, and that a chromosome change, both numerical or structural, constitutional or clonal, is the primary cause of BMFS/AA in a small but certainly not negligible proportion of cases.

Methods

Chromosome analyses were repeatedly performed in the two patients with routine methods and QFQ-banding technique on BM direct preparations and 24-48^h cultures, on PB unstimulated and PHA-stimulated cultures, and on cells from lymphoblastoid cell lines established by Epstein-Barr virus (EBV) infection. Routine methods were also applied for chromosome analysis of the patients' parents and of a sister of patient 2.

FISH was done on metaphases by standard procedures with different probes and libraries to define the chromosome anomalies, both in patients 1 and 2. All probes and libraries used for FISH assays are listed in Table 1.

The a-CGH was performed with the 244 K genome-wide system (Agilent Technologies Inc., Santa Clara, CA, USA), according to the manufacturer's instruction on DNA from PB of patient 1 and her parents, on DNA from BM of patient 2 and her parents.

The DNA was extracted using the Qiagen Flexigene kit (QIAGEN GmbH, Hilden, Germany), and competitor DNA was purchased from Agilent as part of the labeling kit. Slides were scanned using Agilent's microarray scanner G2565CA and microarray images were analysed using Agilent's Feature Extraction 12.0.2.2 software, and by Agilent's Genomic Workbench software (7.0.4.0). All map positions in the results refer to the genome assembly hg19.

The relative expression of the *RUNX1T1* gene was evaluated in both patients on RNA from total BM using Applied Biosystems ABI 7000 real-time thermocycler (Life Technologies Corporation, Carlsbad, California, USA), and the results were compared with RNA from BM of 6 age-matched healthy control subjects who donated haematopoietic cells for transplantation of a relative.

The assay was performed with Applied Biosystems Taqman system: we used #Hs00231702_m1 primers/probe-set for *RUNX1T1* transcript, and #Hs_00824723_m1, for Ubiquitin C (*UBC*), and #Hs02800695_m1, for Hypoxanthine Phosphoribosyltransferase 1 (*HPRT1*), primers/probe-sets as control house-keeping genes, as suggested for analysis on BM by Vandesompele et al. [22]. Relative expressions were calculated by the standard $\Delta\Delta$Ct method [23].

Abbreviations
AA: Aplastic anaemias; a-CGH: Array comparative genomic hybridization; AML: Acute myeloid leukaemia; BM: Bone marrow; BMFS: Bone marrow failure syndromes; CAMT: Congenital amegakaryocytic thrombocytopenia; DBA: Diamond-blackfan anaemia; DEB: Diepoxybutane; EBV: Epstein-Barr virus; FA: Fanconi anaemia; FISH: Fluorescent in situ hybridization; FLI1: Friend leukemia virus integration 1; GFI1: Growth factor-independent 1; IBMFS: Inherited bone marrow failure syndromes; MDS: Myelodysplastic syndrome; MPL: Myeloproliferative leukemia virus oncogene; PB: Peripheral blood; QFQ: Q banding by fluorescence and quinacrine; RPS19: Ribosomal protein S19; RUNX1: Runt-related transcription factor 1; RUNX1T1: Runt-related transcription factor 1, translocated to, 1; SAA: Severe aplastic anaemia; TCPT: Thrombocytopenia Paris-Trousseau type

Acnowledgements
The support of the Fondazione Banca del Monte di Lombardia and of the Associazione Italiana Sindrome di Shwachman (AISS) is gratefully acknowledged.

Funding
Grants from the Associazione Italiana Sindrome di Shwachman (AISS) to EM and RV, and from the University of Insubria to RV, EM and FP made this research possible.

Authors' contributions
GM and EM contributed to chromosome analyses and FISH. RV, AF, MF, AM and CO performed array-CGH end expression studies. LV and FL were responsible for the clinical management of the patients and of the analysis of clinical and haematological data. FL, FP and EM conceived and coordinated the study, and drafted the manuscript. All authors have read and approved the final manuscript.

Competing interests
The authors declare that they have no competing interests.

Author details
[1]Genetica Umana e Medica, Dipartimento di Medicina e Chirurgia, Università dell'Insubria, Varese, Italy. [2]Dipartimento di Onco-Ematologia Pediatrica, Ospedale Pediatrico Bambino Gesù, Roma, Università di Pavia, Pavia, Italy. [3]Istituto di Ricerca Genetica e Biomedica, CNR, Milan, Italy. [4]Unit of Haematopathology, European Institute of Oncology, Milan, Italy. [5]Genetica Medica, Fondazione IRCCS Policlinico S. Matteo e Università di Pavia, Pavia, Italy.

References
1. Parikh S, Bessler M. Recent insights into inherited bone marrow failure syndromes. Curr Opin Pediatr. 2012;24:23–32.
2. Dokal I, Vulliamy T. Inherited aplastic anaemias/bone marrow failure syndromes. Blood Rev. 2008;22:141–53.
3. Shimamura A, Alter B. Patophysiology and management of inherited bone marrow failure syndromes. Blood Rev. 2010;24:101–22.
4. Kojima S, Ohara A, Tsuchida M, Kudoh T, Hanada R, Okimoto Y, et al. Risk factors for evolution of acquired aplastic anemia into myelodysplastic syndrome and acute myeloid leukemia after immunosuppressive therapy in children. Blood. 2002;100:786–90.
5. Marletta C, Valli R, Pressato B, Mare L, Montalbano G, Menna G, et al. Chromosome anomalies in bone marrow as primary cause of aplastic or hypoplastic conditions and peripheral cytopenia: disorders due to secondary impairment of *RUNX1* and *MPL* genes. Mol Cytogenet. 2012;5:39.

6. Noris P, Valli R, Pecci A, Marletta C, Invernizzi R, Mare L, et al. Clonal chromosome anomalies affecting *FLI1* mimic inherited thrombocytopenia of the Paris-trousseau type. Eur J Haematol. 2012;89:345–9.

7. Van Zutven LJCM, van Bever Y, Van Nieuwland CCM, Huijbregts GCM, Van Opstal D, von Bergh ARM et al. Interstitial 11q deletion derived from a maternal ins(4,11)(p14;q24.2q25): a patient report and review. Am J Med Genet Part A. 2009;149A:1468–75.

8. UCSC Genome Browser: Kent WJ, Sugnet CW, Furey TS, Roskin KM, Pringle TH, Zahler AM et al. The human genome browser at UCSC. Genome Res. 2002;12:996–1006. Htpps://genome.ucsc.edu/cgb-bin/hgGateway. Accessed 25 Aug 2017.

9. Kumar R, Cheney KM, McKirdy R, Neilsen PM, Schulz RB, Lee J, et al. CBFA2T3-ZNF652 corepressor complex regulates transcription of the E-box gene HEB. J Biol Chem. 2008;283:19026–38.

10. Zhang L, Tümer Z, Møllgård K, Barbi G, Rossier E, Bendsen E, et al. Characterization of a t(5,8)(q31;q21) translocation in a patient with mental retardation and congenital heart disease: implications for involvement of RUNX1T1 in human brain and heart development. Eur J Hum Genet. 2009;17:1010–8.

11. Lam K, Zhang D-E. RUNX1 and RUNX1-ETO: roles in hematopoiesis and leukemogenesis. Front Biosci. 2012;17:1120–39.

12. Hock H, Hamblen MJ, Rooke HM, Schindler JW, Saleque S, Fujiwara Y, et al. Gfi-1 restricts proliferation and preserves functional integrity of haematopoietic stem cell. Nature. 2004;431:1002–7.

13. Utkus A, Sorokina I, Kucinskas V, Röthlisberger B, Balmer D, Brecevic L, et al. Duplication of segment 1p21 following paternal insertional translocation, ins(6,1)(q25;p13.3p22.1). J Med Genet. 1999;36:73–6.

14. Firth HV, Richards SM, Bevan AP, Clayton S, Corpas M, Rajan D, et al. DECIPHER: *D*atabase of *C*hromosomal *I*mbalances and *P*henotype in *H*umans using *E*nsembl *R*esources. Amer. J Hum Genet. 2009;84:524–33.

15. Allanson J, Smith A, Hare H, Albrecht B, Bijlsma E, Dallapiccola B, et al. Nablus mask-like facial syndrome: deletion of chromosome 8q22.1 is necessary but not sufficient to cause the phenotype. Am J Med Genet Part A. 2012;158A:2091–9.

16. Yuan H, Meng Z, Liu L, Deng X, Hu X, Liang L. A *de novo* 1.6Mb microdeletion at 19q13.2 in a boy with diamond-Blackfan anemia, global developmental delay and multiple congenital anomalies. Mol Cytogenet. 2016;9:58.

17. Maserati E, Minelli A, Menna G, Cecchini MP, Bernardo ME, Rossi G, De Filippi P, Lo Curto F, Danesino C, Locatelli F, Pasquali F. Familial myelodysplastic syndromes, monosomy 7/trisomy 8, and mutator effects. Cancer Genet Cytogenet. 2004;148:155–8.

18. Porta G, Maserati E, Mattarucchi E, Minelli A, Pressato B, Valli R, Zecca M, Bernardo ME, Lo Curto F, Locatelli F, Danesino C, Pasquali F. Monosomy 7 in myeloid malignancies: parental origin and monitoring by real-time quantitative PCR. Leukemia. 2007;21:1833–5.

19. Maserati E, Panarello C, Morerio C, Valli R, Pressato B, Patitucci F, et al. Clonal chromosome anomalies and propensity to myeloid malignancies in congenital amegakaryocytic thrombocytopenia (OMIM 604498). Haematologica. 2008;93:1271–3.

20. Maserati E, Pressato B, Valli R, Minelli A, Sainati L, Patitucci F, et al. The route to development of myelodysplastic sindrome/acute myeloid leukaemia in Shwachman-diamond syndrome: the role of ageing, karyotype instability, and acquired chromosome anomalies. Br J Haematol. 2009;145:190–7.

21. Gazda H, Lipton JM, Willig T-N, Ball S, Niemeyer CM, Tchernia G, et al. Evidence for linkage of familial diamond-Blackfan anemia to chromosome 8p23.3-p22 and for non-19q non-8p disease. Blood. 2001;97:2145–50.

22. Vandesompele J, De Preter K, Pattyn F, Poppe B, Van Roy N, De Paepe A et al. Accurate normalization of real-time quantitative RT-PCR data by geometric averaging of multiple internal control genes. Genome Biol 2002; 3: research0034.1–0034.11.

23. Schmittgen TD, Livak KJ. Analyzing real-time PCR data by the comparative C(T) method. Nat Protoc. 2008;3:1101–8.

Permissions

All chapters in this book were first published in MC, by BioMed Central; hereby published with permission under the Creative Commons Attribution License or equivalent. Every chapter published in this book has been scrutinized by our experts. Their significance has been extensively debated. The topics covered herein carry significant findings which will fuel the growth of the discipline. They may even be implemented as practical applications or may be referred to as a beginning point for another development.

The contributors of this book come from diverse backgrounds, making this book a truly international effort. This book will bring forth new frontiers with its revolutionizing research information and detailed analysis of the nascent developments around the world.

We would like to thank all the contributing authors for lending their expertise to make the book truly unique. They have played a crucial role in the development of this book. Without their invaluable contributions this book wouldn't have been possible. They have made vital efforts to compile up to date information on the varied aspects of this subject to make this book a valuable addition to the collection of many professionals and students.

This book was conceptualized with the vision of imparting up-to-date information and advanced data in this field. To ensure the same, a matchless editorial board was set up. Every individual on the board went through rigorous rounds of assessment to prove their worth. After which they invested a large part of their time researching and compiling the most relevant data for our readers.

The editorial board has been involved in producing this book since its inception. They have spent rigorous hours researching and exploring the diverse topics which have resulted in the successful publishing of this book. They have passed on their knowledge of decades through this book. To expedite this challenging task, the publisher supported the team at every step. A small team of assistant editors was also appointed to further simplify the editing procedure and attain best results for the readers.

Apart from the editorial board, the designing team has also invested a significant amount of their time in understanding the subject and creating the most relevant covers. They scrutinized every image to scout for the most suitable representation of the subject and create an appropriate cover for the book.

The publishing team has been an ardent support to the editorial, designing and production team. Their endless efforts to recruit the best for this project, has resulted in the accomplishment of this book. They are a veteran in the field of academics and their pool of knowledge is as vast as their experience in printing. Their expertise and guidance has proved useful at every step. Their uncompromising quality standards have made this book an exceptional effort. Their encouragement from time to time has been an inspiration for everyone.

The publisher and the editorial board hope that this book will prove to be a valuable piece of knowledge for researchers, students, practitioners and scholars across the globe.

List of Contributors

Jinlei Han, Zhiliang Zhang and Kai Wang
Key Laboratory of Genetics, Breeding and Multiple Utilization of Corps, Ministry of Education, Fujian Provincial Key Laboratory of Haixia Applied Plant Systems Biology, Center for Genomics and Biotechnology, Fujian Agriculture and Forestry University, Fuzhou, Fujian, China

Kai Wang
National Engineering Research Center of Sugarcane, Fujian Agriculture and Forestry University, Fuzhou, China

Sara Peixoto, Joana B. Melo, José Ferrão, Luís M. Pires, Nuno Lavoura, Marta Pinto and Isabel M. Carreira
Cytogenetics and Genomics Laboratory, Faculty of Medicine, University of Coimbra, Coimbra, Portugal

Sara Peixoto and Guiomar Oliveira
Neurodevelopmental and Autism Unit from Child Developmental Center and Centro de Investigação e Formação Clinica, Hospital Pediátrico, Centro Hospitalar e Universitário de Coimbra, Coimbra, Portugal

Sara Peixoto
Department of Paediatrics of the Centro Hospitalar de Trás-os-Montes e Alto Douro, EPE, Vila Real, Portugal

Joana B. Melo and Isabel M. Carreira
CNC.IBILI, University of Coimbra, Coimbra, Portugal

Joana B. Melo and Isabel M. Carreira
CIMAGO - Centro Investigação em Meio Ambiente, Genética e Oncobiologia, Faculty of Medicine, University of Coimbra, Coimbra, Portugal

Guiomar Oliveira
University Clinic of Pediatrics and Institute for Biomedical Imaging and Life Science, Faculty of Medicine, University of Coimbra, Coimbra, Portugal

Guangrong Li, Dan Gao, Hongjun Zhang, Jianbo Li, Hongjin Wang, Shixiao La, jiwei Ma and Zujun Yang
School of Life Science and Technology, University of Electronic Science and Technology of China, Chengdu 610054, China

Edoardo Errichiello, Francesca Novara and Orsetta Zuffardi
Department of Molecular Medicine, University of Pavia, Via Forlanini 14, 27100 Pavia, Italy

Anna Cremante and Annapia Verris
National Neurological Institute IRCCS C, Mondino, Pavia, Italy

Jessica Galli and Elisa Fazzi
Mother-Child Department, Child Neurology and Psychiatry Unit, Spedali Civili, Brescia, Italy

Daniela Bellotti
Department of Molecular and Translational Medicine, University of Brescia, Brescia, Italy

Laura Losa and Mariangela Cisternino
Department of Pediatrics, IRCCS Policlinico San Matteo, University of Pavia, Pavia, Italy

Jelena Filipović, Gordana Joksić and Ivana Joksić
Vinca Institute of Nuclear Sciences, University of Belgrade, Mike Petrovica Alasa 12-14, Belgrade 11001, Serbia

Dragana Vujić
Mother and Child Health Care Institute of Serbia, "Dr Vukan Cupic", Radoja Dakica 6, Belgrade 11070, Serbia

Kristin Mrasek, Anja Weise and Thomas Liehr
Institute of Human Genetics, Jena University Hospital, Friedrich Schiller University, Kollegiengasse 10, Jena D-07743, Germany

Svetlana A. Romanenko, Larisa S. Biltueva, Natalya A. Serdyukova, Anastasia I. Kulemzina, Violetta R. Beklemisheva, Olga L. Gladkikh, Natalia A. Lemskaya, Nadezhda V. Vorobieva, Alexander S. Graphodatsky and Vladimir A. Trifonov
Institute of Molecular and Cellular Biology SB RAS, Novosibirsk, Russia

Svetlana A. Romanenko, Nadezhda V. Vorobieva and Alexander S. Graphodatsky
Novosibirsk State University, Novosibirsk, Russia

Elena A. Interesova
Novosibirsk Branch of the Federal State Budgetary Scientific Institution "State Scientific-and-Production Centre for Fisheries (Gosrybcenter)", Novosibirsk, Russia
Tomsk State University, Tomsk, Russia

Marina A. Korentovich
Federal State Budgetary Scientific Institution "State Scientific-and-Production Centre for Fisheries (Gosrybcenter)", Tyumen, Russia

Harita Ghevaria, Roy Naja, Sioban SenGupta and Joy Delhanty
Preimplantation Genetics Group, Institute for Women's Health, University College London, 86-96 Chenies Mews, London WC1E 6HX, UK

Paul Serhal
The Centre for Reproductive and Genetic Health, 230-232 Great Portland Street, London W1W 5QS, UK

Woori Jang, Hyojin Chae, Myungshin Kim, Yonggoo Kim
Department of Laboratory Medicine, College of Medicine, The Catholic University of Korea, Seoul, Korea

Woori Jang, Hyojin Chae, Jiyeon Kim, Jung-Ok Son, Seok Chan Kim, Bo Kyung Koo, Myungshin Kim and Yonggoo Kim
Catholic Genetic Laboratory Center, Seoul St. Mary's Hospital, College of Medicine, The Catholic University of Korea, Seoul, Korea

In Yang Park
Department of Obstetrics and Gynecology, College of Medicine, The Catholic University of Korea, Seoul, Korea

In Kyung Sung
Department of Pediatrics, College of Medicine, The Catholic University of Korea, Seoul, Korea

Hyojin Chae
Department of Laboratory Medicine, Seoul St. Mary's Hospital, College of Medicine, The Catholic University of Korea, 222 Banpo-daero, Seocho-gu, Seoul 137-701, Korea

Yanyan Zhao, Feng Yu, Ruijuan Liu and Quanwen Dou
Key Laboratory of Adaptation and Evolution of Plateau Biota, Northwest Institute of Plateau Biology, the Chinese Academy of Sciences, Xining 810008, China

Caiyun Wu and Hong Jiang
The Reproductive Medicine Center, Clinical College of People's Liberation Army Affiliated to Anhui Medical University, Hefei, Anhui, China

Caiyun Wu, Hong Jiang and Zhenyi Cao
The Reproductive Medicine Center, 105 Hospital of People's Liberation Army, Hefei, Anhui, China

Liu Wang, Furhan Iqbal, Xiaohua Jiang, Ihtisham Bukhari, Howard J. Cooke and Qinghua Shi
Molecular and Cell Genetics Laboratory, The CAS Key Laboratory of Innate Immunity and Chronic Diseases, Hefei National Laboratory for Physical Sciences at Microscale, School of Life Sciences, University of Science and Technology of China, Hefei, Anhui 230027, China

Liu Wang, Xiaohua Jiang, Ihtisham Bukhari, Howard J. Cooke, Gengxin Yin, Tonghang Guo and Qinghua Shi
Collaborative Innovation Center of Genetics and Development, Fudan University, Shanghai 200438, China

Furhan Iqbal
Institute of Pure and Applied Biology, Bahauddin Zakariya University, Multan 60800, Pakistan

Tonghang Guo
Center for Reproductive Medicine, Anhui Medical University, Affiliated Provincial Hospital, Hefei, China

Gengxin Yin
Anhui Provincial Family Planning Institute of Science Gengxin Yin7and Technology, Hefei, China

Mathew Bloomfield and Peter Duesberg
Department of Molecular and Cell Biology, Donner Laboratory, University of California at Berkeley, Berkeley, CA, USA

Nida Anwar, Aisha Arshad, Muhammad Nadeem, Sana Khurram, Naveena Fatima, Sumaira Sharif, Saira Shan and Tahir Shamsi
National Institute of Blood Disease and Bone Marrow Transplantation (NIBD), St 2/A block 17 Gulshan-e-Iqbal KDA scheme 24, Karachi, Pakistan

Emanuele G. Coci, Armin Stelzner, Hendrik Langen and Joachim Riedel
Center of Social Pediatrics and Pediatric Neurology, General Hospital of Celle, 29221 Celle, Germany

Udo Koehler
Medizinisch Genetisches Zentrum, 80335 Munich, Germany

Thomas Liehr
Institute of Human Genetics, Friedrich Schiller University, Jena University Hospital, 07743 Jena, Germany

Christian Fink
Department of Radiology, General Hospital of Celle, 29223 Celle, Germany

Qin Wang, Weiqing Wu, Zhiyong Xu, Fuwei Luo and Jiansheng Xie
Shenzhen Maternity and Child Healthcare Hospital, 3012 Fuqiang Road, Shenzhen, Guangdong, China

Weiqing Wu, Qinghua Zhou and Peining Li
Department of Genetics, Yale School of Medicine, New Haven, CT, USA

Qinghua Zhou
First Affiliated Hospital, Biomedical Translational Research Institute, Jinan University, Guangzhou, Guangdong, China

Jun Gu, Corrie DeGraffenreid and Kenneth Sterns
School of Health Professions, The University of Texas MD Anderson Cancer Center, 1515 Holcombe Blvd. Unit 0002, Houston, TX 77030, USA

Alexandra Reynolds and Xinyan Lu
Department of Hematopathology, The University of Texas MD Anderson Cancer Center, 1515 Holcombe Blvd. Unit 0350, Houston, TX 77030, USA

Lianghua Fang and Keyur P. Patel
Department of Hematopathology, The University of Texas MD Anderson Cancer Center, 1515 Holcombe Blvd. Unit 0149, Houston, TX 77030, USA

Lianghua Fang
Department of Oncology, Jiangsu Hospital of Traditional Chinese Medicine, Nanjing, Jiangsu, China

L. Jeffrey Medeiros and Pei Lin
Department of Hematopathology, The University of Texas MD Anderson Cancer Center, 1515 Holcombe Blvd. Unit 0072, Houston, TX 77030, USA

Xinyan Lu
Department of Pathology, Northwestern University Feinberg School of Medicine, 303 East Chicago Avenue, Tarry 7-723, Chicago, IL 60611, USA

Renae Domaschenz, Alexandra M. Livernois, Tariq Ezaz and Janine E. Deakin
Institute for Applied Ecology, University of Canberra, Canberra, ACT 2601, Australia

Renae Domaschenz
Present address: John Curtin School of Medical Research, The Australian National University, Canberra, ACT, Australia

Sudha Rao
Discipline of Biomedical Sciences, Faculty of Education, Science, Technology and Mathematics, University of Canberra, Canberra, ACT 2601, Australia

Mathew Bloomfield and Peter Duesberg
Department of Molecular and Cell Biology, Donner Laboratory, University of California at Berkeley, Berkeley, CA 94720, USA

Mathew Bloomfield
Department of Natural Sciences and Mathematics, Dominican University of California, San Rafael, CA, USA

Gang An, Si Ping Liu, Yan Hong Yu and Fang Yang
Nanfang Hospital, Southern Medical University, Guangzhou 510515, Guangdong, China

Gang An, Yuan Lin, Liang Pu Xu and Hai Long Huang
Fujian Provincial Key Laboratory for Prenatal diagnosis and Birth Defect, Fujian Provincial Maternity and Children's Hospital of Fujian Medical University, Fuzhou, Fujian, China

Zuhair N. Al-Hassnan
Department of Medical Genetics, King Faisal Specialist Hospital and Research Centre, Riyadh, Kingdom of Saudi Arabia

Zuhair N. Al-Hassnan, Waad Albawardi, Faten Almutairi, Rawan AlMass, Albandary AlBakheet, Osama M. Mustafa, Laila AlQuait, Zarghuna M. A. Shinwari, Salma Wakil, Osima Al-Nakhli, Balsam AlMaarik, Hana A. Al-Hakami, Maysoon Alsagob and Namik Kaya
Department of Genetics, King Faisal Specialist Hospital and Research Centre, MBC: 03, Riyadh 11211, Kingdom of Saudi Arabia

Mustafa A. Salih and Saeed M. Hassan
Division of Pediatric Neurology, Department of Pediatrics, College of Medicine, King Saud University, Riyadh, Kingdom of Saudi Arabia

Majid Al-Fayyadh
Heart Center, King Faisal Specialist Hospital and Research Centre, Riyadh, Kingdom of Saudi Arabia

Brynn Levy
Department of Pathology and Cell Biology, Columbia University, New York, NY, USA

Majid Al-Fayyadh and Dilek Colak
Department of Biostatistics, Epidemiology and Scientific Computing, King Faisal Specialist Hospital and Research Centre, Riyadh, Kingdom of Saudi Arabia

Zuhair N. Al-Hassnan
College of Medicine, Alfaisal University, Riyadh, Saudi Arabia

Durkadin Demir Eksi
Department of Medical Biology, Alanya Alaaddin Keykubat University, Faculty of Medicine, Antalya, Turkey

Yiping Shen
Guangxi Maternal and Child Health Hospital, Nanning, China
Department of Pathology, Harvard Medical School, Boston, MA 02115, USA
Division of Genetics and Genomics, Boston Children's Hospital, Boston, MA 02115, USA
Shanghai Children's Medical Center, Shanghai Jiaotong University School of Medicine, Shanghai 200127, China

Munire Erman and Meric Bilekdemir
Department of Obstetrics and Gynecology, Akdeniz University, Faculty of Medicine, Antalya, Turkey

Lynn P. Chorich, Megan E. Sullivan, Hyung-Goo Kim and Lawrence C. Layman
Section of Reproductive Endocrinology, Infertility, & Genetics, Department of Obstetrics & Gynecology Medical College of Georgia at Augusta University, Augusta, GA, USA
Department of Neuroscience & Regenerative Medicine, Medical College of Georgia at Augusta University, 1120 15th Street, CA2041, Augusta, GA 30912, USA

Elanur Yılmaz, Guven Luleci and Ozgul M. Alper
Department of Medical Biology and Genetics, Akdeniz University, Faculty of Medicine, 07058 Antalya, Turkey

Anna A. Kashevarova, Elena O. Belyaeva, Nikolay A. Skryabin, atyana V. Nikitina, Stanislav A. Vasilyev, Yulia S. Yakovleva, Nadezda P. Babushkina, Ekaterina N. Tolmacheva, Mariya E. Lopatkina, Renata R. Savchenko, Lyudmila P. Nazarenko and Igor N. Lebedev
Research Institute of Medical Genetics, Tomsk NRMC, Tomsk, Russia

Aleksandr M. Nikonov and Olga V. Plotnikova
Diagnostic Center of the Altai Region, Barnaul, Russia

Yulia S. Yakovleva, Yulia S. Yakovleva, Lyudmila P. Nazarenko and Igor N. Lebedev
Siberian State Medical University, Tomsk, Russia

R. Valli, A. Frattini, M. Fabbri, G. Montalbano, F. Pasquali and E. Maserati
Genetica Umana e Medica, Dipartimento di Medicina e Chirurgia, Università dell'Insubria, Varese, Italy

L. Vinti and F. Locatelli
Dipartimento di Onco-Ematologia Pediatrica, Ospedale Pediatrico Bambino Gesù, Roma, Università di Pavia, Pavia, Italy

R. Valli and A. Frattini
Istituto di Ricerca Genetica e Biomedica, CNR, Milan, Italy

M. Fabbri
Unit of Haematopathology, European Institute of Oncology, Milan, Italy

C. Olivieri and A. Minelli
Genetica Medica, Fondazione IRCCS Policlinico S. Matteo and Università di Pavia, Pavia, Italy

Index

www.ingramcontent.com/pod-product-compliance
Lightning Source LLC
Chambersburg PA
CBHW061256190326
41458CB00011B/3689

* 9 7 8 1 6 3 2 4 1 7 9 9 2 *